MW00844659

McRae's
# ORTHOPAEDIC
# TRAUMA
and Emergency Fracture Management

# Ronald McRae (1926–2012)

Ronald McRae was a consultant surgeon who wrote several outstanding practical handbooks on orthopaedics and fracture management that have been used by medical students and trainee surgeons around the world.

Born in Ayrshire in Scotland, he went on to study medicine at Glasgow University, graduating in 1949. He served as a commissioned medical officer in the Royal Air Force, working mostly in Ely, Cambridgeshire, which met the accident and orthopaedic needs of both servicemen and their families. There he dealt with difficult cases invalided back to the UK from the Middle and Far East, such as polio victims in iron lungs, neglected compound fractures sustained in hostile environments, and cases of bone and joint tuberculosis before the introduction of streptomycin.

When he left the Armed Forces, he returned to Glasgow and was eventually appointed consultant orthopaedic surgeon at the city's Southern General Hospital. The hospital was the first in Scotland to carry out hip replacement surgery and he was closely involved in this development. Given the location of the hospital, he found himself treating accident victims from the numerous local shipyards and the construction of the Clyde Tunnel. While working at the Southern General, he became a lecturer in anatomy at the Glasgow School of Chiropody. His ground-breaking teaching methods later earned him an Honorary Fellowship of the Society of Chiropodists. Following involvement in the treatment of victims of the 1971 Ibrox disaster, he helped develop the principles of major incident trauma management.

Ronald McRae had a love of all things mechanical, which was encouraged by his grandfather, who, like his six brothers, was a marine engineer. Ron established a workshop at his home in Nithsdale Road, Glasgow, where he used his engineering skills to design and make specialised tools to assist in particularly challenging operations, as well as teaching aids. He also built a range of scale models, including an exhibition-quality beam engine, and several gauge 1 live steam locomotives, which he ran on a small track outside his home. This passion continued during his retirement in Gourock.

Ronald McRae was charged with the responsibility of setting up an orthopaedic teaching programme for medical students, something he greatly enjoyed. He became interested in many aspects of teaching technology, and derived great pleasure whenever a teaching aid that he had produced was proved successful. As part of this programme, he prepared scores of handout notes for the undergraduates, produced on a Roneo duplicating machine with many small drawings, each accompanied by a brief text. It was these drawings and accompanying texts that were to form the basis of his best-selling orthopaedic textbooks, which were widely translated. They were also the inspiration behind this book, which closely follows the principles and ideas established by Ronald McRae.

# McRae's
# ORTHOPAEDIC TRAUMA
## and Emergency Fracture Management

## Third Edition

### Timothy O White
**BMedSci, MBChB, FRCSEd (Tr & Orth), MD**

Consultant Orthopaedic Trauma Surgeon,
Royal Infirmary of Edinburgh;
Honorary Senior Lecturer in the Department of
Orthopaedic and Trauma Surgery,
University of Edinburgh

### Samuel P Mackenzie
**BMedSci, MBChB, MRCSEd**

Specialty Trainee in Trauma and Orthopaedics,
Royal Infirmary of Edinburgh;
Honorary Teaching Fellow,
University of Edinburgh

### Alasdair J Gray
**MBChB, FRCS, FCEM, MD**

Consultant in Accident and Emergency
Medicine,
Royal Infirmary of Edinburgh;
College Professor of Emergency Medicine,
University of Edinburgh

Illustrated by Robert Britton

ELSEVIER

Edinburgh   London   New York   Oxford   Philadelphia   St Louis   Sydney   Toronto   2016

# ELSEVIER

Originally published as *Pocketbook of Orthopaedics and Fractures* by Ronald McRae

First edition 1999

Second edition 2006

Third edition 2016

ISBN   978-0-7020-5728-1

International ISBN   978-0-7020-5730-4

**Notices**

*Content Strategist:* Laurence Hunter

*Content Development Specialist and Illustration Manager:* Fiona Conn

*Project Manager:* Louisa Talbott

*Designer:* Christian Bilbow

your source for books,
journals and multimedia
in the health sciences

**www.elsevierhealth.com**

  Working together
to grow libraries in
**Book Aid** developing countries

www.elsevier.com • www.bookaid.org

The publisher's policy is to use **paper manufactured from sustainable forests**

Printed in Poland

Last digit is the print number:   9   8   7   6   5   4   3   2

# Contents

# Preface

The care of the injured patient is a rewarding and fascinating specialty, requiring an understanding of an unparalleled range of anatomy and physiology, practical procedures and surgical techniques. Skilled, coordinated management is vital; trauma is the principal cause of death and disability in the young, while the epidemic of fragility fractures grows inexorably. As trainees, we looked to Ronald McRae's iconic handbook as the authoritative guide to fracture management, with its clear visual depictions and succinct text. In this Third Edition, we have sought to emulate his didactic style whilst re-writing the text and redrawing the illustrations completely, aiming to provide a cutting-edge, contemporary and comprehensive text that covers the full range of musculoskeletal emergencies.

While no single volume can hope to be exhaustive, we hope this *vade mecum* will be a source of clear and immediate reference to the doctor or extended-scope practitioner in the Emergency Department or fracture clinic, as much as to the orthopaedic surgical trainee on call, on the ward or in the operating theatre.

TOW

SPM

AJG

# Dedications and acknowledgements

To Ishbel, Calum, Katie and James for all their love and support, especially during the writing of this book, to my mother Liz and late father Ian, and with thanks to my mentors and colleagues in Edinburgh and Vancouver.

TOW

This book is for my parents, John and Norma. Everything that I have, and everything that I am, is because of them.

SPM

We would like to thank a number of our colleagues who have kindly reviewed the contents of some of the chapters and have provided invaluable advice. While their suggestions have improved the text, any errors remain our own. In particular, we thank CM Robinson (Shoulder girdle chapter), JT Reid (Elbow chapter), P Bates (Pelvis and Acetabulum chapters), A Watts (Wrist and carpus chapter), A McLullich ('Trauma in the elderly' in the Management of the injured patient chapter), A Duckworth (Wrist and carpus chapter) and CW Oliver (Hand chapter).

TOW
SPM
AJG

# Contributors

### Emily J Baird
**MBChB, FRCS (Tr & Orth), MFSTEd**

Consultant Orthopaedic Surgeon, Royal
Hospital for Sick Children, Edinburgh

*Chapter 25 Lower limb paediatric trauma*

### Alexander DL Baker
**MBChB, DipTh, BSc (Hons), MSc, MRCS,
FRCS (Tr & Orth)**

Consultant Orthopaedic Surgeon and Spinal
Specialist, Lancashire Teaching Hospitals
NHS Foundation Trust, Lancashire

*Chapter 14 Spine*

### Alastair Murray
**BSc, MD, FRCS (Tr & Orth), FFST**

Consultant Orthopaedic Surgeon, Royal
Hospital for Sick Children, Edinburgh

*Chapter 23 Principles of paediatric trauma*

*Chapter 24 Upper limb paediatric trauma*

*Chapter 25 Lower limb paediatric trauma*

# Part 1

## General Principles

## Fracture types and patterns

A fracture is any break in the continuity of a bone. The word 'fracture' covers a wide spectrum of possible injuries, from an open, multifragmentary femoral fracture to an undisplaced stress fracture of a metatarsal. Fractures are described in terms of a number of characteristics:

- *aetiology* – the cause of the fracture
- *morphology* – the fracture pattern
- *severity* – the degree of comminution, or involvement of soft tissue or a joint
- *location* – which part of the bone is affected
- *displacement* – how the bone fragments have moved in relation to one another.

### Aetiology

#### *Traumatic fractures*

Injuries are caused by direct or indirect violence; they are the effect of an abnormal force applied to a normal bone.

#### *Pathological fractures (Fig. 1.1)*

Pathological fractures occur within abnormal or diseased bone and are often caused by relatively little violence or energy; they are the effect of a normal force on an abnormal bone. The pathology may be localized to one part of the bone (e.g. a tumour deposit) or generalized (e.g. osteoporosis and osteomalacia).

#### *Insufficiency fractures (Fig. 1.2)*

These are the most common type of pathological fracture, but are often considered separately due to their prevalence. They most often occur as a result of *osteoporosis*, a progressive bone disease characterized by a decrease in bone mineral density (BMD) and deterioration in bone microarchitecture. Common sites of osteoporotic fractures are the hip, wrist,

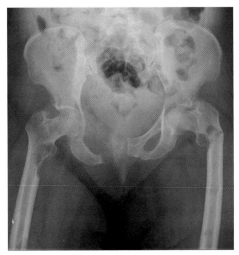

Fig. 1.1 Pathological fracture. This radiograph demonstrates numerous lytic lesions within the subtrochanteric regions of both femora. On the left side there is a pathological fracture.

Normal bone                    Osteoporotic bone

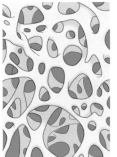 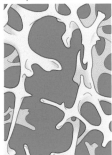

Fig. 1.2 Normal and osteoporotic bone. From Sproat C, Burke G, McGurk M: Essential Human Disease for Dentists (Churchill Livingstone 2006) with permission.

proximal humerus and spine. *Osteomalacia*, in contrast, is bone softening caused by defective mineralization of the matrix. The most common cause is vitamin D deficiency, often resulting from alcohol abuse or renal disease.

### Fatigue (or stress) fractures (Fig. 1.3)

These fractures are the result of the cyclical application of normal forces to normal bone with excessive frequency. These often occur following a change in the level or intensity of activity. Classic examples include the second metatarsal of army recruits (the 'march fracture') and novice long-distance runners. The fracture is typically linear and incomplete. It may be very subtle initially and may be appreciated only after the development of callus, or on magnetic resonance imaging (MRI) or bone scan. An entirely undisplaced fracture is occasionally termed an *infraction*.

## Morphology

### Transverse and oblique fractures (Fig. 1.4)

These fractures are caused by a bending force resulting from a direct blow by a moving object, or by a bone striking a resistant object (such as the ground). Higher-energy transfer will result in a greater number of fragments; a wedge or *butterfly fragment* is produced on the tension side of the bone; while higher energy still will result in a *multifragmentary* (or 'comminuted') fracture. In a segmental (or 'double') fracture there is a separate complete bone segment.

### Spiral fractures (Fig. 1.5)

These are caused by indirect rotational forces. The mechanism of injury is often a simple twist and fall, or a sporting accident, typically to the tibia, humerus or fingers. Spiral fractures may have butterfly fragments or comminution with increasing energy transfer.

### Avulsion fractures (Fig. 1.6)

These fractures are caused by traction from a ligament, tendon or capsular insertion. They can result from explosive muscular contraction (e.g. an anterior inferior iliac spine avulsion caused by rectus femoris whilst kicking; see Fig. 15.14), a violent joint movement (e.g. avulsion of the base of the fifth metatarsal at the peroneus brevis insertion during ankle inversion) or momentary joint dislocation (e.g. a finger joint dislocation).

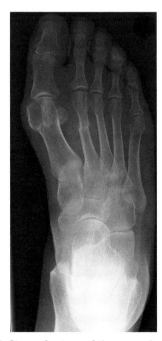

Fig. 1.3 Stress fracture of the second metatarsal.

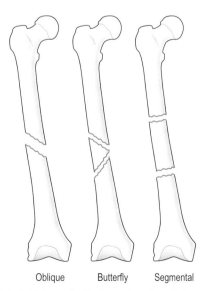

Oblique    Butterfly    Segmental

Fig. 1.4 Oblique, butterfly and segmental fractures.

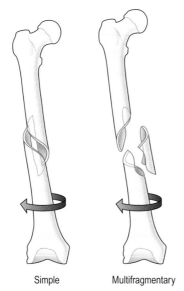

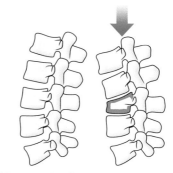

Fig. 1.7 Impaction fracture.

Simple          Multifragmentary

Fig. 1.5 Simple and multifragmentary spiral fractures.

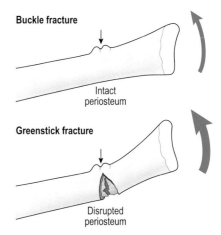

Fig. 1.8 Buckle and greenstick fractures.

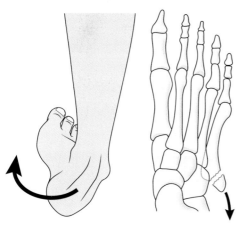

Fig. 1.6 Avulsion fracture.

### Impaction fractures (Fig. 1.7)

These fractures are caused when bone fails in compression. This commonly occurs at a joint (e.g. the tibial plateau in the course of a valgus injury to the knee), or at the humeral or femoral neck (e.g. valgus impacted fractures; see Fig. 17.9), or at calcaneus (after a fall from a

height). A common variant is the *wedge compression* fracture of the spine.

### Paediatric fractures (Fig. 1.8)

Paediatric fractures occur in the immature bones of children, which are far more flexible than adult bones. A *torus (buckle) fracture* occurs when an applied force causes the compression side of a bone to buckle. These injuries are entirely stable. A *greenstick fracture* occurs if the tension side of the fracture also fails, causing the periosteum to tear and the tension cortex to gap. These can be difficult injuries to reduce. Alternatively, *plastic deformation* may result in a bent bone with no other abnormality, often in one forearm bone when the other has fractured. *Physeal injuries* warrant special consideration and are described on page 553.

## Severity

### Open fractures (see Fig. 3.1)

These injuries warrant special consideration because of the markedly greater risk of infection. Open fractures are often described as being *compound*. A fracture is described as *complicated* if there is associated damage to an adjacent structure. *Neurovascular compromise* is particularly important and often requires emergency treatment. The classification and management of open and complicated fractures are described in Chapter 3.

### Intra-articular fractures (Fig. 1.9)

A fracture that disrupts an articular surface is of particular importance, as joint incongruity after union will predispose to post-traumatic arthritis. Marked displacement is an indication for surgical reduction and fixation.

### Comminution (Fig. 1.10)

*Multiple fragments* are indicative of a high-energy injury. There is increased risk of associated injury and complications, including non-union.

### Joint dislocation (Fig. 1.11)

A joint is *dislocated* if there is complete loss of congruity between the articular surfaces. The shoulder and patella are most commonly affected. A joint is said to be *subluxed* if there is loss of congruity but the two surfaces are still in contact. A *transient subluxation* during movement may cause sudden pain and the sensation of something 'slipping out', but often reduces spontaneously such that the joint is *enlocated* at the time of examination.

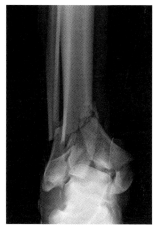

Fig. 1.10 Comminution.

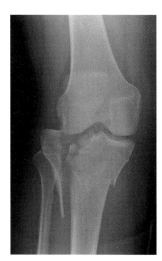

Fig. 1.9 Intra-articular fracture.

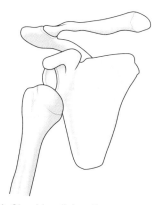

Fig. 1.11 Shoulder dislocation.

### Fracture-dislocation (Fig. 1.12)

This complex injury, comprising a fracture and a dislocation of the adjacent joint, often poses a difficult management challenge. The likelihood of a neurovascular complication is higher. Moreover, closed reduction is often difficult and the attempt can result in further displacement. Open reduction and fracture stabilization are often necessary, and may be required urgently in the presence of neurovascular compromise.

### Sprains (Fig. 1.13)

A sprain is an incomplete tear of a ligament or tendon. The stability of the joint is related to how much of a ligament has torn or become stretched, and many common sprains have classification systems that describe the degree of instability caused (e.g. medial collateral ligament injuries of the knee; p. 431). Inversion injuries of the ankle commonly result in sprains of the lateral collateral ligament complex.

## Location (Fig. 1.14)

The anatomical regions of *skeletally immature* bone are described in relation to the *physis* (growth plate); these are the *epiphysis* (Greek: *epi*, 'upon') and the *metaphysis* (Greek: *meta*, 'adjacent to').

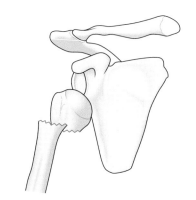

Fig. 1.12 Fracture-dislocation.

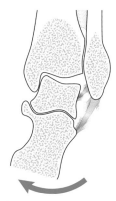

Fig. 1.13 Sprain.

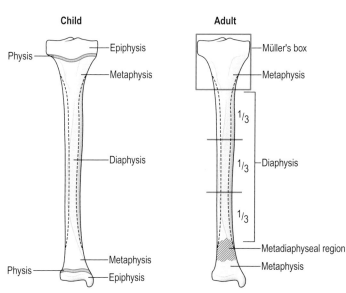

Fig. 1.14 Fracture location in the child and the adult.

In the *skeletally mature* individual, there is no physis or epiphysis, and the entire end region of the bone is termed the metaphysis. The *metaphysis* is composed of cancellous bone, has thin cortices and carries articular cartilage at the joint surface. It is defined as the section fitting within a square 'Müller's box', with sides equal to the widest part of the metaphysis. The *diaphysis* is the portion between the metaphyses. It is tubular with thick cortices and is split into thirds for descriptive purposes. The junction between the diaphysis and the metaphysis is often termed the '*metadiaphyseal region*' and mechanically comprises a vulnerable area where the cortical bone thins and the metaphysis begins to flare.

Some fractures have eponymous labels by virtue of long usage and custom. Examples are the Colles' fracture of the distal 2.5 cm of the radius, which results in a typical 'dinner fork' deformity with dorsal translation and tilt; the Maisonneuve fracture dislocation of the ankle; and the Lisfranc dislocation of the tarsometatarsal joint. These terms are often rather imprecise, not to mention unjust; the named individual commonly was not the first to describe the condition, or often described something completely different!

## Displacement

A fracture that is complete but has not moved is termed *undisplaced* or is said to be in an *anatomical* position. Similarly, a reduction of a displaced fracture to a perfect position is termed an anatomical reduction. A fracture (or an imperfect reduction) that is very nearly anatomical is said to be *minimally* displaced. Fracture *displacement* is described in terms of:

- *length*: distraction/shortening
- *angulation*: *varus/valgus* in the coronal plane and *flexion/extension* in the sagittal plane
- *rotation*: *internal* and *external* rotation
- *translation*: movement anteriorly, posteriorly, medially or laterally.

An image or deformity is described in terms of three standard anatomical planes (**Fig. 1.15**):

- the *transverse* (axial) plane (sections across the body)

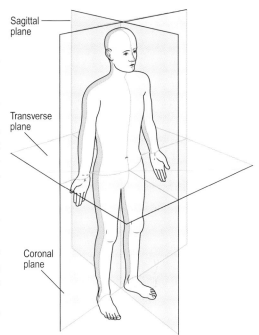

Fig. 1.15 Anatomical planes.

- the *coronal* plane (sections viewed from the front, as you would see if performing a coronation)
- the *sagittal* plane (sections viewed from the side, as you would see if standing in front of an archer (Latin: *sagittarius*)).

### Displacement in length (Fig. 1.16)

Oblique and spiral fractures, and those with significant comminution, displace by *shortening*. Where two fractured bone ends have no contact and have slipped past each other, the fracture is said to be 'off-ended'. Fracture shortening may be accompanied by kinking of adjacent blood vessels, causing vascular compromise. In the Emergency Department, these fractures require reduction by manipulation or traction. Excessive traction will result in the opposite deformity: *distraction*.

### Displacement by angulation (Figs 1.17, 1.18)

This is described by reference to the apex of the fracture. In the coronal plane, a fracture

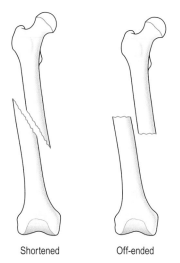

Shortened        Off-ended

Fig. 1.16 Displacement in length: shortened and off-ended fractures.

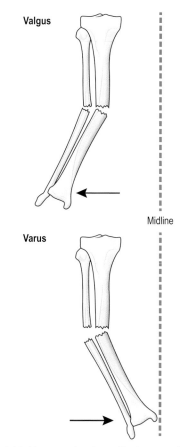

Fig. 1.17 Varus and valgus displacement of fractures.

that has angulated with the apex pointing towards the midline can be said to have medial angulation or to be in *valgus*. A fracture with its apex pointing laterally is said to have lateral angulation or to be in *varus*. In the sagittal plane, a fracture with its apex pointing posteriorly may correctly be said to have pos-terior angulation, to be *apex-posterior*, or to lie in extension or *recurvatum*. Finally, where the apex points anteriorly, the fracture has anterior angulation, is *apex-anterior*, or lies in flexion or *procurvatum*.

At the hand and wrist, alternative terms are often used. The posterior aspect of the wrist is termed *dorsal*, and the anterior aspect is termed *volar*. A Colles' fracture has a clinically obvious bump deformity over the posterior aspect of the wrist, and so, although the frac-ture has volar (anterior) angulation, it is most commonly said to be dorsally *tilted* (see Fig. 4.1). In the foot, the upper surface is termed *dorsal* whilst the underside is *plantar*.

### Displacement by rotation (Fig. 1.19)

A fracture may be rotated *internally* or *exter-nally*. Rotation is usually appreciated more easily on clinical examination than on plain radiographs (or fluoroscopy). Radiographically, rotation is most easily judged by the appear-ance of the two bone ends and therefore radio-graphs of a long bone fracture must include the joint above and the joint below. Uncorrected rotational deformity is often disabling. In the lower limb, rotational deformity will place the foot in an awkward position; in the fingers, it may prevent normal hand function.

### Displacement by translation (Fig. 1.20)

Translation occurs when the fracture surfaces have shifted sideways relative to each other. The displacement is described in terms of the position of the distal fragment. For example, a fracture may be said to have lateral translation, posterior translation, or both lateral and poste-rior translation.

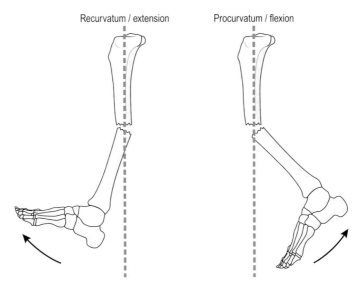

Recurvatum / extension          Procurvatum / flexion

Fig. 1.18 Recurvatum/extension and procurvatum/flexion displacement of fractures.

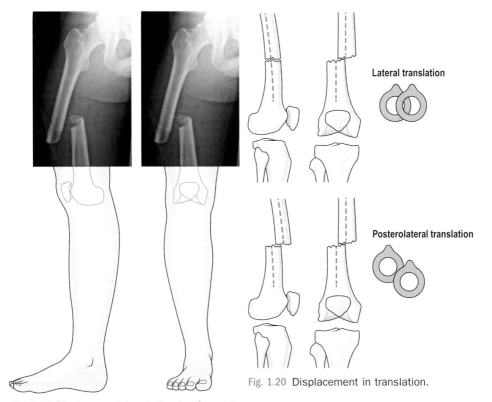

Lateral translation

Posterolateral translation

Fig. 1.20 Displacement in translation.

Fig. 1.19 Displacement in rotation is often not evident radiographically. This radiograph gives no indication of the rotational alignment of the leg.

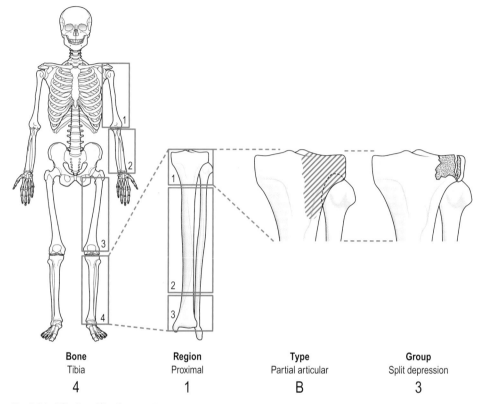

| Bone | Region | Type | Group |
|------|--------|------|-------|
| Tibia | Proximal | Partial articular | Split depression |
| 4 | 1 | B | 3 |

Fig. 1.21 AO classification system.

## Classification systems

Numerous classification systems are used to describe fracture patterns. Many are eponymous and specific to a single injury type, and in this book these are described in the sections related to that region. The Swiss AO group (the Arbeitsgemeinschaft für Osteosynthesefragen or Association for the Study of Internal Fixation (ASIF) has constructed a comprehensive classification of all fractures that is widely used and has subsequently been adopted by other groups, including the Orthopaedic Trauma Association (OTA).

### AO comprehensive classification system

This alphanumeric system is structured and formulaic. It provides a common description of the principal patterns of diaphyseal and meta-

physeal fracture, which is then adapted to specific anatomical regions. The classification follows a common pattern (**Fig. 1.21**):

- The *bone* is first given a number: 1, humerus; 2, radius and ulna; 3, femur; 4, tibia and fibula.

- The *region* of the bone is also numbered: 1, proximal metaphysis; 2, diaphysis; 3, distal metaphysis. The ankle is a special case and is coded 44.

- The fracture *type* is then denoted by a letter: A, B or C. In general, there is a hierarchy of severity and complexity, with A being the simplest fracture that has the best prognosis, and C being the most complex and difficult to manage. The classification of the fracture type is different for the metaphysis and the diaphysis.

- There are then three *groups* within each fracture type: 1, 2 and 3, again numbered in a hierarchy of increasing complexity.
- There are then three *subgroups* within each group: these are denoted by a decimal point and then three numbers, 1, 2 and 3.

The type and group codes are common to most fractures, are easy to commit to memory and are helpful descriptors to use in routine clinical practice. The subgroups have poor inter- and intra-observer reliability and are principally tools for research.

### AO classification of shaft fractures (Fig. 1.22)
The three fracture types are:

- A: simple, two-part fractures
- B: wedge fractures, with some contact between the two principal fragments (remember B = butterfly)
- C: multifragmentary fractures with no contact between the principal fragments (remember C = comminuted).

Within each fracture type, the groups indicate increasing complexity, with 1 indicating a spiral pattern, and 2 and 3 increasing comminution. Spiral types, although they are often quite unstable, are graded lowest because, with their large surface area, they often heal most rapidly.

### AO classification of metaphyseal fractures (Fig. 1.23)
The three fracture types are:

- A: extra-articular
- B: partial articular
- C: complete articular.

This represents increasing difficulty in reduction and fixation. Within each type are groups indicating increasing complexity. Within type B, these usually represent various sagittal and coronal fracture planes, although at either end of the tibia, the B types represent differing degrees of impaction. Within type C, the groups describe increasing comminution of the metaphyseal and articular components of the fracture:

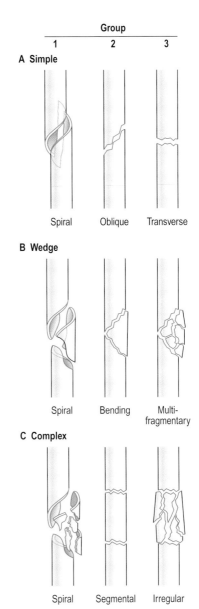

Fig. 1.22 AO classification of diaphyseal fractures.

- C1 is simple metaphyseal, simple articular.
- C2 is complex metaphyseal and simple articular.
- C3 is complex metaphyseal, complex articular.

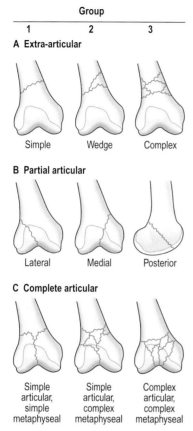

Fig. 1.23 AO classification of metaphyseal fractures.

## ASSESSMENT OF A FRACTURE

## History

In an isolated injury in a physiologically stable patient, history comes first, followed by examination and investigation. The management of the unstable trauma patient is different and is described in Chapter 2.

### History of injury

- *What was the mechanism of injury?* There should be a history of a discrete event, and the exact description will often predict the type of injury present. For example, a blow to the outer aspect of the knee will cause a valgus moment (force), which will commonly result in injury to the medial collateral ligament of the knee in the young (under tension) or a lateral tibial plateau fracture in the elderly (under compression), rather than a medial-sided fracture or medial meniscal injury.
- *How much energy was involved in the injury?* A high-energy mechanism should prompt a careful search for other injuries.
- *What has happened since the injury?*
- *Has the patient been able to bear weight through an injured lower limb?*
- *Are the symptoms improving or deteriorating?*
- *Are there any 'red flag' symptoms?* Ask about symptoms such as progressive, incessant, aching pain that is worse at night and associated with sweats, rigors, malaise or weight loss, which might indicate another pathology such as infection or malignancy (Ch. 6, and Ch. 7 p. 122).

### Medical and drug history

A comprehensive enquiry should include conditions that might alter any surgical plan, including diabetes and anticoagulant drugs.

### Social history

This should cover occupation, hand dominance, degree of social independence, hobbies and sports, and, importantly, smoking and other drugs.

## Examination

Follow the principles:

- **Look**
- **Feel**
- **Move**
- **Neurovascular assessment**

Examine the injured region, including both the joint above and the joint below.

### Look

Inspect the injured part before touching, looking for:

- *Swelling*: initially localized after injury but rapidly become more diffuse.
- *Bruising (contusion)*: may not be present immediately after injury but develops over

hours and days. The location is important: look for seatbelt restraint patterns after a motor vehicle collision, or bruising in the sole of the foot indicating an important structural injury to the hind foot or midfoot.

- *Abrasion*: may be accompanied by ingrained dirt, which has to be removed to avoid permanent tattoo marking.

- *Laceration*: a tearing injury to skin caused by a blunt object such as a hard surface.

- *Incised wounds*: made by a sharp object such as a knife or glass. You should assume that the wound has penetrated to bone until you can demonstrate otherwise.

- *Deformity*: suggests a structural injury. Fracture displacement in any plane may result in excessive skin tension or traction on neurovascular structures, and usually should be reduced (corrected) as a matter of urgency.

### Feel (Fig. 1.24)

Begin palpating distant from the site of injury, usually by excluding injury in the joints above and below, gaining the patient's trust and allowing them to relax the limb gradually. Examine for tenderness and deformity. Where

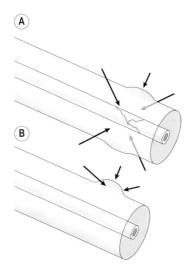

Fig. 1.24 Tenderness. **A**, Bony tenderness arising from a fracture is painful on palpation of the bone from any direction. **B**, In contrast, soft tissue tenderness is only present locally.

there is *tenderness* over a bone, palpate at the same level from another direction to distinguish between bony tenderness (tender on palpation from all directions: **Fig. 1.24A**) and overlying soft tissue injury (tender just over that area: **Fig. 1.24B**). *Deformity* may include a bony prominence or a defect in the contour of a bone, muscle or tendon.

### Move

Gauge the extent of active movement (produced by the patient) and passive movement (performed by the examiner) in the injured joint, and above and below the level of injury. A loss of active movement can result from pain inhibition, a fractured bone, an avulsed or torn tendon, or a neurological injury. Where there is a clear fracture, it is not necessary to perform a detailed examination of range of movement! When there is no history of injury, exquisite pain in a joint that prevents any active or passive movement is suggestive of a septic arthritis.

### Neurovascular assessment

This is mandatory. Assess the limb for colour, temperature and capillary return. Determine the presence and character of pulses distal to the injury and compare these to the uninjured side. Mark the location of palpable pulses with an 'X' to allow comparison later. Determine whether the motor and sensory supplies to the limb are intact and normal (Ch. 3).

## Radiological assessment

### Radiographs

Good-quality radiographs are needed for adequate assessment. Do not accept substandard images. Consider the rule of twos:

- *Two orthogonal views*: Two orthogonal views (taken at 90° to each other: usually an anteroposterior (AP) view and a lateral) of the injured part are required (**Fig. 1.25**).

- *Two joints*: Views of two joints, above and below, are required for a diaphyseal fracture to determine fracture extensions and rotational alignment (see Fig. 1.19). In simple injuries involving just one joint, a single pair of orthogonal radiographs of that joint will usually suffice: for example, for a distal radial fracture. Radiographs of joint injuries may also require other joints to be included in specific circumstances: for example, where there is a suspicion of connected elbow and wrist injuries (see Monteggia and Galeazzi fractures, Chapter 11).

- *Two time points*: Some injuries, such as a scaphoid fracture, may not be visible on the day of injury but may be clear 10 days later when the fracture edges have resorbed.

- *Two limbs*: It is occasionally useful to compare the symptomatic with the asymptomatic side: for example, where the patient has a congenital skeletal deformity. In children, uncertainties relating to the presence of physeal lines should usually be resolved by reference to an atlas rather than by taking additional radiographs.

Some injuries, such as those to the scaphoid, calcaneus or shoulder, have a specific radiographic series that is detailed in the regional chapters. *Traction films* are plain radiographs taken whilst traction is applied distal to a complex injury, often allowing a better appreciation of the fracture configuration. *Stress films* are also occasionally indicated to determine whether a joint is stable or unstable. Sedation or anaesthesia is often required for traction and stress films.

### Ultrasound

This is commonly used to assess the integrity of soft tissues such as the Achilles and quadriceps tendons and the rotator cuff. It is also useful in identifying small joint effusions.

### Computed tomography (CT)

This allows complex bony injuries to be viewed in multiple planes and in three-dimensional reconstruction (**Fig. 1.26**).

### Magnetic resonance imaging (MRI)

This is most useful for assessment of intra-articular and soft tissue abnormalities, and for detecting some occult fractures such as those of the scaphoid and hip (**Fig. 1.27**).

### Aspiration

This is required for the assessment of an acutely painful joint. Aspiration is described in Chapter 6.

### Blood tests

This is useful in the assessment of suspected infection or malignancy and often required for the general medical assessment of the unwell patient or those about to undergo surgery.

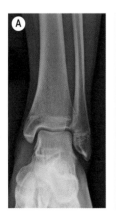
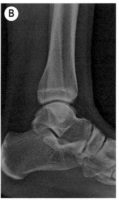

Fig. 1.25 Orthogonal radiographs of the ankle. **A**, AP view. **B**, Lateral view.

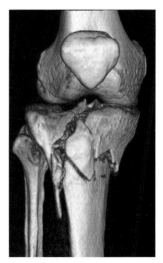

Fig. 1.26 Three-dimensional computed tomogram (3D CT) of a tibial plateau fracture.

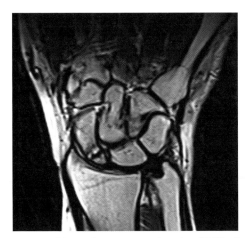

Fig. 1.27 Magnetic resonance imaging (MRI) of a scaphoid proximal pole fracture.

## PRINCIPLES OF FRACTURE MANAGEMENT

The treatment of any fracture comprises three main considerations:

1. *Is the fracture position acceptable or does it need to be reduced?*
2. *Is the fracture stable or does it need to be held?*
3. *When can the patient begin to use and move the limb?*

This can be resolved into the simple paradigm:

**Reduce – Hold – Move**

These factors are intimately related: the method employed to *reduce* a fracture will influence the choice of how to *hold* it (the fixation technique), and this in turn will be influenced by the importance of and difficulty anticipated in allowing the patient to *move* during subsequent rehabilitation. Compare a Colles' fracture with a pilon fracture of the distal tibia. The former can often be reduced closed, held satisfactorily in a cast for 4–6 weeks, and then rehabilitated relatively quickly and simply. Conversely, the pilon fracture can only be reduced open, must be held with absolute stability during healing to ensure final alignment and joint congruence, and has to be rehabilitated slowly with prolonged restricted weight-bearing.

## Reduce

The acceptability of a *fracture position* is dependent on the location of the fracture, the degree of displacement present, and the functional demands of the patient. The acceptable limits of displacement are addressed in the region-specific chapters. Fracture reduction is achieved by either direct (open) or indirect (closed) means.

### Direct reduction

This implies surgical exposure, visualization of the fracture, and anatomical reduction of the key fragments. It is generally required for periarticular fractures where the congruity of the joint surface is important. It is usually accompanied by compression and rigid fixation of the fragments, in the expectation of primary bone healing.

### Indirect reduction

This is accomplished closed (without exposing the fracture), and is achieved with traction and manipulation, which may be a temporary intraoperative manœuvre (such as when femoral nailing) or a definitive strategy (such as when using an external fixator). In periarticular fracture treatment, the application of traction to a distal part of the limb results in *ligamentotaxis* – the reduction of the joint by tension on the surrounding ligaments. This is often imperfect: for example, at the wrist, the volar ligaments are shorter than the dorsal ligaments, and the fracture will often be pulled into dorsal tilt. Equally, some fragments of articular surface have no ligamentous or capsular attachments (often termed *die-punch* fragments) and cannot be reduced at all in this manner.

## Hold

How a fracture is held depends on its degree of stability. *Stability* is clearly a spectrum, but fractures are often described in binary terms.

### Stable fractures

Stable fractures will not displace under physiological loading. This is due to the fracture configuration (e.g. impacted or torus fractures) or regional anatomy (e.g. isolated malleolar fractures of the ankle). They require support only for the comfort of the patient and are usually best treated with removable splintage (orthoses), normally secured with Velcro. This allows the patient to alter the device to allow for the development, and subsequent resolution, of swelling. Orthoses also allow removal for bathing, and for progressive 'weaning' as pain settles and function returns. Common orthoses include 'moon boot' walkers for stable fractures of the foot and ankle, wrist splints for stable distal radial fractures, and mallet splints for fingertip injuries (Fig. 4.27).

### Unstable fractures

Unstable fractures will displace with loading and require stabilization to prevent collapse. Fracture stabilization can be achieved *non-operatively* with splintage or plaster, or *surgically* with the use of a variety of devices including plates, screws, nails and external fixators. The device selected will be influenced by fracture type and location, whether it required a reduction and, if so, whether this was direct or indirect. The type of stabilization provided will, in turn, influence the mechanical environment and how the fracture heals.

### Move

The timing of rehabilitation is a compromise between protecting the fracture reduction through prolonged immobilization and avoidance of load-bearing, and avoiding joint stiffness, muscle wasting and impaired function through early movement.

## BONE STRUCTURE AND HEALING

### Bone anatomy (Fig. 1.28)

Cortical bone is made up of components termed osteons. At the core of the osteon is a central Haversian canal containing blood vessels. Around the canal is a series of concentric lamellae or rings of bone matrix, embedded within which are the bone cells: osteocytes. Adjacent osteons communicate via channels termed Volkmann's canals. Osteons are tightly arranged and overlap, providing cortical bone with its high density. In the diaphysis of a long bone, a ring of cortical bone surrounds a medullary canal containing a central nutrient artery, bone marrow and cancellous bone. In the metaphysis, the cortex is thin, and the architecture

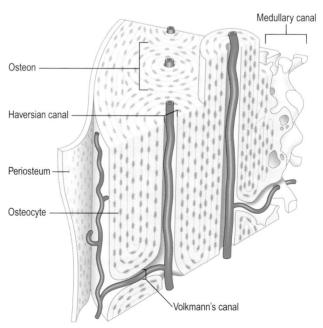

Medullary canal

Osteon

Haversian canal

Periosteum

Osteocyte

Volkmann's canal

Fig. 1.28 Bone micro-anatomy.

comprises delicate trabeculae (Latin: 'beams') of woven bone (Fig. 1.2).

Covering the outer aspect of the cortex is a layer of specialized connective tissue, the periosteum, which is highly vascular and (unlike cortical bone) contains nociceptors. Covering the inner aspect of the cortex is a similar membrane, the endosteum. Both the periosteum and endosteum contain progenitor cells that, after fracture, differentiate into chondroblasts and osteoblasts, which produce callus.

## Fracture healing

The way a fracture heals depends on the amount of movement occurring between fragments, described in *Perren's Strain Theory*. *Strain* is calculated as change in length/original length. Where strain of the tissue at the fracture site is more than 10%, granulation tissue forms; at between 2% and 10%, fibrous tissue forms; while, at under 2%, bone formation is possible. Where there is some movement at the fracture, secondary bone healing occurs, with a gradual transition of tissue types from flexible to rigid as healing progresses. Where there is no movement (i.e. in the artificial situation that exists after rigid internal fixation), bone heals directly with bone.

### Secondary bone healing (healing with callus) (Fig. 1.29)

Under most circumstances, there is movement at the fracture site and bone heals with callus in four phases:

1. *Inflammation* (week 1): The injury causes a haematoma and local inflammation. There is an influx of neutrophils, macrophages and fibroblasts from surrounding soft tissues, and granulation tissue is formed. There is erythema, heat, swelling and pain (rubor, calor, tumor and dolor). The fracture ends are mobile and may grate together (crepitus), causing pain.

2. *Soft callus* (weeks 2–3): The fracture ends die back and an undisplaced fracture, such as one at the scaphoid waist, may become more evident on radiography. The granulation tissue is gradually replaced with fibrous connective tissue (by fibroblasts) and cartilage (by chondroblasts). The fracture ends

**1. Inflammation**: week 1

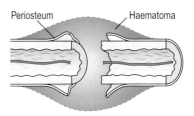
Periosteum          Haematoma

**2. Soft callus**: weeks 2–3

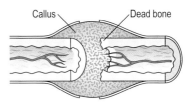
Callus          Dead bone

**3. Hard callus**: weeks 4–12

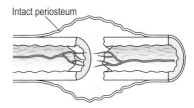
Intact periosteum

**4. Remodelling**: months to years

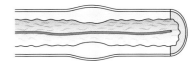

Fig. 1.29  Secondary bone healing.

become 'sticky' and movement is reduced. The fracture can resist shortening but not angulation.

3. *Hard callus* (weeks 4–12): Bone formation (by osteoclasts) begins within the soft callus where the strain is lowest. Bone can be formed in two ways: by intramembranous ossification (which occurs under the periosteum away from the fracture site) and by endochondral ossification (from a cartilage precursor at the fractured bone ends). This progresses centrally across the fracture gap, gradually reducing movement and strain. Calcium is laid down in the matrix

and the callus then becomes visible on radiography. The fracture becomes rigid with this woven bone and is *united* when there is no movement or crepitus at the fracture site. The fracture has *consolidated* once it has completely healed with bridging bone.

4. *Remodelling* (months to years): Creeping substitution replaces the woven bone with lamellar bone (Fig. 1.28). This is the same process as occurs in routine skeletal turnover, as well as in primary bone healing (below). Bone is laid down according to Wolff's Law: the highest density of lamellar bone (and strength) is restored where the load is the greatest. In children, the prominent callus bump shrinks and radiographs can return to normal. In adults, this process is rarely complete.

## Primary bone healing (Fig. 1.30)

If the fracture is reduced and held absolutely rigidly following internal fixation and fracture compression, then the bone heals directly with bone by the same mechanism as intact or woven bone remodels itself. Osteoclasts form a specialized membrane, the 'ruffled border', which adheres to the woven bone, creating Howship's lacunae. Osteolytic enzymes are discharged into the lacunae and bone is resorbed. A 'cutting cone' is formed as the line of

osteoclastic resorption is followed by a trail of osteoblasts, which lay down organized lamellar bone to create a brand-new Haversian system.

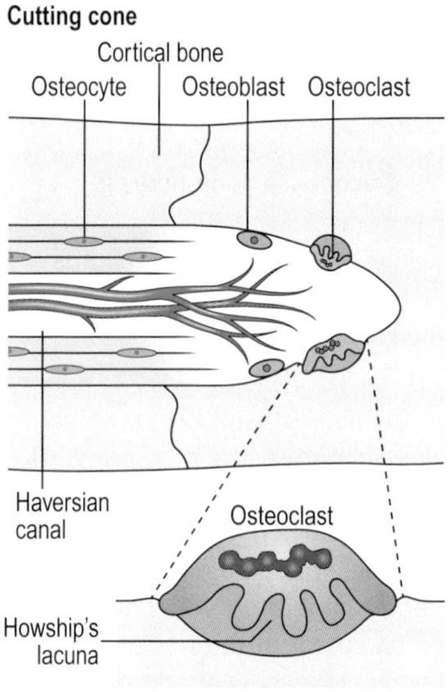

## Assessment of healing

Although bone healing is at the heart of fracture care, determining whether or not a fracture has united is often difficult. In general, a fracture is said to have united when the signs of a fracture have resolved such that:

- there is no local tenderness or heat
- there is no abnormal movement or crepitus
- there is no pain on normal loading
- the radiographs demonstrate that the fracture has healed.

Radiographic fracture healing in itself can be difficult to discern. As a general principle, once the fracture line in three out of four cortices of a long bone has been obliterated or bridged with callus, a fracture is said to have united. In the metaphysis, the presence of bridging trabeculae or a zone of increased bone density indicates union.

# HOW TO PRESENT A RADIOGRAPH

It is important to be able to describe a radiograph clearly and concisely. Classification systems or eponymous terms can quickly define a fracture but, in many circumstances, a methodical description of the points covered in the previous sections is preferable.

Before describing the fracture, it is essential to check the demographics of the radiograph:

- radiographic view provided
- patient name
- date of radiograph
- skeletal maturity – whether the physeal plates closed.

Now describe the 'ABCS' of the fracture:

- **A**dequacy and alignment
- **B**one quality and fracture configuration
- **C**artilage (joint involvement)
- **S**oft tissues.

The following are examples of common injuries and how to describe them.

**Cutting cone**

Cortical bone

Osteocyte    Osteoblast    Osteoclast

Haversian canal

Osteoclast

Howship's lacuna

Fig. 1.30 Primary bone healing.

## Description of a distal radial fracture

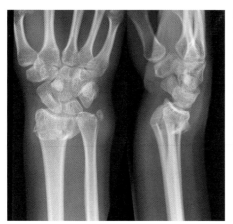

**Figure 1.31** is an AP and a lateral radiograph of the left wrist of Mr T White, taken on the 1st of December. The film is of adequate quality. There is a simple transverse fracture of the left distal radius. There is dorsal tilt of 20°, as well as shortening with some loss of radial height. The fracture is extra-articular and there is minimal soft tissue swelling [*or*: there is a Colles' fracture of the left distal radius].

Fig. 1.31 Distal radius fracture.

## Description of an ankle fracture

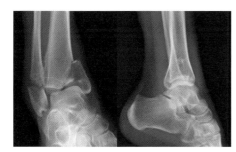

**Figure 1.32** is an AP and a lateral radiograph of the left ankle of Mr SP Mackenzie, taken on the 1st of December. There is a transverse fracture of the distal fibula and an oblique fracture of the medial malleolus of the tibia, with impaction of the medial third of the tibial plafond. There is medial subluxation of the ankle joint, which is no longer congruent. There is moderate soft tissue swelling both medially and laterally [*or*: there is a displaced supination adduction (SAD) fracture of the left ankle].

Fig. 1.32 Ankle fracture 1.

## Description of a hip fracture

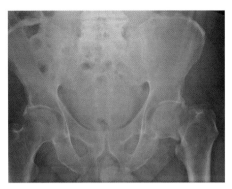

Fig. 1.33 Hip fracture 1.

**Figure 1.33** is an AP radiograph of the pelvis of Mr T White, taken on the 1st of December. It is inadequate because the right proximal femur is not fully visualized. From the limited film, there is an intracapsular fracture of the femoral neck with varus angulation and impaction. Further AP and lateral views of the right proximal femur, and a lateral of the left side, are required to complete the imaging.

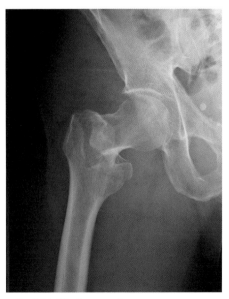

Fig. 1.34 Hip fracture 2.

**Figure 1.34** is an AP radiograph of the hip of Mr SP Mackenzie, taken on the 2nd of December. It shows an intertrochanteric fracture with shortening and varus angulation.

## MAJOR TRAUMA

## The anatomy of the trauma system and team

### The trauma system

A centralized trauma system incorporates several interconnected and coordinated elements. A sophisticated prehospital emergency system, which may include a medical team, allows time-critical interventions such as airway management to be provided at scene. Trauma triage and bypass protocols, based on physiological or injury criteria, allow the rapid transport of the patient to the most appropriate hospital. The major trauma centre will provide rapid and expert resuscitation and definitive management, but must receive a sufficient number of severely injured patients to maintain the expertise of its staff and to justify these sophisticated and expensive services. The acute services are supported by rehabilitation facilities, as well as audit, quality assurance and governance systems. There is evidence that centralized trauma systems can reduce both mortality and morbidity.

### The trauma team

The efficient management of the multiply injured patient relies on the concerted activities of a trained trauma team working together to a common protocol. The sequence of events begins with a pre-alert, and the assembly and preparation of the resuscitation team. In the resuscitation room, the team, directed by an experienced senior doctor, carries out a swift and simultaneous assessment in a standard sequence, aiming to identify and treat life-threatening injuries in order of priority.

## Primary survey

### A – airway with cervical spine control

The airway must be assessed and, if necessary, secured immediately. A patient who is talking coherently is likely to have a patent airway and adequate cerebral oxygenation. However, noisy or absent breath sounds suggest a compromised airway. This is initially addressed by airway positioning, suction, and the use of adjuncts such as an oropharyngeal airway.

Despite simple measures, patients may have persistent airway obstruction or inadequate oxygenation, or may be unable to protect their airway due to a reduced conscious level. They require early definitive airway management, which consists of the placement of a cuffed endotracheal tube which normally requires a rapid-sequence induction of anaesthesia.

Injury to the cervical spine is prevented initially by manual in-line stabilization, followed by the application of a semi-rigid cervical collar, blocks and tape.

### B – breathing with 100% oxygen

Once the airway is secured, high flow oxygen is delivered by facemask with a reservoir bag or via the endotracheal tube, and a rapid evaluation is performed for life-threatening, significant chest injuries. These are recalled using the mnemonic 'ATOM FC':

- **A**irway obstruction
- **T**ension pneumothorax
- **O**pen pneumothorax
- **M**assive haemothorax
- **F**lail chest
- **C**ardiac tamponade

A supine AP chest radiograph will normally be carried out as part of the primary survey (**Fig. 2.3**).

### C – circulation with haemorrhage control

Assess a central pulse for rate and volume, and obtain measurements of blood pressure and peripheral oxygen saturation. Insert two large-bore cannulae and obtain venous blood

**Table 2.1   Grades of hypovolaemic shock**

| Clinical feature | I | II | III | IV |
|---|---|---|---|---|
| Blood loss (mL) | Up to 750 | 750–1500 | 1500–2000 | ≥2000 |
| Blood loss (%) | <15 | 15–30 | 30–40 | >40 |
| Pulse rate (beats/min) | <100 | 100–120 | 120–140 | >140 |
| Blood pressure (mmHg) | Normal | Normal | Decreased | Decreased |
| Pulse pressure | Normal or increased | Decreased | Decreased | Decreased |
| Respiratory rate (breaths/min) | 14–20 | 20–30 | 30–40 | >35 |
| Urine output (mL/hr) | >30 | 20–30 | 5–15 | Negligible |
| Mental status | Slightly anxious | Mildly anxious | Confused | Lethargic |

for cross-match, full blood count, biochemistry, lactate and coagulation screen. Begin intravascular fluid replacement if the patient is shocked.

### Hypovolaemic shock

Hypovolaemic shock is the inadequate perfusion of the central organs due to low circulatory volume. The clinical features associated with the grades of shock are shown in **Table 2.1**. Note that the figures in Table 2.1 are guides; a previously fit young patient may compensate more for hypovolaemia by physiological vasoconstriction, and may not develop clear clinical signs of shock until 2 L of blood have already been lost. The site of the blood loss must be identified and will be in one (or more) of the following areas (**Fig. 2.1**):

1. *Intrathoracic cavity*: Haemorrhage from a great vessel, the pulmonary trunk or an intercostal artery will be manifest as the presence of impaired ventilation, absent breath sounds and frank blood in the intercostal drain. More than 1500 mL in the drain, or the ongoing drainage of 500 mL/hr, is an indication for an exploratory thoracotomy.

2. *Intraperitoneal cavity*: Haemorrhage from a solid organ such as the liver or spleen, or from a mesenteric tear, may result in clinical peritonism. The source of haemorrhage is usually revealed by the trauma CT.

Alternatively, a focused abdominal sonogram for trauma (FAST scan) may reveal intraperitoneal fluid. Where CT or ultrasound is not available, a diagnostic peritoneal lavage (DPL) in the resuscitation room may be considered. If patients do not respond to resuscitation and have signs of abdominal injury (including free fluid on the FAST scan), they should be taken directly to the operating theatre for an exploratory laparotomy.

3. *Retroperitoneal cavity*: Pelvic fractures typically result in extensive bleeding from the low-pressure venous plexus at the back of the pelvis. Bleeding here can track proximally through the retroperitoneal space like smoke rising through a chimney. Arterial bleeding from torn iliac or pelvic vessels, or from the aorta itself, also collects in this space. Retroperitoneal haemorrhage is difficult to detect clinically and must be suspected from the presence of a pelvic fracture. The diagnosis is usually confirmed on CT scan. Where there is any suspicion of a pelvic fracture, a pelvic binder must be applied as part of the primary survey to stabilize the pelvis and minimize further haemorrhage (Figs 15.20 and 15.21).

4. *Thigh compartments*: A closed femoral shaft fracture results in internal haemorrhage involving as much as 2 L of blood, as well

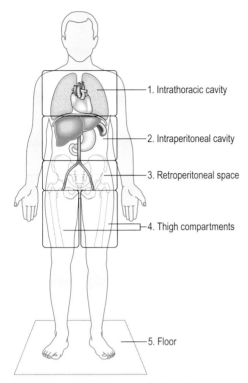

1. Intrathoracic cavity

2. Intraperitoneal cavity

3. Retroperitoneal space

4. Thigh compartments

5. Floor

Fig. 2.1 Sources of haemorrhage after trauma.

as pain and fat embolization. Realignment and immobilization of the limb with femoral traction allows clot to form, minimizing further haemorrhage.

5. *Floor*: Haemorrhage from open wounds can be hard to gauge. An estimate can be made based on reports from the ambulance service and assessment of the volume within splints and dressings and on the floor. Local direct pressure over the bleeding wound, elevation and dressings are required to control blood loss. Brisk arterial bleeding from a limb may require the use of indirect pressure over a major proximal artery. Press the heel of your hand or your fist against the femoral artery at the groin, or use your fingertips to compress the brachial artery against the humerus in the upper arm, where it is felt in the interval between biceps and triceps. In the presence of major limb haemorrhage, application of

a tourniquet is highly effective but at the cost of rendering the limb temporarily ischaemic.

## ⊘ Key point

Substantial ongoing blood loss can be caused by mobile fractures of the pelvis or long bones, as movement impairs clot formation or can dislodge a formed clot. *Skeletal stability is required for haemodynamic stability*, and the application of a binder to the pelvis, and traction or splintage to the long bones, are essential components of the primary survey.

### D – disability

An assessment of central nervous system function is initially made according to the mnemonic AVPU:

- **A**wake
- **V**erbal – the patient responds to verbal orders (such as 'squeeze my fingers')
- **P**ain – the patient reacts to pain
- **U**nresponsive

A more accurate assessment is made with the *Glasgow Coma Scale* (**Table 2.2**).

### E – exposure

Having been undressed for examination, the patient will be at risk of hypothermia, which in turn affects blood clotting, oxygen consumption and conscious level (amongst other factors). The patient should be covered with blankets and, if necessary, warmed.

## Secondary survey

A secondary survey then follows, consisting of a methodical clinical examination from head to foot, in order to detect other injuries. A urinary catheter is placed to allow continued monitoring of fluid balance. Examination should also include the ears and nose, the oropharynx, and the rectum and vagina. Appropriate radiographs are taken as required, depending on the clinical findings. Except

### Table 2.2   Glasgow Coma Scale

| Category | Best response |
| --- | --- |
| **Eye opening** | |
| Spontaneous | 4 |
| To speech | 3 |
| To pain | 2 |
| None | 1 |
| **Verbal*** | |
| Orientated | 5 |
| Confused | 4 |
| Inappropriate words | 3 |
| Incomprehensible sounds | 2 |
| None | 1 |
| **Motor** | |
| Follows commands | 6 |
| Localizes to pain | 5 |
| Withdraws from pain | 4 |
| Abnormal flexion (decorticate) | 3 |
| Abnormal extension (decerebrate) | 2 |
| None | 1 |

*In the intubated patient, add the annotation 't' when scoring verbal response, e.g. 'V-t1'.

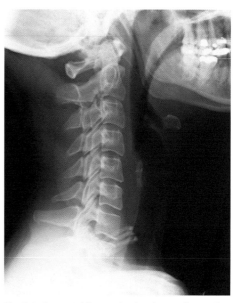

Fig. 2.2 Cross-table cervical spine radiograph.

## Imaging in trauma

### Radiographs

An initial trauma series of three radiographs is classically obtained as part of the primary survey:

- *Cross-table cervical spine (C-spine)*: In addition, a lateral and an open-mouth (odontoid peg) view are often obtained (**Fig. 2.2**).
- *AP chest* (**Fig. 2.3**).
- *AP pelvis* (**Fig. 2.4**).

Some of these plain radiographs may be omitted if an early trauma CT scan is anticipated. Other plain radiographs (usually of the limbs) may be indicated following clinical examination of the patient.

### CT

Subsequently, a CT scan extending from the vertex of the skull to the symphysis pubis ('trauma scan' or 'pan scan') is obtained in order to identify and characterize other injuries. A major trauma resuscitation protocol will usually involve a trauma scan with contrast within 30 minutes of arrival.

where a pelvic injury is suspected (Ch. 15), a log roll is performed to allow inspection of the patient's back, and to remove a spinal board (see Fig. 14.6).

## Tertiary survey

A tertiary survey must be performed after admission, usually on the ward or critical care unit, or following a transfer between centres, in order to exclude other injuries that may have been missed during resuscitation.

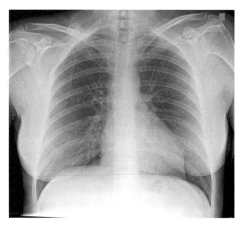

Fig. 2.3 Chest AP radiograph.

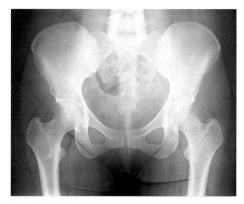

Fig. 2.4 Pelvis AP radiograph.

## INTRAVASCULAR FLUID REPLACEMENT IN MAJOR TRAUMA

Traditional teaching has been for fluid resuscitation to commence with 2 L of crystalloid (Hartmann's solution or Ringer's lactate). However, this can result in systemic cooling, haemodilution, and a rapid rise in blood pressure which may threaten a clot that has formed at the site of injury. Permissive hypotension aims to protect this clot by tolerating a modest reduction in blood pressure during the resuscitation phase provided that the perfusion of the central organs is adequate. Maintenance of a systolic blood pressure of 90 mmHg, which clinically is assessed as the presence of a palpable radial pulse, is usually considered adequate. A more profoundly shocked patient requires fluid resuscitation and improved survival has been demonstrated with early replacement of 'like with like'. This requires early consideration of the use of blood and blood products.

## Blood

The categories of blood issued are:

- *Universal donor O negative blood*: This is available for immediate use in the Emergency Department, allowing blood replacement to begin immediately. The principal restriction with this type of blood is a small incidence of antigen-mediated transfusion reaction.

- *Type-specific blood*: This requires a sample of the patient's blood to be matched in the laboratory for ABO and rhesus group, allowing blood to be issued within 20 minutes. The risk of a transfusion reaction is small.

- *Fully cross-matched blood*. There are numerous other potential antigens, and full cross-matching is a more time-consuming but safer process. Blood can usually be issued in 45 minutes.

Despite the clear advantages of using blood, it is important to bear in mind a number of potential problems associated with blood administration, including hypothermia, transfusion reactions and electrolyte imbalance (particularly hyperkalaemia). Moreover, there are still potential risks involved with contamination and transmission of infection.

## Blood products

Haemorrhage and clotting result in the consumption of clotting products and this, along with haemodilution (from crystalloid administration), hypothermia (which affects enzyme activity in the coagulation pathway) and the development of disseminated intravascular coagulation (DIC), leads to a gradual failure of the coagulation system. This is associated with

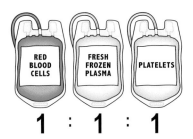

Fig. 2.5 Major haemorrhage pack.

a raised mortality after trauma. Early replacement of clotting products with fresh frozen plasma and platelets, in contrast, improves survival.

## Antifibrinolytic drugs

Tranexamic acid improves survival from haemorrhage if administered early after injury to patients who have suffered significant blood loss.

## Major haemorrhage protocols and packs

Prompt administration of blood and blood products is supported by having a major haemorrhage protocol that allows a single blood sample and request to trigger the release of a standard pack of blood and blood products, and the priority assistance of the Blood Bank and Haematology service. Although local protocols will vary, a typical major haemorrhage pack will usually be available in the resuscitation room within 20 minutes of request and will consist of (**Fig. 2.5**):

- packed red cells
- fresh frozen plasma
- platelets.

## DECISION-MAKING IN TRAUMA

Once the primary survey is under way, the senior doctor in charge of the resuscitation has to begin a complex process of decision-making in order to select the most appropriate disposition for the patient: either for emergency definitive intervention, or for further investigation, or for resuscitation in the ICU. Unnecessary delay in making this crucial decision can result in an extended period in the resuscitation room, delayed definitive treatment and poorer patient outcomes. On the other hand, agreed protocols, well-rehearsed resuscitation team-working and clear communication can allow very rapid definitive intervention.

## Response to resuscitation

The key factor in decision-making is the patient's response to resuscitation as assessed by:

- *physiological values* (pulse, blood pressure, respiratory rate, oxygen saturation, urine output)
- *laboratory measurements* (haemoglobin, coagulation, lactate and base excess).

Whilst individual measurements are important, the trends in these measurements over time are particularly informative. Three terms are used to categorize the response to resuscitation: non-responder, transient responder and responder (**Box 2.1**).

### The lethal triad

The lethal triad is a group of three key physiological abnormalities indicating inadequate resuscitation and increased risk of death (**Fig. 2.6**).

- *Coagulopathy*: indicates consumption of coagulation factors and the hyperstimulation of the inflammatory and coagulation systems.

- *Hypothermia*: occurs from exposure and cold fluid resuscitation, and results in impaired function of a range of enzyme-dependent pathways, including blood clotting.

- *Acidosis*: may reflect inadequate oxygenation (respiratory acidosis) but more commonly indicates occult peripheral tissue hypoperfusion (metabolic acidosis), and is a marker of persistent tissue hypoxia. As a guide some major trauma centres now consider that a lactate of >2.5 mmol/L precludes all but life-saving surgery, whilst a lactate of <2 mmol/L indicates that the patient is adequately resuscitated to undergo surgery. A figure between 2 and 2.5 mmol/L is indeterminate and the direction of a trend over time should be considered.

## Box 2.1 Responses to the fluid challenge

| | |
|---|---|
| **Non-responder** | A patient who has remained shocked despite intravascular filling. The rate of blood loss is greater than the rate of replacement and the patient will exsanguinate unless the source of the blood loss is identified and controlled. The patient is too unstable for further time-consuming investigation and must be taken directly to the operating theatre for surgical haemorrhage control |
| **Transient responder** | A patient who initially improves during resuscitation but whose condition then begins to deteriorate. Again, the rate of haemorrhage outstrips the ability to replace the intravascular volume, and the patient requires emergency surgery |
| **Responder** | A patient who, despite being shocked on admission, improves with resuscitation. Although there are likely to be significant injuries present that may require surgery, the patient is stable enough to undergo further investigation and physiological resuscitation, if required, prior to surgery |

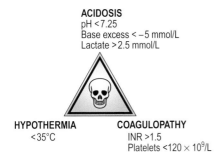

**ACIDOSIS**
pH <7.25
Base excess < −5 mmol/L
Lactate >2.5 mmol/L

**HYPOTHERMIA**          **COAGULOPATHY**
<35°C                         INR >1.5
                              Platelets <120 × 10⁹/L

Fig. 2.6 The lethal triad.

A patient initially taken to the ICU should be taken to the operating theatre for fracture surgery once the elements of the lethal triad have been reversed. Similarly, a patient who was initially stable and who is undergoing surgery, but who then develops elements of the lethal triad, may require suspension of further surgery and a period of resuscitation in the ICU.

### Disposition from the resuscitation room

Options for disposition from the resuscitation room include:

- *Operating theatre*: Non-responders and transient responders to resuscitation usually require emergency surgery to identify and control the source of haemorrhage. The first procedure will be either a thoracotomy, a laparotomy or pelvic packing (Fig. 15.24), depending on clinical assessment of the most likely source of bleeding. A second and a third procedure may then be required in prompt succession. Where there is raised intracerebral pressure or an extradural haematoma, emergency neurosurgery will be required.

- *CT scan*: Most multiply injured patients undergo a 'trauma scan' from vertex to pubic symphysis with intravascular contrast as part of the secondary survey, in order to detect important injuries to the head, trunk and axial skeleton.

- *Interventional radiology*: A small proportion of patients with a single source of haemorrhage detected on CT scan, such as a branch of the internal iliac artery, which may be difficult to control surgically, are suitable for emergency embolization.

- *Intensive care*: Patients who have responded to resuscitation and are haemodynamically stable are none the less often not physiologically normal. They may have ongoing abnormalities in respect of ventilation, acidosis, intravascular filling, coagulation, temperature control and electrolyte balance. A period of further resuscitation in the ICU (summarized as 'wrap 'em up, warm 'em up and fill 'em up') before surgery is beneficial.

## Orthopaedic decision-making: early total care and damage control orthopaedics

Functional recovery from orthopaedic trauma is optimal when the skeleton has been stabilized and the soft tissues have been repaired soon after injury, allowing early rehabilitation and joint movement. However, some reconstructive procedures require subspecialist expertise or specific equipment, and are time-consuming. Lengthy surgery on physiologically compromised patients may worsen their systemic condition. Some surgery, therefore, is best deferred until both the patient and the surgeon are optimally prepared. A number of concepts have been described.

### Early total care

Early total care (ETC) is the definitive stabilization of all long bone fractures within 24 hours of injury once the patient is physiologically stable. It is not usually *immediate* total care. ETC is the most appropriate treatment for the majority of injured patients.

### Damage limitation surgery

Damage limitation surgery or 'damage control orthopaedics' (DCO) is immediate surgery that is required to save life and limb, other reconstructive procedures being deferred until the patient's physiological condition has improved after a period of resuscitation in the ICU. The term is rather loosely employed and there is currently no consensus as to which patients require DCO, or which procedures should be considered. However, procedures that are life- or limb-saving should be considered, even in unstable patients. These include:

- Stabilization of an unstable pelvic ring fracture: This is usually accomplished by application of a binder but may require more complex management.
- Stabilization of a femoral fracture: For those patients who are considered too unstable to undergo nailing, application of either traction or an external fixator ('portable traction') can achieve temporization. Neither technique has shown superiority over the other. Pragmatically, an external fixator may be straightforward to apply if the patient is

in the operating theatre for other reasons, whereas traction (either skeletal or skin traction) may be more easily applied if the patient is in the resuscitation room or in intensive care.

- Decontamination of open wounds.
- Amputation of unsalvageable, dysvascular limbs.
- Decompression of limb compartments for compartment syndrome.

### Early appropriate care

Early appropriate care is the pragmatic concept that unites the entities of ETC and DCO. Patients should undergo as much of their surgery as is safe, as soon as they are physiologically able to cope with such surgery. Life- and limb-saving surgery is prioritized. Ongoing resuscitation in theatre addresses the lethal triad and monitors the patient's response to this. Where patients' physiological condition deteriorates, non-life-saving surgery is suspended for as long as required for further resuscitation to be undertaken, often on the ICU; patients are then returned to the operating theatre as soon as their physiological state allows. Where the patient's physiological condition remains stable or is improving, surgery continues.

## The stress response to trauma

The physiological effects of haemorrhage and resuscitation take place against the background of the body's own stress response. The response is *initiated* by a combination of nociception (afferent pain pathways), local tissue injury (cytokine release) and higher centre (cognitive) responses. This results in the very rapid and complex *activation* of autonomic, immunological, endocrine and haematological responses. Although there is probably a brief initial anergic phase of sympathetic inhibition at the time of injury, the recognized initial *manifestations* of the stress response are tachycardia and tachypnoea, vasoconstriction, pyrexia, a raised white cell count and increased concentrations of hormones such as cortisol, and cytokines such as the interleukins. These systemic features are recognized as the systemic inflammatory response syndrome (SIRS). The aim of this natural response is homeostatic maintenance of blood flow to the core organs, and the mobilization of fat and proteins for injury repair and sustenance of the injured individual. After moderate injury, this response resolves after a few days as the patient recovers.

The magnitude of the response is broadly related to the severity of the injury sustained, modified by genetic predisposition. A proportion of patients develop an exaggerated response with persistent hypoxaemia, peripheral tissue hypoperfusion (identified by a raised lactate and base excess), a hypercoagulable state that may manifest as DIC, fluid retention, and the development of a catabolic state with muscle wastage and negative nitrogen balance. When severe, this results in the multiple organ dysfunction syndrome (MODS). In the lungs, increased membrane permeability and fluid extravasation result in heavy, waterlogged, stiff lungs with impaired oxygen transfer, a condition recognized as acute respiratory distress syndrome (ARDS) (**Box 2.2**). This is compounded when fat and marrow contents have been intravasated from a fracture into the venous circulation. These pass through the right side of the heart to become lodged in the filter of the lungs, exacerbating the ventilation/perfusion mismatch. The criteria for the diagnosis of fat embolism syndrome (FES) are somewhat dated (**Box 2.3**) but represent a recognition of features of ARDS, SIRS, and the shunting of fat and fat breakdown products through the lungs and into the systemic circulation, where they cause petechial haemorrhages. As fat floats, the latter are usually evident on the face and chest. Fat embolism can be detected in 90% of patients with fractures, but FES is rare except after femoral fracture or polytrauma.

### The 'second hit'

During the first 5 days or so of an exaggerated stress response, the immune system is 'primed' to deliver a further increase in response in the face of further stimulation. Surgery during this period can be a potent stimulant and is termed a 'second hit' to the

---

**Box 2.2 Definitions in the stress response to trauma**

| | |
|---|---|
| SIRS | Two or more of: |
| | • Temperature >38°C or <36°C |
| | • Heart rate >90 beats/min |
| | • Respiratory rate >20 breaths/min or $PaCO_2$ <4.3 kPa |
| | • White cell count <4000 or >12 000 cells/mm$^3$ |
| MODS | The presence of altered organ function in an acutely ill patient such that normal homeostatic biological mechanisms cannot be maintained without intervention |
| ARDS | • Hypoxaemia (ratio of arterial $pO_2$ to fraction inspired $O_2$ <26.7) |
| | • Diffuse bilateral pulmonary infiltrates on plain chest radiograph |
| | • No evidence of left atrial hypertension (pulmonary artery wedge pressure <18 mmHg) |

---

immune system. Surgery that is neither life- nor limb-saving may be deferred until the stress response is seen to be resolving, usually towards the end of the first week after injury. Correct timing is judged on the basis of overall physiological progress, as described above. Some specific markers, such as interleukin-6 (IL-6), are abnormally elevated in patients with an exaggerated stress response, and although the role of these markers has yet to be established, they may in future prove to be useful clinical tests as our understanding of the stress response improves.

### Management of the stress response, MODS and ARDS

Whilst there are clear atavistic survival advantages to the stress response, its development in the setting of modern surgery and medicine is often detrimental, and critical

**Box 2.3** Fat embolism syndrome: Gurd and Wilson's diagnostic criteria

One major and four minor criteria are required for diagnosis:

### Major

- Respiratory symptoms, signs and radiographic changes
- Cerebral signs unrelated to head injury or other conditions
- Petechial rash

### Minor

- Tachycardia >110 beats/min
- Pyrexia >38.5°C
- Retinal changes of fat or petechiae
- Renal changes
- Jaundice
- Bloods:

  Acute fall in haemoglobin

  Sudden thrombocytopaenia

  High erythrocyte sedimentation rate (ESR)

  Fat macroglobulinaemia

care management following trauma is principally focused on reversing, or at least minimizing, the effects of hypoxaemia, coagulopathy, fluid retention and nitrogen loss. No specific curative intervention has yet been identified and management is centred on rapid and effective initial resuscitation, *anticipating* a stress response (monitoring the patient carefully in a critical care environment), *supportive therapy* (altered ventilator settings, prone positioning, organ support) and *avoidance* of the 'second hit'.

## ANAESTHESIA AND ANALGESIA

Untreated pain not only is psychologically distressing, but also results in an exaggerated physiological stress response. Effective pain relief is therefore an essential part of trauma

care and encompasses analgesia and anaesthetic techniques.

## Types of anaesthesia

Anaesthesia is the reversible abolition of sensation through the blockade of nerve function by pharmacological agents. Four types of anaesthesia are commonly employed in the Emergency Department:

1. *Local anaesthesia*: infiltration of local anaesthetic agents within the skin or around a peripheral nerve to cause an area of numbness to allow for minor procedures, wound care or suturing. Specific techniques are described below in detail.

2. *Regional anaesthesia*: the use of local anaesthetic agents that are either infiltrated around a nerve(s) or plexus, or injected intravenously distal to a tourniquet (e.g. a Bier's block) to affect an entire body region. With intravenous anaesthetic techniques, neither cardiopulmonary nor central nervous system effects are anticipated or desired. However, systemic effects can occur with, for example, cuff failure and so precautions are required, such as 6 hours of pre-procedure starvation and the availability of resuscitation facilities.

3. *Procedural sedation and analgesia*: the administration of analgesic and anaesthetic agents to provide a brief period of reduced consciousness to allow for the reduction of major fractures or dislocations. Specialist training and facilities are required.

4. *General anaesthesia*: The balanced administration of analgesic, anaesthetic and muscle relaxation agents to induce a more profound reduction in consciousness. This allows extensive control and is useful in resuscitation when a definitive airway has to be established and either extensive investigations or invasive procedures are anticipated.

## Local anaesthetic agents

The most commonly used agents are *lidocaine* and *bupivacaine* (**Table 2.3**), amides that penetrate a nerve cell axon and block the sodium

**Table 2.3   Local anaesthetic doses**

| Agent | Action | Max. dose | Preparations | Max. volume in 70-kg adult | Dose with adrenaline (epinephrine) |
|---|---|---|---|---|---|
| Lidocaine | Short-acting | 3 mg/kg | 1%=10 mg/mL<br>2%=20 mg/mL | 1%: 20 mL<br>2%: 10 mL | 7 mg/kg |
| Bupivacaine | Long-acting | 2 mg/kg | 0.25%=2.5 mg/mL<br>0.5%=5 mg/mL | 0.25%: 80 mL<br>0.5%: 40 mL | Not used |

(Na⁺) ion channels, preventing polarization (see Fig. 3.9). The local anaesthetic is infiltrated into the skin and subcutaneous fat, blocking local cutaneous nerves. Systemic administration can lead to toxicity, with drowsiness, perioral tingling, tinnitus, convulsions and cardiopulmonary arrest. The agents are *contraindicated* in heart block. Effectiveness is *reduced* in infected (and therefore acidic) environments, as this lowers the amount of agent that can enter the axon. In some instances (e.g. when treating scalp lacerations), the addition of adrenaline (epinephrine) can be used to cause local vasoconstriction, reducing local bleeding. Adrenaline must *never be used* in regions with a terminal arterial supply: fingers, ears, lips or external genitalia.

Errors during needle insertion can occur if the tip enters either a major nerve or a vessel. If the needle touches or pierces a nerve, the patient will experience paraesthesia and/or severe shooting pain in the distribution of the nerve. The needle should be withdrawn immediately; under no circumstances should local anaesthetic agents be infiltrated into a nerve. If the needle tip is placed within a vessel, the likelihood of systemic adverse effects is greatly increased and, again, the needle should be withdrawn.

## Preparation for local anaesthesia

Patients should be placed on an examination couch as they may faint during the course of the procedure. Prepare any equipment and

drugs on a separate clean trolley and ensure a sharps disposal box is to hand. Wash your hands and put on gloves before beginning. Arrange for senior support if required.

---

###  Key point

Before injecting local anaesthetic, always pull back on the syringe plunger to check there is no flashback of blood into the chamber. Blood in the chamber means the tip of the needle lies within a vessel, and the needle should be withdrawn to safety or a new trajectory tried. Aspiration should be repeated each time the needle is moved, before injection.

---

### Haematoma block

Injection of local anaesthetic into a fracture haematoma will anaesthetize the periosteum, which may be sufficient to allow fracture manipulation. Patience is essential, as the local anaesthetic will take up to 15 minutes to provide maximal benefit. This is most commonly employed in the reduction of a dorsally tilted distal radius (Colles') fracture.

### Technique (Fig. 2.7)

Firstly, gently palpate the fracture on the dorsal side of the wrist. A bump where the distal fragment has tilted backwards gives a reference for the entry point for the needle. This is followed by thorough skin preparation to avoid introducing infection. Using an aseptic technique, the needle is introduced just proximal to the bump

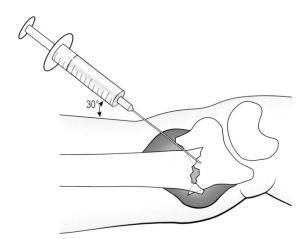

Fig. 2.7 Haematoma block.

at an angle of 30°, directed distally. A small amount of anaesthetic is infiltrated to numb the skin. Advance the needle and infiltrate the tissue with anaesthetic (aspirating each time) as the needle tip moves its way to the fracture site. Pulling back the plunger at this point may result in a small flashback of dark haematoma blood into the syringe chamber, confirming the needle position. Unlike a venous or arterial blood flashback, this is quite acceptable. Slowly infiltrate 10 mL of 1% lidocaine in a fanning motion.

## Regional nerve blockade

Regional nerve blockade provides excellent and reproducible anaesthesia for many procedures in the Emergency Department. The most commonly used techniques allow for anaesthesia to the hand and proximal femur.

### *Sensory nerve supply to the hand*

Sensation to the hand is supplied by the median, ulnar and radial nerves (see Figs 3.17–3.19). Each finger receives four *digital sensory nerves*: two palmar and two dorsal. The palmar digital nerves are larger, more consistent and also more important, as they provide sensation to the finger pulp. They arise in the palm, just proximal to the metacarpal heads, from the common digital nerves of the median and ulnar nerves. The palmar digital nerves run with the digital arteries. The dorsal

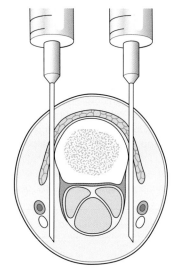

Fig. 2.8 Ring block.

digital nerves are smaller and arise as terminal branches of the radial and ulnar nerves.

### Ring block (digital nerve block)

A ring block provides dense and effective anaesthesia of an entire digit, and aims to block all four digital nerves. For a ring block, 5 mL of 2% lidocaine is required but adrenaline (epinephrine) *must not* be used.

### *Technique (Fig. 2.8)*

Rest the patient's hand on your gloved hand, palm down, and clean the skin with a swab.

The needle is introduced from the dorsal aspect of the base of the finger to one side of the midline. Advance the needle just past the bone of the proximal phalanx until you feel the skin 'tenting' at its volar surface. Do not advance further, as you will risk injuring yourself. Aspirate to ensure the tip is not in a vessel, and then infiltrate local anaesthetic gradually as you withdraw the needle slowly back. Repeat this process on the other side of the phalanx. By passing down both sides of the finger, a ring of local anaesthetic will have been infiltrated and is seen as a characteristic bulge. The ring block will take effect in 10 minutes.

## Metacarpal block

This is useful for slightly more proximal injuries that involve the area over the knuckles and aims to block the common digital nerves. The anaesthetic is infiltrated between the metacarpals and, because two common digital nerves are anaesthetized, the digit and the adjacent halves of the two adjacent digits may be affected. Care must be taken during injection not to place the needle too proximally – the superficial palmar arch lies volar to the metacarpals at the level of Kaplan's cardinal line, which runs from the first web fold in line with the proximal palmar skin crease. A larger volume is required compared to the ring block: 10 mL of 1% lidocaine.

### Technique (Fig. 2.9)
Rest the patient's hand on yours, palm down, and clean the skin with a swab. Palpate the metacarpal heads and necks. The needle is introduced from the dorsal side, between the metacarpal necks, until it 'tents' subcutaneously on the palmar surface of the hand. Aspirate, and then inject slowly as the needle is withdrawn.

## Ulnar nerve block

This block allows a wider region of anaesthesia for injuries that affect the ring and little fingers. The dorsal cutaneous branch of the ulnar nerve, which supplies the back of the hand on the ulnar side, must be addressed with a separate injection.

### Technique (Fig. 2.10)
Ask the patient to flex the wrist. Palpate the flexor carpi ulnaris tendon; the nerve lies deep

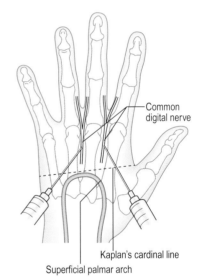

Common digital nerve

Kaplan's cardinal line

Superficial palmar arch

Fig. 2.9 Metacarpal block.

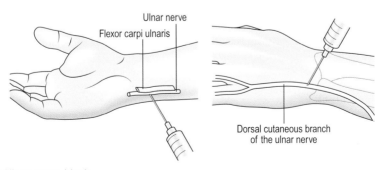

Ulnar nerve

Flexor carpi ulnaris

Dorsal cutaneous branch of the ulnar nerve

Fig. 2.10 Ulnar nerve block.

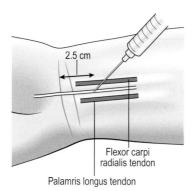

Fig. 2.11 Median nerve block.

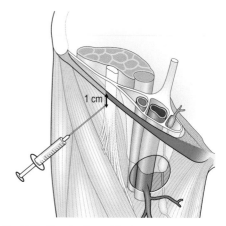

Fig. 2.12 Fascia iliaca block.

to the tendon. After skin preparation, pass the needle transversely behind the tendon towards the radius. The nerve lies at a depth of approximately 10 mm. Aspirate, and then infiltrate 3–4 mL local anaesthetic. To block the dorsal branch of the ulnar nerve, turn the hand palm down and perform a separate subcutaneous injection of 4 mL local anaesthetic, 2 cm distal to the ulnar styloid.

## Median nerve block

Median nerve blocks provide a wide area of anaesthesia over the radial palm and lateral three digits. The nerve is blocked proximal to the carpal tunnel to ensure that the palmar cutaneous branch is included. The key landmarks are the flexor carpi radialis and palmaris longus (present in 85% of the population).

### Technique (Fig. 2.11)

Ask the patient to make a fist and flex the wrist to allow palpation of the flexor carpi radialis and palmaris longus. After skin preparation, insert the needle 2.5 cm proximal to the volar wrist crease between the two tendons. The median nerve is superficial at this level and the depth of injection should be 10 mm. Between 3 and 5 mL of local anaesthetic is used.

## Fascia iliaca block

This provides effective pain relief for injuries to the hip or proximal femur. It may reduce opiate requirements, which is particularly useful in the elderly. Three main nerves contribute to proximal thigh pain: the femoral nerve (anterior), the lateral cutaneous nerve of the thigh (lateral) and the obturator nerve (medial). The nerves lie within and on the psoas and iliacus muscles as they pass under the inguinal ligament, and the fascia iliaca covers this neuromuscular bundle. The three nerves therefore lie in the same fascial compartment and can be blocked with a single injection. In practice, the femoral and lateral cutaneous nerves are reliably blocked while the effect on the obturator nerve is variable. Of note, the femoral branch of the genitofemoral nerve supplies the skin at the groin crease but lies in a different compartment and is unaffected by this method.

### Technique (Fig. 2.12)

With the patient lying supine, palpate the anterior superior iliac spine (ASIS) and the pubic tubercle – the origin and insertion of the inguinal ligament. Imagine the ligament divided into thirds and mark a point 1 cm caudal to (below) the junction of the lateral and middle thirds; this represents the injection site. Now palpate the femoral pulse, which should lie medially by 2–3 cm. Carefully prepare the skin and ready the equipment for aseptic injection. With the non-injecting hand covering the femoral pulse, insert the needle at 90° to the skin. After skin infiltration, tip the needle cranially (upwards) so that the angle between skin and needle is 60°. Advance the needle until two 'pops' are felt. Aspirate, then inject 30 mL of 0.5% bupivacaine. Even though the needle position does not change, aspirate after every 5 mL of local anaesthetic infiltration.

**Key point**

Two fascial planes are crossed by the needle during the fascial iliaca block: the anterior aspect of the fascia lata and the fascia iliaca. Two characteristic 'pops' are felt as the needle tip crosses each plane. Using a short, bevelled needle increases the sensation of the 'pops' and provides confidence that the compartment has been breached.

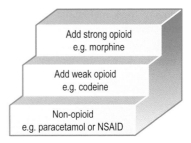

Fig. 2.13 The World Health Organization (WHO) pain ladder. NSAID, non-steroidal anti-inflammatory drug.

## Regional intravenous anaesthesia

Intravenous injection of local anaesthetic distal to a pneumatic tourniquet affords dense anaesthesia. The agent invades the small vascular arcades that surround nerves (vasa nervorum). The tourniquet stops systemic spread of the anaesthetic, thus avoiding cardiopulmonary complications. The tourniquet is therefore the essential piece of equipment in this technique, with many advocating the use of two separate tourniquets placed adjacent to one another in case of equipment failure. A short-acting agent such as prilocaine is used, whose intravenous effects dissipate after 30–40 minutes, after which time the tourniquet can be released safely. This technique should only be performed by those with specific training and experience. Although it can be used in any limb, it is mainly utilized for procedures to wrist or hand, with the tourniquets around the arm; in this case, it is commonly referred to as a 'Bier's block'.

## Analgesia

Analgesia may comprise either oral or intravenous medication, or both. The World Health Organization (WHO) pain ladder provides a stepwise guide to the approach to pain relief (**Fig. 2.13**), beginning with simple preparations such as paracetamol and increasing to weak, and then strong, opiates.

The 'ladder' provides a guide rather than a rigid protocol and, clearly, severe injuries require strong intravenous opiates from the outset. The patient's general health and age should be carefully considered when choosing the dose. Strong analgesics such as morphine are 'titrated to pain', with small aliquots given and allowed to take effect before further doses are given.

## TRAUMA IN THE ELDERLY

As the population ages, the elderly make up an increasingly large proportion of injured patients. Ageing results in reduced bone mineral density, reduced muscle power, impaired balance and slower reflexes, and the majority of fractures in the elderly occur in osteoporotic bone after a fall from standing height. The management of these patients is complicated by a high prevalence of comorbidity and polypharmacy, which may have contributed to the fall and may require optimization before treatment. Elderly patients have reduced physiological reserve and are more susceptible to the complications of recumbency, as well as the physiological insults of surgery. Prompt surgical management should be complemented by intensive medical management. Orthogeriatricians specialize in the perioperative management of older injured patients and are invaluable for optimizing care and rehabilitation. Involvement of physiotherapists and, in most cases, occupational therapists is essential.

## History of the presenting complaint

Enquire about:

- Any pain *before* the fall: Few patients will have had pre-existing pain in the injured region, but it is an important symptom suggesting either a pathological fracture secondary to a metastatic deposit, or a stress fracture.

- The *reason* for the fall: A clear description of events leading to the fall must be obtained. Most occur after a mechanical trip or stumble; however, some patients may complain of chest pain or dyspnoea, or are aware that they blacked out before the fall. The most common precipitants of a low-energy fracture are intercurrent infection (usually of the urinary or respiratory tract), postural hypotension or a transient loss of consciousness. Aim to exclude serious conditions such as myocardial infarction or a pulmonary embolus.

- The *consequences* of the fall: A head injury is common and symptoms of amnesia, severe headache or neurological dysfunction should prompt further investigation. Enquire about anticoagulant medications if the patient has had head trauma. If patients were unable to get up after the fall, ask how long they lay on the floor (a long period lying down can result in rhabdomyolysis, hypothermia, dehydration and electrolyte imbalance) and how they managed to get help. While the patient may be preoccupied with a particularly painful limb injury, enquire about any other areas of discomfort that may also require investigation.

If the patient is unable to recollect the fall or has cognitive impairment, seek a witness account.

## Past medical history

A full and detailed past medical history should be taken from the patient, with corroboration from hospital records and other sources such as the general practitioner. Previous cardiac or respiratory illnesses are particularly important, as assessment of these conditions may be required before anaesthesia. A full, systematic enquiry should be undertaken to help guide investigations (**Box 2.4**).

## Cognitive assessment

Cognitive impairment is common in elderly injured patients, who may have pre-existing dementia (chronic cognitive decline) or delirium (acute-onset impairment, often precipitated by peripheral disorders or by drug adverse effects or withdrawal). A structured cognitive assessment will clarify a patient's level of impairment (which is closely predictive of morbidity and mortality) and their capacity to give consent for an operation, and provides a baseline in case of perioperative deterioration. In patients who attend with impairment, ask relatives or nursing home staff about baseline function. There are a number of rating scales, of which the 'Four As' Test (4AT) is well suited to rapid initial assessment (**Fig. 2.14**). A score of 4 or more suggests delirium or cognitive impairment, and a score of 1–3 suggests possible cognitive impairment, while a score of 0

---

**Box 2.4 Systematic enquiry**

| | |
|---|---|
| Cardiovascular | Pre-existing cardiovascular conditions, chest pain, syncope, palpitations, orthopnoea, exercise tolerance |
| Respiratory | Pre-existing respiratory diseases, sputum, cough, haemoptysis, wheeze, dyspnoea |
| Gastrointestinal | Pre-existing GI diseases, dyspepsia, vomiting, abdominal pain, irregular bowel habit, per rectum blood/mucus, weight loss |
| Genitourinary | Pre-existing disease, dysuria, flow problems, incontinence |
| Neurological | Pre-existing neurological disease, vertigo/dizziness, headache, limb weakness, paraesthesia/sensory deficit |
| General | Personal history of malignancy anywhere, alcohol intake, smoking |

| [1] Alertness | |
|---|---|
| This includes patients who may be markedly drowsy (e.g. difficult to rouse and/or obviously sleepy during assessment) or agitated/hyperactive. Observe the patient. If asleep, attempt to wake with speech or gentle touch on shoulder. Ask the patient to state their name and address to assist rating. | |
| Normal (fully alert, but not agitated, throughout testing) | 0 |
| Mild sleepiness for < 10 seconds after waking, then normal | 0 |
| Clearly abnormal | 4 |
| **[2] AMT4** | |
| Age, date of birth, place (name of the hospital or building), current year. | |
| No mistakes | 0 |
| 1 mistake | 1 |
| 2 or more mistakes/untestable | 2 |
| **[3] Attention** | |
| Ask the patient: "Please tell me the months of the year in backwards order, starting at December." To assist initial understanding one prompt of "what is the month before December?" is permitted . | |
| Achieves 7 months or more correctly | 0 |
| Starts but scores < 7 months / refuses to start | 1 |
| Untestable (cannot start because unwell, drowsy, inattentive) | 2 |
| **[4] Acute change or fluctuating course** | |
| Evidence of significant change or fluctuation in: alertness, cognition, other mental function (e.g. paranoia, hallucinations) arising over the last 2 weeks and still evident in last 24hrs. | |
| No | 0 |
| Yes | 4 |
| 4AT Score | |

**4 or above**: possible delirium ± cognitive impairment
**1–3**: possible cognitive impairment
**0**: delirium or severe cognitive impairment unlikely
    (but delirium still possible if [4] information incomplete)

Fig. 2.14 The 'Four As' Test (4AT) for delirium and cognitive impairment. AMT4, Abbreviated Mental Test with four questions. www.the4AT.com © MacLullich A, Ryan T, Cash H, reproduced with permission.

suggests that the patient is unlikely to have cognitive impairment.

## Social history

The patient's level of dependency (including any pre-fracture family or other care at home) should be defined. Those patients who need help at home are likely to require additional assistance during recovery, while those in a nursing home may be suitable for early transfer back to their place of residence. It is also important to know whether the patient uses any aids for mobilization, such as a walking stick or a frame.

## Drug history

A full drug history and documentation of allergies are essential but special attention should be given to those drugs that may affect surgery.

- *Warfarin and its indication*: Critical indications, such as the protection of a metallic heart valve, will require conversion to a heparin infusion, usually with haematological advice. Non-critical indications, such as prophylaxis for patients with atrial fibrillation, usually will simply require temporary reversal with 1–2 mg vitamin K preoperatively.

- *Clopidogrel and aspirin*: These are not usually stopped preoperatively because of their long half-life, but they may cause the anaesthetist to avoid a spinal anaesthetic.
- *Angiotensin-converting enzyme (ACE) inhibitors*: Stop on admission and restart on day 3 postoperatively to protect renal function. (Do not restart if there is acute kidney injury or hypotension; seek a medical review.)
- *Diuretics*: Generally, these should be withheld perioperatively unless there is prominent congestive cardiac failure. (Do not restart if there is acute kidney injury or hypotension; seek a medical review.)
- *Non-steroidal anti-inflammatory drugs (NSAIDs)*: These should generally be avoided in the elderly, who are more prone to both nephrotoxic and gastrointestinal effects.
- *Beta-blockers*: Continue perioperatively but be aware that they limit the patient's ability to mount a compensatory tachycardia.
- *Antidepressants, antipsychotics, drugs for Parkinson's disease, benzodiazepines and antiepileptics*: These should all be continued, using a nasogastric tube if necessary.
- *Corticosteroids*: If the dose is above 5 mg per day for longer than 2 weeks, additional perioperative steroid is essential to avoid an Addisonian crisis.
- *Oral hypoglycaemics*: These can be withheld on the morning of surgery.
- *Insulin*: A dextrose infusion and a sliding scale of insulin will be required on the day of surgery.

## Examination

A full examination of the cardiopulmonary, gastrointestinal and neurological systems should be undertaken alongside the injury-specific examinations.

## Investigations

Laboratory assessment of the blood count, liver function, renal function, electrolytes (including calcium) and coagulation are required. In fractures of the hip or long bones, a cross-matched sample for possible blood transfusion should be stored.

A plain chest radiograph is required preoperatively. A 12-lead electrocardiogram should be performed in all elderly patients. An echocardiogram may be indicated in patients with a significant history of cardiac failure or valvular heart disease, but this should not delay surgery. Early discussion with the anaesthetist and/or the orthogeriatrician often helps to tailor preoperative investigations and expedite surgery.

## Common medical problems

A review by an orthogeriatrician will often allow complex comorbidities to be addressed quickly.

### Delirium

Delirium is common in elderly patients, affecting more than 40% of hip fracture patients. Early detection and management are important. Treatment involves initial screening for life-threatening acute medical and/or drug causes, and then a more detailed evaluation of precipitants and a tailored management plan are required. Patients with delirium should be reviewed by an orthogeriatrician.

### Dehydration and electrolyte imbalance

Intravenous fluids are commonly required to optimize fluid balance, and additional caution is required in patients with pre-existing cardiac or renal dysfunction. If there is an element of acute kidney injury (failure), stop nephrotoxic drugs, begin a regular fluid-monitoring chart, optimize fluid and oxygen therapy, consider bladder scanning and/or renal ultrasound scan, and consider catheterization.

### Cardiac dysrhythmias

Atrial fibrillation commonly complicates systemic infection in the elderly. Fluid optimization and antibiotic treatment may allow spontaneous cardioversion but pharmacological agents may be required. If the patient is already on a drug such as digoxin or a beta-blocker, a small increase in dose may be required.

## Myocardial infarction

The majority of ischaemic cardiac events in the elderly are non-ST elevation myocardial infarctions (NSTEMI), which are treated by combination antiplatelet therapy. Discussion with a cardiologist is recommended to optimize treatment of the myocardial infarction without risking significant blood loss during surgery.

## Infection

Urinary or respiratory tract infections should be treated empirically and promptly after obtaining urine or sputum specimens.

## Pathological fractures

Where there is a possibility of a pathological fracture, begin with examination of common primary sites (breast, thyroid, neck and axillary lymph nodes, abdomen, prostate). In addition to the routine blood tests listed above, $Ca^{2+}$ level and serum electrophoresis assays are obtained routinely, along with specific tumour marker assays as appropriate. Further imaging should be considered before surgery, including, as a minimum, full-length views of the affected bone. Where the primary is unknown, a skeletal survey or isotope bone scan, and CT of the chest, abdomen and pelvis are often required. Where there is suspicion of a renal tumour (which may be highly vascular), an arteriogram and possibly preoperative embolization may be appropriate. Surgery may need to be delayed.

## Postoperative management

A patient confined to bed is at risk of the complications of recumbency, including:

- infections of the pulmonary and urinary tract
- venous thromboembolism
- wastage of muscle and decreased strength
- joint stiffness and wastage of cartilage
- accelerated osteoporosis
- malnutrition and constipation
- depression and loss of confidence
- pressure sores and ulcers
- delirium.

The process of ensuring that a frail and vulnerable patient rehabilitates as rapidly as possible is complex and requires the coordinated activity of not only surgeons, physicians and nurses, but also occupational therapists, physiotherapists and often a variety of other services; it is a true multidisciplinary endeavour. Early involvement of these groups will help recovery, and allow important tertiary fracture prevention with falls assessment and osteoporosis therapy.

## Analgesia

Elderly patients may not state clearly when they are in pain, especially where there is cognitive impairment. As well as asking patients about pain, observation for signs such as general distress, lack of movement, grimacing and so on is important in pain assessment. Effective analgesia is essential to reduce distress, assist with early mobilization and reduce the risk of delirium. However, many drugs may themselves cause delirium. In the preoperative and early (2 days) postoperative phase, a simple regime of paracetamol and low-dose oxycodone (e.g. 2 mg three times a day+2 mg as required) is often effective. Morphine, codeine and dihydrocodeine are best avoided because of metabolite accumulation when there is renal impairment. Tramadol and nefopam frequently cause significant adverse effects and generally should be avoided.

## Falls and fracture prevention

Following a fragility fracture, patients have a 40% risk of further fragility fractures. During the postoperative period, patients should undergo a falls assessment (including assessments of vision, hearing, cognitive function, and tripping hazards at home). Elderly patients suffering a hip fracture are deemed to have osteoporosis and do not require dual-energy X-ray absorptiometry (DEXA) scanning, but should receive secondary prevention. Patients with other fragility fractures should undergo DEXA scanning and then be offered preventative therapy where appropriate.

## CLOSED SOFT TISSUE INJURIES

A fracture can be thought of as a severe soft tissue injury within which there happens to be a broken bone. Injury to the soft tissues around a fracture will often influence the management of the fracture, and the likelihood of encountering complications. Fractures resulting from a direct blow or high-energy transfer are usually associated with worse soft tissue injury than fractures caused by indirect torsional forces. Some injuries, such as pilon fractures (p. 506), are associated with a particularly vulnerable soft tissue envelope.

## Contusion

A fracture causes internal bleeding, which, unless contained within a joint capsule, gradually tracks to the skin and results in a contusion (bruise) or a haematoma (a collection of blood). The pattern of contusion may be of importance in diagnosis; for example, a calcaneal fracture will often result in a contusion on the sole of the foot. Contusion may take several hours to appear and may not be evident at the time of presentation to the Emergency Department, but may become surprisingly extensive over the course of a few days after fracture.

## Haematoma

A haematoma is a discrete collection of blood within soft tissues. A deep haematoma will result in local swelling and tenderness. A superficial haematoma, particularly in the pretibial region, may compromise skin viability.

## Swelling

The inflammatory reaction to injury causes a local increase in vascular permeability, resulting in tissue swelling and heat. An area of swollen (and often contused) skin will have a reduced capillary circulation and thus a reduced capacity to heal. Surgical incisions placed through such skin will have a higher risk of dehiscence (breakdown). Swelling will regress with rest, intermittent compression and skin cooling (ice packs or cryotherapy devices), and elevation (RICE: rest, ice, compression and elevation). As acute swelling subsides, the skin takes on a wrinkled appearance and regains its elasticity; this is the point at which surgery can safely be performed.

## Tenting

Skin pulled taut over a prominent bone end will have a very localized area of impaired circulation, which is at risk of necrosis and spontaneous breakdown. This converts a closed fracture to an open fracture and greatly increases the chances of infection. Skin tenting must be addressed by reduction of the fracture or dislocation at the time of recognition, and may be an indication for urgent surgery.

## Blisters

The rapid development of swelling can cause a shear injury between the epidermis and dermis. Where this potential space fills with serous fluid, a *clear fracture blister* forms. Where the underlying capillaries of the dermis are breached, the blister will fill with blood and this is termed a *haemorrhagic blister*. In either case, the dermis itself remains intact. Blisters are uncomfortable but will resolve over 10–14 days, and are best left undisturbed if possible. The blister fluid is sterile, but a ruptured or deroofed blister will rapidly become colonized with bacteria. A surgical incision through an area of haemorrhagic blistering takes longer to epithelialize and carries a higher risk of infection.

## Degloving

A degloving injury is a shear injury resulting in a plane of cleavage under the skin, between the subcutaneous fat and the deep fascia. A typical mechanism of injury is one in which the soft tissues of a limb are crushed and deformed by the wheels of a vehicle or the rollers of a piece of machinery. The normal vascular supply to the skin arises directly from its underlying deep fascia, and so a degloving injury results in an impaired blood supply or even complete devascularization of the overlying skin. It is usually unwise to make a surgical incision through an area of degloved and devitalized skin, as the rate of wound dehiscence and infection is extremely high. Of particular note is the Morel–Lavallée lesion, an extensive area of degloving over the hip associated with an acetabular fracture. A high degree of suspicion is required for diagnosis. The skin will be cool and insensate. If the skin has been devascularized, surgical exploration and excision of all non-bleeding skin and fat are required. A large sheet of excised skin can, on occasion, be 'defatted', stored, and used as a full-thickness skin graft.

## OPEN FRACTURES

An open fracture exists where there is a fractured bone and a breach of the dermis in the same limb segment. Even where the open wound is not directly overlying the fracture, it should be assumed initially that there is a direct communication. Prompt and expert management is imperative, as the risk of major complications, particularly infection, is far higher than for a closed fracture.

### Classification
The *Gustilo and Anderson classification* is widely used (**Fig. 3.1**, **Table 3.1**).

## Emergency Department management
An open fracture often results from high-energy trauma, and initial management consists of an ATLS primary survey and then secondary survey (pp. 21-25).

### History
A full history of the circumstances of the injury is required, including a description of the mechanism of injury and the environment to which the bone was exposed, particularly whether this included farmyard waste or immersion in water.

### Examination
- *Look*: The wound should be inspected and assessed. Take a photograph of the wound and then cover it with a simple, sterile, saline-soaked dressing.
- *Feel*: There will be crepitus on passive movement as the fracture is reduced.
- *Move*: There is no advantage to testing movements of adjacent joints, other than those involved as part of the motor nerve tests.
- *Neurovascular assessment*: A careful examination of the distal neurological and vascular supply is required.

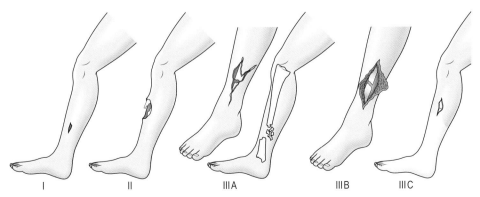

| I | II | IIIA | IIIB | IIIC |

Fig. 3.1 Gustilo and Anderson classification of open fractures. See Table 3.1 for description.

**Table 3.1    Gustilo and Anderson (GA) classification of open fractures**

| Grade | Description |
|-------|-------------|
| I | A wound that is <1 cm in length |
| II | A wound that is >1 cm but <10 cm in length |
| III | A wound of >10 cm in length, or a wound of any size that is associated with: <br> High-energy mechanism of injury or fracture comminution <br> Crushing of the soft tissues <br> Contamination that is extensive or involves farmyard or marine material |
| GA grade III injuries are subdivided according to further criteria: | |
| IIIA | No extensive periosteal stripping or soft tissue loss |
| IIIB | Extensive periosteal stripping and/or inadequate soft tissues remain to allow closure, necessitating flap or graft coverage |
| IIIC | Presence of a vascular injury requiring repair |

## Treatment

- *Intravenous antibiotics*: Give these as early as possible after Emergency Department presentation. The choice of antibiotic will vary, depending on local protocol, but would typically consist of a cephalosporin (cefuroxime 1.5 g three times a day) or co-amoxiclav (1.2 g three times a day). For patients with a penicillin allergy, clindamycin (600 mg four times a day) is an alternative.
- *Heavily contaminated wounds*: Add an aminoglycoside such as gentamicin (1.5 mg/kg three times a day).
- *Anti-tetanus toxoid*: Give this where there is any doubt regarding full immunity.
- *Further cleaning*: No attempt should be made at this stage to remove anything other than gross contamination. Cover with a simple, sterile saline soaked dressing.
- *Splinting/casting*: The limb should be brought out to length and correct alignment, and then splinted or casted.

## Orthopaedic management

Surgery comprises thorough debridement and a form of surgical stabilization, although the latter may not be the definitive method of fixation. While timing is important, the surgical team involved in the management should be experienced in the treatment of such injuries. Surgery can then be considered in two main scenarios: emergency and urgent.

### Emergency surgery indications

Emergency surgery is likely to be required in circumstances involving:

- a wound with gross contamination, or contamination with farmyard or marine material
- a dysvascular limb (p. 58)
- compartment syndrome (p. 45).

### Urgent surgery (<24 hours) indications

All other open fractures should undergo surgical debridement within 24 hours. Although the timing of surgery is important, the expertise of the team performing the operation is probably more important. Where local facilities do not include such expertise, arrangements should be made for expeditious transfer of the patient to an appropriate facility rather than attempting any initial surgery locally. Tibial fractures are at greater risk of complication than other open fractures; Gustilo and Anderson grade III fractures of the tibia should be viewed as particularly urgent, if not necessarily emergency, cases.

## Principles of surgery in open fractures

Open fractures are difficult injuries to treat and may require multiple complex bone and soft tissue reconstructive procedures. Ideally, an initial assessment is made by a plastic surgeon and an orthopaedic surgeon, operating together. In very severe injuries, early consideration should be given to the requirement for a primary amputation (p. 60). The sequence of events will vary, depending on local preference and the nature of the injury, but several stages are required:

### 1. Set-up

Surgery is performed under general anaesthesia and without traction. A *tourniquet* is applied to allow the identification of neurovascular structures and careful assessment of tissue integrity, but this may be deflated during the operation to allow assessment of the capacity of the soft tissue and bone to bleed. An initial '*pre-scrub*' of the limb is performed to remove gross contaminants, such as road grit, glass fragments and plaster of Paris, from the skin. A large bowl of warm saline with aqueous chlorhexidine is useful, as is a nailbrush. The limb is then formally prepared and free-draped to allow complete manoeuvrability.

### 2. Wound debridement

The wound edges are excised and the wound extended, both proximally and distally, far enough for all the traumatized tissue within the 'zone of injury' to be seen and assessed. This will clearly include the fractured bone ends but should also take into account any skin undermining or degloving, and any contamination that has worked its way into deeper tissue planes. The location of these wound extensions must take into account the surgical exposure required for subsequent fracture stabilization, and a possible requirement for plastic surgical flaps and grafts. Working carefully and sequentially through each tissue layer, all contaminated and dead tissue is excised, including skin, fat, fascia, muscle and bone (**Fig. 3.2**). Muscle viability is assessed according to the 'four Cs' (colour, contractility, consistency and capacity to bleed; p. 49). Major peripheral nerves and vessels should be

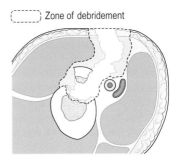

Fig. 3.2 Wound debridement.

identified and protected. The bone ends are then delivered into the wound sequentially and examined. Contamination of the (external) periosteum and (internal) endosteal canal is removed with sharp dissection and curettage. Fragments of bone are subjected to the 'tug test': those that can be removed easily from the wound with forceps are deemed to have insufficient soft tissue attachment to maintain their viability. These fragments of avascular bone pose a substantial risk for later osteomyelitis and are discarded, unless they have a large articular surface component. In this latter situation, it may be decided that the benefits of preserving the fragment outweigh the risks. The soft tissues deep to the bone are also examined and debrided carefully before the bone ends are released back into the wound. Finally, the wound is irrigated extensively with warmed normal saline (around 6 L) at low pressure to remove remaining invisible contaminants, on the premise that '*the solution to pollution is dilution*'. There is no benefit from pulsatile lavage (which forces remaining contaminants deeper into the tissue planes), or from adding antibiotics to the lavage fluid.

### 3. Fracture stabilization

The patient may need to be repositioned on the table – with traction, for example, if intramedullary nailing is planned. The surgical team should rescrub, the limb should be reprepared and redraped, and new instruments should be used. Definitive fracture fixation is performed wherever possible and, provided that debridement has been adequate, internal fixation with an intramedullary nail, or with plate fixation, is optimal. Where there is very extensive contamination – for example, following ballistic or blast injury, there is substantial potential for deterioration in the state of injured tissues over the first few days. In this context, definitive fracture fixation often cannot be performed safely at the first procedure, and temporary external fixation is required. The fixator pins should be placed well away from the wound and any potential sites of later metalwork placement.

### 4. Wound closure

Primary wound closure at the first procedure may be considered where:

- the patient has no significant comorbidities, such as diabetes or immunosuppression
- the patient has been fully resuscitated
- there was no farmyard or marine contamination
- debridement is complete and the residual tissues are healthy
- the fracture has been stabilized
- the wounds can be closed without tension.

Interrupted sutures are preferred to a continuous suture. Drains do not provide any particular benefit, but a low-pressure vacuum dressing applied to the closed wound may help to minimize wound-edge oedema. Where the above criteria cannot be met, the wound is left open and delayed primary closure is performed at the second (or subsequent) procedure.

### 5. Repeated inspection and debridement

Where there is any doubt regarding the viability of the remaining tissues, the wound is left open and dressed. Suitable options include:

- a 'bead pouch' consisting of a string of gentamicin cement beads under an adhesive impermeable dressing
- a vacuum dressing (**Fig. 3.3**).

The patient is then brought back to theatre after 48 hours for a repeat assessment and debridement of the wound. Several such procedures may be required before all tissues of dubious viability have 'declared' themselves.

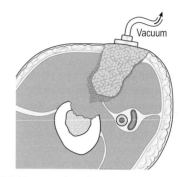

Fig. 3.3 Vacuum dressing.

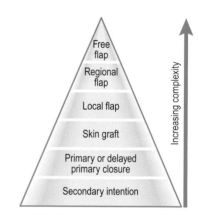

Fig. 3.4 Soft tissue reconstructive ladder.

### 6. Soft tissue reconstruction

Tissue loss or wound oedema may mean that the wound cannot be closed without tension, preventing either primary or delayed primary closure, and soft tissue coverage with a flap or graft is required. This surgery should be performed as soon as practicable, or at least within 6 days. The 'reconstructive ladder' describes the available options for soft tissue coverage in order of complexity (**Fig. 3.4**):

- *Healing by secondary intention*: Where bone, tendon and metalwork have been covered in a healthy fascial envelope, small residual skin defects can be left to granulate. A vacuum dressing may assist in this healing response.
- *Primary closure*: Primary closure of the defect may be possible where two healthy,

viable skin edges can be brought together without tension.

- *Skin graft*: This can be applied to a healthy, vascularized tissue such as muscle or fat, but not directly on to bone or tendon, or over metalwork.

- *Local tissue transfer*: This may be required to cover bone, tendon or metalwork. The flap may contain skin, fat, fascia or muscle, or combinations of these tissues. A local skin flap may have a random pattern (not based on any specific vascular supply) or an axial pattern (based on a defined vascular pedicle). A muscular flap (such as a gastrocnemius flap) is defined according to the site of its vascular pedicle. A split-thickness skin graft (often harvested from the thigh) may then be required to cover the flap or donor site (**Fig. 3.5**).

- *Regional tissue transfer*: Regional flaps are harvested from an area not immediately adjacent to the defect. They are then moved on a vascular pedicle under (or over) an area of intact tissue to cover the defect.

- *Free tissue transfer*: Free tissue transfer of muscle and skin may be required for larger defects. For example, latissimus dorsi or rectus abdominis can be elevated and detached from its vascular supply and then placed in the defect, with a microvascular anastomosis to uninjured local vessels.

### 7. Bone defect reconstruction

There may be a residual defect in the bone after debridement. This should not be grafted primarily and the options are:

- To splint the fracture out to length with either external or internal fixation, with a view to addressing the defect at a later procedure. The defect may be filled with cement to maintain a gap, with a view to filling this later with bone graft.

- To shorten the limb acutely, either definitively (particularly in the upper limb), or temporarily with a view to later lengthening. An acute skeletal shortening can often decrease the effective size and complexity of a soft tissue defect.

The subsequent management of the defect is described in Chapter 7.

## COMPARTMENT SYNDROME

Compartment syndrome is the development of muscle swelling within an indistensible fascial compartment, resulting in increased intracompartmental pressure and tissue hypoperfusion. Left untreated, the tissues within the compartment become ischaemic, dysfunctional and then necrotic (**Fig. 3.6**). Compartment syndrome is therefore a surgical emergency.

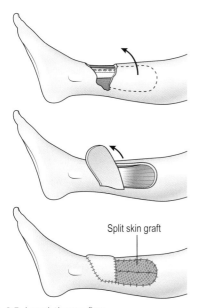

Fig. 3.5 Local tissue flap.

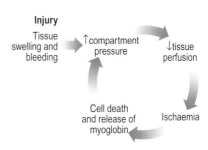

Fig. 3.6 The vicious circle of compartment syndrome.

## Aetiology

Compartment syndrome is caused by:

- *Fractures*: typically, a tibial fracture, but other anatomical sites like the forearm are also at risk, particularly after high-energy injury. Although some damage to the fascial envelope occurs in open fractures, this is rarely enough to decompress the compartment and so open fractures are at risk just as much as closed fractures.

- *Blunt contusion*: to a muscle, such as following a direct blow to the thigh.

- *Haemorrhage*: into a compartment, particularly in patients taking anticoagulants.

- *Extravasation*: caused by irritants or by excess fluid that has been erroneously administrated intramuscularly and can increase the intracompartmental pressure.

- *Reperfusion injury*: following a period of limb ischaemia. Muscle damage resulting in renal injury is termed *crush syndrome* (p. 49). Common scenarios include:

  - following revascularization of a critically ischaemic limb (prophylactic fasciotomies are usually performed)

  - following release from prolonged entrapment

  - following prolonged compression, typically affecting the thighs and buttocks of an individual who has lost consciousness and has remained recumbent in one position for a prolonged period of time: for example, following a drug overdose.

## Emergency Department management

### History and examination

The cardinal features are:

- pain out of proportion to the injury sustained

- pain on passive stretching of the muscles within the affected compartment(s)

- reduced power in the muscles within the affected compartment(s)

- paraesthesia and hypoaesthesia in the distribution of the nerves travelling through the affected compartment(s)

- a feeling of tightness and tension in the muscles in the compartment.

---

##  Key points

- Compartment syndrome may not be immediately obvious and must be considered in order to be diagnosed.

- The symptoms of compartment syndrome are *not* the same as the 'six Ps' of critical ischaemia (Box 3.1, p. 59).

- The presence of a distal pulse does not exclude a compartment syndrome, and loss of the pulse suggests that irreversible damage has already occurred to the nerves and muscle.

- Compartment syndrome is a surgical emergency.

---

## Treatment

- Any constricting circumferential dressings should be split down to skin along their entire length.

- The limb should be placed at the level of the heart (but not into high elevation).

- Any fracture should be realigned, immobilized and splinted.

- Urgent surgical review is necessary, with a view to fasciotomy.

## Orthopaedic management

Where a diagnosis of compartment syndrome is made on clinical grounds, urgent fasciotomy is required without further delay. Where there is no clinical diagnosis of acute compartment syndrome but suspicion remains regarding existing (or potential) limb swelling, the patient should be discussed with a senior colleague and admitted for close monitoring, serial examination and possibly pressure monitoring.

## Pressure monitoring

Monitoring of the pressure within the compartment is a useful adjunct, particularly in the unconscious or obtunded patient. Moreover, intracompartmental pressures tend to rise before the symptoms of the condition present, and continuous pressure monitoring therefore provides an 'early warning' of the development of the condition. The presence of the monitoring equipment, and the requirement for the nurse at the bedside to record the pressure readings every hour, also raise awareness of this important condition, reducing the likelihood of a 'missed' compartment syndrome in all cases at risk. The use of pH monitoring, rather than pressure monitoring, may offer a refinement of this technique once its role has been defined.

### Technique (Fig. 3.7)

Prepare the necessary equipment first:

- cannula, preferably long enough to pass through an incision distant to the fracture (e.g. a 14Ch-gauge spinal cannula), although an intravenous cannula is adequate
- knife, preferably with a pointed no. 11 blade
- local anaesthetic (in the conscious patient)
- sterile saline
- 5 mL syringe
- sterile dressing pack and gloves
- pressure transducer (as for an arterial or central venous pressure line).

All equipment should be opened after hand-washing, using a 'no-touch' technique. The surgeon should then don sterile gloves.

1. Select the entry point. For a tibial fracture, this is over the anterior compartment of the leg (the most commonly affected compartment), 2 cm lateral to the tibial border, and 10 cm away from the fracture (**Fig. 3.7A**). For mid-shaft and distal fractures, the entry point is proximal to the fracture. For proximal fractures, the entry point is distal to the fracture, and the cannula is passed proximally in a retrograde manner.

2. Open the transducer and prime the line with sterile saline, making sure there are no air bubbles. Unlike with an arterial line, a slow, continuous flow of saline is not required through a compartment monitor, as this will increase compartment pressure.

3. Clean the skin, infiltrate with local anaesthetic, and make a stab incision 5 mm long.

4. Prepare the cannula by making a slit at the tip of the catheter to minimize the chance of it becoming blocked with muscle.

5. Pass the cannula through deep fascia at an angle of 45° and into the anterior compartment muscle (**Fig. 3.7B**). Once the fascia has been penetrated, lower the hand so the cannula is at an angle of 20° and then progress it down the leg, running parallel with the tibial border. Stop when the tip comes to lie at the level of the fracture (**Fig. 3.7C**). Withdraw the needle from the cannula.

6. Prime the cannula with 2 mL of sterile saline and attach the pressure transducer. Secure the cannula and tubing carefully to prevent inadvertent displacement. The transducer must be at the level of the fracture (**Fig. 3.7D**).

7. Set the transducer to zero and measure the intracompartmental pressure.

8. Calculate the $\Delta P$ by subtracting the compartment pressure from the diastolic blood pressure. This is the 'perfusion pressure' supplying blood to the compartment, and the $\Delta P$ should be >30 mmHg. The monitor should be left in place to allow repeated measurements, which will establish a trend in pressure.

A persistently low $\Delta P$ gives a diagnosis of compartment syndrome. Where the $\Delta P$ is normal and the trend is a gradual rise (falling intracompartmental pressure) over 12 or more hours after injury or surgery, continuous monitoring can be discontinued.

## Fasciotomy of the leg (Fig. 3.8)

Under general anaesthesia, all four compartments are widely opened to relieve the pressure, the muscle is inspected carefully, and any non-viable tissue is debrided.

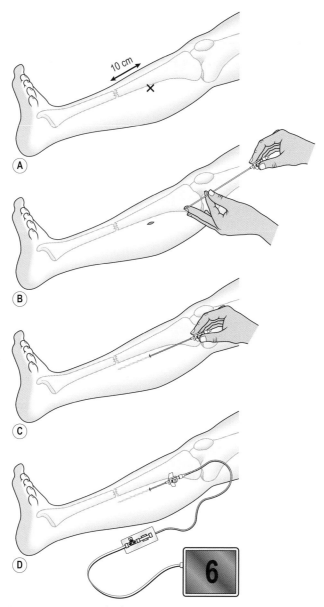

Fig. 3.7 Compartment pressure monitoring.

A tourniquet is applied to allow tissue inspection. The *posterior* and *deep* compartments are addressed through a medial incision placed 3 cm behind the posterior border of the tibia. Blunt dissection through fat avoids injury to the saphenous vein and nerve. The posterior compartment fascia is opened and a finger is introduced at the upper and lower extents of the incision to confirm complete release. The gastrocnemius and soleus muscles are reflected back from the posterior aspect of the tibia until the intermuscular septum is

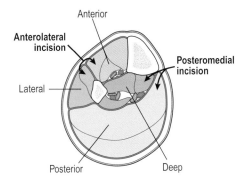

Fig. 3.8 Leg fasciotomies.

encountered. This is then incised longitudinally to expose the deep compartment and, again, complete release is confirmed by palpation. The *anterior* and *lateral* compartments are exposed by a lateral incision placed halfway between the tibial crest and the line of the fibula. Blunt dissection through fat avoids damage to the superficial peroneal nerve, which has a variable course, passing up through the deep fascia of the lateral compartment in the mid-leg to lie in the subcutaneous plane. The anterior compartment fascia is opened longitudinally over the entire length of the muscle belly. The lateral compartment is then released either by opening the intermuscular septum or, more commonly, by making a separate longitudinal incision through the deep fascia. Again, complete release is confirmed by palpation.

The viability of the muscle is confirmed by assessing the *'four Cs' of muscle viability*: colour (pink), contractility (present), consistency (dead muscle can be scooped out with a curette) and capacity to bleed. Muscle that appears healthy externally should be assessed for central necrosis by introducing a large artery clip into the centre of the muscle belly and spreading fibres apart. All dead muscle must be excised. The wounds are left open, and covered with either absorbent or vacuum dressings. The patient is returned to the operating theatre at 48 hours for reassessment and further debridement. The wounds can rarely all be closed at 48 hours and are managed either by gradual closure over the course of repeated operations, or definitively by skin grafting.

## Neglected compartment syndrome

Where the diagnosis of compartment syndrome has been made after a significant delay of 24–48 hours or more, there may be little advantage in releasing or exploring the compartments, as much or all of the muscle will be dead. Moreover, there is a high rate of severe infection after delayed exploration. Delayed joint fusions or an amputation may be preferable.

## CRUSH INJURIES

Soft tissue crushing may follow an obvious traumatic event such as a building collapsing or a person being run over by a vehicle, but may also follow a less dramatic insult such as a prolonged period of immobility following a drug overdose. Even where the injury is closed, crushing often results in surprisingly severe soft tissue injury, including:

- *skin degloving* and devascularization: particularly where there has been a rolling or twisting component to the injury
- *rhabdomyolysis*: the release of breakdown products, including myoglobin and potassium, from damaged, ischaemic muscle
- *crush syndrome*: renal failure, resulting from:

  myoglobin precipitation in the renal glomerular filtrate and blockage of the collecting tubules

  systemic hypovolaemia from fluid loss in the injured muscle
- *reperfusion syndrome*: occurring when the circulation is restored after a prolonged period of ischaemia; the resulting sudden release of muscle breakdown products into the circulation may cause cardiac dysrhythmias and acute renal failure
- *compartment syndrome*: resulting from muscle swelling.

## Emergency Department management

### History and examination

Establish the duration of any long lie (prolonged recumbency) or entrapment. The patient may display the features of shock (Table 2.1). The affected limb will be tense and oedematous with painful muscles. The urine has a typical frothy, tea-coloured appearance.

## Investigation

- The creatine kinase (CK) level is grossly raised.
- Blood chemistry reveals acidosis (low bicarbonate, low pH).
- The urine dipstick is positive for blood (but indicating myoglobin rather than haemoglobin), but there are no erythrocytes on urine microscopy.

## Treatment

Resuscitate the patient with two wide-bore intravenous cannulae and a high-volume crystalloid diuresis. Catheterize and monitor urine output. Disposition should be to a critical care area for monitoring and possibly renal replacement therapy (dialysis).

## Orthopaedic management

Urgent fasciotomy and exploration are sometimes required to reverse any ongoing ischaemic injury, and to debride non-viable muscle to prevent further myoglobin release. Amputation should be considered at an early stage for severely damaged and non-viable limbs, and in the event that the patient has had a tourniquet applied at the scene of injury several hours before, to prevent the crush syndrome that would arise on release of the tourniquet.

## NERVE INJURY

### Anatomy (Fig. 3.9)

A peripheral nerve cell comprises a cell body (**a** on Fig. 3.9), which receives afferent (incoming) impulses via a number of dendritic processes (**b**), and an efferent (outgoing) axon (**c**), which transmits the impulse to the target organ (**d**). The axon is invested in an insulating layer, the myelin sheath (neurolemma, **e**), formed by Schwann cells. Gaps between these cells, known as nodes of Ranvier (**f**), are the sites of the sodium channels where adenosine triphosphate (ATP)-powered ion pumps maintain an electrical gradient in the resting state. An action potential occurs when sodium channels open, resulting in depolarization. The impulse passes rapidly along the nerve by saltatory conduction. Bundles of axons form a fascicle surrounded by perineurium, and multiple fascicles are bound together by the epineurium to form a peripheral nerve (**Fig. 3.10**). Nerves often convey a mixture of motor, sensory and autonomic axons. Various insults, including contusion and pressure, will inhibit nerve function. 'Tenting' of a nerve may be caused by a local area of pressure from a fracture or dislocation, which results in tension on the adjacent segment of nerve (**Fig. 3.11**).

### Classification

The general term *nerve palsy* is used to describe abnormal nerve function after injury. The *Seddon classification* describes three types of

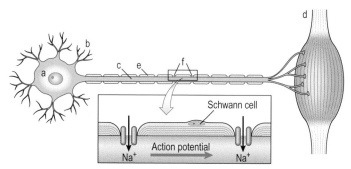

Fig. 3.9 Nerve fibre.

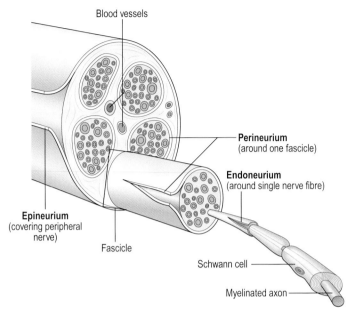

Fig. 3.10 Peripheral nerve.

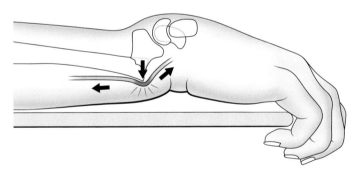

Fig. 3.11 Nerve tenting.

injury (**Fig. 3.12**): neurapraxia, axonotmesis and neurotmesis.

## Neurapraxia

The function of the axon is disturbed by ischaemia following contusion, traction or pressure, and the ion pump ceases to maintain a resting potential, so no impulses are transmitted. For example, 'Saturday night palsy' occurs when individuals fall asleep with their arm over a chair back, exerting pressure against the brachial plexus. The degree of impairment of a peripheral nerve varies, depending on the proportion of the axons within it that are affected. However, the structure of the nerve is unaffected and, once the insult has been removed, the ion pump begins to work and nerve function returns. Note the correct spelling of the word neur-a-praxia, which is derived from Latin and means 'nerve not working'. The commonly used but incorrect term, 'neuro-praxia', is nonsensical, as it conveys precisely the opposite.

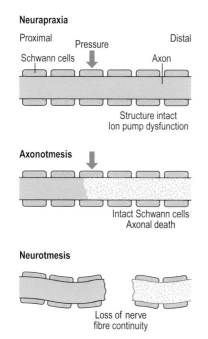

Fig. 3.12  Seddon classification.

### *Axonotmesis*

In a more severe injury, a section of the axon itself is damaged and the segment of axon beyond this point (which is reliant on the cell body for nutrition) dies, in a process termed *Wallerian degeneration*. Nerve function cannot return initially, even after the insult has been removed. However, the myelin sheath remains intact and the axon is able to grow down this 'pipe' to its target organ, where it can re-establish function. Axonal growth occurs at 1 mm a day, and the likely timing of return of function can be estimated by the distance from the injury to the target organ. *Tinel's sign* – a sensation of tingling on light percussion over the regenerating segment – allows assessment of progress. Scarring within the myelin sheath 'pipes' may prevent regeneration of a proportion of the axons in a nerve, and so nerve recovery after axonotmesis is often incomplete.

### *Neurotmesis*

This is complete division of a peripheral nerve, often resulting from a penetrating injury. Regenerating axons have no myelin sheath guide and may form a painful neuroma at the site of injury. Nerve function can only be restored by surgical exploration and repair of the nerve. Thereafter, axons may select the wrong 'pipe' and fail to reach the correct target; others are blocked by scar tissue, and so nerve recovery is usually incomplete. Although repair of individual fascicles may be attempted, an epineural suture repair is generally performed, as it usually results in the same outcome.

## Emergency Department management

This requires the cooperation of the patient. If patients are unconscious or sedated, it is important to know whether they have been seen to move all four limbs at any point after injury.

### History

Gain a full description of the injury mechanism and force. A history of a penetrating injury should be specifically sought. The nature of the symptoms should be carefully detailed, including the presence of paraesthesia (pins and needles), anaesthesia (numbness) or dysaesthesia (altered sensation), and the cutaneous distribution of this. Is weakness present and to what extent? The onset and progression of the symptoms are also important. Symptoms that are improving are likely to continue to do so, while deterioration usually indicates worsening injury.

### Examination

- If you suspect a *spinal or nerve root injury*, assess for defects in a dermatomal and myotomal pattern.

- If you suspect a *peripheral nerve injury*, assess for defects in the distributions of the peripheral nerves.

- Where there is a suspected *brachial plexus injury* (**Fig. 3.13**), a more specialized examination may be required.

### *Nerve root levels: upper limb (Fig. 3.14)*

- *Sensory*: Over the torso, the dermatomes T4 (nipple-level), T10 (umbilicus) and L1 (groin

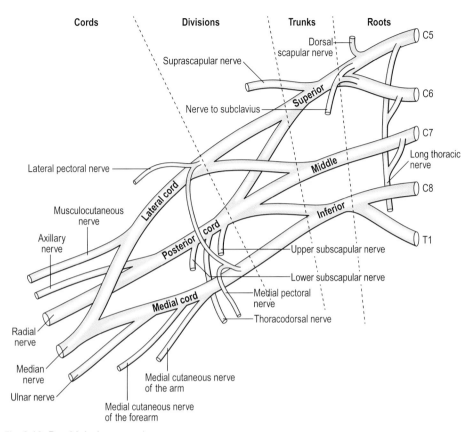

Fig. 3.13 Brachial plexus.

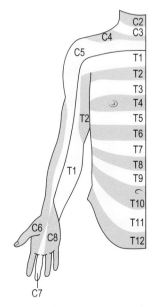

| Movement | Myotome |
|---|---|
| Elbow flexion | C5 |
| Wrist extension | C6 |
| Elbow extension | C7 |
| Finger flexion | C8 |
| Finger abduction | T1 |

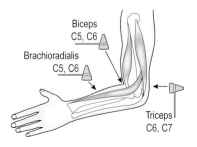

Fig. 3.14 Upper limb nerve root examination.

crease) are constant. In the upper limbs, the distribution is also regular. C6 supplies the radial side of the hand and forearm, the middle finger is C7, and C8 the ulnar side of the hand.

- *Motor*: It is often easiest to memorize a sequence of actions as a rather strange dance: for the cervical roots, flex the elbows (C5), extend the wrists (C6), extend the elbows (C7), flex the fingers (C8), and adduct and abduct the fingers (T1).

- *Reflexes*: Percussion of the biceps tendon and brachioradialis promotes a reflex arc controlled by C5,6. The triceps reflex is C6,7.

### Nerve root levels: lower limb (Fig. 3.15)

- *Sensory*: In the lower limb, the dermatomal orientation is oblique, reflecting the evolutionary rotation of the lower limbs from that of lizard-like external rotation. Note that the

L5 dermatome, supplying the dorsum of the foot and hallux, helpfully coincides with the direction of movement of the motor supply, as does the S1 dermatome over the plantar surface. S2 supplies the back of the knee while S3 supplies the buttock.

- *Motor*: For the lower limbs, there is a more logical sequence of root values for hip flexion (L2), knee extension (L3), ankle eversion (L4), hallux dorsiflexion (L5), and both ankle and hallux plantar flexion (S1).

- *Reflexes*: The knee reflex is controlled by the quadriceps, with the spinal levels L3,4. The ankle reflex test is S1,2.

### Nerve root levels: perineum (Fig. 3.16)

- *Sensory*: S3 supplies the buttock, whilst S3,4 supply the perineum.

- *Motor*: The pelvic floor is memorably supplied by 'S2, 3 and 4, which keep the anus off the floor'. When assessing a patient who

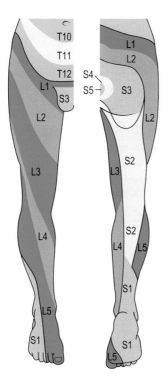

| Movement | Myotome |
|---|---|
| Hip flexion | L2 |
| Knee extension | L3 |
| Ankle dorsiflexion | L4 |
| Hallux extension | L5 |
| Hallux flexion | S1 |
| Ankle plantar flexion | S1 |
| Knee flexion | L5 |

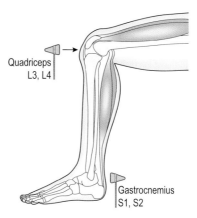

Fig. 3.15 Lower limb nerve root examination.

### Table 3.2  Upper limb peripheral nerves

| Nerve | Unique sensory testing area | Motor testing |
| --- | --- | --- |
| Musculocutaneous | Lateral aspect of forearm | Elbow flexion |
| Axillary | Regimental badge area | Shoulder abduction |
| Median | Pad of index finger | Thumb abduction |
| Ulnar | Ulnar aspect of little finger | Finger abduction |
| Radial | Dorsal aspect of first web space | Wrist extension |

### Table 3.3  Lower limb peripheral nerves

| Nerve | Unique sensory testing area | Motor testing |
| --- | --- | --- |
| Femoral | Anterior thigh | Knee extension |
| Tibial | Plantar aspect of foot | Ankle plantar flexion |
| Superficial peroneal | Dorsum of foot | Ankle eversion |
| Deep peroneal | First web space of foot | Ankle dorsiflexion |

| Movement | Myotome |
| --- | --- |
| Anal tone/contraction | S2, 3, 4 |

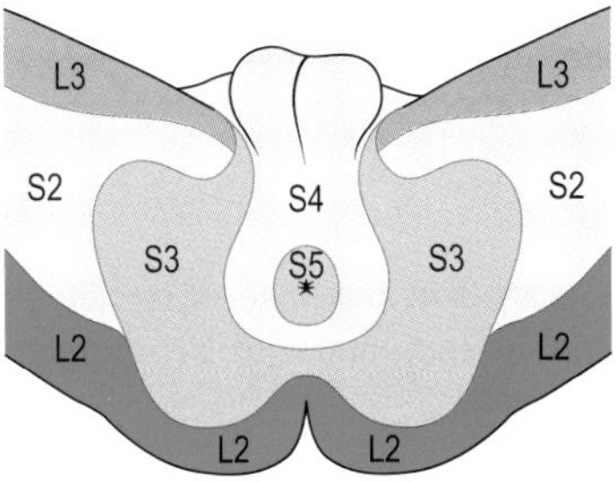

Fig. 3.16 Per-anal nerve root examination.

presents with back or leg symptoms after trauma, a digital rectal examination, in the presence of a chaperone, is recommended. Make note of the anal tone as the digit is introduced. Ask the patient to squeeze your finger; this can initially be difficult for the patient to coordinate. Enquire whether the patient can feel the digit or whether sensation is reduced.

### Peripheral nerve assessment
Note that there is considerable overlap of the peripheral nerve distributions but that there are specific areas that allow unique assessment of only one nerve (**Tables 3.2–3.3**; **Figs 3.17–3.22**).

The severity of a motor injury is assessed according to the Medical Research Council (MRC) grade (**Table 3.4**).

### Treatment
Emergency Department treatment involves identifying the cause and, if possible, limiting the progression of an ongoing nerve injury that is due to a reversible insult. This usually involves the closed reduction of a fracture or dislocation.

### Fracture displacement/joint dislocation
The deformity should be reduced closed under procedural sedation without delay. The limb is then splinted and elevated. If closed reduction is unsuccessful, the fracture may require urgent open reduction in theatre, at which point the

**Sensory**

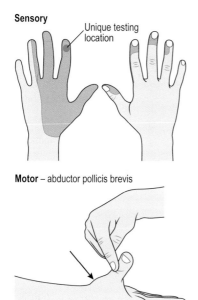

Unique testing location

**Motor** – abductor pollicis brevis

Fig. 3.17 Median nerve examination.

**Sensory**

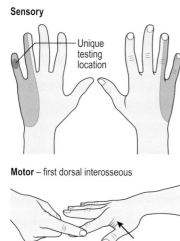

Unique testing location

**Motor** – first dorsal interosseous

Fig. 3.18 Ulnar nerve examination.

nerve should also be explored. Following successful reduction, admit the patient for hourly assessment of limb colour, sensation and movement (CSM) to ensure progressive recovery.

**Sensory**

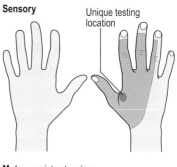

Unique testing location

**Motor** – wrist extension

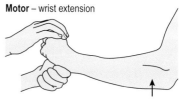

Fig. 3.19 Radial nerve examination.

## ⊘ Key point

It is mandatory to document the neurovascular status of the affected limb before and after attempted reduction. If symptoms develop or worsen after reduction, there may be an iatrogenic nerve injury, which will require urgent intervention.

*Indications for urgent senior review*

- *Failed closed reduction of a fracture or dislocation.*

- *Persisting, worsened or new symptoms after reduction.*

- *Compartment syndrome: This may follow tibial fracture, for example (p. 45).*

- *Specific nerve entrapments: These may be associated with particular fractures, most commonly acute carpal tunnel syndrome after a wrist or carpal injury. Urgent decompression may be required.*

- *Penetrating injuries: Penetrating injuries with nerve lesions suggest a transection that may require exploration.*

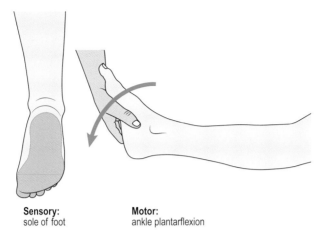

**Sensory:**
sole of foot

**Motor:**
ankle plantarflexion

Fig. 3.20 Tibial nerve examination.

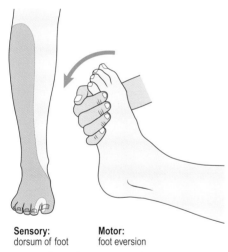

**Sensory:**
dorsum of foot

**Motor:**
foot eversion

Fig. 3.21 Superficial peroneal nerve examination.

| Table 3.4   Medical Research Council (MRC) grades for motor testing: scale for muscle strength | |
|---|---|
| **Grade** | **Muscle activity** |
| 0 | No contraction |
| 1 | Flicker or trace of contraction |
| 2 | Active movement, with gravity eliminated |
| 3 | Active movement against gravity |
| 4 | Active movement against gravity and resistance |
| 5 | Normal power |

## Orthopaedic management

- *Urgent surgery*: required to relieve pressure on a nerve where there is a remediable cause (such as a persistent fracture displacement or joint dislocation, or a compartment syndrome), or where there is the possibility of entrapment of a nerve following initial reduction.

- *Early planned surgery*: required where there is the likelihood of neurotmesis (discontinuity) of a major nerve or plexus. Exploration is likely to require specialist expertise and equipment (such as an operating microscope). Surgery is most successful after a sharp division (e.g. by a knife or glass) and less successful after a traumatic avulsion. Early surgery is *not* usually indicated where the nerve is likely to be in continuity: for example, a radial nerve palsy associated with a humeral shaft fracture. These have a high rate of spontaneous resolution, and

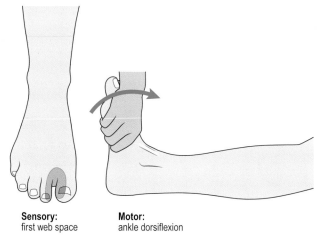

**Sensory:**
first web space

**Motor:**
ankle dorsiflexion

Fig. 3.22 Deep peroneal nerve examination.

observation for a period of 3–6 months is appropriate.

- *Delayed surgery*: may be required where there is a persisting nerve injury in continuity. Debridement, release, cable interposition grafting, nerve transfers or tendon transfers may be considered.

## VASCULAR INJURY

A critically ischaemic limb is a surgical emergency and must be recognized and treated promptly. Causes are (**Fig. 3.23**):

- *Kinking* of a major vessel: particularly where joint dislocation or fracture shortening has occurred (e.g. after a knee dislocation or femoral shaft fracture). Prompt reduction and splintage or traction are required.

- *Arterial spasm*.

- *Arterial puncture*: either by a penetrating injury, from sharp fractured bone ends, or through traction at the time of injury.

- *Intimal dissection*: trauma may result in a tear of the inner layer of the arterial wall – the intima. This may progress after injury, resulting in an intimal dissection and arterial occlusion, which may only become evident some time after admission. Regular reassessment following suspected vascular injury is crucial.

**Arterial spasm**

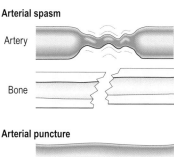

Artery

Bone

**Arterial puncture**

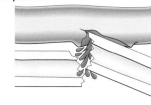

**Intimal dissection**

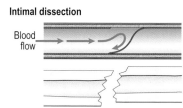

Blood
flow

Fig. 3.23 Causes of vascular injury.

- *Compartment syndrome*: for example, after tibial fracture. The loss of limb vascularity is a late sign of compartment syndrome and suggests that irreparable neuromuscular damage has already occurred. A neglected compartment syndrome may not benefit from urgent fasciotomy and an amputation may have to be considered.

## Emergency Department management

A vascular injury denotes a high-energy mechanism and the patient should initially be managed according to ATLS principles (see Chapter 2).

### Examination

The critically ischaemic limb is identified according to the 'six Ps' (**Box 3.1**).

The adequacy of peripheral circulation is assessed in terms of:

- *Peripheral colour and temperature*: The limb should be generally warm and of the same colour as unaffected extremities.
- *Capillary refill*: Compress the fingernail (or toenail) until the nailbed blanches and then release. A prompt return of a healthy pink colour should be evident within 3 seconds.
- *Peripheral pulses*: Note the presence or absence of the radial pulse in the upper limb and the dorsalis pedis, and posterior tibial pulsations in the lower limb. Mark the site with an indelible 'X' to allow later comparison. Compare the pulse volume with the uninjured side.
- *Doppler wave assessment*: Where the peripheral pulses are weak or absent, a Doppler probe is used to determine whether circulation is present.
- *Ankle–brachial pressure index* (ABPI): This is useful for establishing the adequacy of circulation to the lower limb. Using a sphyg-

momanometer cuff, measure the systolic pressure at which pulsations are first evident (by palpation or Doppler probe) in the upper limb, and then repeat the procedure in the lower limb. The normal ratio of this measurement at the arm divided by that at the ankle is above 0.9.

- *Angiography*: Conventional interventional angiography, or CT angiography with intravascular contrast (CTA), may be helpful:

a. Where there is diagnostic uncertainty: for example, the limb is not critically ischaemic and does not require emergency surgery, but the circulation has at some point been noted to be abnormal and there is the possibility of an intimal tear. This scenario is relatively common after knee dislocation.

b. When the condition of the run-off vessels is suspect, as a part of vascular surgical planning.

c. Where the number of vessels affected is unknown. In the leg, injury to one of the three arteries (anterior and posterior tibial, and peroneal) may be treated conservatively if the other vessels are patent, whereas there is often a preference to intervene if two vessels have been disrupted, even if the 'one-vessel leg' is not critically ischaemic, in order to improve the healing potential and final functional level of the limb.

Angiography is not required in all cases; in the acutely ischaemic limb with an obvious injury such as a knee dislocation or a femoral fracture, the vascular injury will be at the same level and immediate surgical exploration is indicated.

### Treatment

- *Resuscitate the patient*: A shocked patient with a vascular injury may have lost a substantial amount of blood (see Fig. 2.1).
- *Realign and splint the limb*.
- *Make a surgical referral*: Discuss the case urgently with a senior colleague and refer to

the Vascular or Plastic Surgery service, depending on local protocols. The acutely ischaemic limb is a surgical emergency.

## Orthopaedic management

### Vascular repair

Although the sequence of events may vary according to the complexity of the injury and local protocols, surgery is a closely coordinated multidisciplinary procedure and will commonly comprise (**Fig. 3.24**):

- *Extra-anatomical shunt*: An immediate extra-anatomical vascular shunt around the level of the obstruction allows the distal circulation to be restored and limits the warm ischaemic time.

- *Restoration of skeletal stability*: Definitive stabilization is usually preferred, as embarking on this later, after a delicate vascular procedure, risks damage to the graft or repair. However, if reconstruction is likely to be prolonged and complex, a temporary external fixation may be preferred.

- *Vascular repair*: This involves exploration and either grafting or repair. There is a risk of reperfusion syndrome and prophylactic fasciotomies are often performed (see Fig. 3.8).

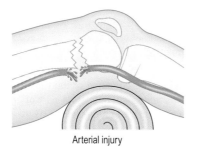

Arterial injury

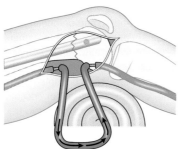

Extra-anatomical vascular shunt

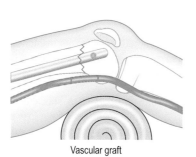

Vascular graft

Fig. 3.24 Extra-anatomical shunt and vascular graft.

## THE MANGLED LIMB

Occasionally, limb injuries may be difficult or impossible to salvage, and consideration of an early amputation is necessary. The clear indications for early amputation are:

- *An incomplete amputation*: The limb is effectively amputated already with no intact crossing neurovascular structures, despite the continuity of a segment of skin or muscle.

- *A critically ill patient*: A patient has compromised physiology, and requires immediate life-saving intervention. Embarking on lengthy and complex reconstructive surgery would add an unacceptable risk to the patient's life ('*life before limb*').

In most other situations, the decision as to whether to amputate immediately or embark on limb salvage is complex and requires consideration of a number of factors:

- the severity of the injury to the bone and soft tissues

- the ischaemic time that has elapsed since injury (more than 6 hours precludes a satisfactory result)

- the patient's age, and physiological and functional state of health

- the likely level of function of a successfully reconstructed limb (which is rarely normal)

- the likely level of function afforded by a prosthesis and the patient's likely ability to cope with this

- the capabilities of the local orthoplastic and rehabilitation services
- the patient's preference (which may not be known if the individual is unconscious).

A number of scoring systems, such as the Mangled Extremity Severity Score (MESS), have been described but none is predictive of outcome. Of importance, it is clear that an insensate foot at presentation can often recover sensation later and that this is not in itself an indication for amputation. Pragmatically, the best outcome is likely where:

- The initial assessment is made by two experienced orthopaedic or plastic surgeons together.
- An inevitable amputation is performed immediately.
- An equivocal decision to amputate is deferred. Initial debridement and spanning stabilization are performed and the patient and/or relatives are consulted at the first opportunity.

## SIGNPOST INJURIES

Some injuries indicate the likely presence of other injuries and should prompt a careful reassessment. These include:

- one injury above the level of the clavicles, indicating the possibility of another, such as a head or cervical spine injury
- one spinal fracture, indicating a 10% probability of another spinal fracture at another level
- a scapular fracture, indicating a high level of energy transfer and the possibility of a thoracic injury, such as a lung contusion or pneumothorax
- a knee dislocation, suggesting a high chance of popliteal artery and common peroneal/tibial nerve injury
- a knee injury from a 'dashboard strike', suggesting a possible femoral, hip or acetabular fracture, a hip dislocation and a sciatic nerve injury (see Fig. 17.33)
- a calcaneal fracture, following a fall from a height, suggesting the possibility of another fracture in sequence such as a pilon fracture, or injury to the tibial plateau, hip, acetabulum or spine (see Fig. 22.26).

# Closed management of fractures

Many commonly encountered fractures are managed non-operatively. A clear understanding of the principles of closed fracture reduction, and effective external support with plaster, splints or orthoses, is central to orthopaedic trauma practice. Fracture management, whether open or closed, follows the sequence:

**Reduce – Hold – Move**

## REDUCE: CLOSED REDUCTION

Many fractures are in a perfectly acceptable position at the time of presentation and do not need to be reduced. However, a closed reduction is indicated where the fracture position is *not* acceptable and requires either urgent or definitive reduction.

## Urgent reduction

Where there is skin, soft tissue or neurovascular compromise, the displacement should be reduced on recognition. Even when initial appearances are satisfactory, be aware of the development of swelling over the first few hours after injury, resulting in progressive soft tissue compromise. If later definitive surgical reduction is planned, an urgent reduction may not have to be absolutely anatomical.

## Definitive reduction

Many fractures (e.g. Colles' fractures) are treated definitively with closed reduction and cast immobilization. Often the reduction can be performed on a planned basis within a few days. Appropriate analgesia or anaesthesia is required (Chapter 2).

## Reduction manœuvres

A fracture may be displaced by any combination of shortening, impaction, translation, angulation and rotation (Chapter 1). Fracture reduction requires a clear understanding of the morphology and displacement of the fracture,

and the sequence of steps that will be required to correct each of these deformities. A Colles' fracture is a common example and is used here to illustrate the principles of closed reduction. A Colles' fracture is an extra-articular distal radius fracture with dorsal tilt, shortening (impaction), loss of radial inclination and radial translation (**Fig. 4.1**). The reduction must reverse each of these deformities and will require the following:

### Disimpaction with traction

The interstices (spikes) of each fragment may be impaled within the other and the fragments cannot be moved until separated. Firm traction in the line of the limb will allow disimpaction (**Fig. 4.2**). Ensure that you have a firm grip on the distal part of the limb, being careful of areas of frail or injured skin. It is possible to cause tears or even degloving, particularly over the dorsum of the hand in the elderly; grasp the thumb and fingers as shown. An

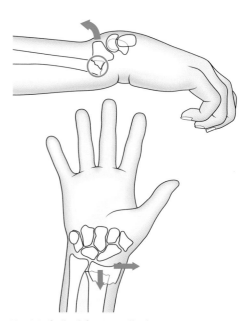

Fig. 4.1 Colles' fracture displacement.

assistant is needed to apply counter-traction. You will often feel a gentle 'give' as the two fragments separate. Successful disimpaction is confirmed if the distal fragment can be moved when gently held between thumb and forefinger (**Fig. 4.3**).

## Unlocking the fragments by exaggeration of the deformity

Once the fracture has been disimpacted, reduction may still be prevented by bone spikes or soft tissue interposition (**Fig. 4.4A**). The interstices of the fractured surfaces are like the teeth of a cog; exaggerating the deformity will allow these to be disengaged and the cortex to be realigned. Place your thumbs over the fracture to act as a fulcrum; extend at the fracture and feel the dorsal cortices of the fragments align with your thumbs (**Fig. 4.4B**). Now continue to apply traction and flex the distal fragment back into place again using the thumbs to ensure the dorsal cortex is now

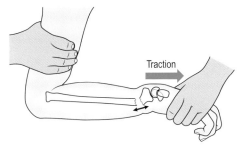

Fig. 4.2 Disimpaction with traction.

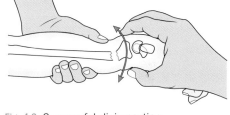

Fig. 4.3 Successful disimpaction.

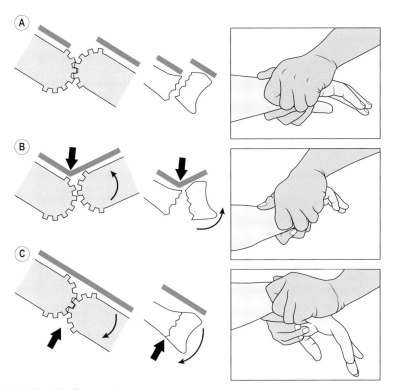

Fig. 4.4 Unlocking the fragment.

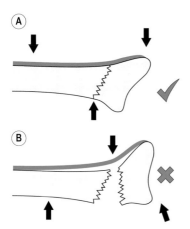

Fig. 4.5 Reduction with periosteal hinge.

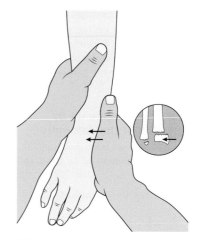

Fig. 4.6 Lateral pressure corrects remaining radial translation.

re-aligned (**Fig. 4.4C**). At the same time, apply ulnar deviation to correct the fracture translation. A common mistake, particularly in casting distal radius fractures, is to apply excessive traction during reduction and application of the cast, only for the reduction to be lost once the traction is released. Similarly, a position of excessive flexion (the 'cotton loader' position) is unacceptable, as this is associated with a high rate of acute carpal tunnel syndrome. Fracture reductions that are not maintained by the position detailed above are intrinsically unstable and not amenable to closed management.

### Reduction with the aid of the periosteal hinge

The fragments are now realigned. If the soft tissues – in particular, the periosteum – remain intact, reduction is greatly assisted. The periosteal hinge will prevent over-reduction, and will stabilize the fracture if three-point pressure is maintained (**Fig. 4.5A**). Note the effect of applying this pressure in the incorrect place (**Fig. 4.5B**).

### Assessment

The reduction is assessed clinically. The limb should be correctly aligned and rotated. Pay close attention to the dorsal skin, which can become trapped during the reduction; it should move freely over the bone. If deformity remains – in particular, translation – then further disimpaction is required. Apply a lateral force whilst repeating the exaggeration and reduction stages (**Fig. 4.6**).

### Positioning for cast application

The fracture will usually slip unless it is now supported promptly. Hold the thumb in one hand. The other hand holds three fingers and maintains gentle traction with the hand pronated, and the wrist in slight ulnar deviation and flexion (**Fig. 4.7**). The use of excessive traction, or an exaggerated position of flexion (Fig. 12.17), must be avoided. A wrist backslab is now applied (see p. 68).

### HOLD: PRINCIPLES OF CAST MANAGEMENT

The cast is an important tool for the treatment of many orthopaedic injuries. The ubiquitous plaster of Paris (gypsum, calcium sulphate) is versatile, easy to handle and strong, and is widely used in Emergency Departments, although it is rather heavy. Synthetic casting materials (fibreglass or polypropylene) are lighter and more commonly used for definitive cast management, but they are more technically demanding to use and are

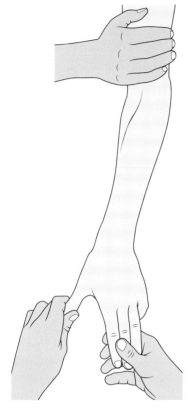

Fig. 4.7 Maintaining control during application of a cast or backslab.

## Table 4.1 Backslabs and their common indications

| Slab | Common indications |
| --- | --- |
| **Upper limb** | |
| U-slab | Humeral shaft fracture |
| Above-elbow | Distal humerus fracture |
| | Elbow dislocation |
| | Forearm fracture |
| Wrist | Distal radius fracture |
| | Scaphoid fracture |
| Volar hand slab | Metacarpal and phalangeal fracture |
| Thumb spica | Base of thumb fracture |
| | Thumb metacarpophalangeal joint injury |
| **Lower limb** | |
| Above-knee | Tibial plateau fracture |
| | Tibial shaft fracture |
| | Knee dislocation |
| Below-knee | Ankle fracture |
| | Foot injury |

not recommended for general use in the Emergency Department.

Casting material is used in two principal ways: to create a split (a backslab) or a full cast.

## Backslabs

The backslab is applied to one side of the injured limb to act as a splint. The casting material is usually provided in 'slabs' several layers thick. This type of splint cannot provide three-point fixation but is commonly favoured during the acute phase of injury, as it is relatively straightforward to apply in the Emergency Department and can be removed simply with scissors in the event of constriction. It is often asserted that the bandages supporting a backslab 'allow for swelling' but this cannot be relied on.

## Full casts

Casting material is wound circumferentially around a limb to provide support. The layers are built up, one on the other, until the cast attains the desired strength. A full cast can be moulded to shape, allowing three-point fixation, and provides better fracture support than a backslab. Casts require a little more experience to apply, and are rather more difficult to remove in the event of swelling and circulatory compromise.

## BACKSLABS

Backslabs are simple to make and provide effective, safe splintage of painful injuries. Common backslabs and their indications are listed in **Table 4.1**. The immobilization of hand injuries with backslabs, splints and taping is described separately in Chapter 13.

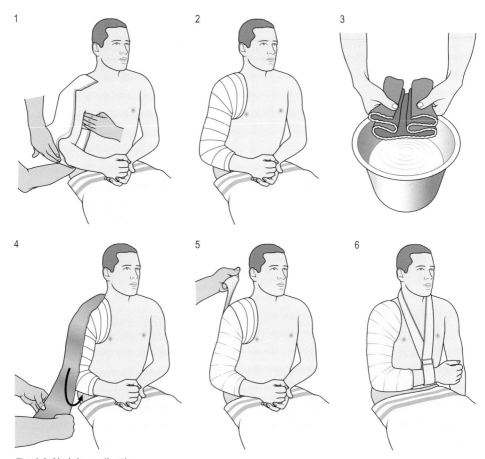

Fig. 4.8 U-slab application.

## Application of a U-slab (Fig. 4.8)

U-slabs are used for the immobilisation of humeral shaft fractures. Although cumbersome they provide excellent pain relief.

### Preparation

- 15-cm width plaster slab, eight layers thick.
- Stockingette.
- Soft wool rolls.
- Bucket of tepid water.
- Ring removal from the patient's fingers.

Patients are placed either in a chair or on an examination trolley, and should support their own wrist with the elbow flexed to 90°. Sedation is rarely necessary, but the procedure can be uncomfortable and adequate analgesia is required. Time is critical as the plaster will cure within a few minutes of wetting. Everything must be prepared and to hand, and both you and your assistants must have a clear understanding of the steps involved in application.

### Technique

1. *Measure plaster slab*: Cut eight thicknesses of 15-cm plaster slab so that it stretches from a hand's-breadth below the axilla, down the inside of the arm, around the elbow and back up over the point of the shoulder.

2. *Apply wool*: Stockingette is not generally used in U-slab application. Apply the wool roll around the limb two thicknesses in depth, except over the prominences of the

elbow, where two extra turns are needed. This padding should extend from the top of the shoulder, over the lateral clavicle, to a point one-third of the way down the forearm.

3. *Wet slab*: Concertina the slab and immerse in tepid water for 4 seconds. Squeeze out the excess water.

4. *Apply slab*: The slab runs from a position *on top* of the shoulder, down the lateral aspect of the arm, under the flexed elbow, and then up the inner side of the arm, ending a hand's-breadth from the axilla. A U-slab that does not pass across the top of the shoulder is at risk of gradually slipping down the arm.

5. *Apply bandage*: Secure the slab with a crepe bandage, firmly enough to prevent the slab from falling off but avoiding constriction. Depending on the level of the fracture, gentle moulding can be used to resist the dominant deforming forces.

6. *Perform safety checks*: The arm is supported in a collar-and-cuff. Check that no skin is exposed to plaster to avoid burns. Check that the skin on the medial aspect of the arm and chest wall is adequately protected with padding. Ensure that neither the moulding nor the application of the cast has resulted in impairment of the distal pulse, capillary return or sensation. Any change in the condition of the limb implies possible entrapment of neurovascular structures within the fracture or an excessively tight cast, and the U-slab must be removed.

7. *Repeat radiographs*: It is mandatory to obtain repeat radiographs after cast application. An unsatisfactory result can be addressed with a repeat attempt.

## Above-elbow backslab (Fig. 4.9)

Above elbow backslabs are used in a variety of injuries around the elbow and forearm (**Table 4.1**).

### *Preparation*

- 15-cm width plaster slab, eight layers thick.
- Stockingette.
- Soft wool rolls.
- Bucket of tepid water.
- Ring removal from the patient's fingers.

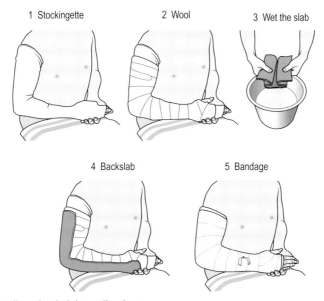

1 Stockingette    2 Wool    3 Wet the slab

4 Backslab    5 Bandage

Fig. 4.9 Above-elbow backslab application.

Patients are placed either in a chair or on an examination trolley, and should support their own wrist with the elbow flexed to 90° and the forearm in mid-rotation (thumb pointing up). Sedation is rarely required for this procedure but again adequate analgesia, assistance and planning are required. Cut eight thicknesses of 15-cm plaster slab so that it stretches from the mid-humerus to the metacarpal necks. A small 5-cm transverse cut is made in each side of the slab where it will curve around the elbow, to allow folding rather than crumpling of the slab edges.

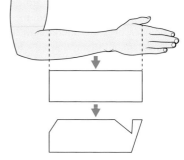

Fig. 4.10 Colles' backslab preparation.

### Technique

1. *Apply stockingette*: Stockingette is applied from the level of the axilla to the fingers, to allow sufficient length to fold over at the ends. Cut a hole for the thumb.

2. *Apply wool*: Apply two turns of wool roll, except over the prominences of the elbow, where two extra turns are needed. This padding should extend from the mid-humerus to the metacarpal heads.

3. *Wet slab*: Concertina the slab and immerse in tepid water for 4 seconds. Squeeze out the excess water.

4. *Apply slab*: The slab runs down the posterior aspect of the arm from the mid-humerus to rest on the ulnar aspect of the hand. If necessary, the limb can be gently realigned at this stage.

5. *Apply bandage*: Secure the slab with a crepe bandage, firmly enough to prevent the slab from falling off but avoiding constriction. The arm is supported in a collar-and-cuff.

6. *Perform safety checks*: Check that no skin is exposed to plaster to avoid burns. Check that the skin on the medial aspect of the arm and chest wall is adequately protected with padding. Ensure that neither the moulding nor application of the cast has resulted in impairment of the distal pulse, capillary return or sensation. Any change in the condition of the limb implies possible entrapment of neurovascular structures within the fracture or an excessively tight cast.

7. *Repeat radiographs*: It is mandatory to obtain repeat radiographs after cast application. An unsatisfactory result can be addressed with a repeat attempt, provided the anaesthetic is still effective.

## Wrist backslab (Colles' backslab)
### Preparation (Fig. 4.10)
- 8–10-cm width plaster slab, eight layers thick.
- Stockingette.
- Soft wool roll.
- 8-cm diameter bandage.
- Bucket with tepid water.
- Ring removal from the patient's fingers.

Time is critical, as the patient will be uncomfortable, the assistant will gradually tire, the fracture may displace gradually, and the plaster will cure within a few minutes of wetting, whether or not you have completed the backslab! Everything must be prepared and to hand, and both you and your assistant must have a clear understanding of the steps involved in application. The plaster slab should be around 10 cm in width and 6–8 layers thick. Cut this to extend from the metacarpal heads to the upper forearm, stopping three fingers'-breadths short of the elbow crease. Cut out a 'V' shape for the thumb and round off the edges.

### Technique (Fig. 4.11)
1. *Apply stockingette*: A layer of stockingette is applied to protect the skin. Measure from elbow to fingertips, as it will shorten when

1 Stockingette    2 Wool    3 Wet slab    4 Slab    5 Bandage

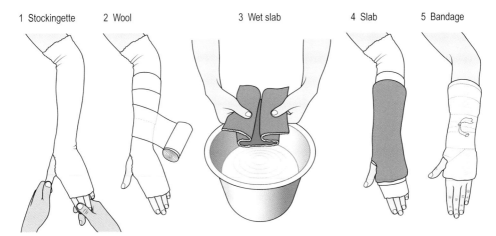

Fig. 4.11 Colles' backslab application.

applied. Cut a hole for the thumb, ensuring there is no constriction.

2. *Apply wool*: Apply wool roll to provide padding and allow for swelling. Two thicknesses should be applied by covering half of the preceding layer with each successive turn. An extra turn is required over the bony prominences at the wrist, and at both the proximal and distal ends. Place a small piece of wool padding around the base of the thumb, as this is the most common site of later abrasion from a plaster edge.

3. *Wet slab*: Keep hold of both ends of the slab and concertina it between your hands. Immerse it completely for 4 seconds in tepid water. Hot water will accelerate the exothermic reaction, reducing the setting time and increasing the risk of burns. Lift the slab out and compress it gently between your hands to expel excess water.

4. *Apply backslab*: Place the backslab on the patient, such that the metacarpal heads are just clear of the backslab, with the 'V' overlying the base of the thumb. Then run the slab up the dorsum of the forearm, slightly towards the radial side. Check that the plaster of Paris is not touching the skin directly, as it can cause a serious thermal burn while curing.

5. *Apply bandage*: Fold over the ends of the stockingette and wool to leave padded edges that allow free elbow, finger and thumb movement (**Fig. 4.12**). Apply the bandage firmly enough to hold the backslab snugly in place but without constriction. At each end the bandage should overlap the folded-back stockingette to give a neat, padded finish. Once the backslab is covered, tear the bandage longitudinally and tie it around the top of the backslab. Alternatively, secure the end with a small piece of wetted plaster slab. Support the backslab while the plaster 'goes off' and hardens.

6. *Perform safety checks*: Check that the edges of the backslab at the fingers, thumb and forearm are covered with wool and stockingette, as unprotected edges of cured plaster are hard and abrasive. Check that the elbow, fingers and thumb are free and able move to at least 90°. Trim any excess plaster or bandage as required to alleviate constriction and allow movement. Check the colour and capillary refill time of the fingers. Assess sensation over the index fingertip (median nerve), dorsum of the index finger metacarpophalangeal joint (radial nerve) and ulnar side of the little finger (ulnar nerve).

7. *Repeat radiographs*: It is mandatory to obtain repeat radiographs after cast application. An unsatisfactory result can be

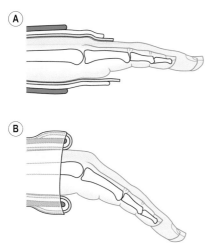

Fig. 4.12 Folding over the stockingette in a Colles' backslab application. **A**, The stockingette and wool should be applied generously beyond the metacarpophalangeal joints, but the plaster should not extend beyond the metacarpal necks. **B**, The stockingette and wool can then be folded back to offer protection against the abrasive plaster edges, allowing free metacarpophalangeal joint movement.

addressed with a repeat attempt, provided the anaesthetic is still effective.

## Below-knee backslab

For ankle and foot immobilization, a below-knee backslab is required. At least one assistant is required to hold the leg (**Fig. 4.13A**), but the use of a thigh support will make the procedure more comfortable for all concerned (**Fig. 4.13B**).

### Preparation

- Stockingette.
- Soft wool roll.
- 15-cm width plaster slab, eight layers thick.
- 10-cm width plaster, four layers thick (stirrup).
- 12-cm diameter bandage.
- Bucket with tepid water.

The backslab can be measured on the uninjured limb and extends from the metatarsal

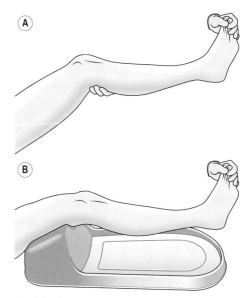

Fig. 4.13 Below-knee backslab leg position.

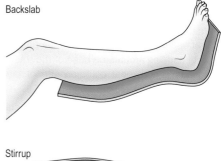

Backslab

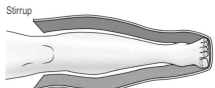

Stirrup

Fig. 4.14 Below-knee backslab preparation.

heads to a point just above the widest part of the calf muscle belly. A second length of plaster, used as a side support, is referred to as the stirrup (**Fig. 4.14**). It should be twice the length of the backslab and can be thinner to reduce the weight of the cast.

## Technique (Fig. 4.15)

1. *Apply stockingette*: Stockingette is measured generously from the toes to the patella to allow for shortening, as it is stretched during application.

2. *Apply wool*: Use two turns of wool bandage, with additional padding at the bony prominences of the ankle and fibular head, as well as the top and bottom of the slab.

3. *Apply backslab*: Wet the slab as described above. With the assistant providing support behind the knee and holding the great toe, the backslab is applied from the metatarsal heads to the top of the calf muscle belly.

4. *Apply stirrup*: The stirrup is then quickly applied, running down the inside of the leg, under the heel, and up the outside.

5. *Apply bandage*: The stockingette and wool are now folded back over the plaster while checking at the same time that no areas of skin are exposed directly to plaster (which will otherwise cause a thermal burn). Apply the bandage, being sure to cover the folded ends of the stockingette. The sole of the foot can now be rested conveniently against your abdomen. Pushing forwards gently, while supporting either side of the leg, encourages the knee to bend and ensures that the ankle is in a neutral position as the plaster cures. Some moulding may be required as the plaster cures to ensure that any fracture reduction is maintained.

---

### ⊘ Key point

Obtaining a neutral (plantigrade) ankle position is essential, as it indicates that the ankle is reduced, and allows for appropriate radiographic evaluation of the ankle joint. Below-knee backslabs are commonly applied poorly with the ankle in an equinus position (plantar flexion). This is often due to inadequate attention to detail and to application of the cast when the knee is straight; gastrocnemius is thus under tension and this pulls the foot into equinus.

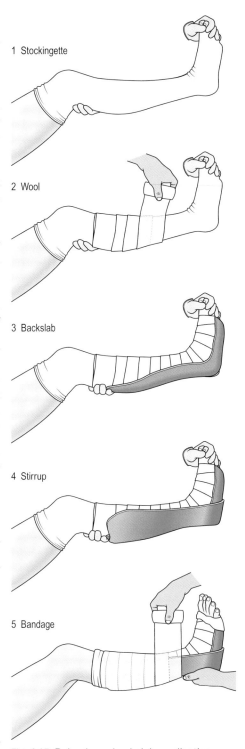

1 Stockingette

2 Wool

3 Backslab

4 Stirrup

5 Bandage

Fig. 4.15 Below-knee backslab application.

6. *Safety checks*: Check for complete padding between the casting material and the skin to avoid abrasions, especially behind the calf and at the metatarsal heads. Check that the toes are all exposed and have adequate capillary refill. It is a common error for the little toe to be 'lost' and compressed in the backslab. Ask the patient to move the toes. Check sensation on the dorsum of the foot (superficial peroneal nerve), first web space (deep peroneal nerve) and on the sole (tibial nerve) (see Figs 3.20-22).

7. *Repeat radiographs*: Obtain check radiographs to confirm that an adequate reduction has been maintained.

### Above-knee backslab

For tibial fractures and injuries about the knee, an above-knee backslab is required. This can be an uncomfortable procedure and requires appropriate analgesia or possibly procedural sedation. Holding the limb during the procedure is awkward and *at least two* assistants are needed: one to support the foot and the fracture, the second to support the thigh and the back of the knee (**Fig. 4.16**). Aligning the patella with the first web space of the foot ensures correct rotation. The knee must be flexed to *30°* when the plaster sets.

#### Preparation
- Stockingette.
- Soft wool roll.
- 15-cm width plaster slab, eight layers thick.
- 10-cm width plaster, four layers thick (stirrup).

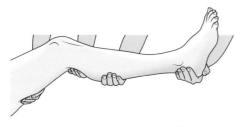

Fig. 4.16 Above-knee backslab position.

- 12-cm diameter bandage.
- Bucket of tepid water.

Casting material should be measured (on the uninjured side) to extend from metatarsal heads to three-quarters of the way up the thigh. A stirrup is also used in an above-knee plaster and should be twice the length of the backslab, but can be made of a thinner slab width.

#### Technique
1. *Apply stockingette*: The stockingette is measured from the tips of the toes to the groin; it will shorten as it stretches around the limb and should be cut at least 30 cm longer.

2. *Apply wool*: Use two turns of wool bandage along the shafts of the tibia and femur, with additional padding at the bony prominences of the ankle and fibular head, as well as the top and bottom of the slab.

3. *Apply backslab*: Once the slab is wet, place one end at the level of the metatarsal heads, where your assistant will hold it with a finger. Smooth the slab into place under the foot and heel, and behind the calf. Support the back of the calf whilst your assistant moves their second hand back into place behind the backslab. Run the backslab up the back of the knee and thigh, again supporting the limb while the second assistant moves hand positions to accommodate the plaster.

4. *Apply stirrup*: The backslab is liable to failure at the ankle and knee, and will need to be reinforced with a side stirrup. This can be applied as one large, U-shaped piece of plaster (twice the length of the backslab but only four layers thick), or as one stirrup to each side. If there are any obvious weak points, further support can be provided by adding smaller pieces where necessary.

5. *Apply bandage*: The stockingette and wool are now folded back over the plaster. At the same time, check that no areas of skin are exposed directly to plaster (which will otherwise cause a thermal burn). Apply the bandage, being sure to cover the folded

ends of the stockingette. The sole of the foot can be conveniently rested against your abdomen. Check that the patella and first web space are aligned. Support the limb while the plaster cures to ensure that the ankle remains in neutral, and the knee at 30° of flexion. Elevate the limb on pillows, providing an extra pillow behind the knee.

6. *Perform safety checks*: Check for complete padding between the casting material and the skin to avoid abrasions, especially behind the thigh and at the metatarsal heads. The most common errors are to leave exposed, rough plaster behind the thigh and to fail to support the metatarsal heads. Check that the toes are all exposed and have adequate capillary refill. It is common for the little toe to be 'lost' and compressed in the backslab. Ask patients to move their toes. Check sensation on the dorsum of the foot (superficial peroneal nerve), first web space (deep peroneal nerve) and on the sole (tibial nerve) (see Figs 3.20-22).

7. *Repeat radiographs*: Obtain check radiographs to confirm that an adequate reduction has been maintained.

---

###  Key point

An important component of tibial shaft fracture immobilization is maintenance of correct rotational alignment. A below-knee backslab, although it covers the fracture, will not stop the foot rotating externally around the long axis of the tibia, causing soft tissue tension and compromise. An above-knee plaster that is straight at the knee is no better. However, if the ankle is in neutral and the knee is bent to 30°, the Z-shaped backslab is unable to rotate around the tibia (**Fig. 4.17**).

---

### Reinforcement techniques

The backslab will be greatly strengthened by additions that increase its cross-sectional depth. Additional strips of plaster slab can be

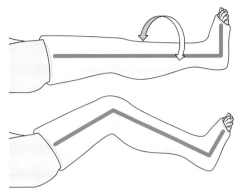

Fig. 4.17 Above-knee backslab or cast: the importance of a Z-shape.

placed to either side of the backslab. At the ankle, this is best achieved with a stirrup (see Fig. 4.13). At the knee and thigh, side slabs are effective. In the upper limb, the cast can be girdered by pinching up a section of the slab (see Fig. 13.13).

## FULL CASTS

Full casts provide circumferential fracture support, allow three-point moulding, and are used for the definitive management of many fractures. A full cast is not recommended for acute treatment in the Emergency Department. A wrist cast is used below as an example to demonstrate the principles. The application of a full ankle cast for the management of unstable ankle fractures is detailed in Figure 21.22.

### Preparation
● Plaster rolls: 8-cm width for upper limb, 15-cm for lower limb.
● Stockingette.
● Soft wool roll.
● Bucket of tepid water.
● Ring removal from the patient's fingers.

As for backslab application, time is critical, as the patient will be uncomfortable, the assistant(s) will gradually tire of holding the limb, the reduction may displace, and the plaster will cure within a few minutes of wetting it! Everything must be prepared and to hand,

1 Stockingette    2 Wool    3 Wet roll    4 Plaster    5 Bandage

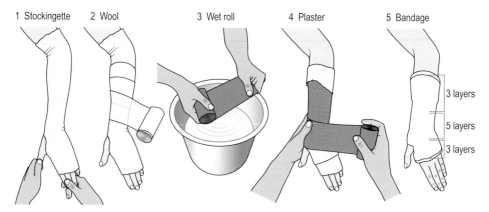

3 layers

5 layers

3 layers

Fig. 4.18 Full-cast technique.

and both you and your assistant(s) must have a clear understanding of the steps involved in the procedure. Remove the wool and casting material from their wrappers. Use a 10-cm bandage for a wrist fracture and 15-cm for an ankle.

### Technique (Fig. 4.18)

1. *Apply stockingette*: A layer of stockingette is applied to protect the skin. Measure from elbow to fingertips, as it will shorten when applied. Cut a hole for the thumb, ensuring there is no constriction.

2. *Apply wool*: Apply wool roll to provide padding and allow for swelling. Two thicknesses should be applied by covering half of the preceding layer with each successive turn. An extra turn is required over the bony prominences at the wrist, and at both the proximal and the distal ends. Place a small piece of wool padding around the base of the thumb, as this is the most common site of later abrasion from a plaster edge.

3. *Wet plaster*: Hold the roll in one hand and the tail in the other to prevent it becoming lost in the mass of wet bandage. Place it in tepid water for a few seconds until bubbles stop rising. Remove the bandage and squeeze gently between your hands to remove excess water, keeping hold of the tail.

4. *Plaster roll technique*: Place the tail of the bandage against the limb, with the bandage roll uppermost. The cast is most conveniently started at the straightest part of the limb – just above the wrist for a Colles' cast, or above the ankle for a below-knee cast. Unroll the bandage in your hand for a length of 20 cm, and then, using only sufficient tension to compress the wool to half-thickness, bring your hand under and round the limb to complete one turn, passing the roll from one hand to the other and back again as you do so. Use the other thumb to catch the bandage edge to make neat tucks and ensure a smooth fit.

5. *Complete plaster*: After each layer of bandage, smooth down the surface to exclude trapped air and consolidate the separate layers of bandage into one mass of plaster. Two or three layers of plaster are needed over the shaft of the limb, and four or five to reinforce the wrist joint. Take care with the area around the base of the thumb, where it is easy to form an abrasive edge. The bandage should be trimmed before it turns through the narrow space at the web of the thumb. Check that the plaster of Paris is not directly touching the skin, where it can cause a serious thermal burn while curing. Roll the stockingette and wool back over the edge of the plaster before applying the last turn of the bandage at either end so that

the rolled edge of the stockingette and wool provide a neat and padded end.

6. *Safety checks*: Check that the edges of the cast at the fingers, thumb and forearm are covered with wool and stockingette, as unprotected edges of cured plaster are hard and abrasive. Check that the elbow, fingers and thumb are free to move to at least 90°. If there is any restriction, trim the cast as required. Check the colour, capillary return and sensation of the skin, as for a Colles' backslab.

7. *Repeat radiographs*: Obtain check radiographs to confirm that the position of the fracture has been maintained.

## Moulding and three-point fixation

At the time of fracture, the periosteum at the tension side of the fracture is torn, while the periosteum at the compression side usually remains intact. In a Colles' fracture, as the fragment tilts dorsally, the volar periosteum is torn while the dorsal periosteum is unharmed. This intact dorsal periosteal hinge can be exploited in order to improve the stability of the casted fracture (**Fig. 4.19**).

During casting, pressure is applied on the volar aspect of the wrist at the level of fracture to act as a fulcrum (**1** on Fig. 4.19). Pressure is then applied on the dorsal side of the wrist, both proximally (**2**) and distally (**3**) to the fracture. As the pressure is applied, the dorsal periosteum comes under tension, providing some compression on the volar side as it rests against the fulcrum; this is termed *three-point fixation*. The moulding is maintained until the plaster has set.

Pressure applied over a small area will result in high pressure under the plaster and skin compromise, so apply pressure with the heel of the hand and thenar eminence to create as broad an area as the size of the bone will allow. Three points of pressure require three hands and an assistant is therefore essential. Ensure that the assistant also uses the flat of the hand to avoid a pressure point. Over a larger area (while holding the back of the thigh, for example), the assistant should ease their hand gently back and forth to avoid local indentation. A well-moulded cast is never perfectly flat on its exterior surface; a bent cast is required to maintain a straight bone. The adequacy of three-point pressure can be gauged from the final radiographs by assessing where the wool padding has been compressed.

## Synthetic casts

Synthetic casting materials, such as fibreglass or polypropylene, are lighter and stronger than plaster of Paris, and are resistant to water damage. Indeed, with some synthetic padding materials, a cast can be immersed completely in water (e.g. for water sports) and will dry out without causing maceration. Synthetic casts are therefore usually preferred in the fracture clinic setting.

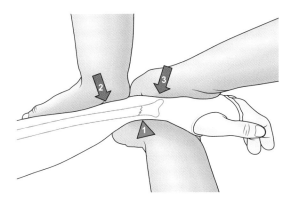

Fig. 4.19 Three-point fixation.

Some experience is required for the safe use of synthetic casting materials, however. They generally mould less well than plaster of Paris and the edges are more abrasive; application is therefore more demanding. The wet casting material is often highly irritating to the skin during application, and gloves should be worn routinely. Cast removal can be more difficult than with plaster of Paris; thus where swelling is anticipated after injury, it is usually not appropriate to use a synthetic material.

## LIMB ELEVATION

### Upper limb

Oedema and bruising are gravity-dependent and appropriate support of an injured limb is essential to aid comfort and limit swelling. This can be achieved in a number of ways:

- actively placing the injured hand on the contralateral shoulder as much as possible (**Fig. 4.20A**)
- collar-and-cuff
- broad arm sling
- elevation sling
- Bradford sling.

### Collar-and-cuff

The simplest adjunct to elevation is the collar-and-cuff; a loop of padded fabric is paced around the affected wrist and around the back of the neck (**Fig. 4.20B**). The collar-and-cuff

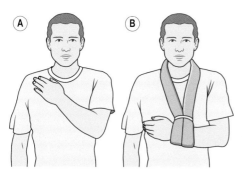

Fig. 4.20 Limb elevation. **A**, Placement of the hand on the contralateral shoulder. **B**, Collar-and-cuff.

does not support the elbow and this is particularly useful in fractures of the proximal humerus, where the weight of the arm will provide gentle traction to the fracture (Fig. 9.7). If a collar-and-cuff has been provided, this should be positioned to keep the hand and wrist above the level of the elbow; a dependent position must be avoided.

### Broad arm sling

Certain injuries, such as clavicle fractures and acromioclavicular joint sprains, are more comfortable in a sling that provides elbow support. If a collar-and-cuff is used in these circumstances, the weight of the arm can cause discomfort. A broad arm sling supports the arm from elbow to wrist. To apply a broad arm sling (**Fig. 4.21**):

1. Place the patient's hand across the abdomen, with the elbow flexed at 90°. Place a triangular bandage under the patient's forearm and shoulder, with the apex towards the elbow and the hypotenuse hanging vertically.

2. Bring the lower point of the triangle up and over the elbow and around the patient's neck to meet the other corner; tie a reef knot behind the patient's neck.

3. Secure the loose apex of the triangle behind the point of the elbow with a safety pin.

### Elevation sling

This secures the hand in a position of elevation as it rests on the contralateral shoulder, and is used in hand injuries. To apply an elevation sling (**Fig. 4.22**):

1. Place the patient's hand on their contralateral shoulder. Place a triangular bandage over the forearm and shoulder, with the apex towards the elbow and the hypotenuse hanging vertically.

2. Bring the lower point of the triangle up and under the elbow and across the patient's back, and tie a reef knot just behind the shoulder (not over the fingers).

3. Secure the apex of the triangle behind the point of the elbow with a safety pin.

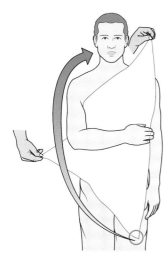 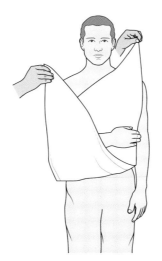 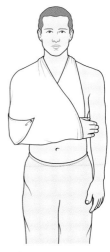

1 Place the patient's arm across the abdomen. Place a triangular bandage under the forearm and shoulder, with the apex towards the elbow, and the hyponenuse hanging vertically.

2 Bring the lower point of the triangle up and over the elbow and around the patient's neck to meet the other corner and tie a reef knot.

3 Secure the loose apex of the sling with a safety pin.

Fig. 4.21 Application of a broad arm sling.

Avoid the use of a broad arm sling or collar-and-cuff for hand injuries; these allow the hand to hang down in a dependent position and cause constriction at the wrist, exacerbating the development of swelling.

Inpatients with swelling should be provided with a Bradford sling (see below).

## Bradford sling

Inpatients with injuries to the hand, wrist or forearm can conveniently be treated with a Bradford elevation sling. This method is useful after casting and also when elevation is required to treat excessive swelling from infection or injury. Proprietary models are available but this sling can be created conveniently at the bedside with a pillowcase, string and a drip stand (**Fig. 4.23**):

1. Hold a pillowcase with its opening towards the ceiling.

2. Pinch one lower corner, then invaginate it so that it lies within the opposite corner.

3. Bring the top corners neatly together.

4. This creates a sling that is open at the top and along one side. Rest the patient's elbow in the newly formed corner.

5. Tie string to the top of the pillowcase and then attach it to a drip stand for support.

This sling is highly effective but the patient may develop a feeling of stiffness in the shoulder and require short periods of movement outside the sling for comfort. The height of the drip stand can be changed to allow the patient's elbow to rest on the bed/chair arm for support.

## Lower limb

Lower limb injuries require elevation such that the foot is above the level of the heart, whether in bed or in a chair. Resting in a chair with the leg at hip level will tend to lead to the development of swelling. Pillows or the use of an elevation frame (Braun frame) are all that is required to achieve a satisfactory position.

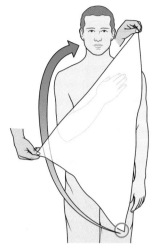

1 Place the patient's hand on their contralateral shoulder. Place a triangular bandage over the forearm and shoulder, with the apex at the elbow and the hyponenuse hanging vertically.

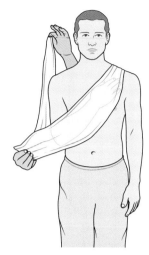

2 Bring the lower point of the triangle up and under the elbow and across the patient's back to a reef knot behind the shoulder (not over the fingers).

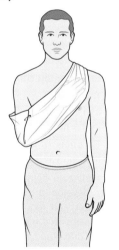

3 Secure the apex of the triangle behind the point of the elbow.

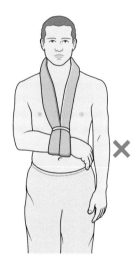

Avoid this dependent position which encourages hand swelling

Fig. 4.22 Application of an elevation sling.

## CAST AFTERCARE

### Routine care

Patients should be provided with verbal and written instructions regarding care of their cast. This should include instructions:

- to watch for signs of constriction (pain, excessive swelling, discoloration, paraesthesia or numbness) and to return immediately if there is any cause for concern

- to move the adjacent joints; fingers and toes should be kept supple and mobile, and the elbow and shoulder (or hip and knee)

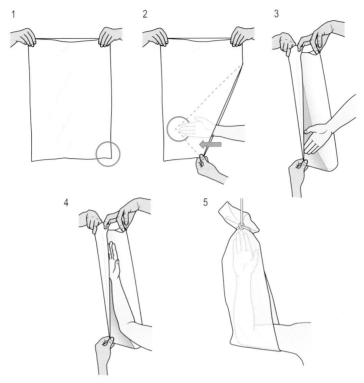

Fig. 4.23 Application of a Bradford sling.

should be moved and stretched throughout their full range several times a day (e.g. for 5 minutes every waking hour)

- to keep the cast clean and, importantly, dry; water under the cast will result in macerated skin

- not to push anything down inside the cast in order to scratch or for any other reason

- to keep the affected extremity elevated.

## Cast removal

### Cast constriction

Where there is any question of circulatory compromise, the situation requires urgent assessment and intervention. Where compromise is mild, with modest swelling and some moderate discomfort, place the limb in high elevation and reassess after 15–20 minutes. If there is improvement, persist with elevation. If there is

severe or persisting compromise, the backslab or cast must be splint down to skin or removed.

 **Key point**

Where there is significant swelling, discoloration, excessive pain or any new neurovascular abnormality, or where a period of elevation as been unsuccessful in relieving symptoms, *the cast must be split from end to end and from surface to skin*. The loss of fracture position is a secondary concern in this situation.

### Backslab removal (Fig. 4.24)

To remove a backslab, cut through the encircling bandages, wool and stockingette until skin is fully exposed, using bandage scissors to prevent skin injury. Ease back the edges of the plaster shell until it is clear that it is not constricting the limb in any way. Where there are surgical dressings or swabs that have hardened with blood clot, these can also cause constriction and must be elevated carefully.

## Plaster saw (Fig. 4.25)

A complete cast must be split along its length completely using a plaster saw or shears. A plaster saw has an oscillating (not rotating) blade and is highly effective, but can cause burns or skin lacerations if used incorrectly.

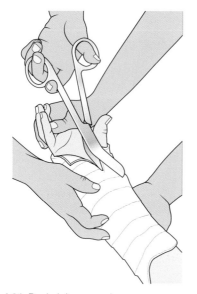

Fig. 4.24 Backslab removal.

Ensure that the blade is sharp and undamaged. Select a line for the cut that is well padded underneath with wool and not over any bony prominence. The volar aspect of the wrist and forearm, and the area over the anterior compartment of the leg are convenient. Alternatively, a lower limb cast can be bivalved (divided completely into two sections with two longitudinal saw cuts) to release the limb completely. Warn the patient that the noise of the saw and vacuum attachment is considerable. Cut down through the plaster at one level. The noise of the saw will change and you will feel a loss of resistance as soon as it is through. Bring the blade back to the surface, move it 2 cm along and repeat. Do not slide the saw laterally in shallow cuts; the cutting movement must be up and down. If the patient complains of pain, reassess your technique; you may be 'plunging' beyond the cast material and you risk burning or cutting the skin. Once the cast has been divided along its entire length, use plaster spreaders to separate the edges of the cast, and then cut all the padding and soft dressings down to skin along the entire length of the cast.

## Plaster shears

Plaster shears are inserted at one end of the cast between the casting material and the wool, with the lower handle placed parallel to the limb or even a little depressed. Lift up the upper handle and push the shears forwards

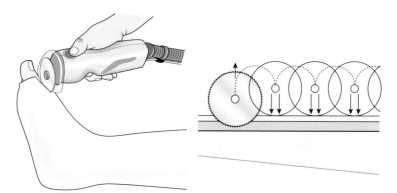

Fig. 4.25 Using a plaster saw.

with the lower handle so that the plaster fills the throat of the shears. Maintain a slight pushing force and perform the cutting action with the upper handle, moving it up and down like a beer pump. Use plaster spreaders to separate the edges of the cast, and then cut all the soft dressings down to skin along the entire length of the cast.

Once the cast has been split, the patient will usually report prompt relief. Elevate the limb as above. If the symptoms resolve rapidly, a crepe bandage is wrapped lightly around the split cast to prevent it from falling off, and to act as a splint.

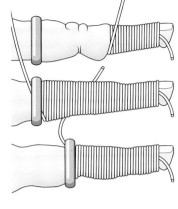

Fig. 4.26 Ring removal.

##  Key point

Where splitting the cast or backslab has not alleviated the patient's symptoms, urgent senior review is required. Possible diagnoses include:

- compartment syndrome
- vessel entrapment
- arterial dissection.

*Delay is limb-threatening.*

## Cast checks in the outpatient clinic

Each time a patient attends the outpatient department with a cast, ask yourself three questions to ensure the cast remains safe and of benefit to the patient:

1. *Is the cast comfortable?* Where the patient complains of pain or skin compromise, the cast should be removed or a window cut in it to allow adequate examination. The plaster window should then be replaced; otherwise, the skin can swell through the window, resulting in local injury on the sawn edge of the plaster. Exchange of plaster for an orthosis should be considered.

2. *Is the cast loose?* Casts will usually loosen as the underlying limb swelling abates. A loose cast does not offer any fracture support and movement causes skin abrasion. Assess looseness by attempting to move the plaster proximally and distally, noting its excursion in either direction. If loose, the cast should be exchanged, unless there is concern that the risk of losing a difficult reduction during exchange is greater than the risk of it slipping in a loose cast.

3. *Does the cast allow adjacent joint movement?* Where the patient has restricted movement, the cast should be trimmed or replaced as appropriate.

## Ring removal

The patient's rings should be removed as soon as possible after injury, before the development of swelling. A tight ring can usually be eased off with oil or washing-up liquid. A recalcitrant ring can be coaxed off by compressing the finger distally with twine and then easing the ring distally (**Fig. 4.26**). Otherwise, a ring cutter may be required.

## ORTHOSES

Orthoses are often far more convenient than a cast, as they allow the patient to adjust the tightness of the device, remove it for washing

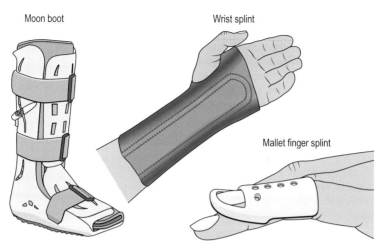

Fig. 4.27 Orthoses.

and skin care, and, in the lower limb, walk with comparative ease. For self-limiting, stable injuries, and after surgical fracture stabilization, an orthosis also allows patients to 'wean' themselves gradually from the device as their level of comfort returns. For these reasons, moon boots (walker boots), hinged knee braces, wrist splints and mallet splints are usually preferred over casts wherever possible (**Fig. 4.27**).

Fractures are managed according to the paradigm in Chapter 1:

**Reduce - Hold - Move**

Non- operative treatment is appropriate for the majority of fractures, but where the fracture cannot be adequately reduced, the reduction cannot be held, or there is a substantial functional advantage to early movement, operative management should be considered.

The aims of operative fracture management are to reduce and stabilize the fracture so as to restore the alignment of the limb, control pain, and allow early movement and rapid return of function. The benefits of accurate reduction and early rehabilitation must be weighed against the inherent risks of anaesthesia, surgery and implantation of foreign material. Successful fracture surgery demands a clear understanding of biomechanics and the effect of surgical intervention on the biology of fracture healing.

## REDUCE: CLOSED OR OPEN FRACTURE REDUCTION

If a fracture needs to be reduced anatomically (e.g. a displaced intra-articular fracture), this will usually imply the requirement for an *open reduction*. An open reduction allows direct visual assessment of the fracture, and the application of bone clamps that can make the reduction more straightforward. An open reduction is usually followed by internal fixation with compression using screws and plates, or a tension band technique.

In contrast, *closed reduction* is employed where the aim is restoration of length, rotation and alignment, such as in the treatment of most long bone fractures. Reduction must be achieved using traction and closed manipulation, and is assessed radiographically. A closed reduction avoids exposure of the fracture site, minimizing further soft tissue stripping and the

potential for both devascularization of the fracture fragments and the introduction of infection. For periarticular injuries, traction is applied through ligamentotaxis (tension on the periarticular ligaments and joint capsule), which allows some realignment of the joint. However, this is rarely perfect and cannot address 'die-punch' intra-articular fragments with no ligamentous attachment (Fig. 12.11).

## HOLD: CONSTRUCT STABILITY

Construct stability is the *ability of a fixed fracture to resist displacement*, and is determined by both the intrinsic stability of the fracture pattern and the type of implant used to fix it. The degree of fracture stability achieved after internal fixation is described in terms of two theoretical mechanical environments: absolute stability and relative stability. These two types of stability aim to exploit a different type of fracture healing (Figs 1.29 and 1.30).

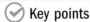
### Key points

- Absolute stability implies primary bone healing (without callus).
- Relative stability implies secondary bone healing (with callus).

### Absolute stability

Absolute stability is achieved where the fracture fragments are compressed and held rigidly so that there is no movement at the fracture site under physiological load. This allows primary bone healing. It is commonly used following the open anatomical reduction and fixation of intra-articular injuries. *Compression* is a key concept in achieving absolute stability and has two effects: *mechanically*, it brings the bone fragments into contact and allows the interstices of the fracture to 'lock' together, thus stabilizing the fracture; and *biologically*, it causes piezoelectric stimulation, promoting osteogenesis (Wolff's Law). At surgery, fracture compression can be achieved *temporarily* using clamps and other devices, and *definitively* with the use of fixation techniques such as:

- a lag screw (any screw that produces compression across a fracture)
- compression plating
- tension band wiring.

## Relative stability

Relative stability is achieved in a construct that allows a small amount of motion ('micromotion') at the fracture site. This results in secondary bone healing with callus.

The concept is employed with closed methods of fracture treatment, and where closed reduction and percutaneous fixation have been employed, such as with:

- intramedullary nails
- external fixators
- bridge plating.

## Selection of surgical technique

In reality, stability is a continuum and the many types of fracture pattern and methods of fracture stabilization available provide a limitless variety of different mechanical environments that are not yet fully understood. A general hierarchy of increasing stability is given in Fig. 5.1.

## Factors influencing construct stability

### Moment arm (Fig. 5.2)

The stability of a construct is influenced by the location of the fixation device in relation to the mechanical axis of the bone. Thus an intramedullary nail that is placed within that axis, or a circular frame that is centred on the axis, is intrinsically stable (**Fig. 5.2A**). A plate that is placed on the bone surface results in a short moment arm. If the plate is placed on the tension side of a bone (e.g. on the anterior or lateral cortex of the femur rather than the medial or posterior cortex), and if the opposite

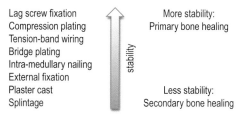

Lag screw fixation
Compression plating
Tension-band wiring
Bridge plating
Intra-medullary nailing
External fixation
Plaster cast
Splintage

stability

More stability:
Primary bone healing

Less stability:
Secondary bone healing

Fig. 5.1 The scale of stability.

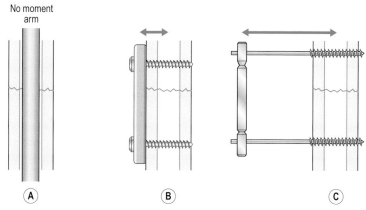

No moment
arm

(A)　　　　　(B)　　　　　(C)

Fig. 5.2 Moment arm.

cortex is intact, then this does not pose a problem (**Fig. 5.2B**). However, if the opposite cortex is deficient, the moment arm will tend to cause the construct to collapse. An external fixator has a greater moment arm and thus even less stability (**Fig. 5.2C**). External fixators are therefore usually insufficient for definitive stabilization of femoral or tibial fractures.

### Fracture comminution (Fig. 5.3)

Stability is also determined by fracture configuration. An *A-type* transverse mid-shaft fracture of a long bone with interlocking interstices, which has been reduced anatomically, is intrinsically stable; when fixed with a well-fitting intramedullary nail, the bone and implant construct is highly stable. When the patient stands on this leg, part of the body weight is supported by the bone (through the fracture) and part through the nail. The nail is therefore said to be *load-sharing*. In contrast, a *C-type* comminuted fracture at the same level has no intrinsic stability, and if the patient were allowed to take full weight immediately, the nail would be *load-bearing*. In between these extremes, a *B-type* fracture with a transverse area of contact will be load-sharing and stable after nailing, whereas a spiral or oblique B-type fracture may be vulnerable to shortening initially. To protect the implant, full weight-bearing may be delayed in type B and C fractures until some callus has begun to form.

## HOLD: IMPLANT CHOICE

Holding a fracture in the reduced position is achieved through the use of surgical implants of various types, each offering different advantages. The following are commonly used:

- **Screws**
- **Plates**
- **Fixed-angle devices and locked plates**
- **Tension band wire**
- **External fixators**
- **Intramedullary nails.**

## Screws

### Anatomy of a screw (Fig. 5.4)

A screw is a device that converts a rotational force (torque) into a longitudinal one (compression). A screw has a head and a shaft. The socket of the head has a specific shape to accommodate a screwdriver, most commonly a hexagon or a star. Note that, although the top of the head is flat, the under-surface is hemispherical. The shaft of the screw has a solid core and a thread. The separation of the threads is termed the pitch: this is the distance advanced when the screw is turned once. Screws may have cutting flutes to allow them to be self-tapping.

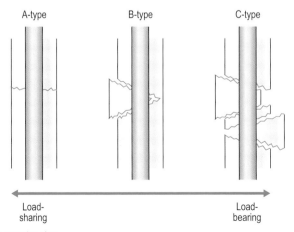

Fig. 5.3 Fracture comminution.

## Types of screw

Screws may be described according to either their form or their function (**Box 5.1**). In terms of *form* (shape), a cortical screw has a relatively small diameter and pitch, suitable for gripping dense cortical bone, whilst a cancellous screw has a larger diameter and pitch, which provide a better grip in more porous cancellous bone (**Fig. 5.5**). Cancellous screws may have thread along their whole length (fully threaded) or only a section at the tip (partially threaded). They may have a central cannulation that allows them to be placed over a guide wire. A locking screw has threads in the head as well as the shaft, allowing it to engage with specialized plates. A variable-pitch screw compresses two fragments together as it is tightened and is often used for scaphoid fixation (see Fig. 12.31). Screws are commonly referred to according to their outer diameter, the most common sizes being 3.5 mm and 4.5 mm. These are part of standardized sets of instruments and implants designed by the Swiss AO

### Box 5.1 Screw form and function

| | |
| --- | --- |
| **Form** (description of its shape) | Cortical |
| | Cancellous |
| | Partially threaded |
| | Fully threaded |
| | Self-tapping |
| | Cannulated |
| | Locking screw |
| | Variable pitch |
| | Size (e.g. 2.7 mm, 3.5 mm, 4.5 mm) |
| **Function** (description of how it is used) | Lag screw |
| | Compression screw |
| | Position screw |
| | Blocking screw |

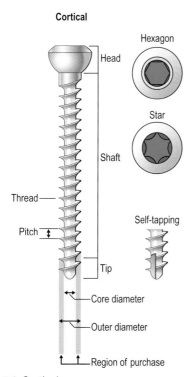

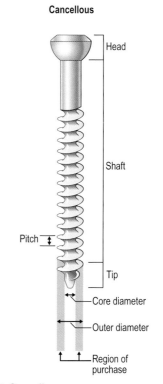

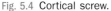

Fig. 5.4 Cortical screw.

Fig. 5.5 Cancellous screw.

## Table 5.1 Common AO screw diameters and drill sizes

| Screw type | Compact set | | Small fragment set | | Standard (large) fragment set | |
|---|---|---|---|---|---|---|
| | Cortical | Cortical | Cortical | Cancellous | Cortical | Cancellous |
| Screw thread diameter (mm) | 1.5 | 2 | 3.5 | 4.0 | 4.5 | 6.5 |
| Drill bit – gliding hole | 1.5 | 2 | 3.5 | – | 4.5 | – |
| Drill bit – pilot hole | 1.1 | 1.5 | 2.5 | 2.5 | 3.2 | 3.2 |
| Tap | 1.5 | 2 | 3.5 | 4.0 | 4.5 | 6.5 |

group (the Arbeitsgemeinschaft für Osteosynthesefragen or Association for the Study of Internal Fixation (ASIF)), and a working knowledge of the components of these sets is essential (**Table 5.1**).

In terms of *function*, there are many uses to which a screw may be put, irrespective of its shape. A *lag screw* is any screw used to compress two fragments together. *Compression* and *position screws* are terms used in plating. *Blocking* and *locking* screws are terms used with reference to intramedullary nailing.

### Inserting a screw (Fig. 5.6)

1. Use a *drill bit* with a guide to drill a pilot hole in the bone. The drill size corresponds to the core diameter of the screw to be used (see Table 5.1).

2. Use a *depth gauge* to measure the length of screw required.

3. Place a *tap* through the drill guide and use it to cut a threaded channel in the bone. The shape of the tap corresponds to the type of screw to be used; cortical and cancellous taps are different. As the tap cuts through the bone, it produces *swarf* (bone dust), which is forced up and out along the flutes of the tap. This must be released during the process of tapping by turning the tap anticlockwise half a turn for every three clockwise turns of advancement. In practice, most screws are now *self-tapping* and this step is often not necessary.

4. Insert the screw with the hex screwdriver.

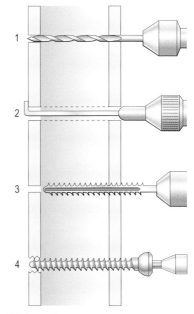

Fig. 5.6 Inserting a screw.

## Inserting a cortical lag screw (Fig. 5.7)

1. To compress two fragments of bone together, the screw threads must grip one fragment only, whilst the screw head pulls down on the other fragment. This is achieved by drilling a larger 'gliding' hole first. The diameter of the gliding hole is the same as the thread diameter of the screw and so the threads do not grip this hole.

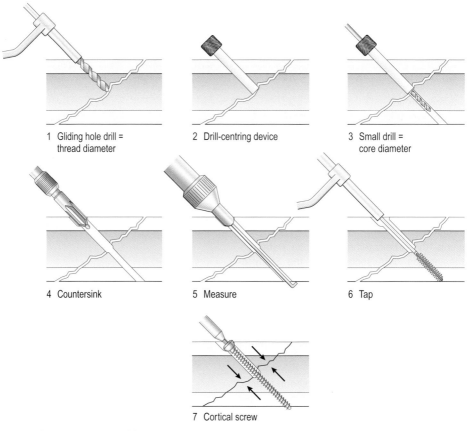

1  Gliding hole drill =
   thread diameter

2  Drill-centring device

3  Small drill =
   core diameter

4  Countersink

5  Measure

6  Tap

7  Cortical screw

Fig. 5.7 Inserting a cortical lag screw.

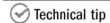 **Technical tip**

Inordinate amounts of time can be wasted during the process of screw insertion when, in moving from one step to another, an instrument fails to find the correct trajectory to pass smoothly through the drill hole. Focus entirely on your trajectory throughout the whole process and do not take your eyes off the bone; the scrub nurse must place the instrument in your hand without you needing to turn to look. Keep one instrument in the correct trajectory at all times; thus when the drill is removed, keep the drill guide in place until the depth gauge is poised, ready to be inserted. Then leave the depth gauge in place until the screw is mounted and again poised for insertion.

2. Place a drill-centring device (the 'top hat' or the smaller end of the double-ended drill guide) in the gliding hole.

3. Use the smaller-diameter drill bit (corresponding to the core diameter of the screw) to drill the far cortex.

4. Use a countersink to cut a shallow groove in the cortex to accommodate the shape of the screw head. If the countersink is not used, the rounded head of the screw has a very small contact area with the flat surface of the cortex and can cause a crack in the bone as it is tightened.

5. Use the depth gauge to measure the screw length.

6. Tap the far cortex.

7. Insert the screw. The lag screw is usually protected by a neutralization plate.

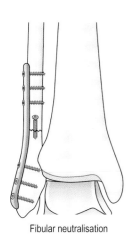 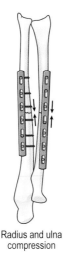 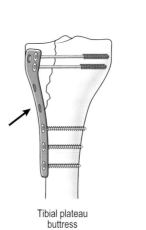 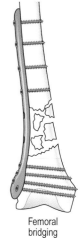

Fibular neutralisation | Radius and ulna compression | Tibial plateau buttress | Femoral bridging

Fig. 5.8 Plate types.

## Box 5.2 Plate types

| | |
|---|---|
| **Function** | Compression |
| | Neutralization (protection) |
| | Buttress |
| | Bridging |
| **Form** | Dynamic compression (DCP) |
| | Locking compression (LCP) |
| | LC-DCP (low contact) |
| | Plate size (e.g. 3.5 set, 4.5 set, 1/3 tubular) |
| | Locking plates |
| | Site-specific plates (e.g. proximal humerus) |
| | Shaped plates (e.g. t-plate, clover-leaf) |

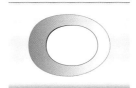

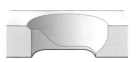

Fig. 5.9 Dynamic compression plate: contoured slot.

## Plates

A plate is a device applied to the exterior of a bone to maintain alignment and reduction during bone healing (**Fig. 5.8**). Like screws, plates are described according to either their form (shape) or their function (**Box 5.2**). There are four key possible functions of a plate. A neutralization (or protection) plate is used in conjunction with a lag screw, to control the shear or torsional forces between bone fragments that would otherwise cause the lag screw to fail (e.g. ankle fracture fixation). A compression plate is used to compress two bone fragments together, and is typically used for diaphyseal fractures. A buttress plate is used to resist shear forces, typically at the metaphyses, whilst a bridging plate is used to span areas of comminution.

### Compression plating
*Dynamic compression plate (DCP)*
The DCP has specially contoured slots that allow interfragmentary compression in diaphyseal fractures (**Fig. 5.9**). The plate is first secured to one of the bone fragments; a central drill guide (with a green-coloured collar) is used to drill the pilot hole before a screw is inserted (**Fig. 5.10**). This screw does not exert any

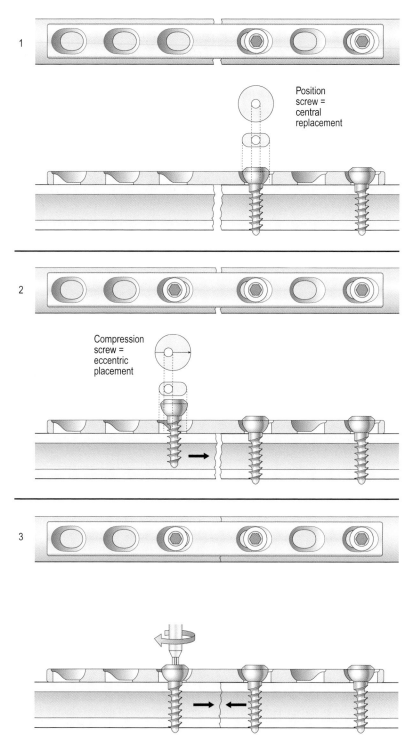

Fig. 5.10 Dynamic compression plate technique.

compression and is termed a position screw (**1** on Fig. 5.10). Attention is then turned to the other end of the plate and the other bone fragment. An offset drill guide (with a gold-coloured collar) is used to drill an eccentric drill hole (**2**). As the screw (termed a compression screw) is tightened, the head is forced down the sloping contour of the hole and slides along the plate (**3**). The fragment of bone gripped by this screw is thereby pulled along the plate, compressing the fracture.

### DCP: plate contouring and positioning (Fig. 5.11)

Applying a straight DCP will compress the near cortex but will result in some gapping of the far cortex as the fracture is compressed. This is avoided by using the plate benders to *pre-bend* the plate; 1–2 mm of concavity is sufficient. This is easily assessed by placing the now-bent plate on top of the (straight) bending tool and assessing the gap between the two. Apply the plate as above, and as the compression screws are tightened, the far cortex is compressed first, and then the near cortex, resulting in an even distribution of compressive force across the fracture.

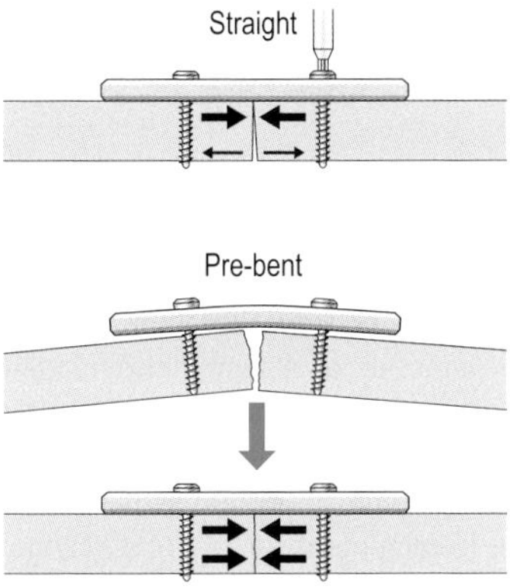

In many anatomical sites the bone is not straight and then the plate may need to be contoured to fit flush. Even site-specific plates are only contoured to fit the 'average' bone and may require modification. The positioning of a plate is usually determined by the surgical approach; however, metal plates function best under tension and so in the femur, where high forces are generated in weight-bearing, a plate must be positioned laterally or anteriorly rather than medially or posteriorly. In the upper limb, six cortices (three screws) on either side of a fracture are required for secure fixation; in the lower limb, eight cortices are required.

Fig. 5.11 Plate contouring.

### DCP: oblique fractures (Fig. 5.12)

Where a fracture is oblique, it can be fixed with a lag screw and neutralization plate. However, a more powerful compression can be obtained by use of a DCP. The plate should be secured to one fragment with position screws to form an 'axilla' (**1** on Fig. 5.12). By inserting compression screws into the free fragment it is compressed into this axilla (**2**), and can then be compressed further by insertion of a lag screw. Beware: if the plate is incorrectly placed at the outset to form an obtuse angle (**3**), using compression screws will only result in displacement (**4**).

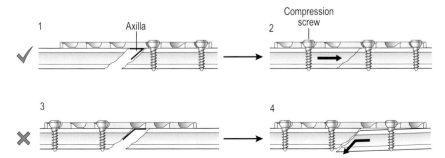

Fig. 5.12 Oblique fracture compression. See text for details.

### *Compression devices*

Compression can also be achieved by using other standard instruments (**Fig. 5.13**). The Verbrugge clamp has two tips, one of which is notched to grip a screw; the other is pointed and is placed within a plate hole. When the knob is twisted, the fracture is compressed. The ingenious articulated compression device also requires a unicortical screw for purchase, and can achieve substantial interfragmentary compression.

### Neutralization plating

A neutralization (or protection) plate is used to protect a lag screw. The lag screw is very

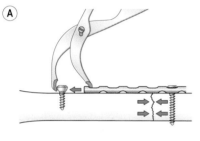

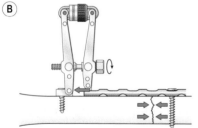

Fig. 5.13 Compression devices. **A**, Verbrugge clamp. **B**, Articulated compression device.

powerful, in that it provides very substantial interfragmentary compression, but it is vulnerable to failure if the fracture is subjected to angulatory or torsional forces. By adding a plate to the construct, these forces can be 'neutralized'. The actual plate selected depends on the location: when fixing a lateral malleolus, the neutralization plate would usually be a 1/3 tubular plate (see Fig. 5.8); in the forearm, a 3.5-mm DCP would be used; in the femur, a 4.5-mm off-set holed DCP would be required.

### Buttress plating

Some periarticular fractures, such as a Smith's fracture (see Fig. 12.13) of the distal radius, or unicondylar tibial plateau fractures, tend to displace through shear, and are most effectively fixed by buttress or 'anti-glide' plating (**Fig. 5.14**). A buttress plate holds the reduction of the apex of the fracture, which maintains the stability of the fragment and allows compression at the joint surface. In some fracture types, the buttress plate may also be used to achieve the reduction.

### Bridge plating

In some situations, it is either not possible, or not desirable, to expose all the fracture fragments and lag or compress them together. The many fragments of a highly comminuted fracture in the shaft or metadiaphyseal region of a long bone are often better left undisturbed so as not to jeopardize their vascularity. Following fracture realignment, a plate is fixed to the proximal and distal fragments, passing over or

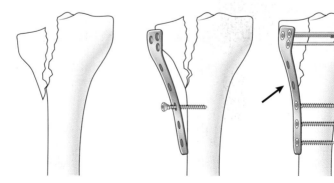

Fig. 5.14 Tibial buttress plate.

'bridging' the comminuted fracture region (see Fig. 5.8). As the fracture does not need to be exposed, the plate can be implanted percutaneously, with an incision only at each end for the screws. *Locking plates* (a description of form) are often used for bridge plating (a description of function). Bridging produces a long segment of plate that is unsupported between the two sets of attachment to bone. This is slightly flexible and, as it provides the conditions of relative stability, the fracture heals with callus.

## Fixed-angle devices and locked plates

In certain circumstances, particularly where a fracture has occurred in the region between the metaphysis and the diaphysis of a long bone (a metadiaphyseal fracture), a standard plate is at risk of failure, as the screws in the cancellous bone of the metaphyseal fragment may rotate in the plate. In contrast, a fixed-angle device can obtain a powerful grip on this fragment whilst maintaining the orientation of the

---

 **Key point**

It is important to understand the function of plates (and other implants) and to be clear on how they should be used and what effect they will have on fracture healing. In the example in **Figure 5.15A**, a bridge plate (relative stability technique) has been used to fix a femoral fracture. This would have been perfectly appropriate for this fracture (although a nail would have been a good alternative), and healing with callus could have been anticipated. However, the addition of a lag screw (absolute stability technique) has confused the issue: there has been insufficient movement for the formation of callus but too much movement for primary bone healing. The failure of this construct was inevitable, as the fracture did not unite (**Fig. 5.15B**). Revision fixation with compression, rigid fixation and absolute stability was successful (**Fig. 5.15C–D**).

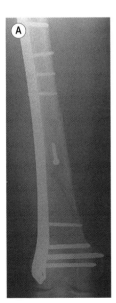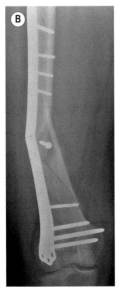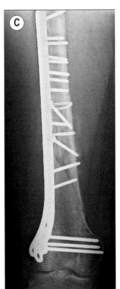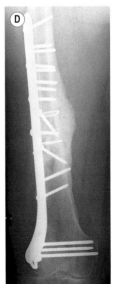

Fig. 5.15 Mixed plate principles.

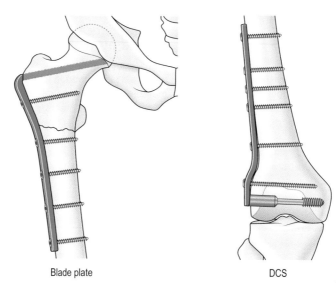

Blade plate                    DCS

Fig. 5.16 Fixed-angle devices. DCS, dynamic condylar screw.

joint surface (**Fig. 5.16**). The *blade plate* has been used for many decades, particularly for proximal and distal femoral fractures, and still has a valuable role in revision and salvage fixation, and to secure osteotomies. The procedure requires the insertion of a seating chisel into the metaphyseal fragment to prepare a channel. The blade of the plate is then seated in this channel. Careful attention to detail is required, as any inaccuracy in placing the seating chisel in any plane will result in a deformity when the plate is secured to the shaft. Conversely, judicious placement of the blade can allow very powerful correction of an existing deformity. The *dynamic condylar screw (DCS)* is used for the same indications; it is inserted with the aid of a jig and is technically easier. A dynamic hip screw (DHS) is the most commonly used fixed-angle device and is used for intertrochanteric hip fractures (p. 365). Its specific design allows for both angle-stable fixation and controlled linear collapse. These traditional fixed-angle devices all require an open reduction.

## Locked plating

Locked plates are the mechanical successors to blade plates. By linking the screw heads and the plate together, the construct becomes a fixed-angle device. The principal indications for locked plating are:

- *Osteoporotic bone:* where there is poor grip from standard screws
- *Metadiaphyseal fractures:* where the orientation of a joint must be maintained, particularly where there is fracture comminution.

Because the components of the locked plate can be assembled after insertion, this type of fixation also lends itself to **M**inimally **I**nvasive-**P**ercutaneous **P**late **O**steosynthesis (MIPPO). The mechanics of a locked plate are quite different from those of a conventional plate. In conventional plating, the screws compress the plate against the bone and construct stability relies on the friction generated by this compression. If the fracture does not heal, the screws will gradually loosen until the friction between the plate and bone is lost and the construct fails. This occurs progressively because the screws move independently from each other and the plate. Sequential radiographs will often show that successive screws develop areas of loosening and lysis, and then back out until the whole construct fails (**Fig. 5.17**).

In comparison, a locked plate system does not allow independent movement of the screws. The locked screws must all fail simultaneously and catastrophically, destroying the entire volume of bone around and between them

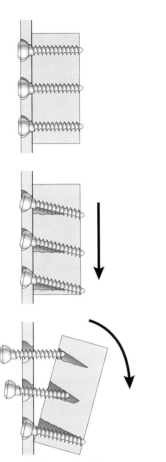

Fig. 5.17 Non-locking screw failure.

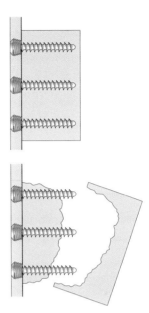

Fig. 5.18 Locking screw failure.

(**Fig. 5.18**). This requires far more energy and thus locked plates offer mechanically far superior bone fixation, particularly in metaphyseal cancellous bone.

As a locked plate does not rely on friction with the bone, the plate can sit away from the surface. This is sometimes described as being 'internal external fixation' and may offer an advantage in terms of preserving the soft tissue attachments to the fracture fragments. The plate can be introduced through a small incision and pushed down under skin or muscle, without extensive exposure (or stripping) of the soft tissues.

There are a number of *disadvantages* to locked plating. The cost is often an order of magnitude greater than the equivalent conventional plate. The MIPPO technique requires considerable expertise; the fracture must be reduced indirectly rather than under direct vision, and high rates of malreduction occur with inexpert use. If locked screws are used on both sides of the fracture, the construct can be very rigid, and even a very small fracture gap with no movement can lead to a delayed union or non-union. Finally, the threads of the screw head or plate may deform if over-tightened (so-called 'cold welding'). This may prevent it from being unscrewed again, and if removal of the metalwork is later required, the screw head or plate may have to be physically burred or cut out.

## Tension band wire

Certain fractures may be difficult to fix with plates either because the fragments are fragile (such as at the olecranon or occasionally the medial malleolus) or because they are subject to high-tension loads (such as at the patella and olecranon); in this case, a tension band wire (TBW) technique is mechanically

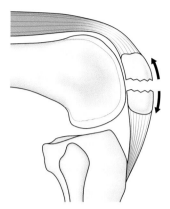

Fig. 5.19 Forces at a patella fracture.

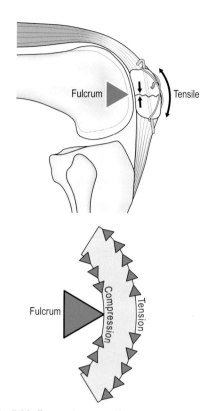

advantageous (**Fig. 5.19**). Tension band wiring uses straight k-wires to prevent fragment translation, and then a fine, flexible wire to exert compression and resist distraction forces. At the olecranon and patella, the other side of the joint (the trochlea of the distal humerus and the femur, respectively) represents a fulcrum. The oblique orientation of the distracting muscular forces around this fulcrum, resisted by the TBW, results in the generation of a compressive force at the joint surface (**Fig. 5.20**). This compression helps to stabilize the fracture at the joint surface (by locking the interstices of the fracture together) and promotes fracture healing. However, if there is a significant defect or comminution at the joint surface, the fracture will not resist compression and the construct will fail. An additional advantage of the TBW technique is that the flexible wire is placed through the insertion of a tendon or ligament, which may be stronger than in the small, frail bone fragment itself, particularly in osteoporotic bone.

Compression is achieved by twisting the flexible wire with pliers. Rather than twisting a loose wire, it is preferable to pull the wire to tighten it, and then twist it to hold the position: *pull to tighten, twist to hold*. The angle of pull is crucial in order to achieve the correct 'double helix' arrangement of wire; pulling unequally to one side will result in a mechanically weak construct (**Fig. 5.21**). Gauging the tension also

Fig. 5.20 Forces in a patella tension band wire.

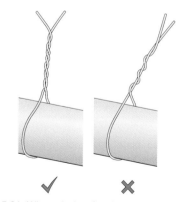

Fig. 5.21 Wire-twisting for the tension band wire technique.

requires experience: too loose and the fracture will gap with time and movement; too tight and the wire may break during twisting. When the shiny wire surface starts to look dull, the wire is reaching its tensile limit.

# External fixators

External fixators may be used for:

- Temporary stabilization of an injury: In this situation the external fixator is employed as 'portable traction'. Indications include temporizing where there is a significant soft tissue injury overlying a fracture or a joint dislocation that prevents early definitive fixation.

- Temporary stabilization of a multiply injured patient, where definitive fixation of, for example, a femoral fracture is prevented by physiological compromise such as the 'lethal triad' (Fig. 2.6).

- Definitive fixation of some juxta-articular fractures, such as at the distal radius.

- Definitive treatment of complex fractures, non-unions or malunions: The fixators used for this specialized treatment are generally ring fixators using the Ilizarov method (see Fig. 5.23).

## Temporary external fixation

### Mechanical stability (Fig. 5.22)

The simplest and most stable construct is summarized as 'Near–near, far–far and add a bar'. Two pins are placed in each fragment: one near the fracture and one as far from it as the anatomy and bar length will allow. The pins must be placed parallel to each other and are linked by a bar (**a** on Fig. 5.22). Increasing stability is achieved by using thicker pins (**b**), moving the bar closer to the bone (**c**), adding further pins and bars (**d**), and placing further pins and bars in other planes and then linking these with cross-struts (**e**). Pins intended for long-term use may be coated with hydroxyapatite to allow bony ingrowth and increased longevity. Pin loosening and infection are more likely where there has been thermal bone necrosis, and so pilot holes should be drilled prior to pin placement.

### Anatomical considerations

Pin placement must not cause additional complications. In particular:

- Safe anatomical corridors must be used to avoid nerve or vessel injury. Pins are placed through stab incisions where the bone is subcutaneous (such as the anteromedial surface of the tibia, Fig. 20.30), but a small incision and formal dissection may be required in some regions where the pins are passed in close proximity to a major structure (such as the lateral humeral fixator, where the proximal pins are close to the axillary nerve, and the distal pins close to the radial nerve).

- Muscle transfixion should be avoided wherever possible.

- Pin placement must not compromise subsequent definitive surgery. In particular, pin sites should be kept well away from the site of planned surgical incisions and definitive implants.

## Ring external fixation

A ring fixator provides both multiaxial stability and the opportunity to move bone segments gradually over time, correcting length and angulation, and applying either compression or distraction. In acute trauma, this technique is principally indicated for the treatment of severe soft tissue and bone loss, particularly in tibial fractures. Acute shortening of the limb may allow primary wound closure, avoiding complex plastic surgical reconstruction. Limb length is then restored with subsequent gradual distraction osteogenesis. Periarticular fractures are also amenable to ring fixation, as fine wires achieve powerful purchase in small fragments; locking plates, and nails with very proximal and distal locking options, are often preferable, however, as they carry a lower likelihood of intra-articular infection. Ring fixators are highly versatile in experienced hands and are particularly effective in limb reconstruction and salvage surgery.

The fixator is constructed from *fixation elements* (half-pins and tensioned fine wires) and *connecting elements* (rings, arches and rods). Whilst the classic Ilizarov technique achieves bone transport using the gradual adjustment of threaded rods and nuts, the Taylor spatial frame uses a system of six articulated struts (**Fig. 5.23**).

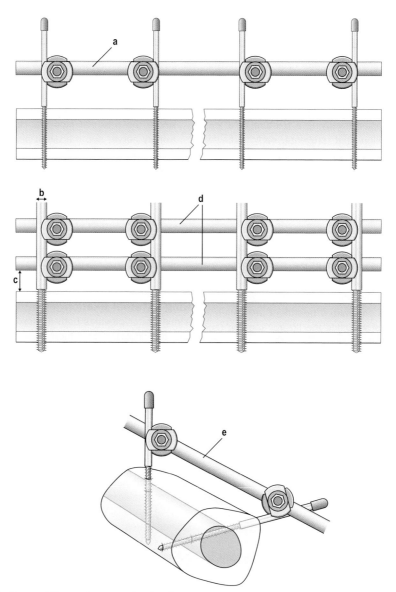

Fig. 5.22 External fixator. See text for details.

## Intramedullary nails

Intramedullary nailing is the standard of care for most diaphyseal fractures of the lower limbs, and there are expanding indications for nailing in periarticular fractures and in many injuries of the upper limbs. The principles of nailing comprise the following:

- Indirect fracture reduction, often using a traction device, aims to restore length, angulation and rotation, but not a perfect cortical reduction.

- Percutaneous surgery is performed via small incisions placed away from the fracture. The fracture site is not exposed and the periosteum is not disturbed in closed

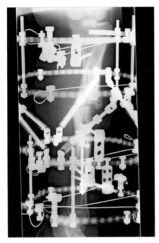

Fig. 5.23 Taylor spatial frame.

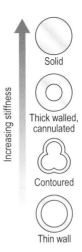

Fig. 5.24 Factors affecting nail rigidity.

fractures, which protects the vascular supply to the fractured bone ends, improving fracture *healing potential* and reducing the risk of *infection*.

- The nail controls translation and angulation.
- The cross-screws control length and rotation.
- Some movement (micromotion) occurs at the fracture site, allowing callus healing.
- The biomechanical strength of the nail usually allows immediate or early weight-bearing.

## Biomechanics

Nails are highly stable by virtue of their position within the bone (as close as possible to the mechanical axis and minimizing the moment arm), particularly where the construct is load-sharing (Fig. 5.3). Nails are flexible enough to allow some micromotion but must be rigid enough to avoid being bent. Nail rigidity increases with (**Fig. 5.24**):

- greater diameter (exponentially as related to $r^4$)
- greater wall thickness
- a contoured cross-sectional shape
- solidity (most nails are cannulated for ease of use and this makes them more flexible).

*Material* is also important: titanium is inherently more flexible (it has a lower Young's modulus) than steel. Finally, flexibility is related to the *working length*, which is the distance over which the nail is coupled to the bone. There are two ways in which a nail can be coupled to bone: by tight contact between the nail and the cortex, and by the use of cross-screws. The first intramedullary nails did not use cross-screws and relied on tight contact between the nail and the endosteal surface of the thickened diaphyseal segment of the bone (referred to as the isthmus) (**Fig. 5.25A**). This resulted in a relatively short working length, and the technique was effective only in mid-shaft fractures. The development of reaming allowed the medullary canal of the bone to be widened (**Fig. 5.25B**), creating a longer segment of cortical bone with a uniform internal diameter. This allowed a thicker nail to be passed, with a greater area of cortical bone contact and therefore an increased working length, thus extending the range of fractures that could be nailed (**Fig. 5.25C**). In contemporary locked nailing, the area of cortical bone contact remains important but the working length is now the distance between the two sets of cross-screws, allowing all but periarticular fractures to be nailed (**Fig. 5.25D**). The cross-screws also control length (preventing fracture shortening) and rotation.

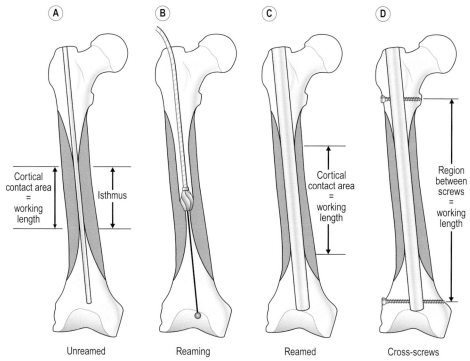

Fig. 5.25 Nail working length and reaming.

## Set-up

Correct set-up on the operating table is essential for a smooth nailing procedure. The precise position will depend on the bone to be nailed and the surgeon's preferred technique, but clear planning is vital and should include access to the entry point, location of the incision, space for movement of the instruments without contamination of the lights or other equipment, and access for the image intensifier.

## Entry point and trajectory

The correct entry point and guide-wire trajectory are the key to intramedullary nailing. The incision should not lie directly over the entry point but usually a few centimetres away, following the oblique path the guide wire will follow as it passes through skin, fat and muscle through to the entry point and then down the centre of the bone. The bony entry point defines how the reduction is achieved and maintained, and should not introduce any unwanted deformity

(e.g. see Fig. 17.30, showing a poor entry point in cephalomedullary nailing).

## Reaming

The process of reaming has a number of beneficial effects:

- *Increased working length*: The canal is enlarged, allowing a larger (and therefore stiffer and stronger) nail to be placed, with a greater working length (**Fig. 5.25**).

- *Increased blood flow at the fracture site*: Although the endosteal (centrifugal) blood supply is obliterated, the periosteal (centripetal) blood supply is stimulated and overall vascularity at the fracture site increases.

- *Bone grafting*: Bone reamings are forced into the fracture gap, providing autogenous bone graft. Bone healing is faster with reamed than unreamed nails.

There are drawbacks to reaming, which must be borne in mind:

- *Thermal necrosis*: Local heat is generated by the reamer, and if it is blunt or spins without advancing, this can cause a region of thermal bone necrosis. It is important to keep the reamer tip moving to allow the local blood supply to cool the bone. Where a reamer will not advance easily, a slow pumping action can help the tip to advance. A tourniquet should not be used.

- *Fat intravasation*: Intramedullary instrumentation displaces fat and bone marrow from the endosteal canal into the venous system, where it travels to the lungs, causing fat embolism. In predisposed patients, this can result in fat embolus syndrome and acute respiratory distress syndrome (Ch. 2). The greatest embolization is caused by the first instrument to enter the bone, usually the guide wire, and there is little difference between reamed and unreamed nails. Where fat embolus syndrome is a concern, damage control orthopaedics should be considered.

### Blocking screws

Nails are very effective at maintaining longitudinal alignment in shaft fractures where there is a tight cortical fit. In fractures at the proximal and distal metaphyses, however, the nail does not fit tightly into the cortex, but sits within relatively weak cancellous bone like a 'broomstick in a bucket'. This can result in fracture displacement and malunion. One technique used to avoid this is to insert *blocking screws*, also known as *poller screws*, from the German word for a traffic bollard, indicating a solid structure that forces redirection of travel. This technique is most commonly used in the treatment of proximal tibial shaft fractures (see Fig. 20.26).

## MOVE: ACTIVITY RESTRICTION AND WEIGHT-BEARING

Ideally, all methods of fracture management would afford the patient full use of the affected limb immediately after treatment. In practice, however, certain injuries require the patient to limit limb function to protect the construct and avoid displacement during fracture healing. Activity restrictions relate to weight-bearing status or the range of movement at a particular joint. Restrictions should not be prescribed lightly, as they can prolong hospital stay, cause the patient inconvenience and increase total recovery time.

## Range of motion

Restrictions may be recommended on the range of movement allowed and on the way that movement occurs. The restriction should be documented in terms of an arc of motion, e.g. 0–90° of knee flexion. The restriction may be enforced by the prescription of a brace that allows only this range of movement.

- *Active movements*: The joint is moved by the patient's own muscular effort only. The patient will generally limit these movements to those that do not cause pain. Active movement may be restricted, particularly where a muscle insertion has been repaired, e.g. tuberosity fractures at the shoulder.

- *Active assisted movements*: Patients are allowed to assist their own joint movement by support or effort with their other limbs. This may allow a greater range of movement than can be achieved by active movement alone if muscles are weak, or alternatively may protect muscle insertion repairs.

- *Passive movements*: The joint is mobilized by another person.

- *Resisted movement*: Movement exercises work against resistance (such as lifting weights or using an elastic band device) in order to build muscle.

## Weight-bearing

Restrictions on weight-bearing are used to protect the fixation of fractures in the lower limb. Restricted weight-bearing requires the patient to support the body weight on an uninjured (or at least unrestricted) leg and crutches. This is inconvenient and may not be possible after multiple injuries. In the elderly or cognitively impaired patient, this is often impractical and should be avoided wherever possible. Factors influencing the need for restricted weight-bearing include:

- *Fracture comminution*: If there is no cortical apposition after reduction, the fixation device is load-bearing (see Fig. 5.3) and may fail earlier through fatigue.

- *Poor bone quality*: Osteoporotic bone may fail around an implant.

- *Use of an implant*: It is usually necessary to protect a lower limb plate or a monolateral external fixator. Nails and circular frames usually allow immediate full weight-bearing.

- *Articular involvement*: Intra-articular fractures are particularly vulnerable to displacement.

The options for weight-bearing restriction are:

- *Non-weight-bearing*: The affected limb does not touch the floor during ambulation. It may rest on the floor during sitting or lying down but no force passes through the limb.

- *Partial weight-bearing*: Some weight is passed through the limb during ambulation. This is inexact and requires patient training and careful compliance. In practice, it often results in patients putting as much weight through the limb as they find comfortable.

- *Toe-touch weight-bearing*: Special consideration is given to fractures around the acetabulum. Non-weight-bearing would initially seem desirable; however, the weight of the entire lower limb is supported by muscle contraction around the hip and this generates powerful joint reaction forces across the injured joint. To avoid this, patients are permitted to have the toes and ball of the foot resting on the floor during ambulation.

## ACUTE ARTHRITIS

Acute atraumatic pain and swelling of a joint is a common presentation to the Emergency Department. Examination and investigation are focused on differentiating **septic arthritis** from the large number of differential diagnoses. Prompt diagnosis of septic arthritis is important; rapid joint destruction results from enzymes released from bacteria, as well as free radicals and other chemicals from the lymphocyte and macrophage response, and profound septic shock may develop, especially in elderly or immunosuppressed patients, who can deteriorate rapidly.

## Differential diagnoses of acute monoarthritis

There are numerous possible aetiologies, which are conveniently recalled using the 'surgical sieve' acronym for all diseases – 'CAT IN BED = VIP':

- **C**ongenital
- **A**cquired:
  - **T**rauma: *direct or indirect trauma, effusion or haemarthrosis*
  - **I**nfection: septic arthritis
  - **N**eoplasia: bone, soft tissue or haematological malignancy
  - **B**iochemical: crystal arthropathy (gout and pseudogout)
  - **E**ndocrine: diabetic joint disease (Charcot joint)
  - **D**egenerative: exacerbation of osteoarthritis
  - **V**ascular: haemophiliac haemarthrosis
  - **I**nflammatory: autoimmune/rheumatoid disease
  - **P**sychogenic.

## Emergency Department management

### History

- *Septic arthritis*: This often develops spontaneously, but there may be a history of predisposition (diabetes, rheumatoid arthritis, immunosuppression, prosthetic joint) or of a source of infection (penetrating injury, insect bite, recent surgery). Patients will report pain that has 'red flag' features: it is severe, constant, throbbing and worsening (see Box 7.1, p. 122). There may be symptoms of systemic inflammation (sweats and rigors, anorexia or malaise).

- *Trauma*: Ask about recent falls, knocks or unaccustomed activity.

- *Degenerative arthritis*: Was there pre-existing mechanical pain in the affected joint that may have been aggravated by a recent event or activity?

- *Biochemical causes*: Ask about a history of gout in this or other joints.

- *Inflammatory arthropathy*: Is there a personal or family history suggestive of inflammatory joint disease? Some 10% of new cases of rheumatoid arthritis present as a knee monoarthritis. Ask about symptoms of polyarthritis, particularly involving the small joints of the hands, the cervical spine and the temporomandibular joint. Ask about skin and nail changes suggestive of psoriasis. If there are symptoms of recent GI upset, iritis or urethritis, consider Reiter's syndrome (the patient 'can't see, pee or bend the knee').

### Examination

- *Look*: The patient with a septic arthritis often looks unwell, and has a fever and tachycardia.

- *Feel*: A superficial joint will be hot, swollen and tender. Deep joints, such as the hip, are not palpable.
- *Move*: Attempted passive movement of a septic joint is exquisitely painful, such that the patient will not tolerate more than a few degrees of motion.

## Investigation

Blood tests will demonstrate a raised inflammatory profile (raised white cell count, erythrocyte sedimentation rate (ESR) and C-reactive protein (CRP)). The key investigation is joint aspiration; the techniques for specific joints are described on page 109–114. A careful aseptic technique is important in order not to contaminate the specimen. Avoid penetrating skin that is injured or cellulitic. Aspirate as much fluid as possible and note whether it is purulent, clear or blood-stained, or is frank blood (a haemarthrosis). Send the specimen for urgent microscopy and culture. This investigation drives subsequent treatment but a false negative result may occur if antibiotics have been given prior to the aspiration. The key positive findings are the presence of bacteria (sepsis) or crystals (gout). Other laboratory findings may also offer a guide to diagnosis (**Table 6.1**).

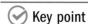 **Key point**

Joint aspiration must be performed before antibiotics are given, except in the situation of life-threatening systemic sepsis.

## Orthopaedic management

If the patient is systemically unwell, begin empirical intravenous *antibiotics* immediately after aspiration; otherwise, wait for the results of the urgent microscopy. The definitive treatment of a septic major joint is *urgent surgical lavage*, which can be both life-saving and joint-saving. The hip joint is usually washed out using an open approach, whereas many other joints, including the knee, shoulder and ankle, can be washed out arthroscopically. Subsequent management will be guided by the patient's response, as judged by clinical improvement and inflammatory indices. Further joint washout may be required at 24 or 48 hours. The duration of intravenous and subsequent oral antibiotic treatment will depend on the organism and its sensitivities, and is guided by local microbiological advice, but is typically at least 8 weeks in duration. In the long term, there remains the risk of late reactivation of infection, and of accelerated degenerative arthritis.

### Infection of prosthetic joints

These differ from infections of native joints in several respects:

- The risk of infection of an arthroplasty is higher and the local clinical signs are less pronounced. A higher index of suspicion is required.
- Patients with a septic prosthetic joint may be more unwell, and may deteriorate faster, than an otherwise healthy patient with a septic native joint. They may require fluid resuscitation, early empirical antibiotic treatment and emergency joint lavage.

| Table 6.1   Laboratory investigation of joint fluid | | | |
|---|---|---|---|
| **Criteria** | **Normal** | **Inflammatory** | **Septic** |
| Colour | Straw-coloured | Yellow | Yellow or green |
| Clarity | Clear | Opaque | Opaque |
| White blood cells/μL | <200 | 1000-50 000 | 50 000-200 000 |
| Polymorphonuclear cells | <25% | >50% | >75% |

- The risk of inoculating infection into a sterile joint is higher; when planning a diagnostic aspiration, consideration should be given to carrying out the aspiration in an operating theatre environment.
- An infected prosthesis will usually require extensive revision surgery. Deep tissue samples are usually taken for culture at the time of initial surgery, as identification of the infecting organism is crucial to the likelihood of successful eradication. If the patient is systemically well, avoid commencing empirical antibiotics prior to surgery.

## CELLULITIS

Cellulitis is a superficial infection of the skin. It is characterized by the cardinal features of inflammation: *rubor*, *calor*, *tumor* and *dolor*: erythema, warmth, swelling and pain.

## Emergency Department management

### History

Ask about the time of onset, and whether there was a precipitating breach in the skin from a wound, insect bite or injection site. Is the patient immunosuppressed by diabetes, disease (such as AIDS), or drugs? Is there systemic upset (fever, rigors, malaise, anorexia)? Has the patient received any treatment to date?

### Examination

- *Look*: Expose the entire limb and check for the cardinal signs of inflammation. Ascending lymphangitis – a tracking cellulitis along the superficial lymphatic system – can suggest a more severe infection. Comment on the quality of the skin. Is it normal, or is it vulnerable hypovascular skin from scarring or venous stasis (haemochromatosis or lipodermatosclerosis)?
- *Feel*: Palpate gently over the affected area to detect induration (thickened, oedematous skin) or fluctuance (suggestive of an underlying abscess). Palpate for regional lymphadenopathy in the groin or axilla.

- *Move*: Assess the ranges of movement of adjacent joints to exclude a septic arthritis.

## Investigation

Take blood for inflammatory indices (full blood count (FBC), ESR, CRP) and culture.

## Orthopaedic management

Most superficial cases of cellulitis with no systemic upset are diagnosed on clinical grounds alone and are managed in the community with oral antibiotics. Indications for further investigation and admission for intravenous antibiotics include failure of oral antibiotic treatment, and immunocompromise or systemic upset.

## Treatment

The organism is most commonly a staphylococcus or a streptococcus, and empirical treatment is usually intravenous flucloxacillin (1 g)+benzylpenicillin (1.2 g) four times a day, although local policies may vary.

---

 **Key point**

For all cases of infection, mark the periphery of the erythematous area with an indelible marker to allow later comparison.

---

## NECROTIZING FASCIITIS

This is a life- and limb-threatening, rapidly progressive infection that is a surgical emergency. The infection infiltrates the subcutaneous fat and underlying muscle fascia, causing necrosis (tissue death). The fascial plane then allows rapid propagation of the infection. This condition should be suspected in any unwell patient with infection; the external clinical features may initially be subtle, and regular review is needed to appreciate the rapid development of the condition. The infection is polymicrobial, often including streptococci, staphylococci, Clostridia and Bacteroides. Clostridia are gas-forming organisms that cause *gas gangrene*.

## Emergency Department management

### History

The patient will report rapidly progressive swelling and often severe pain. There is commonly a history of intravenous drug abuse or immunocompromise.

### Examination

- *Look*: The patient will usually be systemically unwell with a fever, tachycardia and possibly hypotension. The limb will be swollen and erythematous. The necrotic tissue is in the fascia deep to skin and so the skin itself may initially look normal. Later it may become discoloured and blistered.
- *Feel*: The limb will be tender to touch. There may be subcutaneous crepitation from gas in the tissues. A cardinal feature is damage to the cutaneous nerves, producing a localized area of numbness overlying the infection.

### Treatment

Urgent senior review is mandatory. Establish intravenous access and take blood for an FBC, urea and electrolytes (U&E), inflammatory indices, lactate, group and save, and culture. Mark out the affected area with an indelible pen. Begin fluid resuscitation and empirical high-dose intravenous antibiotics. *Triple therapy* with flucloxacillin (2 g), benzylpenicillin (2.4 g) and clindamycin (1.2 g) is recommended, although local protocols will vary. Time-consuming imaging has little part to play.

## Orthopaedic management

### Debridement

Treatment is emergency surgical debridement. The area of necrotic tissue expands very rapidly. At surgery, an incision is made well proximal to the clinically affected area and the fat and fascia are carefully inspected. If there is any evidence of fat or fascial necrosis with, for example, tracking fluid in the tissue planes, the incision needs to be made further proximally. Once a clearly normal level has been identified, wide excision of skin, fat and fascia is performed. Practically, this often requires an amputation. The specimen must be sent for pathological and microbiological analysis.

### Postoperative management

The patient requires critical care monitoring with high-dose intravenous antibiotic treatment. Regular review and clinical examination are required, and if there is evidence of disease progression at the excisional margins, further excision is necessary. Once the patient's condition has stabilized, soft tissue coverage can be contemplated (Fig. 3.4).

## ABSCESSES

An abscess is a discrete collection of pus, which is usually amenable to surgical drainage. A small, pointing skin abscess or paronychia can usually be lanced satisfactorily in the Emergency Department and then managed in the community with oral antibiotics. Deeper collections may require further investigation and radiographic or surgical drainage.

### History

The patient will report localized pain and swelling. Ask about the duration of the infection, a history of penetrating injury, and immunosuppression.

### Examination

- *Look*: There will often be a clearly demarcated area of skin inflammation, and possibly a pointing abscess. Look for signs of spreading infection (lymphangitis, lymphadenopathy) and systemic sepsis.
- *Feel*: A subcutaneous abscess will be palpable as an area of *fluctuance*. Place your thumb and index finger on either side of the swelling and then press down over the centre of the swelling with your other index finger. You will feel the swelling 'bulge' to each side between the examining thumb and finger, confirming the presence of fluid. A deeper abscess may be indistinct or entirely impalpable.

## Investigation

Imaging is often required to distinguish between a diffuse infection and a discrete abscess. Ultrasound allows good visualization and additionally permits the sonographer to place a needle into the abscess for aspiration. MRI scanning may be required for deeper abscesses and helps to delineate the anatomy for surgical drainage.

## Treatment

The surgical adage applies to most situations: 'pus about: let it out'. Where the patient is systemically unwell, drainage may need to be performed urgently. In common with other infections, empirical antibiotics should be withheld until a specimen for microbiological analysis has been obtained, unless the patient is systemically unwell.

## Psoas abscess

This is an uncommon but important surgical diagnosis. The patient presents with deep hip, groin or iliac fossa pain, and often with systemic sepsis. On examination, the hip is irritable with pain on attempted extension. The abscess is too deep to be palpable and plain radiographs of the hip are unremarkable. The diagnosis is usually revealed by an MRI or ultrasound scan of the pelvis. Treatment is drainage, either by radiographically directed needle aspiration or by surgery.

## MUSCLE INFECTION

Muscle is usually resistant to bacterial infection by virtue of its excellent blood supply, and so muscle infections are rare and constitute a cause for concern. Infective myositis may be bacterial, fungal or parasitic, and acute or chronic.

## Acute infective myositis

This is an emergency condition very similar to necrotizing fasciitis and should be managed in the same manner. A region of swollen, painful muscle is evident. Request creatine kinase levels for evidence of muscle breakdown. The systemically unwell patient requires rapid resuscitation, senior review and, often, surgical debridement.

## BONE INFECTION (OSTEOMYELITIS)

Osteomyelitis is generally a more indolent infection than an acute infection in the skin, muscle or joints. Patients may present with an erythematous painful area that may be difficult to differentiate from cellulitis.

## Classification

Cierny and Mader have classified both the infected host and the stage of the disease.

### Host

*Class A: normal host*
- Physiological, metabolic and immune functions are normal.
- There is an association with a much better prognosis.

*Class B: impaired host*
- The patient is immunocompromised, either locally (Bl), systemically (Bs), or both (Bls).
- Local factors include peripheral vascular disease, venous stasis or lymphoedema.
- Systemic factors include smoking, hypoxaemia, chronic renal failure, malignancy, diabetes or immunosuppressive drugs (e.g. steroids).
- The goal is to address any remediable factors.

*Class C: health of host does not allow full treatment*
- Treatment poses a greater risk than the infection itself.
- Surgery may not be possible because of the patient's debilitated or immunocompromised status.

### Disease (*Fig. 6.1*)

*Type 1: medullary osteomyelitis*
- Disease is limited to the medullary cavity.
- It is often caused by a solitary organism.

Type I: Medullary

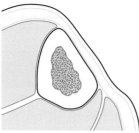

Type II: Superficial

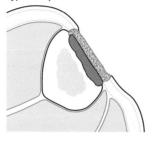

Type III: Localized

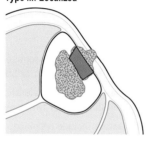

Type IV: Diffuse

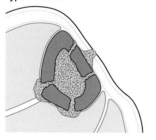

Fig. 6.1 Cierny and Mader classification of osteomyelitis.

## Type 2: superficial osteomyelitis
- There is involvement of the cortex.
- The cause is often an adjacent soft tissue infection.
- Exposed, infected outer necrotic surface of bone is observed at the base of a soft tissue wound.
- Local ischaemia is seen.

## Type 3: localized osteomyelitis
- There may be involvement of both the medulla and cortex, but the bone generally remains stable, as the infection does not involve its entire diameter.

## Type 4: diffuse osteomyelitis
- Disease is extensive.
- It may occur on both sides of a non-union or a joint.
- There is involvement of the entire thickness of the bone, with loss of stability.

A segment of dead bone is termed a *seque-strum*. In chronic cases this may be walled off with surrounding live new bone, termed an *involucrum*. There may be a connecting *sinus* between the sequestrum and the skin surface.

# Emergency Department management
## History
There will often be a history of a precipitating open fracture or previous surgery. Patients will complain of localized pain, which often has 'red flag' features: it is chronic, worsening, aching, not related to activity and worse at night. It may be associated with systemic features of malaise, sweats, rigors and anorexia.

## Examination
The features will depend on the anatomical site. Where the soft tissue coverage is thin, such as over the anteromedial tibia, there is often induration, tenderness and the cardinal signs of infection. In deeper locations, such as the femur, the skin may be normal and the only indication may be a discharging sinus.

## Investigation

- *Blood tests*: FBC, ESR, CRP and blood culture.
- *Wound swab*: Swabs taken from the skin surface or the mouth of a sinus usually reveal contaminants rather than the organism causing the deep infection, and are rarely worthwhile.
- *Plain radiographs*: In the initial phase of osteomyelitis there may be no visible changes on plain radiographs. Later, bone resorption and a periosteal reaction are usually seen.
- *CT*: This is particularly useful in detecting an island of dead bone (sequestrum), which can lie within an involucrum of reactive live bone.
- *MRI*: Bone oedema is readily apparent and the extent of the infection can be defined.

## Treatment

*Avoid starting empirical antibiotics* unless the patient is systemically unwell. The key to successful treatment of osteomyelitis (as for septic arthritis) is identification of the causative organism(s). This usually requires a bone biopsy, and often laboratory culture, before definitive antibiotic therapy can be instituted.

## Orthopaedic management

This is a specialized area of practice. Depending on the organism, the site, and the presence or absence of a fracture or orthopaedic implants, treatment may be surgical excision, antibiotic eradication or suppression.

## JOINT ASPIRATION AND INJECTION

All joints in the body are accessible by needle and can therefore be aspirated for the purposes of diagnosis, or injected as a means of treatment. However, one should not enter a joint lightly, as there is a risk of introducing infection. Scrupulous aseptic technique must be observed.

 **Key point**

Do not aspirate a joint through cellulitic, abraded or psoriatic skin. This runs the risk of inoculating bacteria into the joint.

## Consent for joint aspiration

Document your discussion of the potential complications; the most important is septic arthritis (1 : 40 000). You must give clear instructions for the patient to return immediately, should symptoms develop. Other complications from aspiration might include neurovascular injury (from the needle) and a small scar. If injecting local anaesthetic peripherally, warn the patient of possible transient extremity numbness afterwards, and the importance of avoiding sharp, hot or very cold objects until sensation returns to normal. If injecting steroid, warn of a risk of septic arthritis, and the possibility of lipodystrophy (local skin dimpling) or loss of pigment.

## Set-up

Essential equipment includes:

- sterile dressing pack that includes a pot or tray for preparation and irrigation solutions, swabs, and a small drape with a hole in the centre
- skin preparation such as chlorhexidine
- 10-mL syringe
- 21-gauge needle (green)
- sterile gloves
- sterile sample pots
- small dressing.

Optional equipment includes:

- local anaesthetic: skin or intra-articular infiltration
- steroid: intra-articular injection
- three-way tap: allows easier drainage of large effusions.

## Procedural steps

For the aspiration of any joint, the patient should be comfortably positioned. Palpate the joint and identify the bony landmarks used as reference for needle insertion. It is often helpful to mark these in ink. Then:

1. Wash your hands: pre-preparation.

2. Open the dressing pack without touching the contents, and in a sterile fashion place the needle, syringe and sample pot into the sterile field.

3. Pour skin preparation into the sterile pot.

4. Open the glove packet and place on to a clean surface.

5. Wash your hands: pre-procedure.

6. Apply the sterile gloves.

7. First skin preparation: starting at the planned point of needle insertion, apply a swab soaked in skin preparation to the skin and clean a large area. Work your way outwards in a circular fashion.

8. Second skin preparation: repeat the above procedure.

9. Allow the skin to dry: this completes the antiseptic action of the skin preparation.

10. Apply a sterile drape with a centre hole over the insertion site.

11. Aspirate the joint without touching the needle.

12. Place the fluid in the sterile container for microscopy and plating. If you have more than 5 mL of fluid, consider sending the remainder in blood culture bottles.

13. Telephone the laboratory to ensure the sample is expected and will be dealt with expeditiously.

14. Ensure needles are disposed of correctly and apply a dressing.

# Injection of steroid

*Contraindications and cautions* include the following:

- any joint where there is a risk of infection
- timescale within 3-6 months of planned joint replacement
- active tuberculosis, ocular herpes or acute psychosis
- pregnancy (in the first 16 weeks)
- allergy
- anticoagulant medication/bleeding diathesis.

# The shoulder (glenohumeral) joint (Fig. 6.2)

The glenohumeral joint is readily accessible from the posterior aspect of the shoulder. The

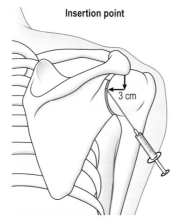
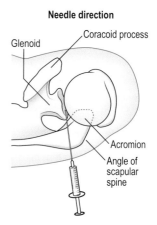

Fig. 6.2 Shoulder joint aspiration.

**Needle direction**

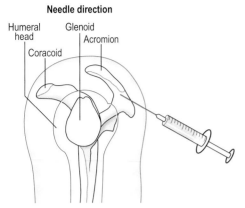

Fig. 6.3 Subacromial space injection.

**Insertion point**

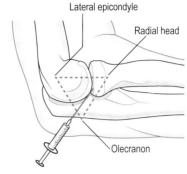

Fig. 6.4 Elbow aspiration.

patient should sit upright in a chair with the whole shoulder exposed. Identify the acromion, the scapular spine and the coracoid process.

**Insertion point** The needle should be inserted in the sulcus between the acromion and humeral head, which is found 3 cm medial to the end of the acromion, below the scapular spine.

**Needle direction** Place your finger on the coracoid process anteriorly, and aim towards it to pass between the glenoid and the humeral head. The joint is relatively deep through subcutaneous tissue and the external rotators. Aspiration of fluid confirms entry to the joint, but in the case of a dry tap, a repeat aspiration under ultrasound guidance may be indicated.

## The subacromial space (Fig. 6.3)

The subacromial space is not a common site of infection but it is often injected with steroid to alleviate the symptoms of rotator cuff impingement or calcific tendonitis. It lies between the supraspinatus and the underside of the acromion. The patient should sit upright in a chair. The landmarks are similar to those for accessing the glenohumeral joint.

**Insertion point** The needle is inserted 1 cm below the acromion.

**Needle direction** The needle does not head towards the coracoid process but rather aims to travel directly under the acromion. After entering the skin at a perpendicular angle, the needle tip is aimed upwards by lowering the hand to the floor. Aim for a point 2 cm medial to the lateral end of the acromion.

## The elbow joint (Fig. 6.4)

The elbow joint is accessible from its lateral aspect. The elbow is held in 90° flexion. Identify the lateral epicondyle, the olecranon and the radial head (which is felt to move during forearm rotation). There is a triangular 'soft spot' between these landmarks, which may exhibit a fullness if there is a particularly large effusion.

**Insertion point** The needle is inserted in the soft spot between the lateral epicondyle, radial head and olecranon.

**Needle direction** Aim the needle towards the middle of the antecubital fossa.

## The wrist joint (Fig. 6.5)

Although the joint is readily palpable, access can be challenging and only a small amount of fluid may be present. Place the patient's forearm on a table, palm down. A small crepe bandage can be placed under the wrist to allow some flexion.

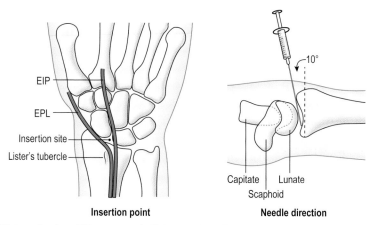

Fig. 6.5 Wrist aspiration. EIP, extensor indicis proprius; EPL, extensor pollicis longus.

***Insertion point*** The needle is inserted on the dorsal aspect of the wrist joint, distal to the palpable prominence of Lister's tubercle, between the extensor pollicis longus and extensor indicis tendons.

***Needle direction*** Angle proximally by 10° to mirror the volar tilt of the distal radius. The needle may strike the distal radius or the carpus, but simply 'walk' the tip distally to enter the joint.

## The hip joint (Fig. 6.6)

The hip joint is too deep to be palpated directly and it is preferable to be guided by imaging, either fluoroscopy or ultrasound. Local anatomical landmarks assist needle placement. The femoral pulse, found at the mid-inguinal point (between the anterior superior iliac spine and pubic symphysis), lies directly over the hip joint. Some 3 cm lateral to the pulse lies the femoral nerve. A finger should be kept over the femoral pulse during needle insertion to ensure it is protected.

***Insertion point*** The needle is inserted immediately below the groin crease, just lateral to the femoral pulse.

***Needle direction*** The needle aims to reach the junction of the femoral neck and head. The needle should be aimed 30° medially. In the event of a dry tap, the injection of radiopaque contrast confirms that the needle is within the

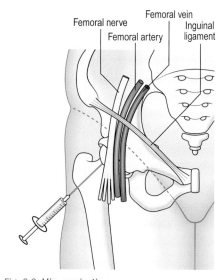

Fig. 6.6 Hip aspiration.

joint. The contrast forms a 'halo' around the head–neck interface (**Fig. 6.7**).

## The knee joint

### Aspiration (Fig. 6.8)

There are a number of needle placement options. The knee joint cavity extends proximally behind and above the patella (into the suprapatellar pouch). A lateral approach for knee aspiration, with the needle entering the patellofemoral joint, avoids any soft tissue blocking the needle, which can result in a 'false

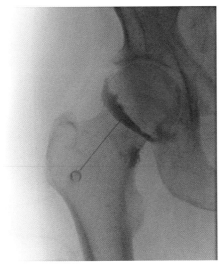

Fig. 6.7 Hip injection: the 'halo' sign.

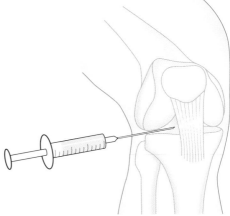

Fig. 6.9 Knee injection.

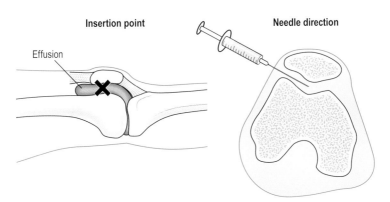

Fig. 6.8 Knee aspiration.

negative' tap when aspiration is attempted from other directions. Place the patient supine on an examination couch with a straight knee. Palpate the sulcus behind the lateral edge of the patella.

***Insertion point*** The needle is inserted in the sulcus between the lateral edge of the patella and the femoral condyle.

***Needle direction*** Aim medially, transversely and slightly posteriorly, parallel to the patello-femoral joint.

## Injection (Fig. 6.9)

For injection, an anterolateral approach is preferred. With the knee held at 90° of flexion, palpate the soft spot within a triangle bordered by the patella tendon medially, the tibial plateau inferiorly, and the femoral condyle laterally.

***Insertion point*** The needle is inserted in the centre of the 'soft spot'.

***Needle direction*** Aim for the centre of the intercondylar notch, directing the needle parallel to the tibial plateau (90° to the tibial shaft) and

Insertion point                    Needle direction

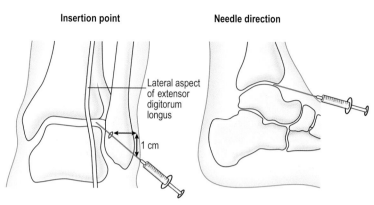

Fig. 6.10 Ankle aspiration.

slightly medially to avoid the articular surface of the condyle.

## The ankle joint (Fig. 6.10)

The patient is positioned supine on an examination couch. Palpate the lateral malleolus, and then ask the patient to extend the toes to allow palpation of the lateral aspect of the extensor digitorum longus tendon.

*Insertion point* The needle is inserted 1 cm proximal and medial to the tip of the lateral malleolus, lateral to the extensor tendons.

*Needle direction* The needle should be aimed at 45° to the skin and directed proximally and medially.

## NON-UNION

### Definition

Non-union is the failure of a fracture to heal within the expected time frame for that fracture. The actual time to union will clearly vary with factors such as the age of the patient and the fracture location and severity, and so there is no universally accepted time point for fracture union. The most commonly cited specific definition is that of the US Food and Drug Administration (FDA), which, for research purposes, identified a non-union as failure of a fracture to heal by 9 months, with no radiographic progression in healing seen in the previous 3 months. Clinically, non-union is identified by ongoing pain, movement, deformity and crepitus at the fracture site. In the lower limb, the most important feature is persistent pain on weight-bearing. *Delayed union* is a slower than expected progression towards union.

### Aetiology

Factors that delay bone healing may relate to the patient, the fracture or any surgery that has been performed:

- *Patient factors*: These include: *age* (children's fractures heal far more rapidly than adults') and, very importantly, *smoking*. The presence of *systemic disease* can delay fracture healing, including diabetes (can double time to union), peripheral vascular disease, severe malnutrition, anaemia and hypothyroidism. Some *drugs*, including non-steroidal anti-inflammatories (NSAIDs) and corticosteroids, may delay fracture healing. Some *antibiotics*, including ciprofloxacin and rifampicin, also delay bone healing, which may exacerbate the problem if prescribed for infection around a fracture.
- *Fracture factors*: These include *which bone* it is (the femoral shaft takes 20 weeks to unite, a metacarpal 6 weeks), and *which part* of the bone is affected (e.g. fractures of different parts of the scaphoid). Union time is also greatly affected by the *vascularity* of the fractured fragments. Vascularity is reduced in high-energy, open, comminuted fractures with marked displacement, stripping and bone loss, and in fractures complicated by vascular injury. Local *infection* will delay fracture healing.
- *Surgeon factors*: These also relate to the vascularity of the bone around the fracture, and the surgical technique undertaken. Non-unions are more common where there has been extensive *soft tissue stripping*, and failure to provide appropriate stability. This is usually *inadequate stabilization*, resulting in excessive fracture movement that prevents the natural progression from a flexible granulation tissue to rigid bone. Alternatively, where a relative stability construct has been chosen, an ill-considered lag screw may result in *excessive* stability, which can prevent callus formation. The presence of a *fracture gap*, resulting from inadequate reduction, predisposes to non-union. Most importantly, the introduction of *infection* greatly increases the likelihood of a non-union.

### Types

Non-unions are classically viewed as being one of two types (**Fig. 7.1**):

- *Hypertrophic non-union*: a mechanical problem due to inadequate fracture stability. It is the most common cause of non-union, and is addressed by increasing fracture stability, usually by compressing the non-union site.
- *Atrophic non-union*: a biological problem due to reduced or absent fracture healing activity, which may relate to any of the causative factors outlined above. It is relatively uncommon, but is addressed by excision of

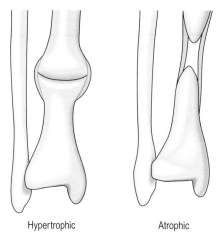

Hypertrophic            Atrophic

Fig. 7.1 Types of non-union.

the fibrous non-union tissue and introduction of bone graft or another osteo-inductive agent (see below).

## Diagnosis

Diagnosis is based on the *clinical features* of ongoing pain, loss of function and (in the lower limb) inability to weight-bear, as well as tenderness, mobility and crepitus at the fracture site. *Radiographic features* are a persistent fracture gap with the absence of bridging callus or trabeculae. Standard plain radiographic views may be insufficient to demonstrate this in complex fractures, and oblique projections and often a CT scan are invaluable.

Initially, it is important to distinguish a sterile non-union from an *infected non-union*. Enquire about infected or leaking wounds, the provision of antibiotics or the requirement for multiple surgeries. Exclude 'red flag' symptoms of throbbing persistent pain that is not activity-related but is often nocturnal, and any associated systemic symptoms such as sweats and weight loss (see Box 7.1). Obtain blood for a full blood count (FBC) and measurement of erythrocyte sedimentation rate (ESR) and C-reactive protein (CRP).

## Management

**Sterile non-union** is approached in a number of ways, depending on the cause and on which

bone is affected. Non-unions of the tibia and femur that have been nailed are usually treated successfully with exchange-nailing. Other fractures are generally compressed and plated, and familiarity with devices such as the blade plate and compression devices is invaluable (see Figs 5.13 and 5.16). Occasionally, in the presence of a true atrophic non-union, additional fracture stimulation with autogenous bone graft or a graft substitute is used. Graft and graft substitutes are defined by their mechanical and biological properties:

- *Osteoconductive* materials are biologically inert but provide a scaffold on which host bone can grow. They are principally used where mechanical support is required. Materials include calcium sulphate (the same material as plaster of Paris) and calcium phosphate cements and ceramics (such as hydroxyapatite, the same material that makes up the inorganic matrix of bone).

- *Osteo-inductive* agents are synthetically produced members of the transforming growth factor β super-family, such as bone morphogenic proteins. They are intercellular messengers that stimulate transformation of cell types seen in secondary bone healing. The optimal role of these expensive agents has yet to be defined.

- *Osteogenic* material is that which intrinsically contains all the components required to form new bone. Fresh autogenous bone graft not only is osteoconductive and osteo-inductive, but also contains the cell types that form new bone. Autogenous graft is most commonly harvested from the iliac crests. More graft can be obtained from the femoral canals using a reamer-irrigator-aspirator (RIA), which collects the endosteal bone for implantation. In smaller bones, local graft may reduce the morbidity associated with graft harvest: for example, graft from the distal radius in wrist and hand non-unions.

**Infected non-union** is best dealt with by an expert, in a centre familiar with this complex problem. Complex, staged surgery with multiple deep tissue samples for microbiological analysis, followed by extensive excision of dead, infected bone and prolonged systemic antibiotic treatment, is required.

## INFECTION

Acute infection after orthopaedic trauma surgery is often a very significant problem and usually results in prolonged antibiotic treatment, repeated attendances for wound care, delayed fracture healing and often complex revision surgery. Outcomes are usually much worse than in patients without complications. There are two principal strategies: infected fracture fixation implants and infected arthroplasty implants.

### Infected fracture fixation implants

Where there is an un-united fracture, it is often most prudent to attempt to identify and suppress the causative organism and await fracture union, and then deal with the much easier problem of eradicating infection from an intact bone later. Management can be complex but will usually include:

- Assessment of blood indices of inflammation.
- Tissue samples for microbiological analysis: Superficial wound swabs are often misleading, and deep samples are much more reliable. They may be obtained at the time of debridement, or if a deep collection is aspirated.
- Wound debridement: Early recognition of infection and wound dehiscence or leak is managed with surgical debridement and lavage and either resuturing or application of a negative-pressure dressing.
- Antibiotic treatment: This usually consists of broad-spectrum empirical antibiotics given after tissue samples have been taken, which can be refined according to culture results.
- Further debridement and removal of all metalwork after fracture union.

Occasionally, this fails to suppress the infection, and then more aggressive debridement is required. If the implant has to be removed before fracture healing, an external fixator is usually required to maintain stability.

### Infected arthroplasty implants

In the presence of a joint prosthesis, every attempt must be made to eradicate the infection at an early stage. This may consist of:

- an initial decompression of pus and joint washout in an acutely sick patient
- a single-stage revision, involving removal of the implant, the taking of deep tissue specimens, extensive excision of all infected tissue and then implantation of a new prosthesis
- a multiple-stage revision, involving an initial debridement, followed by a 'fallow period' with no implant (or a spacer device) and antibiotic treatment, with staged further debridements and finally reimplantation.

## MALUNION

### Definition

Malunion is healing of a fracture in a non-anatomical position. This may result from inadequate initial reduction, or from subsequent loss of reduction, which may itself relate to inadequate initial stabilization of the fracture.

### Assessment

The consequences of malunion will depend on a number of factors:

- *Patient factors*: The age and functional requirements of the patient will dictate how symptomatic the malunion is. Deformity that would be entirely unacceptable in a young, athletic individual may be quite asymptomatic in an elderly, sedentary person.
- *Location* of the malunion: An intra-articular step is more likely to be symptomatic, and to result in deformity and functional restriction, than a step of the same size in the shaft of a bone. Intra-articular malunions often lead to accelerated post-traumatic osteoarthritis (PTOA). The morphology is often complex and these cases require careful assessment and occasionally an

intra-articular osteotomy and reduction. An angular deformity that causes loss of the normal mechanical axis in the lower limb will often cause pain, instability and PTOA at the knee or ankle. The closer the malunion is to the joint, the greater its effect on the overall mechanical axis.

- *Severity* of the malunion: Clearly, the more deformed the fracture, the more likely it is that the patient will complain of a cosmetic and functional impairment.

## Management

A deformity that results in pain, loss of function or the likelihood of progressive PTOA may justify (revision) surgery. This will entail careful planning, judicious osteotomies and then secure fixation, followed by functional rehabilitation.

## BONE DEFECTS

Traumatic bone loss can occur either at the moment of injury or after debridement. The management of a bone defect will depend principally on its size:

- *Defects <2 cm*: A diaphyseal defect <2 cm in length and affecting only 50% of the bone circumference will usually fill in spontaneously without further surgery, although this capacity may be reduced by the factors that tend to produce non-union.

- *Defects between 2 cm and 6 cm*: A segmental defect up to 6 cm in length will usually require bone grafting, particularly in the tibia.

- *Defects >6 cm*: A defect >6 cm in length often requires bone transport (**Fig. 7.2**).

There are four principal surgical strategies for major bone defects:

1. *Shorten the limb definitively*: This can be performed at the time of initial debridement of an open fracture, and often simplifies any soft tissue defect, allowing primary wound closure. It is useful particularly in the upper limb, where asymmetrical limb lengths rarely cause a functional problem. In the lower limb, a modest definitive shortening, with subsequent use of a shoe raise, may avoid having to subject a patient to further surgery.

2. *Acutely shorten the limb and then lengthen later*: A circular frame allows acute shortening and correctional angulation of the limb. This can simplify a soft tissue defect and may even allow primary closure. The length and alignment of the limb can then be restored using an Ilizarov technique. Two strategies for lengthening the bone are possible:

   a. shortening and compressing the fracture acutely and then later lengthening through a corticotomy at a different site (distraction osteogenesis)

   b. bone transport (**Fig. 7.2**) – returning the soft tissues to length acutely, leaving a

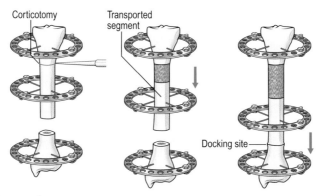

Corticotomy    Transported segment

Docking site

Fig. 7.2 Bone transport.

gap at the fracture site, and then transporting bone from a distant corticotomy into the defect, before 'docking' with the other fragment.

In the femur, lengthening can be achieved with a lengthening nail, or with a monoaxial external fixator over a nail.

3. *Shorten the other limb*: Where there is leg length inequality after bone loss, it may be simpler, quicker and more predictable to shorten the other limb. This can be done using an intramedullary saw and percutaneous osteotome, with nailing and institution of immediate weight-bearing (**Fig. 7.3**).

4. *Splint the limb to length and address the defect later*: If the fracture is fixed definitively after initial (or repeat) debridement – for example, with a nail or plate, a segmental defect can be addressed once the soft tissue envelope has stabilized, around 6 weeks later. The defect can be filled with allograft or graft substitute (see above). The *Masquelet technique* (**Fig. 7.4**) involves placing a cement block in the defect at the time of initial debridement (**Fig. 7.4B**). A membrane then develops around this spacer (**Fig. 7.4C**), and when the cement is removed, there remains a convenient vascularized defect, which is then packed with bone graft (**Fig. 7.4D**). This may allow the successful management of tibial defects up to 20 cm in length.

## HETEROTOPIC OSSIFICATION

### Definition

Heterotopic ossification (HO) is the formation of bone within tissues that are not usually the site of bone formation, particularly muscle. It is often accompanied by the rapid healing of fractures with exuberant callus.

### Aetiology

The cause of HO is unknown, but it tends to form in the context of periarticular muscle damage and is most commonly encountered after head injury, spinal injury or burns. It is also associated with acetabular fractures and elbow dislocations, and even with elective hip arthroplasty. Extensile approaches to the external aspect of the acetabulum are associated with a higher incidence than the ilioinguinal approach. Development is sporadic and there is presumably an element of genetic predisposition. The hip joint is most commonly affected, followed by the shoulder and elbow.

### Clinical features

The HO mass may develop rapidly after injury and be palpable within just a few weeks. It may result in a restriction in joint movement. Plain radiographs will demonstrate calcification in the soft tissues (**Fig. 7.5**).

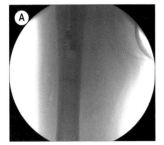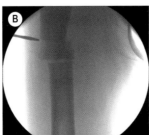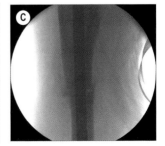

Fig. 7.3 Femoral shortening. **A**, An intramedullary saw is used to perform two corticotomies. **B**, These may need to be completed with a percutaneous osteotome. **C**, An intramedullary nail is used to stabilize the newly shortened femur.

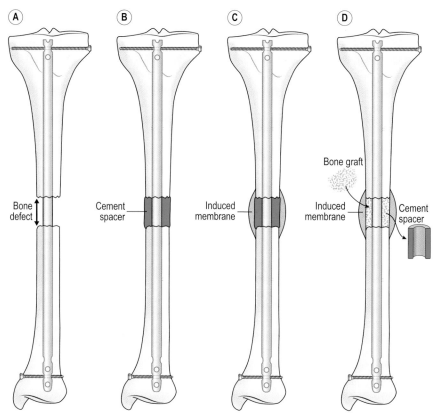

Fig. 7.4 The Masquelet technique.

## Prophylaxis

Both NSAIDs (in particular, indometacin) and radiotherapy have been used to prevent the development of HO. The efficacy and safety of NSAIDs is unclear, particularly in the context of head injury (where haemorrhage is a concern) and fractures (non-union). There is more evidence for the effectiveness of radiotherapy after acetabular surgery, but there are also clear potential adverse effects and practical difficulties, and there is a lack of consensus as to its most appropriate application.

## Management

Patients with symptoms of painful impingement or restricted joint movement may benefit from the excision of HO. This is performed after the heterotopic bone becomes fully mature, at between 6 and 18 months post injury. The risk of recurrence is higher in immature HO and where there are ongoing cognitive or neuromuscular effects of head or spinal injury.

# COMPLEX REGIONAL PAIN SYNDROME

## Definition

Complex regional pain syndrome (CRPS) is an inappropriate pain response to a tissue injury. The pathophysiology of the condition is incompletely understood.

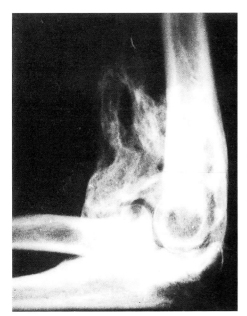
Fig. 7.5 Heterotopic ossification.

## Clinical features

The key features of this condition are as follows:

- There is usually a *precipitating injury*, which is frequently relatively minor, such as a wrist fracture.
- Unremitting, severe *pain* follows. This is often burning, and characterized by hyperaesthesia (excessive sensitivity) and allodynia (the perception of pain following a non-painful stimulus such as stroking).
- There are associated *objective abnormal signs* involving oedema, sweating, skin texture and colour, hair growth and nail appearance.
- These are accompanied by objective *radiographic features* of periarticular osteoporosis.
- There are often *psychological features* associated with the development of chronic pain.
- CRPS is most common in middle-aged women and smokers.

CRPS is defined by the International Association for the Study of Pain as having two subtypes:

- CRPS type 1: arises without any evidence of a precipitating nerve lesion. This condition has also been termed reflex sympathetic dystrophy (RSD), Sudek's atrophy or algoneurodystrophy.
- CRPS type 2: arises after an identifiable partial nerve injury. It is also termed causalgia.

There are *three stages* of CRPS, although patients rarely experience these stages in a predictable sequence or time frame:

1. *Stage one*: also termed 'hot' or acute CRPS. There is severe, burning pain, muscle spasm and joint stiffness with rapid local hair and nail growth. There is vasospasm with altered colour and temperature of the skin and sometimes hyperhydrosis (increased sweating). This stage may resolve spontaneously within a few weeks.

2. *Stage two*: also termed 'cold' CRPS. There is intense pain and oedema. Local hair growth diminishes, nails become cracked and brittle, and there is osteopaenia and muscle atrophy.

3. *Stage three*: considered an irreversible endstage. The pain becomes unremitting and may involve the entire limb. There is marked muscle atrophy and flexor tendon contracture, with severely limited mobility and function. There is marked osteopaenia.

## Management

Eighty-five per cent of patients will experience a substantial improvement in their symptoms over a period of 2 years with treatment. There are four principal components to the treatment of CRPS:

1. *Analgesia*: A spectrum of drugs is used, including simple paracetamol, NSAIDs, opiates, analogues of gamma-aminobutyric acid (GABA, the principal inhibitory central nervous system transmitter) such as gabapentin, and antidepressants.

2. *Physiotherapy*: This will maintain and improve the range of movement.

3. *Psychological techniques*: Patients are advised to stay as active as possible, and

to use the affected limb and joints as normally as possible. Relaxation, desensitization and cognitive behavioural therapy (CBT) exercises are taught. Specific techniques include 'pain exposure' physiotherapy, which aims to address psychosocial and avoidance behaviours and to reduce 'catastrophization' by loading and stretching joints whilst demonstrating that this is safe and does not harm the body. Mirror box therapy (looking at the normal side in a mirror and perceiving it to be the injured side) is reported to be effective.

4. *Spinal cord stimulation*: An implanted stimulator can be effective in refractory cases.

## PATHOLOGICAL FRACTURES

## Definition

A pathological fracture classically results from a normal force acting on an abnormal bone. There are a number of possible pathologies, including, of course, osteoporosis (fragility fracture), as well as osteomalacia, Paget's disease and osteogenesis imperfecta. However, it is particularly important to identify pathological fractures arising from bone tumours.

## Aetiology

Bone tumours may be benign or malignant, and may be primary or secondary. Primary tumours in bones and joints can arise from any of the tissue types present in the skeleton, including bone (e.g. osteoscarcoma), cartilage (e.g. chondrosarcoma), connective tissue (e.g. fibrosarcoma), synovium and blood (e.g. lymphoma, myeloma). Most primary bone tumours, both benign and malignant, occur in children and young adults, while in patients over the age of 40 a secondary metastasis is far more common. The most common malignancies that metastasize to bone are lung, breast, renal, thyroid and prostate. Renal metastases may be highly vascular, and it is usually prudent to obtain preoperative angiographic embolization of the lesion prior to surgery.

**Box 7.1** Red flag symptoms suggestive of major pathology (infection or malignancy)

- Age <20 or >55 years
- Lack of significant history of trauma, or pre-existing local pain
- Nocturnal pain
- Pain that is constant, progressive or non-mechanical in nature
- Constitutional symptoms (fever, night sweats, rigors, weight loss, anorexia)
- Symptoms suggestive of a primary malignancy (e.g. haemoptysis, altered bowel habit)
- History of previous malignancy
- History of immunosuppression (steroid use, drug abuse, human immunodeficiency virus (HIV))

## Clinical features

### History

There are a number of elements in the history that should arouse suspicion. These are termed 'red flags' (**Box 7.1**).

### Examination

Examine the affected site for local swelling and inflammation that is more marked than would be expected for the injury sustained. Enquire as to whether the patient had noticed any local abnormality prior to the fall. Where there is a suspicion of malignancy, there should be a specific examination of the regions that are particularly associated with bony metastases, including the chest, neck, breasts, abdomen, prostate and sites of lymphadenopathy.

### Blood investigations

Where there is any suspicion of malignancy, routine blood tests should include not only FBC, urea and electrolytes (U&Es) and liver function tests (LFTs) but also bone biochemistry (alkaline phosphatase, calcium, phosphate) and serum electrophoresis. Urine should be sent to

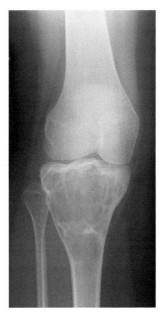

Fig. 7.6 Juxta-articular lesion of the proximal tibia, which is expansile and lytic; however, there is some reactive sclerosis at the margins of the lesion.

be tested for Bence Jones proteins to assess for myeloma. Specific tumour marker assays may be helpful where indicated.

## Radiological assessment

### Plain radiographs

Plain radiographs of the injured region, including full-length views of any affected bone, are obtained initially (**Figs 7.6–7.8**). Inspect these carefully for signs of a lesion at the site of the fracture and in the remainder of the bone. Apply *Enneking's four questions*:

1. Where is the lesion? Is it in the cortex or medulla? The diaphysis or metaphysis (or epiphysis)?

2. What is the lesion doing to the bone? Is it causing bone resorption (lytic) or bone deposition (sclerotic)? Is it expansile or erosive? Is the zone of transition between the lesion and surrounding normal bone sharp or diffuse (rapidly permeative)?

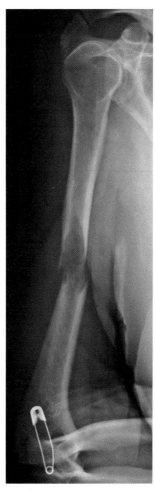

Fig. 7.7 Mid-shaft lesion of the humerus, which is lytic and destructive, with no bone reaction.

3. What is the bone doing to the lesion? Is there a cortical reaction (Codman's triangle)? Is there an area of reactive sclerosis around the lesion (suggests slow progression) or is there no reaction around an area of lysis (suggests rapid progression)?

4. Are there any special features? Many tumours have typical radiographic appearances that, while not always diagnostic, are often helpful.

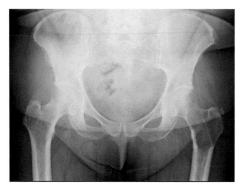

Fig. 7.8 Proximal femoral lesion, which is lytic, with no bone reaction.

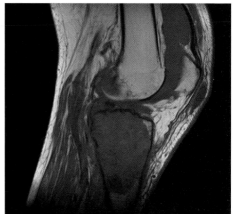

Fig. 7.9 Sagittal MRI appearances of the lesion in Figure 7.6.

## Bone scan

A radioisotope bone scan is helpful in the context of a suspected metastatic lesion in identifying other metastases, and occasionally the primary site of the tumour. It is more accurate than a skeletal survey of plain radiographs of the limbs.

## CT of the chest, abdomen and pelvis

Axial images of the trunk may help to identify a primary source, and to stage a disseminated malignancy where this is not clear from the history.

## MRI

Axial images of the tumour itself help to establish its margins, stage the tumour, and allow planning for definitive excision if appropriate (**Fig. 7.9**).

## Orthopaedic management

Management depends on the nature of the tumour:

- *Benign tumour*: An expert may be confident in diagnosing an entirely benign lesion such as a fibrous cortical defect or enchondroma on the basis of the plain radiographic appearances alone. Management, particularly in children, is then usually non-operative. Occasionally, a fracture through a benign lesion will result not only in satisfactory fracture healing, but also in resolution of the

lesion itself, although this is by no means as predictable as commonly supposed.

- *Potentially curable tumour*: This implies that the lesion is a single primary bone tumour or, occasionally, a solitary metastasis. In this situation, further investigation and management should only be undertaken within a specialist multidisciplinary musculoskeletal tumour service. Axial imaging, including a CT of the chest, abdomen and pelvis, and an MRI of the tumour, will determine the boundaries and stage of the tumour. A biopsy will then provide a tissue type and grade, and a programme of treatment may be formulated, which may include neoadjuvant (before surgery) chemotherapy or radiotherapy. Surgery is then planned as a curative resection with either ablation (amputation) or reconstruction of the limb.

- *Metastasis with life expectancy of >1–2 years*: Many malignancies, even with widespread metastases, can be suppressed or palliated such that the patient can expect to survive for a year or more. This is a rapidly developing field and expert advice from a sarcoma or oncology service is necessary. *Pathological fractures secondary to malignancy will rarely heal*, and in this situation, trauma implants may well fail before the patient dies, exposing them to further pain and the possibility of difficult salvage

**Table 7.1    Mirel's criteria**

| | Score | | |
|---|---|---|---|
| | **1** | **2** | **3** |
| Site | Upper limb | Lower limb | Peritrochanteric |
| Pain | Mild | Moderate | Functional |
| Lesion | Blastic | Mixed | Lytic |
| Size | $<\frac{1}{3}$ | $\frac{1}{3}-\frac{2}{3}$ | $>\frac{2}{3}$ |

Size refers to the circumferential cortical involvement of the lesion
Score >8 suggests prophylactic fixation

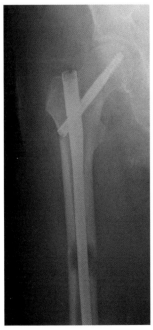

Fig. 7.10 Mid-shaft femoral metastasis in a patient with very limited life expectancy, treated with an intramedullary nail.

surgery. In this situation, excision of the tumour and replacement with an endoprosthesis are often preferred.

● *Metastasis with life expectancy of <1–2 years*: In this situation, a trauma implant is likely to outlast the patient, and palliative surgery to stabilize the fracture with minimal surgical morbidity is required. For example, long bone fractures are best nailed percutaneously (**Fig. 7.10**). The use of suction drainage or an RIA during reaming may reduce lung embolism and metastatic spread. After plating, cement augmentation, using polymethylmethacrylate cement within the lesion, will increase biomechanical strength.

● *Impending fracture*: Occasionally, the patient will present with an intact bone that has been compromised by the presence of a tumour. The likelihood of a pathological fracture is assessed according to Mirel's grading system (**Table 7.1**). Where a fracture is inevitable or even likely, prophylactic fixation or replacement is required. The choice of whether to use a trauma implant or endoprosthesis is made as above.

# Part 2

## Specific Injuries by Region

# 8 Shoulder girdle

## GENERAL PRINCIPLES

### Anatomy

The shoulder girdle consists of the clavicle, scapula and proximal humerus, and their associated ligaments and muscles (**Fig. 8.1**).

### The clavicle

The clavicle (Latin: 'small key') is an irregular S-shaped strut that holds the scapula and shoulder joint in a functional position away from the chest wall. It articulates through true synovial joints with the manubrium of the sternum medially (the sternoclavicular joint, SCJ) and the acromion of the scapula laterally (acromioclavicular joint, ACJ). It is also stabilized by the coracoclavicular (CC) ligaments, the conoid and the trapezoid, which insert into the coracoid process of the scapula.

The clavicle is remarkable in its development and maturation. Firstly, it forms by intramembranous ossification in the same way as the flat bones of the skull, in contrast to other bones, which form by endochondral ossification. Secondly, its medial physis is the last to close – at up to 25 years of age.

### The scapula

The scapula (Latin: 'shoulder') has a complex three-dimensional shape consisting of (**Fig. 8.2**):

- *Blade (or body)*: the triangular, flattened region that articulates with the thorax. The anterior (deep) surface is covered by the subscapularis muscle, one of the four rotator cuff muscles.

- *Spine*: a projection that runs horizontally across the posterior aspect of the blade, forming two fossae, which are the origins of the supraspinatus (above) and the infraspinatus and teres minor (below), the remaining three rotator cuff muscles. It terminates in the acromion.

- *Acromion* (Greek: *akros*, 'highest', and *omos*, 'shoulder'): a continuation of the scapular spine that extends to the highest and most lateral point of the shoulder. It is the site of origin of the deltoid muscle and serves to protect the glenohumeral joint and cuff muscles.

- *Coracoid process* (Greek: 'raven's beak'): an anterior protrusion that is the origin of the short head of biceps and the brachialis

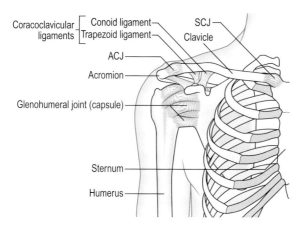

Coracoclavicular ligaments — Conoid ligament — Trapezoid ligament
ACJ
Acromion
Glenohumeral joint (capsule)
SCJ
Clavicle
Sternum
Humerus

Fig. 8.1 Anatomy of the shoulder girdle. ACJ, acromioclavicular joint; SCJ, sternoclavicular joint.

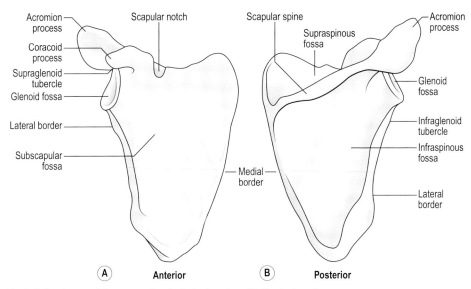

Fig. 8.2 Anatomy of the scapula. **A**, Anterior view. **B**, Posterior view.

muscles, and the insertion of the CC ligaments.

- *Glenoid* (Greek: 'socket'): a shallow, saucer-shaped projection from the lateral aspect of the scapula, deepened by a fibrocartilaginous labrum, which articulates with the humeral head. The glenoid is orientated anteriorly by around 30°.

### *The superior shoulder suspensory complex*

The superior shoulder suspensory complex (SSSC) is an osseoligamentous ring comprised of the glenoid, coracoid, acromion and distal clavicle, with their ligamentous stabilizers, the ACJ and CC ligaments (**Fig. 8.3**). It is supported on the 'struts' of the clavicle and scapular blade, and maintains the normal stable relationship between the upper limb and thorax.

### The proximal humerus

The anatomy of the proximal humerus is described on page 159.

## Clinical assessment of the painful shoulder

### History

Define the reason for presentation: has there been an acute definable injury or is this an

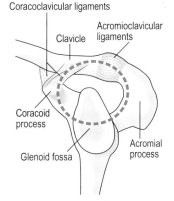

Fig. 8.3 The superior shoulder suspensory complex.

atraumatic or recurrent complaint? A high-energy mechanism of injury, such as a motor vehicle collision or fall from a height, suggests the possibility of other associated injuries and the requirement to assess and manage these first (p. 21).

A localized shoulder injury most commonly follows a simple fall on to an outstretched hand or arm, or a blow to the point of the shoulder. An injury involving excessive external rotation and abduction of the shoulder suggests an anterior shoulder dislocation (p. 146), whilst an epileptic seizure or electrocution raises the possibility of a posterior shoulder dislocation (p. 152).

Patients with an *atraumatic presentation* should be assessed for acute monoarthritis (p. 103). Features of systemic upset with fever and malaise may indicate septic arthritis. Severe atraumatic shoulder pain with no systemic upset should raise the possibility of a calcific tendonitis (p. 157) or frozen shoulder (p. 158). Enquire about previous injuries, operations or problems with the affected shoulder. The medical history is often relevant; for example, diabetes mellitus is commonly implicated in frozen shoulder.

## Examination

Pain and inability to move the shoulder normally are common in a range of shoulder pathologies and it is important to consider the possible differential diagnoses that relate to the structure of the shoulder:

- *Bone*: fracture of the proximal humerus, scapula or clavicle. There will be localized bony deformity, tenderness and crepitus, and the fracture will be evident radiographically.
- *Joint*: dislocation of the glenohumeral joint. There will be a typical squared-off appearance and an abnormal radiograph.
- *Capsule*: frozen shoulder. There will be pain and restriction in both active and passive movement.
- *Muscle*: rotator cuff tear. There will be pain and weakness with a reduction in active, but not passive, movement.

- *Nerve*: brachial plexus injury. There will be weakness and reduction in active movement, as well as abnormalities in sensation and reflexes.
- *Pain inhibition*: a diagnosis of exclusion. It can suggest septic arthritis, subacromial bursitis or calcific tendonitis.

## Look

Inspect the patient's shoulders and upper limbs from the front and back, looking in particular for:

- *Symmetry*: An asymmetrical contour suggests a significant skeletal injury, most commonly a shoulder joint dislocation. Muscle wasting around the shoulder suggests a pre-existing abnormality.
- *Bruising*: Often this is initially absent after injury but quite dramatic bruising evolves over the first 12 hours. Patients may worry unnecessarily unless they are warned about this.
- *Abrasions*: These are common after injury. Inspect carefully to ensure that the dermis is not breached, which implies an open fracture.

## Feel (Fig. 8.4)

Palpate the skeleton of the shoulder girdle systematically. Begin at the SCJ (*a* on Fig. 8.4) and work laterally along the clavicle (*b*) to the ACJ (*c*), and then around the acromion (*d*) and along the scapula spine (*e*). Then work down over the humeral head (*f*) to the shaft and then the biceps tendon (*g*). Note localized bony

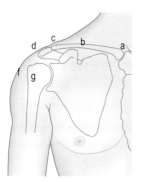
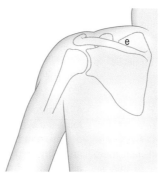

Fig. 8.4 Clinical examination of the shoulder: sequence of palpation.

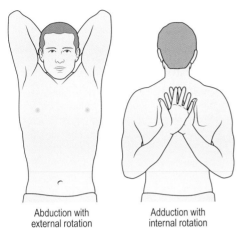

Abduction with
external rotation

Adduction with
internal rotation

Fig. 8.5 Screening movements.

tenderness and abnormalities of contour. Examine the neck and elbow.

### Move

- *Active movements* (**Fig. 8.5**): The patient initially performs *screening movements* with both arms simultaneously. Firstly, assess abduction and external rotation: holding the palms facing anteriorly, the patient takes the upper limbs through a full range of abduction, and then flexes the elbows to bring the fingertips to the interscapular region. Compare which cervical or thoracic level can be touched with each hand. If there is a restriction, note the ability to touch the mouth, ear and occiput. Now test adduction and internal rotation: the patient brings the thumbs into the interscapular region as high up the back as possible. Compare which thoracic level is reached with each hand. If there is restriction, note the ability to touch the trochanter, sacrum or lumbar level.

- *Passive movements*: Where there has been any restriction in these screening ranges of movement, carefully measure formal passive movements of each limb in turn, noting the range of abduction, external rotation and internal rotation in each shoulder. Limitation due to pain is important, but a solid block to movement suggests

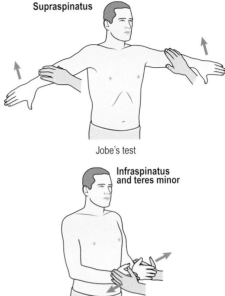

Jobe's test

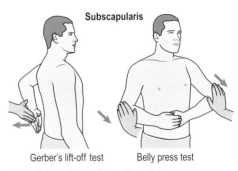

Resisted external rotation

Subscapularis

Gerber's lift-off test          Belly press test

Fig. 8.6 Rotator cuff testing. Active movements are performed by the patient (orange arrows) to test each component of the rotator cuff. These movements are resisted by the examiner.

a significant injury such as a shoulder dislocation.

- *Resisted movements* (**Fig. 8.6**): Assess power in each of the intrinsic (rotator cuff) muscles.

  - *Supraspinatus – Jobe's test*: Ask the patient to abduct the arms to 90° in the plane of the scapula (30° forwards). Now ask them to rotate the arms internally so that the thumbs are pointing to the floor. Place your hands on the patient's elbows and push down, comparing the ability to resist this force with injured and uninjured arms. Inability to adopt this position, or weakness, suggests supraspinatus pathology. Anterosuperior shoulder pain in this position, which is eased with external rotation of the arms (thumbs up), is indicative of supraspinatus tendonitis (also called subacromial bursitis: this is the 'empty can' test)

- *Infraspinatus and teres minor – resisted external rotation*: Ask the patient to tuck the elbows into the sides and hold the forearms parallel to the floor in front of them, and then to resist your attempt to push their hands together. Weakness is indicative of infraspinatus and/or teres minor pathology.

- *Subscapularis – Gerber's lift-off test or belly press test*: Gerber's lift-off test is performed by asking the patient to place the backs of their hands on to their buttocks, to lift them 10 cm posteriorly and away from the buttocks, and then to resist your attempts to push them forwards. In patients who are unable to assume this position due to pain or stiffness, the belly press test is a useful alternative. The patient places the hands over the umbilicus and pushes the elbows forwards, thus internally rotating the shoulders. Assess their ability to hold this position against resistance as you push their elbows posteriorly. Weakness in these positions is indicative of subscapularis pathology.

### Neurovascular assessment

Assess the sensory and motor supply to each of the peripheral nerve distributions of the upper limb, paying special attention to the axillary, median, radial and ulnar nerves (see Figs 3.17–19). Assess the radial pulse and capillary return to the finger nailbeds. If radiating neurology from the cervical spine is suspected, or a brachial plexopathy, testing of the

individual myotomes and dermatomes is indicated (see Fig. 3.14).

## Radiological assessment of the painful shoulder

### Radiographs

Because of the complex osteology of this region, no single radiographic projection shows either the true shape or the true position of any of the bones of the shoulder girdle. Each of the bones can also be obscured by the thorax and ribs. A number of views are described, which show, to various degrees of advantage, the greater tuberosity, the lesser tuberosity, the glenoid, the coracoid and the acromion (**Fig. 8.7**).

- *Anteroposterior (AP) view of the shoulder*: The beam is orientated in the sagittal plane. This shows the clavicle, ACJ, acromion and proximal humerus well. However, the glenoid projection is oblique.

- *True AP view of the shoulder*: The beam is orientated in the plane of the glenoid to show a true AP view of this joint. This allows better assessment of the integrity of the glenoid and congruity of the shoulder joint.

- *Axillary view*: This provides a 'top-down' view through the shoulder and gives a clear image of the humeral head and the glenoid, as well as the relationship between the two. To obtain this type of radiograph, the patient has to be able to abduct the arm to approximately 45°, which may be impracticable after an acute injury. In these circumstances, the modified axial view is an acceptable substitute.

- *Modified axial view*: The patient's arm rests in a sling. The patient leans back 30° over the cassette while the beam is directed from above.

- *Scapular Y view*: This shows the SSSC and glenoid en face, as well as the scapula blade. It is a direct lateral view of the shoulder, with the anteversion of the scapula accounted for by internally rotating the beam by 30°.

The clavicle is seen on the AP views of the shoulder but can be defined more clearly

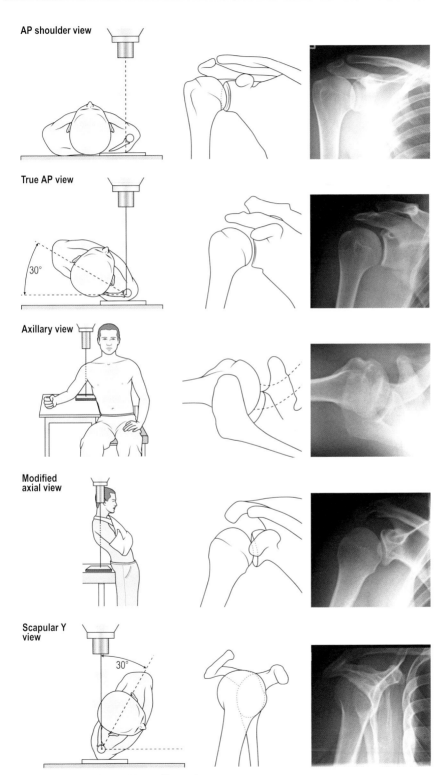

Fig. 8.7 Types of shoulder radiograph.

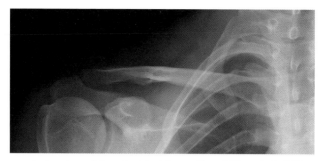

Fig. 8.8 An anteroposterior view of the clavicle taken with a 20° cephalad tilt.

by tiling the X-ray beam towards the head (**Fig. 8.8**):

- *A 20° cephalad tilt view of the clavicle*: This reduces the overlap between the clavicle, and the scapula and thoracic cage.

### Shoulder trauma series

For most presentations with shoulder pain, a standard trauma series of two radiographs is usually adequate:

- *AP shoulder* and
- Either an *axillary view* or a *modified axial*.

Depending on the circumstances and the clinical scenario, a true AP view of the glenohumeral joint or a 20° cephalad tilt view may then also be obtained. The scapula-Y view is occasionally chosen, according to local preferences.

### CT

A CT scan is often required to assess bony injuries to the shoulder girdle clearly.

### CLAVICLE

Fractures of the clavicle are common, and result either from a direct blow or, more commonly, from transmitted forces after a fall on to the shoulder. Deformity is usually clear, with shortening and depression of the lateral fragment (under the weight of the arm), and proximal displacement of the medial fragment.

## Classification

### Robinson (Edinburgh) classification

The Robinson (Edinburgh) classification defines clavicle fractures in terms of location (indicated by a number), degree of displacement (given a letter), and involvement of adjacent joints or degree of comminution of the shaft (given a number) (**Fig. 8.9**):

- Location of the fracture:
    1. medial fifth (5% of clavicle fractures)
    2. central three-fifths (80%)
    3. lateral fifth (15%)
- Degree of displacement:
    A. undisplaced
    B. displaced
- Involvement of adjacent joints and the degree of comminution present:
    1. simple/undisplaced/extra-articular
    2. comminuted/segmental/angulated/ intra-articular.

## Emergency Department management

### Clinical features

- The patient usually presents with a history of having fallen on the shoulder.
- The patient will be aware of pain, and often crepitus, at the fracture site, and will usually present supporting the elbow with the other hand.
- There may be a clear deformity of the clavicle (**Fig. 8.10A**). Assess whether the skin overlying a spike of bone has been tented and is at risk of breaking down. Skin that is puckered or hitched on to the spike is at particular risk. If there is tenting, gently move the skin over the fracture site; if it is

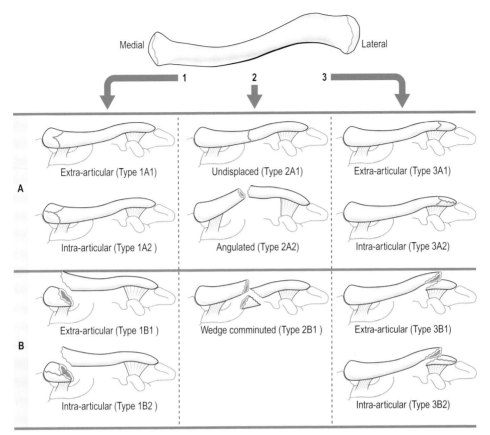

Fig. 8.9 The Robinson (Edinburgh) classification of clavicle fractures.

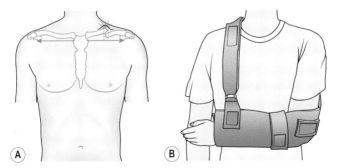

Fig. 8.10 Clavicle fracture. **A**, The shortening of the fracture results in an asymmetrical appearance and tenting. **B**, A poly sling provided to support the elbow.

mobile, the skin is less likely to become compromised.

- Compare injured and uninjured sides. Shortening is indicated by a reduced distance between the SCJ and the ACJ on the injured side (**Fig. 8.10A**).

- Identify clear localized tenderness and deformity at the fracture. Exclude any other bony tenderness of the SCJ, ACJ, scapula or proximal humerus.

- The patient will be unwilling to move the shoulder, but check that there is active shoulder abduction to at least 45° (excludes a major rotator cuff tear).

- Exclude injury to the joints above (SCJ and cervical spine) and below (shoulder and elbow).

## Radiological features
- AP clavicle
- 20° cephalad view (**Fig. 8.11**).

Note the location of the fracture and whether there is comminution or a large butterfly fragment.

## Closed reduction
Attempts at closed reduction of the fracture are not recommended, as the position will not be maintained and there is a danger of damaging adjacent neurovascular structures. Similarly, there is no advantage in applying a figure-of-eight bandage or other forms of strapping around the shoulders.

## Immobilization and reassessment
Provide a sling that will give support to the elbow (Fig. 4.21 and **Fig. 8.10B**). No formal immobilization is required. Repeat the assessment of neurovascular status after sling application.

## Inpatient referral
- Significant tenting.
- Skin compromise.
- Neurovascular compromise.

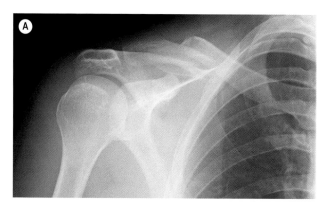

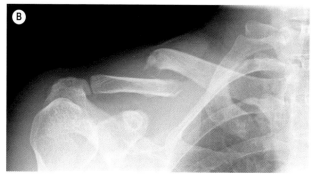

Fig. 8.11 A 2B1 clavicle fracture. **A**, A standard AP view of the clavicle. **B**, 20° cephalad tilt view.

## Outpatient follow-up

- All clavicle fractures should be referred to the fracture clinic.

## Patient instructions

- The sling is only to provide comfort and the patient is encouraged to use the elbow, wrist and hand on the affected side.
- Patients may find sleeping on their back with extra pillows more comfortable.
- Sleeping with a T-shirt worn over the sling helps to minimize movement.

# Orthopaedic management

The indications for surgery remain contentious. The majority of midshaft clavicular fractures (Robinson type 2) will heal rapidly with conservative treatment. Medial fractures (Robinson type 1) are discussed with SCJ injuries (p. 142). Displaced lateral end clavicle fractures (Robinson 3B) have a higher rate of non-union and are discussed in conjunction with ACJ injuries (p. 139). Only a minority of patients (<10%) will experience problems that would justify intervention:

- *Symptomatic non-union*: This typically affects those with highly comminuted shaft fractures, as well as smokers and the elderly.
- *Symptomatic malunion*: This occurs where there is a prominent bone spike (which is particularly troublesome in patients who wear rucksacks regularly: e.g. soldiers). In these patients, a simple excision of the spike is adequate. A less well understood issue is that of 'shoulder ptosis'. Where there is significant clavicular shortening, the scapula will sag forwards and the plane of the glenoid will angle anteriorly. Some patients experience a shoulder girdle ache subsequently. Assessing shortening is difficult; plain radiographs are notoriously imprecise and clinical measurement (by comparison of the distance between the SCJ and ACJ on injured and uninjured sides) is often most accurate. Advocates of early clavicle surgery cite avoidance of this 'ptosis ache' (as well as the avoidance of non-union) as the rationale for operating.
- *Cosmetic appearance*: Some patients are distressed by the appearance of a bone spike or a shoulder ptosis, although this alone should not be an indication for surgery.

## Complications of surgery

The complications of surgery are principally related to the thin soft-tissue coverage of the clavicle and include infection, wound dehiscence, prominent metalwork and division of the supraclavicular nerves, with a resulting area of numbness distal to the incision. In addition, the subclavian artery and vein, the brachial plexus and the apex of the lung are very close to the underside of the clavicle, and major complications can occur during drilling or screw placement.

## Indications for surgery

The indications for surgery represent a weighing up of the relative risks of experiencing a problem against the likelihood of complications. Ten ORIFs are required to avoid one symptomatic non-union. There is little current consensus.

Indications for surgery include:

- open fractures
- impending skin breakdown/tenting
- severe shortening
- severe comminution
- symptomatic non-union (late)

## Surgical techniques

An open reduction with plate fixation remains the most commonly performed procedure (**Fig. 8.12**). A superior plate position is technically easiest, whereas anterior plating allows positioning of the metalwork in a less vulnerable position under the skin. Intramedullary nailing is also described. Because of the serpentine shape of the clavicle, titanium elastic nails and various articulating devices have been used.

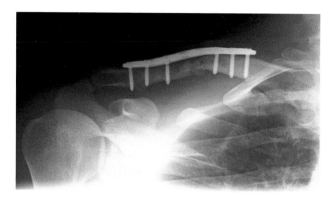

Fig. 8.12 Clavicle plating.

## SURGICAL TECHNIQUE: Clavicular plating

### Surgical set-up

Patient positioning is most commonly supine on a radiolucent table, with a bolster between the scapulae to aid the regaining of clavicular length. The upper limb is draped free. A beach-chair position may be preferred, as it allows the weight of the upper limb to be used as traction.

### Incision

A 12-cm oblique incision is made. Placing this directly over the clavicle makes access easy but may cause an uncomfortable scar and increases the risk of infection if there is dehiscence. Placement of the incision 2 cm anterior to the leading edge of the clavicle may be preferred. Alternatively, a more oblique incision parallel to Langer's lines may improve scar appearance and comfort. Infiltration of the skin with local anaesthetic and adrenaline (epinephrine) prior to making the incision can reduce haemorrhage.

### Approach

The skin is incised and elevated. The clavicle is palpated carefully beneath the platysma muscle. Incise the platysma and its overlying fascia with diathermy directly on to the clavicle. The subclavian artery and vein, and the brachial plexus, are directly deep to bone and extreme caution is required when dissecting around or drilling through the clavicle.

### Open reduction

The fracture ends are identified, cleared and reduced, then temporarily stabilized with wires and reduction clamps.

### Internal fixation – absolute stability

Lag screw compression is used wherever possible. If there is a large butterfly fragment, additional lag screws can be used. Smaller 2.7-mm screws may be useful for smaller fragments. A contoured, low-profile plate is applied. Take special care not to 'plunge' the drill after breaching the far cortex.

### Postoperative restrictions

Movement: Shoulder movement is restricted to pendular exercises for 6 weeks. Instruct the patient to allow the shoulder to hang down freely whilst leaning forwards, and let the shoulder move gently backwards and forwards in the manner of a pendulum. Full active movement at the elbow is encouraged.

Weight-bearing: Patients are allowed to use their hand for feeding themselves but instructed not to lift anything heavier than a glass of water until union.

## Outpatient management

Non-operatively treated patients can be encouraged to mobilize their shoulder as soon as comfortable without restrictions, whereas operatively treated patients will need to observe surgical restrictions for 6 weeks.

| Outpatient management summary | | | |
|---|---|---|---|
| Week | Examination | Radiographs | Additional notes |
| 1 | (Operatively treated fractures) Wound check Neurovascular status | AP clavicle | Commence pendular exercises |
| 8 | | AP clavicle | If clinical and radiographic union, then discharge to physiotherapy |

Further assessments at 4-week intervals if required for delayed union

Average time to union = 6–8 weeks

## COMPLICATIONS

### Early

Local    Wound complications: There is poor soft tissue coverage of clavicle plates and the wound is prone to dehiscence and infection

Numbness: Division of, or injury to, the supraclavicular nerves usually leaves an area of numbness over the anterior chest

### Late

Local    Non-union: This occurs in 10% of conservatively managed clavicle fractures. If there is ongoing pain, surgery is indicated

Malunion: Patients with a prominent bony spike may elect to have this excised. The indications for surgery of a shortened clavicle remain unclear

The most common concerns after surgery relate to wound complications (see Box). The most common complications of non-operative treatment are non-union or malunion, and corrective surgery may be required to achieve an acceptable reduction and union.

## ACROMIOCLAVICULAR JOINT

ACJ dislocations, and very distal fractures in the lateral fifth of the clavicle, typically follow a blow to the outer aspect of the shoulder. The injury is defined by the extent of involvement of the ligaments surrounding the ACJ and the coracoclavicular (conoid and trapezoid) ligaments.

## Classification

### Rockwood classification

The Rockwood classification describes six grades of injury (**Fig. 8.13**):

I.  Sprain of the ACJ without displacement. Radiographs are normal.

II. Rupture of the ACJ ligaments but the coracoclavicular (CC) ligaments remain intact. The displacement is less than the width of the clavicle.

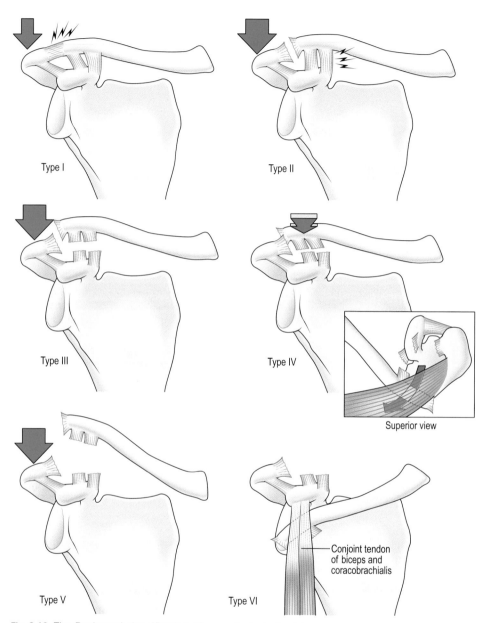

Type I

Type II

Type III

Type IV

Superior view

Type V

Type VI

Conjoint tendon
of biceps and
coracobrachialis

Fig. 8.13 The Rockwood classification of acromioclavicular injury.

III. Rupture of both the ACJ and CC ligaments. The resulting displacement is more than the width of the clavicle.

IV. Rupture of the ACJ and CC ligaments with displacement of the clavicle posteriorly through trapezius.

V. Rupture of the ACJ and CC ligaments with gross displacement of the ACJ and detachment of deltoid and trapezius.

VI. Subcoracoid displacement of the clavicle.

## Emergency Department management

### Clinical features

- There is usually a prominence of the outer end of the clavicle and a sag to the shoulder girdle.

- There is localized tenderness to palpation over the ACJ and the prominence can be partially reduced with firm pressure.

- Confirm active abduction to 45° (to exclude a massive cuff tear) and examine the neck and elbow.

### Radiological features

- *AP clavicle 20° cephalad view*: This view allows adequate assessment of the ACJ. Follow the inferior cortex of the clavicle to ensure it is in line with the inferior aspect of the acromion. If this relationship is lost, the ACJ has been injured.

- *Axillary view*: This view will confirm whether there has been a posterior displacement of the lateral clavicle (Rockwood type IV).

- *Weight-bearing stress films*: These may increase the degree of deformity but do not usually change management and are not, therefore, routinely indicated.

### Closed reduction

Closed reduction is not effective and is not indicated.

### Immobilization and reassessment

Provide a sling to give elbow support (Fig. 4.21).

### Inpatient referral

This is rarely required but is considered if there is:

- neurovascular dysfunction
- skin compromise
- Rockwood grade V–VI.

### Outpatient follow-up

- Grade I ACJ disruptions do not routinely require follow-up.

- Grade II–III ACJ disruptions should be referred to the fracture clinic.

## Orthopaedic management

### Non-operative

- *Type I and II injuries*: These invariably heal without surgical intervention and usually with excellent functional results. A small proportion of patients later develop symptomatic ACJ arthritis or instability, and eventually require late lateral clavicle resection and/ or stabilization (Weaver–Dunn procedure).

- *Type III injuries*: These remain controversial. Late symptomatic instability and pain are more common than with types I and II, but there is little evidence that surgical intervention improves functional outcome.

### Operative

- *Type IV, V and VI injuries*: These are extremely rare and are treated by surgical reduction and stabilization.

### Surgical techniques

Several successful techniques are recognized for stabilizing injuries at the lateral end of the clavicle, and are effective for both ACJ injuries and intra-articular fractures of the lateral clavicle. These all involve fixation of the clavicle to either the acromion or the coracoid. In contrast, direct transfixion across the ACJ with k-wires has led to life-threatening migration of broken wire fragments into the great vessels and must be avoided.

#### *Acromion fixation*

The traditional fixation device is the hook plate, which engages with the underside of the acromion (**Fig. 8.14**). It is extremely robust but

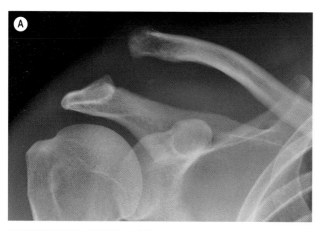

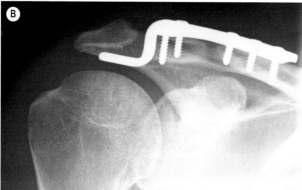

Fig. 8.14 Acromioclavicular joint stabilization. **A**, A Rockwood grade V injury. **B**, Fixation with a hook plate.

has a high rate of rotator cuff irritation, and usually requires removal after healing.

### Coracoid fixation

Robust fixation can also be obtained into the coracoid. The use of a single screw (Bosworth technique) has largely been supplanted by the use of tapes and sutures or, more recently, suture button devices.

## Outpatient management

The majority of patients are assessed for other injuries to the shoulder, and are then discharged with reassurance and instructions regarding active mobilization. Surgically treated patients will usually have restrictions on activity for up to 8 weeks.

## STERNOCLAVICULAR JOINT

Injuries to the sternoclavicular joint are rare, and follow a direct blow to the outer aspect of the shoulder. The injury may be a dislocation of the joint or, under the age of 25, may be a transphyseal fracture, usually Salter–Harris type 2 (Fig. 23.3).

## Classification

- *Anterior displacement*: This results in a prominent, swollen region at the SCJ.
- *Posterior displacement*: This is potentially more hazardous, as pressure from the dislocated medial end of the clavicle may result in dyspnoea or dysphagia.

# Emergency Department management

## Clinical features

- Ask about dyspnoea and dysphagia.

- There may be a prominent, swollen region at the SCJ. Some venous engorgement in the neck or respiratory distress may also be present.

## Radiological features

It is notoriously difficult to obtain adequate plain radiographs of the SCJ, and a CT or MRI scan is often required.

## Closed reduction

Closed reduction is most appropriately performed in the operating theatre.

## Immobilization

Provide a collar-and-cuff for patients with anterior SCJ disruptions.

## Outpatient follow-up

- Sprains of the SCJ are commonly referred to the fracture clinic.

## Inpatient referral

- All posterior dislocations should be discussed with an orthopaedic surgeon.

- If there is any suggestion of obstruction at the root of the neck, consult urgently with a senior colleague.

# Orthopaedic management

## Non-operative

*Anterior SCJ dislocations* require no acute intervention and are managed with reassurance, advice, a collar-and-cuff and rapid, active mobilization.

## Operative

*Posterior dislocations* may require operative reduction and stabilization. The proximity of the great vessels makes surgery in this region potentially hazardous, and an experienced senior surgeon, possibly assisted or supported by a cardiothoracic surgeon, is required.

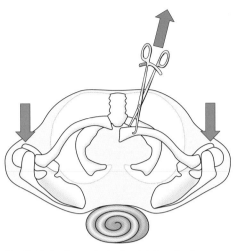

Fig. 8.15 A sternoclavicular joint reduction manoeuvre.

Closed reduction under anaesthesia may be possible by placing a bolster between the scapulae and retracting the shoulder (**Fig. 8.15**). A pair of reduction forceps applied to the clavicle through stab incisions will assist with manoeuvring the medial end anteriorly. If successful, the reduction is usually stable and no further treatment is required. If closed reduction is unsuccessful, an open reduction will be required. The medial end of the clavicle is then most conveniently stabilized with transosseous sutures or with a tendon allograft repair. Wires must be avoided, as there is a tendency to fragmentation and migration. Careful reassessment after reduction is required to exclude complications.

## COMPLICATIONS

### *Early*

| Local | Arterial compression |
|---|---|
| | Venous compression or laceration |
| | Oesophageal injury |
| | Pneumothorax |
| | Tracheal/laryngeal oedema |

## SCAPULA

Fractures of the scapula are rare, accounting for <1% of all fractures, but are none the less important, as more than half are associated with other injuries, including fractures to the clavicle or ribs, a pneumothorax, pulmonary contusion or neurovascular injury. Most fractures of the scapular blade, spine or acromion are managed conservatively. Surgery may have a role in displaced fractures of the *glenoid* and glenoid neck but clear indications have not yet been defined.

###  Key point

Scapula fractures are suggestive of high-energy trauma. Have a high index of suspicion for other shoulder girdle fractures or associated injuries to the thorax, including ribs, lungs, great vessels and brachial plexus.

## Classification

### Ideberg classification

The Ideberg classification of glenoid fractures recognizes six types (**Fig. 8.16**):

I. avulsion fracture of the anterior margin of the glenoid

II:

IIA. transverse fracture through the glenoid fossa exiting inferiorly

IIB. oblique fracture through the glenoid fossa exiting inferiorly

III. oblique fracture through the glenoid exiting superiorly, often associated with an ACJ injury

IV. transverse fracture exiting through the medial border of the scapula

V. combination of a type II and type IV pattern

VI. severe comminution of glenoid surface.

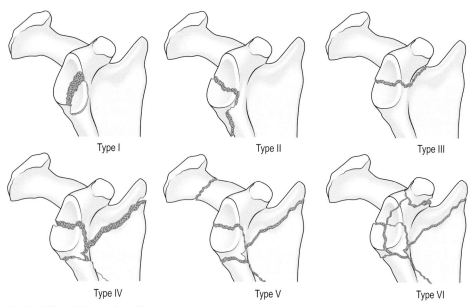

Fig. 8.16 The Ideberg classification of glenoid fractures.

## Emergency Department management

### Clinical features

- There is usually a history of a high-energy injury. If so, assess the patient with a full primary and secondary survey (see Chapter 2).

- Ask about other sites of pain and be aware of a high incidence of intrathoracic pathology.

- The patient will present supporting the injured limb. There is usually little to see, although there may be swelling in the region of the scapula body.

- There is often little to feel other than swelling; the muscle and fascia around the scapula act as a very effective splint.

### Radiological features

- *AP chest radiograph*: This is important to assess for other thoracic and shoulder girdle injuries. Many scapular fractures are recognized on this film initially.

- *Trauma series of the shoulder*: This will reveal the scapular fracture but it is often difficult to define it fully on plain films alone.

- *CT scan*: This can be invaluable for understanding the fracture, a three-dimensional reconstruction being particularly helpful in defining extra-articular or intra-articular components.

### Closed reduction

A closed reduction is not indicated.

### Inpatient referral

- Glenoid or scapular neck fractures.

- Exclusion or management of associated injuries.

### Outpatient follow-up

- Patients with fractures that affect the scapular blade only are provided with a sling or collar-and-cuff for comfort and are referred to the fracture clinic.

## Orthopaedic management

### Operative

Indications for surgery remain controversial, as functional recovery after scapula fracture is usually good. However, proposed indications include:

- Scapular neck fractures resulting in severe displacement of the glenoid.

- Type I glenoid fractures involving >25% of the glenoid rim, to prevent recurrent anterior instability.

- Type II glenoid fractures in which there is humeral head subluxation.

- Incongruity of the glenoid associated with fracture types III–VI.

- 'Floating shoulder' injuries: those that involve two or more components of the SSSC (see Fig. 8.3). The most common combination is a scapular neck fracture with a clavicle shaft fracture. Isolated fixation of the clavicle may be sufficient to realign and stabilize the scapular component of the injury.

- Isolated acromial fractures that cause subacromial impingement.

### Surgical approach

Exposure of the scapula neck and body is usually via the *posterior approach* to the shoulder. Surgery is performed in the lateral or prone position. The incision is along the spine of the scapula and allows the deltoid to be detached from the scapular spine. The internervous approach lies between infraspinatus (suprascapular nerve) and teres minor (axillary nerve); separating these muscles exposes the neck of the scapula and posterior capsule of the shoulder joint.

The *anterior approach* to the shoulder allows access to the anterior aspect of the glenoid and is described on page 138.

## SCAPULOTHORACIC DISSOCIATION

Scapulothoracic dissociation is a rare but very severe upper limb injury, which inevitably follows a high-energy, uncontrolled distraction force. It is effectively a closed fore-quarter amputation with dissociation of the shoulder girdle from the thoracic cage, usually complicated by severe injury to the brachial plexus and axillary artery. There may be associated fractures of the shoulder girdle.

## Emergency Department management

### Clinical features

- There is usually a history of a high-energy injury. Ask about other sites of pain and carry out a full primary and secondary survey.
- There will be marked swelling in the region of the shoulder.
- Complete vascular occlusion will result in the 'six Ps' (see Box 3.1).
- The patient will be unable to move the injured shoulder.
- Careful assessment of the brachial plexus and limb vascularity is required.

### Radiological features

- *Chest radiograph*: Lateral displacement of the scapula on the injured side when compared to the uninjured side on chest radiograph is pathognomonic.
- *Shoulder trauma series*.
- *Vascular investigations*, such as CT angiography: These may be required.
- *MRI*: This is helpful for assessing the brachial plexus and nerve roots.

### Immobilization

Apply a sling to support the injured limb, and provide opiate analgesia.

### Inpatient referral

All scapulothoracic dissociations require urgent orthopaedic review. There is no specific Emergency Department reduction or treatment.

## Orthopaedic management

Emergency surgical exploration and repair of any vascular injury may be required. Major fractures should be stabilized at the same time. The planned reconstruction of the brachial plexus injury is complex and will depend on the

nature, level and severity of the injury. Appropriate options include exploration, grafting, nerve transfers, tendon transfers, joint fusions and, not infrequently, amputation.

| COMPLICATIONS | | |
|---|---|---|
| ***Early*** | | |
| Local | | Neurovascular injury: 90% of patients have an associated plexus or vascular injury |
| ***Late*** | | |
| Local | | Flail limb: occurs in 50% |
| | | Amputation: performed acutely in 20% |
| General | | Death: 10% of patients die of associated injuries |

## ANTERIOR SHOULDER (GLENOHUMERAL) DISLOCATION

Shoulder dislocations are a common presentation to the Emergency Department and comprise up to half of all joint dislocations.

*Anterior dislocation* is the most common (90%) and typically occurs in 'at risk' populations, (particularly young men), engaged in 'at risk' pursuits (including contact sports, skiing and cycling) in which the shoulder is placed in the 'at risk' position of abduction and external rotation, and then pushed further beyond its stable range (**Fig. 8.17**). However, 50% of anterior dislocations occur in the elderly and are associated with rotator cuff tears.

## Anatomy of shoulder stability

The congruity of the glenohumeral joint is maintained by both static and dynamic stabilizers (**Fig. 8.18**):

### Static stabilizers

- *Bone shape (**a** on Fig. 8.18)*: The glenoid provides a shallow concave surface for the humeral head to articulate. This provides far

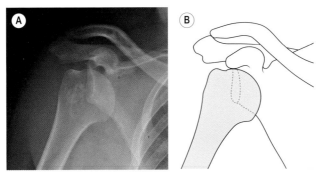

Fig. 8.17 Anterior dislocation of the shoulder. **A**, AP radiograph. **B**, The humeral head lies anterior to the glenoid and inferior to the coracoid.

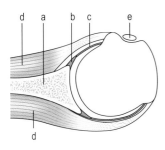
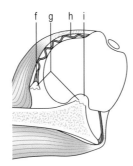

Fig. 8.18 Pathoanatomy of shoulder dislocation.

less stability than the acetabulum of the hip, as the glenoid socket is shallow and shaped like a saucer.

- *Labrum* (**b**): This fibrocartilaginous rim markedly increases the glenoid depth.

- *Joint capsule* (**c**): The anterior capsule acts as a restraint at terminal external rotation.

- *Capsular ligaments*: These thickenings of the joint capsule have been identified as the superior, middle and inferior glenohumeral ligaments.

- *Vacuum effect*: This is produced by the intact closed joint.

### Dynamic stabilizers

- *Rotator cuff muscles* (**d**): The supraspinatus, infraspinatus, teres minor and subscapularis form a cuff of muscle that encloses the glenohumeral joint. Contraction of these muscles results in 'concavity compression', which maintains shoulder congruence and stability throughout movement.

- *Long head of biceps brachii* (**e**): The long head of biceps arises from the superior glenoid rim within the shoulder joint. It then travels over the anterosuperior aspect of the humeral head before passing though the bicipital groove between the greater and lesser tuberosities. Its position above and anterior to the humeral head acts to resist anterior dislocation.

## Pathoanatomy of shoulder instability

Dislocation results in a combination of one or more injures to the structures of the shoulder (see Fig. 8.18):

- *Labrum* (**f**): A Bankart lesion is an avulsion of part of the anterior labrum.

- *Glenoid* (**g**):
  - A bony Bankart lesion is a glenoid rim avulsion fracture, bearing the anterior labrum.

- In recurrent dislocation there is often progressive glenoid bone loss as the humeral head passes over the glenoid rim.
- *Joint capsule* (**h**):
  - There may be stretching of the anterior capsule.
  - Avulsion of the joint capsule from the glenoid rim, or occasionally the humerus, may occur.
- *Humeral head* (**i**): A Hill–Sachs lesion is an impaction fracture of the posterior humeral head as it is compressed against the anterior glenoid after dislocation. This occurs acutely in 25% of shoulder dislocations but is seen in 75% of recurrent dislocations where an 'engaging' Hill–Sachs lesion increases the likelihood of further dislocation.
- *Rotator cuff*: Tears of the rotator cuff tendons occur in 40% of patients over 40 years of age and 60% of patients over 60 years.
- *Brachial plexus*: This most commonly manifests as an axillary nerve palsy. Motor testing is limited initially by pain but sensory deficit is demonstrated in 50% of dislocations. Electromyography (EMG) studies show that some degree of axillary nerve injury is virtually ubiquitous.

## Emergency Department management

### Clinical features

- Ask about the mechanism of injury; this will typically be external rotation in a position of shoulder abduction. For a first-time dislocation there will usually have been a high-energy mechanism related to sport or a fall.
- Previous episodes of instability increase the likelihood and ease of dislocation. Patients with regular 'habitual' dislocations can often sublux and reduce their shoulders at will.
- A patient with an acute traumatic shoulder dislocation will be in clear pain with

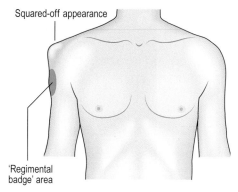

Fig. 8.19 Clinical appearance of anterior shoulder dislocation.

muscular spasm and will present supporting the shoulder.
- The shoulder has a typical 'squared-off' appearance, with prominence of the acromion but without the usual rounded contour of the humeral head beneath it (**Fig. 8.19**).
- Where the appearance is not conclusive (e.g. in the obese patient), palpate the two sides simultaneously. There will be a clear asymmetry between the two shoulders, with loss of the usual convexity under the acromion on the affected side, and a sense of fullness anteriorly.
- Perform a careful neurovascular assessment. An axillary nerve palsy results in numbness in the 'regimental badge' area (Fig. 8.19).

### Radiological features

- *Shoulder trauma series*: This may be too uncomfortable for the patient and so will not be practicable; a plain AP view may demonstrate the diagnosis sufficiently to allow a closed reduction to be performed, with the remaining radiographs being obtained later. Care should be taken to assess for an undisplaced humeral neck fracture or an associated fracture of the greater tuberosity (**Fig. 8.20**). A fracture dislocation (dislocated head with a humeral neck fracture) can also occur and requires surgical management.

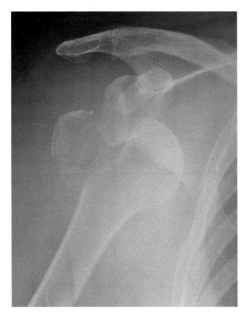

Fig. 8.20 Anterior shoulder dislocation with greater tuberosity fracture.

## Closed reduction

Closed reduction in the Emergency Department is indicated in shoulder dislocations with no humeral neck fracture, with or without an isolated tuberosity fracture. Dislocations with a humeral neck fracture are not amenable to closed reduction in the Emergency Department. Closed reduction is most effective and comfortable the earlier it is performed after dislocation. Procedural sedation is often required. Several successful methods have been reported (and re-reported with variations) but none has shown convincing superiority over another.

## ✓ Key point

Closed reduction of anterior shoulder dislocation does not require the application of huge force. Slow, controlled movements that allow the musculature to relax will result in successful reduction. Excessive force can lead to fractures of the humerus (particularly in the elderly) or to brachial plexus injuries.

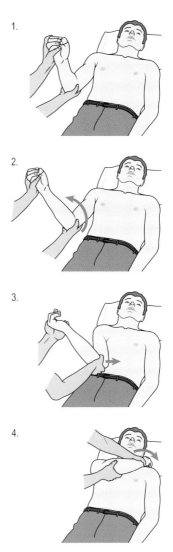

Fig. 8.21 Kocher's technique for closed reduction of an anterior shoulder dislocation.

### Kocher's technique (Fig. 8.21)

Illustrations of this technique are evident in Egyptian hieroglyphics; it is over 3,000 years old. Patients lie supine on the couch with the clinician standing by their side. In the example of a right shoulder dislocation:

1. *Hand position*: The clinician takes the patient's elbow in the right hand and the wrist in the left.

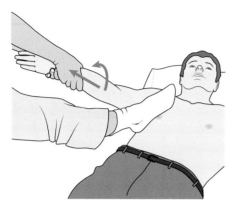

Fig. 8.22 The Hippocratic method for closed reduction of anterior shoulder dislocation.

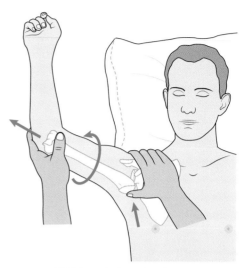

2. *External rotation*: Without applying traction, the humerus is externally rotated slowly and gently until resistance is reached. The arm can usually be rotated to 70–90°.

Fig. 8.23 Milch's technique for closed reduction of anterior shoulder dislocation.

3. *Lifting and adduction across chest*: Maintaining the external rotation, the humerus is then lifted forwards to the front of the chest.

4. *Internal rotation*: Finally, the shoulder is rotated internally to bring the hand to the opposite shoulder.

Relocation can occur during any point of the described manœuvre.

### Hippocratic method (Fig. 8.22)

Hippocrates, the father of medicine, described this classic technique. The patient is placed supine. A stockinged foot is placed in the patient's axilla, resting between the chest wall and the humeral head. The wrist is grasped in both hands, with gentle traction and external rotation applied to the arm. Traction is maintained for several minutes to allow muscle relaxation. The surgeon's foot then acts as a fulcrum as the arm is adducted, allowing the humeral head to be levered laterally, back into the joint. The foot must not be used to apply forceful counter-pressure against the ribs or into the axilla.

### Milch's technique (Fig. 8.23)

This technique was first described by Sir Astley Cooper. The patient is placed supine. For a right

shoulder dislocation, the surgeon places his or her right hand over the dislocated humeral head at the axilla. The patient's wrist is then grasped firmly with the other hand or by an assistant, and the arm slowly and gradually abducted fully. Once it is above the patient's head, gentle external rotation and traction are applied to the wrist, whilst lateral pressure is simultaneously applied to the head of the humerus.

### Stimpson's technique (Fig. 8.24)

Following the administration of effective analgesia, the patient is placed prone, with the arm hanging vertically down over the edge of the couch, and a 4-kg weight is tied to the wrist. With muscle relaxation, the shoulder spontaneously reduces after 10–15 minutes.

### Immobilization and reassessment

The patient is provided with a sling or collar-and-cuff for comfort. Shoulder immobilizers with chest or waist straps may provide additional support and comfort. A careful reassessment is then mandatory:

- *Repeat radiographs*.
- *Rotator cuff*: Full testing of the cuff muscles may be limited by discomfort. However, a

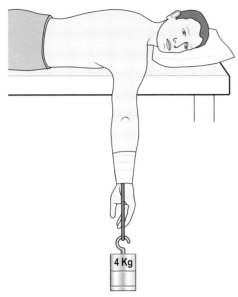

Fig. 8.24 Stimpson's technique for closed reduction of anterior shoulder dislocation.

massive tear should be excluded by asking the patient to demonstrate adduction to 45°.

- *Neurovascular assessment*: Document a full repeat neurovascular assessment; symptoms of paraesthesia may improve quickly. A new deficit raises the possibility of iatrogenic injury and warrants urgent senior review. A patient with a significant brachial plexus palsy should be referred to the regional brachial plexus service.

### Inpatient referral
- Patients with a neurological deficit should be discussed with the orthopaedic service.
- Surgery is rarely required urgently but may be indicated in the case of:
  - irreducible acute dislocation
  - fracture dislocation.

### Outpatient follow-up
All shoulder dislocations require orthopaedic follow-up to allow full assessment of the cuff, further neurovascular examination, and discussion about surgical intervention.

### Patient instructions
- Rest, interspersed with gentle pendular exercises, is indicated for 2 weeks.
- Active movements of the elbow, wrist and hand should begin immediately.
- An active range of shoulder movement is commenced under physiotherapy supervision, with gradual progression to resisted rotator cuff exercises.

## Orthopaedic management
### Non-operative
The majority of first-time dislocations are managed non-operatively with early active movement and physiotherapy.

### Operative
*Urgent surgery*
Surgery is rarely required urgently but is indicated where the shoulder remains dislocated and there is neurovascular compromise.

*Planned surgery*
Surgery may be required within a few days for:

- *Irreducible dislocations or fracture dislocations without neurological compromise*: Careful monitoring is required and urgent intervention may be necessary if the clinical condition deteriorates.

- *Displaced greater tuberosity fractures*: Most fractures of the greater tuberosity will reduce when the humeral head is relocated. If the fracture remains displaced, the supraspinatus will remain defunctioned and open reduction and internal fixation should be considered.

- *Acute rotator cuff tears*: Patients who fail to demonstrate normal rotator cuff function should be investigated with ultrasound or MRI. An acute cuff tear in a young patient is an indication for acute repair.

- *Acute prophylactic stabilization*: This is occasionally recommended after a first dislocation in an individual with a high chance of re-dislocation. Risk factors are age <35 years and an intention to return to contact sport. More commonly, surgery is

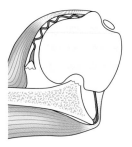
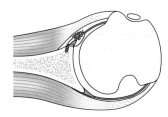

Fig. 8.25 Surgical stabilization of an anterior shoulder dislocation.

recommended as an *elective procedure for recurrent instability* after two or three dislocations. Surgery is dictated by the extent of glenoid bone loss:

*<25% glenoid erosion*: Instability can be addressed by soft tissue reconstruction only. This is commonly performed arthroscopically. The Bankart lesion is reduced back to the glenoid rim and secured with a line of suture anchors. An anterior capsular advancement and plication addresses capsular stretching (**Fig. 8.25**).

*>25% glenoid erosion*: Instability is not amenable to soft tissue reconstruction alone. A bony glenoid augmentation is required. The Bristow–Latarjet procedure uses the tip of the coracoid process, which is detached and then fixed with screws on to the antero-inferior glenoid rim. This functions by deepening the glenoid rim and allowing the coracobrachialis muscle to act as a dynamic sling around the humeral head.

*Late presentation*

After around 3 weeks, closed reduction of a dislocation may prove impossible, and open reduction and stabilization are required. In the very elderly and frail, a late dislocation may be accepted and left untreated if there is no pain, and if the loss of shoulder movement is not causing any significant functional restriction.

## POSTERIOR SHOULDER DISLOCATION

Posterior dislocations account for less than 10% of shoulder dislocations (**Fig. 8.26**). Half

of these occur as a result of abnormal unopposed muscular forces, typically during an epileptic fit or electrocution, and half follow a direct, posteriorly directed blow to the shoulder or arm.

## Emergency Department management

### Clinical features

- Enquire about a fit and any other injuries (e.g. to the tongue) that may have arisen.
- If there is a history of electrocution, there is an additional concern regarding cardiac dysrhythmia, burns, internal muscle injury and compartment syndrome.
- There is usually a less dramatic deformity than with an anterior dislocation.
- The limb may be quite comfortable in the sling position of adduction and internal rotation.
- Importantly, the patient will not be able to demonstrate any external rotation.

### Radiological features

- *AP view of the shoulder*: The 'light bulb sign' indicates full internal rotation of the humeral head with loss of the normal contour of the greater tuberosity, which is projected over the humeral head. There is loss of the usual congruence of the glenohumeral joint.
- *Modified axial view* (**Fig. 8.27**): This is obligatory and usually diagnostic, showing the displaced humeral head, and often a reverse Hill–Sachs impaction fracture of the anterior humeral head.
- *CT*: This should be obtained if there is any remaining doubt.

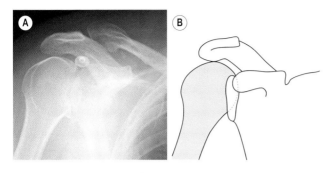

Fig. 8.26 Posterior dislocation of the shoulder. **A**, AP radiograph; note the 'light-bulb sign' of an abnormal contour of the humerus. **B**, The humeral head lies behind the glenoid.

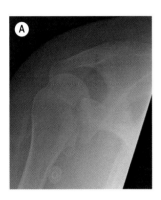
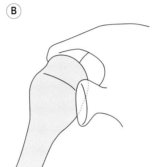

Fig. 8.27 Posterior dislocation of the shoulder. **A**, Modified axial radiograph (same patient as in 8.26). Note the impaction fracture of the anterior humeral head. **B**, This view demonstrates the dislocated position of the humeral head behind the glenoid far more clearly than the AP view.

##  Key point

Posterior shoulder dislocation is one of the most commonly missed diagnoses in the Emergency Department, with very significant functional consequences for the patient. The crucial features are:

- loss of external rotation on clinical examination
- posterior displacement on the axillary or modified axial view; the dislocation cannot be excluded on the basis of the AP radiograph alone.

## Closed reduction (Fig. 8.28)

Procedural sedation is required, although a formal general anaesthetic with muscle relaxation may be necessary. This can be a difficult manœuvre. The patient is supine with the arm held by the side.

1. Traction is applied to the arm with some internal rotation.

2. The shoulder is flexed and adducted, while further internal rotation is added.

3. Direct pressure to the humeral head from behind can facilitate reduction.

4. Once it is unlocked, the humerus is externally rotated gently. Do not attempt a forceful external rotation if the shoulder remains locked.

### Immobilization and reassessment

The patient is provided with a sling or collar-and-cuff for comfort. If there is a large engaging reverse Hill–Sachs lesion (impaction of the anterior humeral head), the arm can be splinted in neutral to prevent internal rotation, but this is not usually successful in the long term and, if there is recurrent instability, the patient will require surgical stabilization. A careful reassessment after reduction is mandatory and is identical to the steps listed for anterior dislocation above.

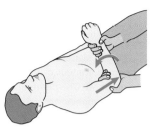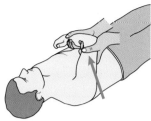

Fig. 8.28 Reduction of a posterior shoulder dislocation.

1 Traction and internal rotation

2 Flexion and adduction

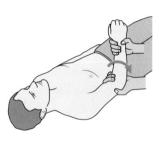

3 Direct posterior pressure

4 External rotation

## Inpatient referral

- Neurovascular compromise mandates inpatient referral.
- Surgery is rarely required urgently but may be indicated in the case of:

  irreducible acute dislocation

  fracture dislocation.

## Outpatient follow-up

All shoulder dislocations require orthopaedic follow-up to allow full assessment of the cuff, further neurovascular examination, and discussion about surgical intervention.

## Patient instructions

- Rest, interspersed with gentle pendular exercises, is indicated for 2 weeks following the injury.
- Active movements of the elbow, wrist and hand should be encouraged.
- An active range of shoulder movement is commenced under the guidance of a physiotherapist, with gradual progression to active and resisted rotator cuff exercises under physiotherapy supervision.

# Orthopaedic management

## Non-operative

In common with anterior dislocations, the majority of posterior dislocations are managed non-operatively with early movement and physiotherapy.

## Operative

### Urgent surgery

Surgery is rarely required as an emergency but is indicated where the shoulder remains dislocated and there is neurovascular compromise.

### Surgery within 48 hours

Prompt surgery is indicated in the case of:

- irreducible posterior dislocation
- fracture dislocation.

### Planned surgery

Planned surgery is indicated in the case of:

- *Persisting acute instability*: If the shoulder dislocates beyond neutral rotation, the cause is usually a large engaging reverse Hill–Sachs lesion and surgical stabilization is required. Surgery aims to fill the defect in the humeral head to prevent engagement. The McLaughlin technique is a transfer of the lesser tuberosity (and its attached subscapularis) into the defect. Larger defects may require a segment of femoral head allograft or a hemiarthroplasty.

- *Displaced lesser tuberosity fragment*: This is relatively common with this injury pattern and is usually reduced and fixed.
- *Recurrent instability*: Later reconstruction with a soft tissue labral repair or a posterior glenoid bone-block may be required.

## INFERIOR SHOULDER DISLOCATION (*LUXATIO ERECTA*)

Inferior dislocation (*luxatio erecta*) is rare (<1%) and follows hyperabduction of the shoulder. Inferior dislocation invariably presents with neurovascular compromise (**Fig. 8.29**).

## Emergency Department management

### Clinical features

- Presentation is with a very characteristic 'salute' position of high abduction and forward elevation, and the patient will be in considerable pain.
- The patient will be unable to adduct the shoulder.

### Radiological features

- *Shoulder trauma series*: Diagnosis does not usually present a challenge; however, an associated fracture is common. Distinguish

a simple dislocation (with or without an isolated tuberosity fracture) from a fracture dislocation (with a humeral neck fracture).

### Closed reduction (**Fig. 8.30**)

Closed reduction of a simple dislocation is performed under procedural sedation:

1. Traction is performed in the line of the abducted limb, with a sheet around the patient's chest providing counter-traction.
2. The arm is then gradually adducted.

### Immobilization and reassessment

The same steps as for anterior glenohumeral dislocation should be followed post reduction.

### Inpatient referral

- Patients with a neurological deficit should be discussed with the orthopaedic service.
- Surgery is rarely required urgently but may be indicated in the case of a fracture–dislocation or neurovascular compromise.

### Outpatient follow-up

All shoulder dislocations require orthopaedic follow-up to allow full assessment of the cuff, further neurovascular examination, and discussion about surgical intervention.

### Patient instructions

- Rest, interspersed with gentle pendular exercises, is indicated for 2 weeks following the injury.
- Active movements of the elbow, wrist and hand should be encouraged.
- An active range of shoulder movement is commenced under the guidance of a

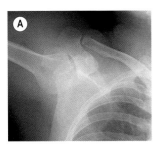

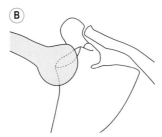

Fig. 8.29 Inferior dislocation of the shoulder (*luxutio erecta*). **A**, AP radiograph. **B**, The humeral head is inferior to the glenoid and the humerus is fixed in abduction.

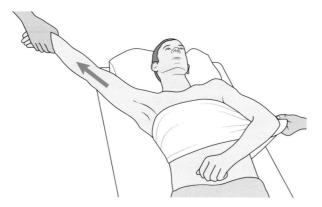

Fig. 8.30 Reduction of an inferior shoulder dislocation (*luxatio erecta*).

physiotherapist, with gradual progression to active and resisted rotator cuff exercises under physiotherapy supervision.

## Orthopaedic management

Surgery is rarely required but is indicated in the case of:

- irreducible inferior dislocation; this may be caused by the humeral head passing through a button-hole in the inferior capsule
- fracture dislocation.

## ROTATOR CUFF TEARS

The four rotator cuff muscles serve to stabilize the glenohumeral (shoulder) joint and assist in initiating movement. The tendons, inserting into the tuberosities of the humeral head, are vulnerable to injury, and cuff tears are common. There are two principal groups:

1. *Chronic degenerative tears*: These arise commonly as part of the normal ageing process, as a result of the gradual accumulation of multiple 'microtrauma' tears and impaired healing. Old age, repetitive overhead activity, diabetes, smoking, previous subacromial impingement symptoms and a hooked acromion predispose to degenerative tears. The cuff tendons in such patients may be thin and attenuated, making surgical repair of degenerative tears difficult or impossible.

2. *Acute traumatic tears*: A defined injury, such as a shoulder dislocation or a fall on to the outstretched arm or shoulder, may result in an acute cuff tear. Where the cuff tendon has been normal prior to injury, there is a greater chance of successful repair.

## Emergency Department management

### Clinical features

- Establish whether there is a history consistent with pre-existing cuff disease, and the circumstances surrounding the injury.
- The shoulder may look entirely normal.
- There may be tenderness at the rotator cuff insertion. Identify the outer edge of the acromion process and press firmly anterior to, and below, this point. Better access to this point is achieved by delivering the insertion point anteriorly, by shoulder extension and internal rotation.
- The cardinal feature of a cuff tear is weakness. Assess the rotator cuff muscles as described above (Fig. 8.6). The weakness may be only partial, and in a small cuff tear or a 'balanced' massive cuff tear (where there are small remaining areas of functioning cuff anteriorly and posteriorly) some shoulder movement is still possible.
- A careful skeletal examination is required to confirm that the weakness is not due to a fracture or dislocation.

- A careful neurological assessment is important to confirm that the weakness is mechanical (from a cuff tear), not neurological (from a nerve or plexus palsy).

### Radiological features
- *Shoulder trauma series*: should be obtained to exclude a fracture or dislocation.
- *Ultrasound scan*: provides confirmation of a cuff tear and its dimensions where the expertise and facilities exist.
- *MRI scan*: also provides excellent images of the rotator cuff where expert ultrasonography is not available.

### Outpatient referral
Provide analgesia and a collar-and-cuff. The patient should be referred for orthopaedic review and consideration of rotator cuff repair, which is optimally performed within four weeks of injury, before the cuff retracts and becomes scarred down.

## CALCIFIC TENDONITIS

Calcific tendonitis is a degenerative condition affecting patients aged 30–60 years; it is characterized by the gradual accumulation of a granular, paste-like calcium deposit in the supraspinatus tendon. For reasons that are not entirely clear, calcific tendonitis can present as an emergency with acute severe shoulder pain.

## Emergency Department management

### Clinical features
- The onset of severe pain is atraumatic.
- There may be a background history of degenerative subacromial bursitis, with shoulder pain during overhead activities.
- The patient will remain systemically well with normal observations.
- Examination will reveal a reduced range of active movement in the shoulder.
- The key differential diagnosis is a septic arthritis, which is characterized by systemic features (p. 103).

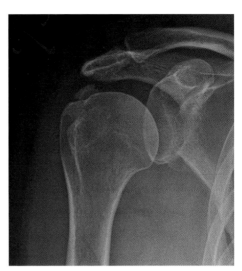

Fig. 8.31 Calcific tendonitis.

### Radiological features
- *Shoulder trauma series*: A characteristic calcific deposit will be evident on the AP shoulder radiograph, and this can be confirmed on ultrasound (**Fig. 8.31**).

### Inpatient referral
Very occasionally, patients require admission for symptomatic control and exclusion of other causes of shoulder pain.

### Outpatient follow-up
Calcific tendonitis is managed with reassurance, oral analgesia (particularly anti-inflammatory medication) and physiotherapy. Patients may be referred back to their GP or to an elective shoulder clinic.

## Orthopaedic management

Management is almost always non-operative in the first instance. Patients with severe symptoms can be offered subacromial steroid injections or ultrasound-guided barbotage (the agitation and lavage of the deposit with saline). Patients with severe and unremitting pain may be offered surgical subacromial decompression and debridement of the calcific deposit.

## FROZEN SHOULDER (ADHESIVE CAPSULITIS)

Frozen shoulder is an inflammatory condition of the shoulder capsule resulting in pain, contraction and shoulder stiffness. It can present as an emergency with the rapid onset of severe shoulder pain and restricted movement. There may be an identifiable traumatic precipitant. Frozen shoulder following a significant injury (such as a proximal humeral fracture) is termed adhesive capsulitis.

The natural history of frozen shoulder is that it passes through three phases, eventually resolving spontaneously after many months or years.

- *Freezing phase* (3 months): There is increasing pain (often worse at night) and worsening restriction in movement.

- *Frozen phase* (6 months): The pain is less severe but movements remain very limited.

- *Thawing phase* (12 months): Pain eases further and the range of movement gradually returns to normal.

## Emergency Department management

### Clinical features

- Any history of injury is usually trivial and there may be no injury at all.

- Predisposing conditions include diabetes mellitus, hypercholesterolaemia and Dupuytren's disease.

- Patients will complain of severe shoulder pain and will have a globally restricted range of both active and passive movement: in particular, loss of external rotation. However, they will remain systemically well.

### Radiological features

- *Shoulder trauma series*: Exclude any skeletal abnormality. There are no diagnostic radiographic features.

### Outpatient follow-up

Frozen shoulder is managed with reassurance, oral analgesia (particularly anti-inflammatory medication) and physiotherapy. Patients may be referred back to their GP or to an elective shoulder clinic.

## Orthopaedic management

Management is almost always non-operative in the first instance. Patients with severe symptoms can be offered glenohumeral steroid injections. Individuals with severe and unremitting pain and stiffness may be offered a distension arthrogram, a manipulation under anaesthesia (MUA) or a surgical capsular release.

## GENERAL PRINCIPLES

## Anatomy

### Proximal humerus

The proximal humerus comprises four major parts (corresponding to the four developmental ossification centres), which are important in describing the anatomy of, and injuries to, this region (**Fig. 9.1**):

1. anatomical head
2. greater tuberosity
3. lesser tuberosity
4. shaft.

The *anatomical head* bears the articular surface of the proximal humerus, which articulates with the glenoid. An understanding of the precise orientation of the anatomical head is important when reconstructing proximal humeral fractures; although the head is directed predominantly medially, note that it is also orientated superiorly by 130°, and anteriorly by 30°. Lateral to the anatomical head are the greater and lesser tuberosities, which are separated by the *bicipital groove*. The *greater tuberosity* is at the lateral aspect of the head, and is the site of insertion of three of the four rotator cuff muscles: supraspinatus, infraspinatus and teres minor. The *lesser tuberosity* is placed more anteriorly and is the site of insertion of the remaining rotator cuff muscle, subscapularis. The four rotator cuff muscles are principally responsible for maintaining stability of the glenohumeral joint. They are active stabilizers (p. 146), producing 'concavity compression' during shoulder movements. When the tuberosities fracture, they tend to displace with retraction and defunctioning of their attached rotator cuff muscles. In effect, a displaced tuberosity fracture is equivalent to a massive rotator cuff tear. The anatomical head and the tuberosities make up the *surgical head* of the humerus. The *surgical neck* of the humerus lies at the junction of the surgical head and the shaft.

Whilst the rotator cuff muscles (termed *intrinsic muscles*) are responsible for stability, the larger *extrinsic muscles* produce the powerful movements of the shoulder. The deltoid arises from the scapula and clavicle and inserts into the deltoid tuberosity. Pectoralis major and teres major insert into the lateral and medial edges of the bicipital groove respectively, whilst latissimus dorsi is remembered as the 'lady between two majors' as it inserts into the floor of the groove.

### Nerves around the proximal humerus

The *brachial plexus*, surrounding the *axillary artery*, is placed just medial to the coracoid process and the attached conjoint tendon (formed by coracobrachialis and the short head of biceps) (**Fig. 9.2**). This relationship is important in avoiding inadvertent neurovascular injury during surgery, as the surgeon should always stay lateral to the coracoid process. The plexus gives off several nerves that travel in close approximation to the shoulder skeleton. In particular, the *axillary nerve* arises from the posterior cord of the plexus, travels through the quadrilateral space (bounded by teres minor above, teres major below, long head of triceps medially and the humerus laterally) to arrive at the surgical neck of the humerus, accompanied by the posterior circumflex humeral artery (**Fig. 9.3**). Here the nerve and artery run deep to deltoid, and the nerve gives terminal branches innervating deltoid (and teres minor) and providing sensation to the skin in the 'regimental badge' area (see Fig. 8.19). The axillary nerve is vulnerable to injury in shoulder dislocations or fractures, and in the course of a deltoid-splitting approach.

### Vascular supply to the humeral head

The vascular supply to the proximal humerus arises from the anterior and posterior

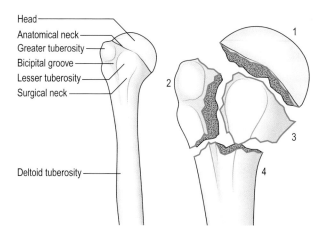

Head
Anatomical neck
Greater tuberosity
Bicipital groove
Lesser tuberosity
Surgical neck

Deltoid tuberosity

1
2
3
4

Fig. 9.1 Osteology of the proximal humerus.

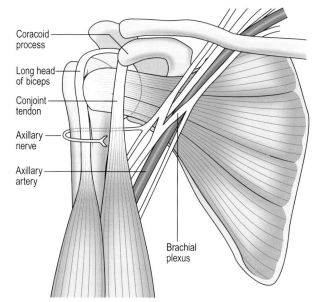

Coracoid process

Long head of biceps

Conjoint tendon

Axillary nerve

Axillary artery

Brachial plexus

Fig. 9.2 Structures around the proximal humerus.

circumflex humeral arteries, both branches of the axillary artery (**Fig. 9.4**). The anterior artery – and in particular its ascending (arcuate) branch, which runs in the bicipital groove – has long been held to be most important, although recent studies have suggested the posterior artery (which runs with the axillary nerve) is predominant. Additional vascular supply arises from the tendon insertions into the two tuberosities and the periosteum, particularly at the calcar of the medial neck. Avascular necrosis may follow a displaced proximal humeral fracture, and affects the anatomical head

particularly in displaced four-part fractures where it loses all vascularized attachments.

## Humeral shaft

The humeral shaft is coded 1–2 in the AO universal fracture classification system (Fig. 1.21), and is that portion between the 'Müller's boxes' of the proximal and distal metaphyses (see Fig. 1.14). It is effectively cylindrical in shape in the mid-shaft, gradually flattening and flaring out into the supracondylar ridges just above the elbow distally. There are two muscular compartments (anterior and posterior)

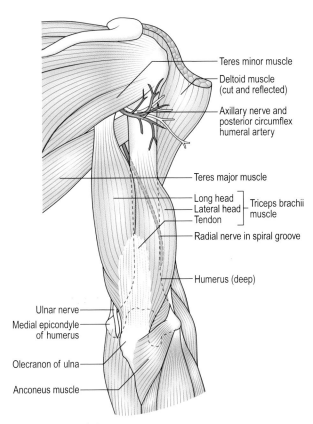

Teres minor muscle

Deltoid muscle
(cut and reflected)

Axillary nerve and
posterior circumflex
humeral artery

Teres major muscle

Long head
Lateral head    Triceps brachii
Tendon          muscle

Radial nerve in spiral groove

Humerus (deep)

Ulnar nerve

Medial epicondyle
of humerus

Olecranon of ulna

Anconeus muscle

Fig. 9.3 Posterior compartment of the arm.

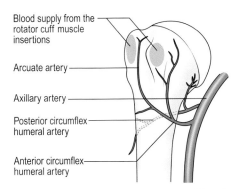

Blood supply from the
rotator cuff muscle
insertions

Arcuate artery

Axillary artery

Posterior circumflex
humeral artery

Anterior circumflex
humeral artery

Fig. 9.4 Vascular supply to the humeral head.

separated by medial and lateral intermuscular septa.

## Anterior compartment of the arm (Fig. 9.5)

The anterior compartment contains the biceps (Latin: 'two-headed') muscle. This arises from two heads: the superior lip of the glenoid (long head) and the coracoid process (short head, along with coracobrachialis). It crosses the shoulder joint and passes distally to cross the elbow joint as well, before inserting into the bicipital tuberosity of the radius. It acts to supinate the forearm and flex the elbow, thus both driving in the corkscrew and pulling out the cork. Lying deep to biceps is the rather larger brachialis muscle, which has a broad origin over the anterior humerus and inserts into the coronoid process of the ulna. The biceps, coracobrachialis and the medial two-thirds of brachialis are all innervated by the musculocutaneous nerve, which arises from the lateral cord of the brachial plexus (see Fig. 3.13), penetrates coracobrachialis, and runs through the anterior compartment between biceps and brachialis. The lateral third of brachialis is innervated by the radial nerve. Thus the internervous plane allowing access to the

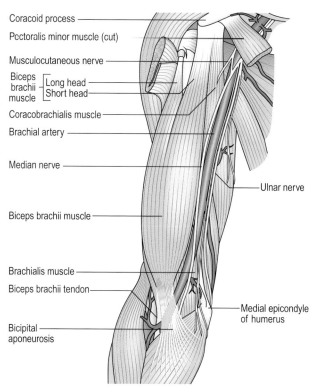

Coracoid process

Pectoralis minor muscle (cut)

Musculocutaneous nerve

Biceps
brachii ⎰Long head
muscle ⎱Short head

Coracobrachialis muscle

Brachial artery

Median nerve

Ulnar nerve

Biceps brachii muscle

Brachialis muscle

Biceps brachii tendon

Medial epicondyle
of humerus

Bicipital
aponeurosis

Fig. 9.5 Anterior compartment of the arm.

anterior aspect of the humerus lies *through* the belly of brachialis muscle, splitting the lateral third from the medial two-thirds. The median and ulnar nerves pass through the anterior compartment but do not supply any muscles at this level. The median nerve lies adjacent to the brachial artery, medial to biceps. The ulnar nerve passes unprotected down the medial aspect of the arm before traversing the medial intermuscular septum and passing posterior to the medial epicondyle, where it is vulnerable to injury.

## Posterior compartment of the arm (see Fig. 9.3)

The posterior compartment contains the triceps (Latin: 'three-headed') muscle, which has a broad origin from the scapula and the posterior aspect of the humerus, and passes distally across the elbow to an insertion into the olecranon process of the ulna. The three heads have somewhat confusing names. The long

head arises from the infraglenoid tubercle of the scapula and is the most medial. The lateral head arises from the dorsal surface of the humerus, lateral and proximal to the groove of the radial nerve. The medial head is deep to the lateral and long heads, and arises distal to the spiral groove, from the posterior aspect of the humerus and from the medial and lateral intermuscular septa. The triceps muscle is innervated by the radial nerve, which arises from the posterior cord of the brachial plexus and passes through the triangular space of the axilla into the posterior aspect of the arm. Here it travels with the profunda brachii artery in the spiral groove, descending and passing medially to laterally until it passes through the lateral intermuscular septum and into the anterior compartment, where it travels between brachialis and brachioradialis into the forearm. The radial nerve is vulnerable to injury at two sites in particular: at the posterior shaft of the humerus and at the elbow. In the spiral groove it rests directly against the humerus, and fractures of the shaft (particularly at the junction of the middle and distal thirds, the Holstein–Lewis fracture (see Fig. 9.17), or instruments being placed during fracture fixation, can injure the nerve. At the elbow, the nerve is at risk during an anterior approach to the distal humerus. The internervous plane is within brachialis whereas dissection lateral to this muscle exposes the radial nerve, which is concealed between brachialis and brachioradialis. In the posterior approach to the humerus, dissection through triceps is an anatomical exercise in locating and protecting the nerve.

## Clinical assessment of the painful arm (humerus)

The clinical assessment of the painful shoulder is described on page 129.

### History

Define the reason for presentation: has there been an acute definable injury? A high-energy mechanism of injury, such as a motor vehicle collision or fall from a height, suggests the possibility of other associated injuries and a requirement to assess and manage these first (Ch. 2).

A localized arm injury most commonly follows a simple fall on to an outstretched hand or arm, a direct blow to the arm, or a twisting injury to the limb. Enquire about previous injuries, operations or problems with the affected limb.

### Examination

#### Look

The patient will be in pain and will present supporting the limb with the other hand. There will be little swelling, and no bruising initially, but after a few hours extensive, deep bruising may develop, which will track down through the arm and around the elbow. Open wounds or skin tenting (an impending open fracture) will require urgent surgical attention. Skin puckering, particularly anterolaterally, can suggest muscle interposition within the fracture, where it may interfere with fracture healing. Proximal humeral fractures rarely display clinical deformity but those fractures affecting the shaft often appear significantly displaced.

#### Feel

There is likely to be instability and crepitus as the limb is realigned. Palpate the shoulder and elbow to exclude concurrent injury.

#### Move

Formal testing of shoulder or elbow movement will prove painful while providing limited information. Hand and wrist movements to assess neurological function are sufficient in the acute setting.

#### Neurovascular assessment

Assess sensory supply to each of the peripheral nerve distributions of the upper limb, paying special attention to the axillary, median, radial and ulnar nerves (see Figs 3.17–3.19). Assess the radial pulse and capillary return to the finger nailbeds. If a brachial plexopathy is suspected, testing of the individual myotomes and dermatomes is indicated (see Fig. 3.14).

The most common neurological abnormality in mid-shaft humeral fractures is a radial nerve palsy, occurring in 10% of cases. Major arterial injury is rare, but may present as a pulsatile expanding haematoma. The classical signs of an acutely dysvascular limb (Box 3.1) are rare, as there is a rich collateral circulation.

## Radiological assessment of the painful arm (humerus)

### Radiographs

- *Anteroposterior (AP) view of the humerus*: This is a full-length view, which should include both the shoulder and the elbow. If there is suspicion of an intra-articular extension, further formal views of the affected joint are required.

- *Lateral humerus*: This view must be obtained with caution. If only the distal fragment is rotated by the radiographer (by moving the forearm), the proximal fragment will not move and the rotation will occur at the fracture site, causing significant discomfort and the risk of soft tissue damage. The X-ray plate must be placed between the patient's arm and chest, and the entire X-ray beam rotated. Alternatively, a trans-thoracic view will show displacement but requires a high dose of ionizing radiation.

## PROXIMAL HUMERAL FRACTURES

Fractures of the proximal humerus are common, representing 5% of all adult fractures. The majority are stable injuries, occurring in elderly osteoporotic individuals after low-energy falls. The majority can be treated non-operatively. A small proportion – those with more severe comminution or instability, or those occurring in high-demand individuals – may benefit from operative treatment, although the selection of those fractures requiring surgery remains contentious.

## Classification

### Neer classification (Fig. 9.6)

Proximal humeral fractures are classified according to the number of parts involved. A part is displaced only if it is >1 cm translated or >45° rotated. A part displaced less than this, even if fractured, is not counted, strictly speaking. Fractures are described as being minimally displaced, or two-, three- or four-part. Fracture-dislocations are a more severe injury and are considered separately.

Some fracture types are not classifiable according to Neer and yet are important to recognize. The valgus impacted fracture usually has an intact periosteal hinge medially and, despite considerable displacement of the anatomical head, can be reduced by surgical leverage on this hinge; it may have a reduced risk of avascular necrosis.

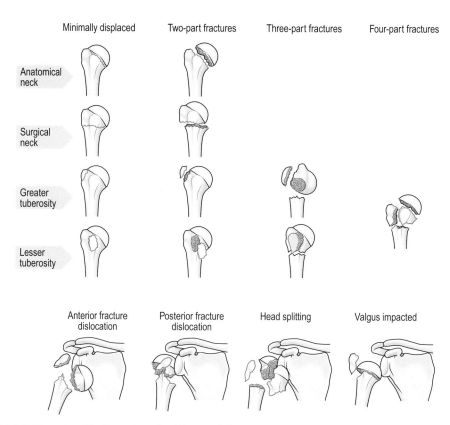

Fig. 9.6 Neer classification of proximal humeral fractures.

# Emergency Department management

## Clinical features

- The patient will present holding the affected arm close to the chest with the wrist supported by the contralateral hand.

- There will be little swelling, and no bruising initially, but after a few hours extensive, deep bruising may develop, which will track down through the arm and around the elbow.

- Skin puckering anterolaterally can suggest that the deltoid has become interposed within the fracture, where it may interfere with fracture healing.

- The patient will not be able to demonstrate active comfortable movement of the shoulder.

## Radiological features

- *AP and modified axial shoulder radiographs*: Assess the humeral head to ensure the glenohumeral joint is congruent, as a fracture dislocation should not be manipulated in the Emergency Department. On the modified axial view, pay close attention to the location of the greater tuberosity, which is commonly retracted posteriorly as well as superiorly.

- *CT*: A CT scan is invaluable in planning surgical reconstruction of complex fractures.

## Closed reduction (Fig. 9.7)

Formal closed reduction is not required, although fractures of the proximal humerus (**Fig. 9.7A**) tend to realign over time as a result of the traction afforded by the weight of the arm, if the wrist is supported in a collar-and-cuff (**Fig. 9.7B**).

## Immobilization and reassessment

This is a painful and awkward fracture, and there is no form of cast that is of benefit. The wrist is supported with a collar-and-cuff and a shirt is worn over the arm for the first few weeks. Repeat the assessment of neurovascular status.

## Inpatient referral

- Open fracture.

- Neurovascular compromise.

- Fracture dislocation of the humeral head.

## Outpatient follow-up

- Patients with proximal humerus fractures are reviewed in the fracture clinic. This allows planned surgery if required.

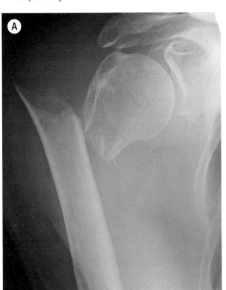 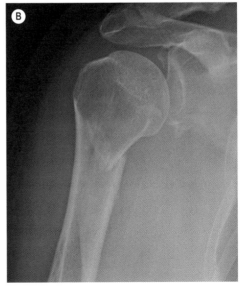

Fig. 9.7 Closed reduction with collar-and-cuff: proximal humeral fractures. **A**, The initial alignment. **B**, Realignment resulting from the weight of the arm when the wrist is supported.

## Patient instructions

- Patients should be advised to remove their wrist from the cuff several times a day and begin pendular exercises immediately, as well as mobilizing the elbow, wrist and hand. They should progress to shoulder exercises as soon as their level of comfort allows.

- In the early stages after fracture, pain control can be difficult. Patients may find it most comfortable to sleep in a chair for the first 2 weeks or so, with a shirt over the arm to prevent movement when turning.

- Patients should be warned that significant bruising down to the elbow, forearm and hand can occur. Gentle movements of these joints limits swelling.

## Orthopaedic management

Many patients with non-operatively treated, displaced fractures none the less enjoy very satisfactory functional recovery. In contrast, those with operatively treated, anatomically reduced fractures often do not regain a normal shoulder; stiffness, weakness and discomfort are all common. The indications for surgery therefore remain contentious.

### Non-operative

Most fractures (90%) can usually be treated *conservatively* including:

- one-part fractures
- impacted fractures of the surgical neck without severe angulation
- two-, three- and four-part fractures with <30° angulation of the articular surface, and good cortical contact with the shaft
- any other fracture pattern with relevant patient factors: old age, low functional requirements, diabetes, renal disease, alcohol abuse, psychiatric condition, dementia.

### Operative
#### *Absolute indications for surgery*
Fewer than 1% of fractures require urgent surgery. These may include:

- open fractures
- fracture-dislocations
- fractures with associated vascular injury.

### *Relative indications for surgery*
Only a minority (around 10%) of fractures are likely to benefit from surgery to reconstruct or replace the humeral head, including:

- two- or three-part fractures where the greater tuberosity is displaced by >1 cm
- 'off-ended' two-part fractures of the surgical neck (see Fig. 1.16)
- two-, three- or four-part fractures where the articular surface has displaced by >30°
- head-splitting fractures (may require a hemiarthroplasty).

### Surgical techniques
Several reconstructive options are available:

- *Percutaneous fixation*: Some fractures are amenable to closed reduction through traction and percutaneous manipulation with wires and levers, and percutaneous screw fixation.

- *Open reduction and internal fixation* (**Fig. 9.8**): A variety of plates have been used, with a recent preference for site-specific locking plates that achieve a powerful hold in osteoporotic bone.

- *Nailing*: Intramedullary nails with multiple proximal locking options have been used successfully for stabilization of proximal humeral fractures and offer the attraction of percutaneous implantation.

- *Arthroplasty* (**Fig. 9.9**): Certain fractures are not amenable to fixation due to a high level of articular comminution or poor bone stock, particularly in elderly patients. In these circumstances, a primary hemiarthroplasty should be considered.

### *Plating of the proximal humerus*
The most commonly performed procedure is an open reduction and plate fixation, through either a deltopectoral or a deltoid-splitting

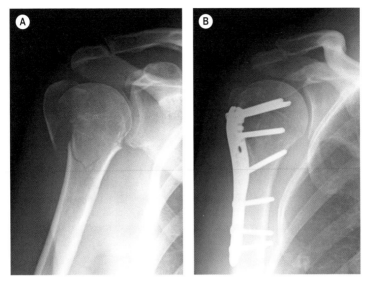

Fig. 9.8 Proximal humerus fracture: open reduction and internal fixation. **A**, Displaced four-part fracture. **B**, Anatomical reduction and internal fixation.

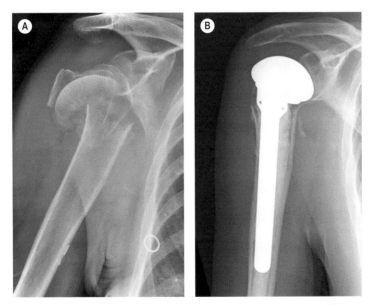

Fig. 9.9 Hemiarthroplasty. **A**, Displaced four-part fracture with poor bone stock. **B**, Replacement with a hemiarthroplasty.

approach. The deltopectoral approach is extensile and is performed through the internervous plane. However, it approaches the humeral head from the front, and exposure of the posterior aspect, in particular the greater tuberosity, can be difficult. In contrast, the deltoid-splitting approach allows better exposure of the greater tuberosity and fracture, but requires careful identification and protection of the axillary nerve.

## SURGICAL TECHNIQUE: Proximal humeral plating – deltopectoral approach

### Surgical set-up (Fig. 9.10)

Patient position may be supine on a radiolucent table, with the upper limb draped free. Alternatively, a beach-chair position may be preferred, as it allows the weight of the upper limb to provide traction. Rehearse obtaining adequate AP and modified axial fluoroscopic images before preparing and draping the patient.

### Orthopaedic equipment

- Pre-contoured site-specific plate with corresponding set
- 1.6-mm k-wires

### Incision (Fig. 9.11)

Place the flat of your hand over pectoralis major and allow your fingertips to locate the edge of that muscle at the deltopectoral interval. The coracoid process is felt at the superior end of the interval. The interval passes obliquely across the front of the shoulder towards the deltoid insertion. The incision is 15 cm along this line between the coracoid and the deltoid tuberosity.

### Approach (Fig. 9.12)

Internervous plane: This approach exploits the interval between the deltoid muscle (axillary nerve) and pectoralis major (lateral and medial pectoral nerves).

The deltopectoral interval is identified; it can usually be seen as a streak of fatty tissue, within which lies the cephalic vein. Dissect bluntly to the medial side of the vein, tying off tributaries as required (**Fig. 9.12A**). Medially, the conjoint tendon (the common origin of coracobrachialis and short head of biceps) is an important landmark. It marks the safe boundary of the surgical field, as the axillary artery and the brachial plexus lie medial to the tendon (**Fig. 9.12B**). The musculocutaneous nerve enters the tendon posteriorly, 5 cm below the tip of the coracoid, and excessive traction on the tendon will result in injury. The clavipectoral fascia lies deep to pectoralis major, overlying subscapularis and the conjoint tendon, and is incised in line with the lateral edge of the conjoint tendon. The insertion of pectoralis major traverses the wound where it inserts on to the lateral aspect of the bicipital groove; it can be released partially at its superior edge. Any adhesions under the acromion and deltoid are cleared with a finger and the fracture fragments are identified. The insertion of deltoid can be elevated to expose the lateral aspect of the humerus for plate positioning. In the base of the wound is the subscapularis muscle, the lower edge of which marks the level of the axillary nerve.

### Open reduction (Fig. 9.13)

The fracture fragments are identified and cleared. The two tuberosities are secured with braided non-absorbable, transosseous sutures (**Fig. 9.13A**). This allows the tuberosities to be drawn apart, and 'opening the doors' will reveal the anatomical head of the humerus. The head is elevated and reduced with wires or osteotomes, being careful to preserve any medial soft tissue hinge. Successful reduction requires anatomical alignment of the medial calcar, and correction of the orientation of the articular surface out of varus or valgus. The distal fragment usually needs to be brought laterally to complete the reduction, and a bolster in the axilla can provide an invaluable fulcrum. The reduction is held temporarily with k-wires. There is usually a residual defect, which should be filled with structural bone graft or bone substitute. The 'doors are closed' by bringing the tuberosities together and tying the transosseous sutures to each other (**Fig. 9.13B**).

## Internal fixation – absolute stability (Fig. 9.14)

A contoured locking plate is then applied to the lateral aspect of the humerus. The plate should not sit proud of the superior edge of the greater tuberosity, as it will cause impingement. A lower position also allows the lowest locking screws to sit just above the calcar and penetrate deep into the head, where they have the best purchase.

### Postoperative restrictions

Movement: Shoulder movement is restricted to pendular exercises for 6 weeks. Instruct the patient to allow the shoulder to hang down freely whilst leaning forwards, and let the shoulder move gently backwards and forwards in the manner of a pendulum for washing. Full active movement is permitted at the elbow, wrist and fingers.

Weight-bearing: Patients are allowed to use their hand for feeding themselves but instructed not to lift anything heavier until union.

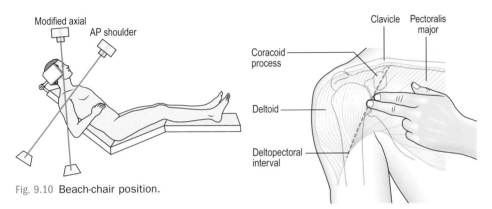

Fig. 9.10 Beach-chair position.

Fig. 9.11 Deltopectoral incision.

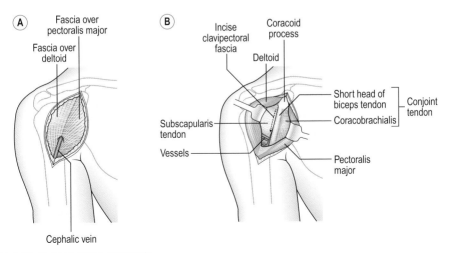

Fig. 9.12 Deltopectoral approach.

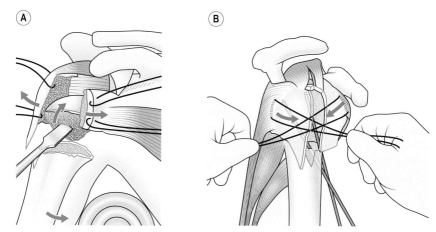

Fig. 9.13 Open reduction of a proximal humerus fracture.

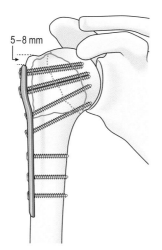

Fig. 9.14 Internal fixation of a proximal
humerus fracture.

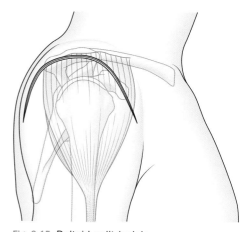

Fig. 9.15 Deltoid split incision.

## SURGICAL TECHNIQUE: Proximal humeral plating – deltoid-splitting approach

### Incision (Fig. 9.15)

The sabre incision is centred on the outer aspect of the acromion and extends in Langer's lines anteriorly and posteriorly towards the axilla.

### Approach (Fig. 9.16)

There is no internervous plane. The anterior fibres of deltoid are supplied by the axillary nerve passing from posterior to anterior, at the surgical neck of the humerus. The nerve, and the accompanying posterior circumflex humeral artery, must be identified and preserved to prevent denervation of the anterior deltoid.

The raphe is identified as a yellow stripe of connective tissue commencing near the anterolateral corner of the acromion (**Fig. 9.16A**). This raphe is split over a distance of 6 cm. The deltoid can be released more proximally by sharp subperiosteal dissection of the tendon from the anterior acromion. The surgeon's finger is placed through the split and advanced distally along the lateral surface of the humerus until it encounters the axillary nerve, which is felt as a bundle of transverse fibres around 8 cm distal to the acromion, rather than one discrete structure. These are marked with a vascular loop and protected.

### Open reduction
The tuberosities are identified and secured with transosseous sutures to allow retraction and exposure of the anatomical head (**Fig. 9.16B**). Then the head is reduced before the 'doors are closed' as before.

### Internal fixation – absolute stability
The plate is positioned by sliding it down the lateral aspect of the humerus under the axillary nerve. The head of the humerus is addressed above the nerve, and screws are placed into the humeral shaft below the nerve. Shaft screws can be placed either through the existing split, or through a separate deltoid split distal to the nerve.

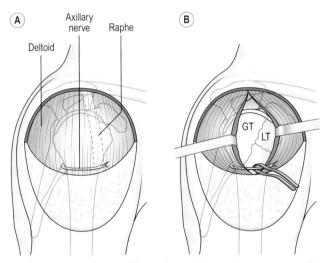

Fig. 9.16 Deltoid split approach. See text for details. GT, greater tuberosity; LT, lesser tuberosity.

## Outpatient management

### Conservatively treated proximal humerus fracture

| Outpatient management summary | | | |
|---|---|---|---|
| **Week** | **Examination** | **Radiographs** | **Additional notes** |
| 1 | Neurovascular status<br>Wound check<br>Check for skin puckering | AP shoulder<br>Modified axial view | Begin pendular exercises |
| 6 | Rotator cuff assessment | AP shoulder<br>Modified axial view | Begin active exercises when tuberosities have united |
| 12 | | AP shoulder<br>Modified axial view | If there is radiological and clinical union, discharge to physiotherapy |

Further assessments at 4-week intervals if required for delayed union

Average time to union = 8 weeks

### Surgically managed proximal humerus fractures

These may have a different outpatient regime, which is prescribed by the operating surgeon.

## COMPLICATIONS

### *Early*

Local Neurovascular injury: The brachial plexus, and the axillary artery and its branches are at risk during injury or surgery to the proximal humerus

Loss of reduction: Osteoporotic or comminuted bone is at risk of collapse, and this may result in locking screws in the subarticular region sitting 'proud' within the joint

Infection: This may involve the shoulder joint itself and can be very challenging to salvage

Nerve injury: The axillary nerve is particularly vulnerable to intraoperative injury in the course of a deltoid-splitting approach, resulting in diminished sensation in the 'regimental badge' area and weakness of forward elevation and abduction of the shoulder. The musculocutaneous nerve is at risk where coracobrachialis has been retracted forcefully, resulting in weakness of elbow flexion

General Intrathoracic or axillary injury: Inadvertent penetration of wires or drill bits beyond the humeral head may cause injury to the lung apex (resulting in a pneumothorax), the axillary vessels or brachial plexus

## COMPLICATIONS... cont'd

### Late

Local
Non-union: This particularly affects two-part surgical neck fractures where there has been soft tissue interposition

Malunion: This is particularly troublesome if the greater tuberosity becomes displaced, leading to defunctioning of supraspinatus and shoulder impingement

Avascular necrosis: Segmental necrosis of devascularized anatomical head fragments is common after displaced fractures. This is usually a radiographic finding in an asymptomatic patient, and spontaneous revascularization commonly occurs; however, if there is collapse of the head, a salvage hemiarthroplasty may be required

Adhesive capsulitis: Shoulder stiffness (frozen shoulder) is common after injury and surgery, and is minimized by early active shoulder movements. After fracture union, active-assisted and passive stretching is usually successful. Recalcitrant cases are treated by a distension arthrogram in which radiographic contrast and saline are injected into the shoulder joint under pressure, resulting in capsular disruption

## HUMERAL SHAFT FRACTURES

Humeral fractures have a typical bimodal distribution of older women (as a result of a simple fall on to the arm) and younger men (as a result of sport or a direct blow). Most are simple A-type spiral or transverse fractures, and <5% are open.

Like the femur and tibia, the humerus is a long, tubular bone. Unlike the lower limb bones, however, it is smaller, well covered in vascularized muscle, is not weight-bearing, and is regularly subjected to rotational, rather than axial, forces. These biomechanical characteristics mean that the management of humeral fractures is rather different.

## Classification

### AO classification
Humeral shaft fractures are classified according to the AO classification of diaphyseal fractures (see Fig. 1.22).

### Eponymous fractures
The *Holstein–Lewis fracture* is considered separately, as it occurs in the distal third of the humerus at the level where the radial nerve transverses the lateral intermuscular septum (**Fig. 9.17**). At this level, the nerve is unable to yield to movement of fractured bone ends and is injured in 25% of cases, compared with 10% overall incidence with humeral shaft fractures.

## Emergency Department management

### Clinical features
- The patient will be in pain and will be supporting the arm, which may be deformed. There may be swelling and some shortening of the arm.
- Bruising may not be present at the time of presentation.
- Any abrasions should be assessed and an open fracture excluded.

- There is likely to be instability and crepitus as the limb is realigned. Assess the shoulder and elbow.
- A careful assessment of radial nerve function should be made; it is abnormal in 10% of cases (see 'Complications' below). Major

arterial injury is rare but may present as a pulsatile expanding haematoma. The signs of an acutely dysvascular limb (see Box 3.1) are rare, as there is a rich collateral circulation.

### Radiological features

- *AP and lateral humerus radiographs*: These should include the joint above (shoulder) and the joint below (elbow). Fractures of the humeral shaft have characteristic displacement, which is dictated by the level of the fracture in relation to the insertion of deltoid.

  *Proximal to deltoid insertion*, the proximal fragment is pulled into adduction by the action of pectoralis major and latissimus dorsi, whilst the distal fragment is lateralized and shortened by deltoid.

  *Distal to deltoid insertion*, the proximal fragment is abducted by deltoid, whilst the distal fragment is medialized and shortened by the muscles of the anterior and posterior compartments.

### Immobilization and reassessment (Fig. 9.18)

There are three options for the initial treatment of humeral fractures:

- *U-slab*: This is used to protect and splint the fracture acutely (see p. 66 and **Fig. 9.18A**).
- *Hanging cast*: This may be used for definitive management, applying traction through gravity in order to realign the fracture. It is now rarely used, as it is awkward and

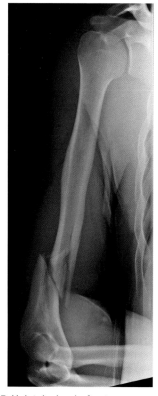

Fig. 9.17 Holstein–Lewis fracture.

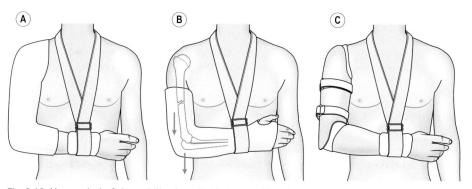

Fig. 9.18 Humeral shaft immobilization. **A**, U-slab. **B**, Hanging cast. **C**, Functional brace.

requires considerable patient compliance. Displaced fractures usually undergo surgery while minimally displaced fractures are suitable for functional bracing (**Fig. 9.18B**).

- *Functional (Sarmiento) brace*: This is preferable for most fractures. An initial U-slab is replaced by a functional brace at around 2 weeks after injury. The brace can be removed for washing, and the tightness can be adjusted as swelling subsides (**Fig. 9.18C**).

After applying any form of immobilization, repeat the assessment of neurovascular status and obtain repeat radiographs.

### Inpatient referral
- Open fractures.
- Neurovascular compromise.

### Outpatient follow-up
- Mid-shaft humerus fractures are reviewed in the fracture clinic within a week.

### Patient instructions
- Those patients with a U-slab should be warned of the potential of plaster complications. This cast provides comfort but can prove heavy and awkward.
- Encourage movements of the hand and wrist.

## Orthopaedic management
### Non-operative
Most humeral fractures are treated non-operatively in a functional brace and heal in around 9 weeks. Around 10% should be considered for surgery.

### Operative
Indications for surgery include:

- Open fractures.
- Multiple trauma.
- Dysvascular limb or expanding haematoma.
- Severe displacement. Acceptable limits will clearly depend on the functional requirements of the patient, but as a rule of thumb, up to 30° of angulation in any direction and 3 cm of shortening are acceptable.
- Segmental or intra-articular fractures.

## Surgical techniques
There are three options for surgical stabilization of the humerus:

1. *Open reduction and internal fixation with plate and screws* (see page 85 and **Fig. 9.19**): This is the most commonly performed procedure. It allows direct anatomical reduction and compression of the fracture. It does not involve disturbance of either the shoulder or the elbow. The most common surgical approaches to the humerus are:

   a. Posterior: This allows excellent exposure of the distal humerus and is described below. It does not allow proximal extension to the shoulder.

   b. Anterolateral: This is an extension of the deltopectoral approach described above. In the middle and distal thirds of the humerus, the bone is covered by brachialis, and the internervous plane is between the lateral third (radial nerve) and medial two-thirds (musculocutaneous nerve) of the muscle.

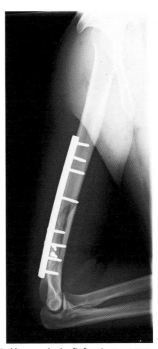

Fig. 9.19 Humeral shaft fracture: open reduction and internal fixation.

2. *Antegrade nailing*: This may be preferred in segmental fractures (which would otherwise require an extensive exposure and soft tissue dissection) and in pathological fractures. Surgery is performed in the beach-chair position. A small incision is made just lateral to the acromion. The deltoid is split and the supraspinatus tendon is opened with sharp dissection. The entry point is identified at the margin of the articular cartilage with fluoroscopic assistance. A sequence of drills and reamers is used to prepare the canal before implantation of the nail. The nail is cross-locked proximally and distally. *Hazards* include the necessity for the proximal end of the nail to be buried to prevent subacromial impingement and cuff irritation. *Shoulder pain* from cuff irritation is the principal complication of this technique. The proximal locking screws are in close proximity to the axillary nerve, the distal screws to the median nerve and brachial artery.

3. *Retrograde nailing*: This technique aims to minimize the insult to the shoulder and rotator cuff by employing an entry point distally at the olecranon fossa. The entry point is narrow and there is a risk of fracture propagation and *elbow pain*.

## SURGICAL TECHNIQUE: Humeral shaft plate fixation – posterior approach

### Surgical set-up (Fig. 9.20)
The patient is placed in the lateral decubitus position, with the injured arm uppermost and the elbow flexed over a prop. Supports are placed on the pelvis to secure the patient. Rehearse the fluoroscopic manœuvres required to obtain adequate images.

### Incision (Fig. 9.21)
The incision is longitudinal, along the posterior aspect of the arm. Length and starting point are defined by the fracture position.

### Approach (Fig. 9.22)
Internervous plane: There is no true internervous plane, as the approach splits triceps, all of which is usually considered to be supplied by the radial nerve. However, because of the proximal innervation this does not result in any denervated muscle.

After sharp dissection through the subcutaneous tissue, the triceps fascia is brought into view. The fascia is incised in line with the wound, directly over the muscle. Identify the interval between the long and lateral heads of triceps and dissect bluntly between the two. A pair of Langenbeck retractors is ideal for this task (**Fig. 9.22A**). The radial nerve is identified and protected as it courses with the profundus artery in the spiral groove. Sharp dissection is used to complete the separation of the long and lateral heads distally. The radial nerve is gently mobilized so that the medial head of triceps can be split safely, and cut is made down to bone in the midline to expose the humerus and fracture (**Fig. 9.22B**).

### Open reduction
The fracture ends are cleared and reduced. Temporary stabilization is effected with bone-holding forceps.

### Internal fixation – absolute stability (see Fig. 9.19)
The fracture and any butterfly fragments are lagged. A 4.5-mm dynamic compression plate is usually selected, although a 3.5-mm dynamic compression plate is appropriate for a small humerus. Aim to achieve 6–8 cortices (3–4 screws) above and below the fracture.

### Postoperative restrictions
Movement: Free movement of the shoulder and elbow are initiated early.

Weight-bearing: Patients are allowed to use their hand for feeding themselves but instructed not to lift anything heavier until union.

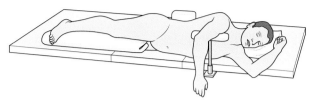

Fig. 9.20 Lateral decubitus position.

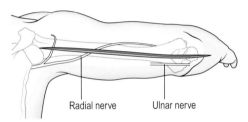

Fig. 9.21 Posterior humerus plating: incision.

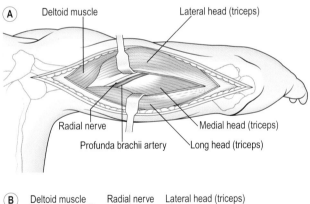

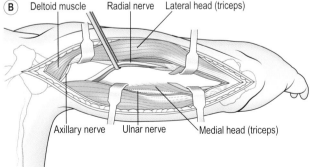

Fig. 9.22 Posterior humerus plating: posterior approach.

## Outpatient management

### Non-operative management of humeral shaft fractures

| Outpatient management summary | | | |
| --- | --- | --- | --- |
| **Week** | **Examination** | **Radiographs** | **Additional notes** |
| 2 | Neurovascular status<br><br>Removal of U-slab | AP and lateral humerus | Apply functional brace<br><br>Allow pendular movements of the shoulder, full movements of elbow |
| 8 | | AP and lateral humerus | Commence physiotherapy<br><br>Reduce use of collar-and-cuff |
| 12 | | AP and lateral humerus | Allow unrestricted movements<br><br>If there is radiological and clinical union, discharge to physiotherapy |
| Further assessments at 4-week intervals if required for delayed union | | | |
| Average time to union = 9 weeks | | | |

### Operative management of humeral shaft fractures

| Outpatient management summary | | | |
| --- | --- | --- | --- |
| **Week** | **Examination** | **Radiographs** | **Additional notes** |
| 1 | Neurovascular status<br><br>Wound check | AP and lateral humerus | Impose no limitation on active movement but allow restricted weight-bearing |
| 10 | | AP and lateral humerus | Allow unrestricted movements<br><br>If there is radiological and clinical union, discharge to physiotherapy |
| Further assessments at 4-week intervals if required for delayed union | | | |
| Average time to union = 9 weeks | | | |

## COMPLICATIONS

### Early

Local    Radial nerve injury: A radial nerve palsy at presentation is not an indication for surgical exploration. An evolving nerve palsy, or one that arises after surgery, should usually be explored. Most radial nerve palsies are lesions in continuity (neurapraxia or axonotmesis; p. 50) and resolve spontaneously over 3–4 months

Vascular injury: The brachial and profundus arteries are at risk during injury and surgery, but a dysvascular limb is very rare because of the rich collateral circulation

### Late

Local    Non-union: This occurs in up to 10% of cases. Open reduction and internal fixation may be required

Malunion: Although evident radiographically, this is usually functionally irrelevant, as the range of movement at the shoulder will compensate for the deformity

## LONG HEAD OF BICEPS RUPTURE (PROXIMAL INJURY AT THE SHOULDER)

Rupture of the long head of biceps may present in one of two ways:

- *Attritional rupture*: This occurs in elderly patients as a component of rotator cuff tendonopathy. The degenerate long head of biceps has often been a source of pain prior to injury and complete rupture may actually provide symptomatic relief.

- *Traumatic rupture*: This occurs in younger patients during heavy weight-lifting. There is a history of a sharp pain and occasionally an audible 'pop'. Bruising gradually evolves over a few hours.

## Emergency Department management

### Clinical features
- The 'Popeye' appearance arises because the muscle belly of the long head, no longer held to length by its tendon, contracts to form a short and bulging muscle belly in the mid-arm (**Fig. 9.23**).

- Confirmation should be sought that the swelling arises from the biceps muscle belly and not, for example, skin or bone.
- Palpation will establish whether the biceps tendon insertion into the radius remains intact, and other injuries to the shoulder, humerus and elbow should be excluded.

### Radiological features
- *AP and modified axial shoulder radiographs*: These may be required to exclude a bony injury.
- *Ultrasound scan*: The diagnosis is usually evident on clinical examination but an ultrasound scan may be useful where there is uncertainty.

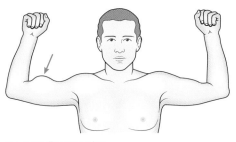

Fig. 9.23 Popeye sign.

## Immobilization

Provide a collar-and-cuff, and analgesia, for comfort.

## Outpatient referral

- Patients should be referred for assessment of the rotator cuff and consideration of a biceps tenodesis (surgical suturing of the long head of biceps to the bicipital groove of the humeral head).

# BICEPS TENDON AVULSION (DISTAL INJURY AT THE ELBOW)

At the elbow, the biceps tendon can be avulsed from its insertion into the bicipital tuberosity of the radius. Patients are typically men over the age of 35 engaged in body-building or heavy lifting manœuvres.

## Emergency Department management

### Clinical features

- There will be prominence of the biceps belly, although this is not usually so marked or well defined as a long head of biceps rupture. Bruising is usually minimal.
- There will be tenderness just above the elbow crease and a tender fullness over the biceps belly.
- An attempt should be made to define whether the biceps tendon is present or absent. Start with the uninjured side and, with the elbow flexed, press your fingertip into the medial side of the antecubital fossa; slide it laterally, feeling for the well-defined edge of the biceps tendon. Compare this with the injured side: a clear absence of the tendon with pain is diagnostic.
- The patient will still be able to demonstrate active elbow flexion, as brachialis remains intact.

### Radiological features

- *AP and lateral elbow radiographs*: These may be required to exclude a bony injury.
- *Ultrasound scan*: The diagnosis is usually evident on clinical examination but an ultrasound scan may be useful where there is uncertainty.

### Immobilization

Provide analgesia and a collar-and-cuff for comfort.

### Inpatient referral

The patient should be referred to Orthopaedics for consideration of repair of the injury, as approximately half of the supination strength and one-third of elbow flexion strength are lost.

## Orthopaedic management

Most injuries occur in working-age men and are suitable for repair. The procedure is performed under general anaesthesia. A transverse incision is made at the antecubital fossa. The tract of the avulsed tendon is usually evident and a finger can be passed through it to touch the exposed bicipital tuberosity. The avulsed tendon end is retrieved and secured with whip-stitches. A drill hole (or holes) is (are) placed at the tuberosity and the tendon is secured with a suture button device, suture anchor or transosseous sutures.

## GENERAL PRINCIPLES

## Anatomy

### Distal humerus (Fig. 10.1)

The distal humerus is an anatomically complex region in which the cylindrical humeral *shaft* gradually flattens out to form the medial and lateral *supracondylar ridges*, which then terminate in the medial and lateral *condyles*. The most prominent points of the condyles are termed the *epicondyles*. Between the two supracondylar ridges are two fossae: anteriorly is the *coronoid fossa*, which accommodates the coronoid process of the ulna in full elbow flexion, and posteriorly is the *olecranon fossa*, which accommodates the olecranon process in full elbow extension (**Fig. 10.2**). Each fossa is filled with a fat pad, which, in the presence of a haemarthrosis, floats out into the joint and can be perceived as a triangular filling defect on a lateral elbow radiograph (the sail sign; see Fig. 10.7). The condyles bear the articular surfaces of the humerus, which project distally and anteriorly at 45°, and are slightly angled to give around 6° of physiological valgus at the elbow. The distal humerus articulates with the ulna via the *trochlea* (Latin: 'pulley'), and with the radial head via the *capitellum* (Latin: 'small

head'). Mechanically, the distal humerus is described as having medial and lateral *columns*, separated by the 'tie arch' of the articular component.

### Proximal radius and ulna

The olecranon has a saddle-shaped articular surface that conforms closely with the trochlea of the distal humerus, imparting considerable stability to the elbow joint. The anterior process is termed the coronoid (Greek: 'raven's beak'; see Fig. 11.1). On the lateral side of the olecranon is the radial notch, which articulates with the radial head (see Fig. 10.23). The triceps tendon inserts into the olecranon, and the brachialis muscle and anterior joint capsule

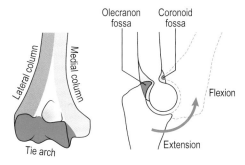

Fig. 10.2 Distal humerus: functional anatomy.

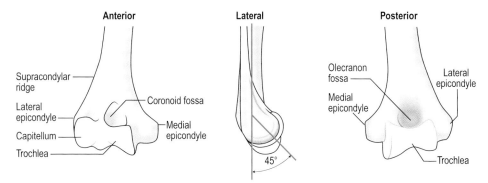

Fig. 10.1 Distal humerus: osteology.

into the coronoid. The proximal radius has a short cylindrical head, which rotates against the capitellum, and within the radial notch of the ulna, during pronation and supination. It is restrained in this articulation by the annular ligament. The bicipital tuberosity of the radius is the insertion point of the thick biceps tendon.

### Neurovascular anatomy

The brachial artery passes medial to the biceps tendon to cross the elbow joint before dividing into the radial and ulnar arteries. It has a rich collateral circulation at the elbow; there may be distal perfusion and normal capillary return even after complete occlusion (or division) of the artery.

Each of the three peripheral nerves of the upper limb crosses the elbow and enters the forearm between the two heads of a muscle:

- The *median nerve* travels medial to the brachial artery and passes between the two heads of pronator teres to gain access to the space between flexor digitorum profundus and flexor digitorum superficialis. It gives off the anterior interosseous nerve (AIN). The AIN supplies the radial half of flexor digitorum profundus, flexor pollicis longus and pronator quadratus, thus allowing the formation of the 'OK' sign of a circular ring between thumb and index finger; the loss of this movement suggests an AIN palsy. The median nerve proper continues to supply most of the superficial flexor compartment of the forearm, before passing through the carpal tunnel (see Fig. 12.3) to supply the LOAF muscles of the hand (lateral two *lumbricals, opponens pollicis, abductor pollicis brevis* and *flexor pollicis brevis*). The median nerve is most commonly injured in supracondylar fractures of the humerus and in conditions affecting the carpal tunnel (p. 259).

- The *ulnar nerve* travels intimately behind the medial epicondyle of the humerus, where it is easily injured, to pass between the two heads of flexor carpi ulnaris (which it supplies). It then passes through the forearm (also supplying the ulnar half of flexor digitorum profundus), before passing through

Guyon's canal at the wrist (see Fig. 12.3) to supply the intrinsic muscles of the hand.

- The *radial nerve* crosses the elbow joint anterior to the lateral epicondyle between brachialis and brachioradialis, where it divides into the radial nerve proper (sensory) and the posterior interosseous nerve (PIN; motor). While the radial nerve continues distally under brachioradialis, the PIN passes through the supinator muscle and winds around the radius to reach the posterior compartment of the forearm, which it supplies. The PIN is in danger during dissection around the proximal radius. When an anterior approach is adopted, the forearm must be supinated to take the PIN laterally. When a lateral approach is adopted, the forearm is pronated to carry the PIN anteriorly and medially (see Fig. 10.20).

## Clinical assessment of the painful elbow

### History

Define the reason for presentation: has there been an acute definable injury or is this an atraumatic or recurrent complaint? A high-energy mechanism of injury, such as a motor vehicle collision or fall from a height, suggests the possibility of other associated injuries and the requirement to assess and manage these first (see Ch. 2).

A localized elbow injury most commonly follows a simple fall on to an outstretched hand or the point of the elbow. The patterns of fractures around the elbow are classically related to the elbow flexion angle at the time of injury, although the patient will often not recall the precise sequence of events:

- Radial head and coronoid fractures typically occur at flexion angles of less than 80° (i.e. an outstretched arm).

- Olecranon fractures occur following a fall on to an elbow held at around 90° of flexion.

- Distal humerus fractures are seen when the flexion angle exceeds 110°.

Patients with an *atraumatic presentation* of elbow joint pain should be assessed for an acute monoarthritis (p. 103). Features of systemic upset with fever and malaise may indicate a septic arthritis. Enquire about previous injuries, operations or problems with the affected elbow, and obtain a medical history.

## Examination

### Look

Examine the elbow circumferentially, assessing for swelling, deformity and, later, bruising. Assess any skin abrasion or laceration, and consider the possibility of an open fracture or penetrating intra-articular injury.

### Feel

Gently palpate the shoulder and humerus, and then move down to the elbow.

Palpate the bony landmarks of the elbow. Palpation of the posterior aspect of the flexed elbow reveals an *inverted equilateral triangle* with apices at the medial and lateral epicondyles, and the point of the olecranon (**Fig. 10.3**). Disruption of this triangle suggests a displaced fracture or dislocation. Locate the lateral epicondyle and then move distally to identify the radiocapitellar articulation and the *radial head*. With the examining thumb on the radial head, gently pronate and supinate the forearm, and assess radial head movement, crepitus and pain. Palpate the subcutaneous border of the olecranon. Finally, palpate the forearm and wrist for deformity and tenderness.

### Move

Confirm the range of movement from full extension (0°) to full flexion (150°). With the elbow held at 90°, assess the range of pronation (80°) and supination (80°) (**Fig. 10.4**).

### Neurovascular assessment

Conduct a thorough assessment of sensation and power in the distributions of the median, radial and ulnar nerves (see Figs 3.17–3.19). Palpate the radial pulse and check the capillary refill to the fingernails. Major arterial injury is rare but may present as a pulsatile expanding haematoma. The classical signs of an acutely dysvascular limb (Box 3.1) are rare, as there is a rich collateral circulation.

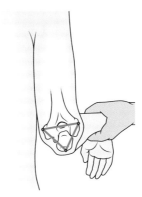

Fig. 10.3 Elbow examination: feel.

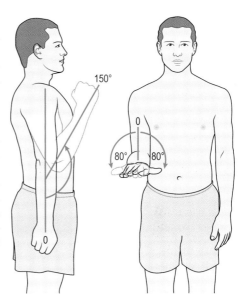

Fig. 10.4 Elbow examination: move.

## Radiological assessment of the painful elbow

### Radiographs

- *AP view of the elbow* (**Fig. 10.5A**): The elbow is held in extension with the forearm fully supinated.

- *Lateral view of the elbow* (**Fig. 10.5B**): The elbow is held at 90° of flexion with the forearm fully supinated. The trochlea and capitellum are superimposed and the joint space is visible.

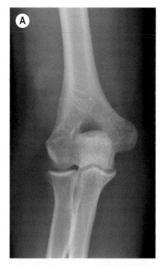

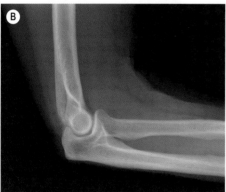

Fig. 10.5 Normal elbow radiographs. **A**, AP view. **B**, Lateral view.

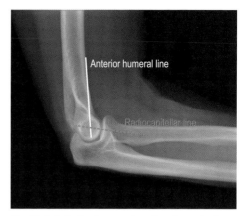

Fig. 10.6 Anterior humeral and radiocapitellar lines.

against the cortex. However, a haemarthrosis results in elevated fat pads that give the characteristic appearance of a ship that has raised its sails. This indicates the likelihood of a fracture being present, even if the fracture itself cannot be discerned on the radiograph. The most common occult fracture is an undisplaced radial head or neck fracture.

## CT

CT scans may assist in the evaluation of and preoperative planning for intra-articular distal humerus fractures.

Interpretation of the films is assisted by referring to specific radiographic features:

- The *radiocapitellar line* (**Fig. 10.6**): A line drawn through the centre of the radial neck should pass through the centre of the capitellum in any view.
- The *anterior humeral line* (**Fig. 10.6**): A line drawn along the anterior cortex of the humerus in the lateral view should transect the capitellum.
- The *sail sign* (**Fig. 10.7**): The anterior and posterior fat pads may be just discernible in a normal lateral radiograph as dark lines

## DISTAL HUMERAL FRACTURES

Distal humeral fractures account for less than 1% of all fractures in adults but are often complex and challenging. There is a classical bimodal distribution of men in their second or third decade who have suffered high-energy injuries, and older osteoporotic women who have had a simple fall.

## Classification

### AO classification

The AO classification of distal humeral fractures follows the standard pattern of assessing injuries as extra-articular, partial articular or complete articular (**Fig. 10.8**). Fractures with a

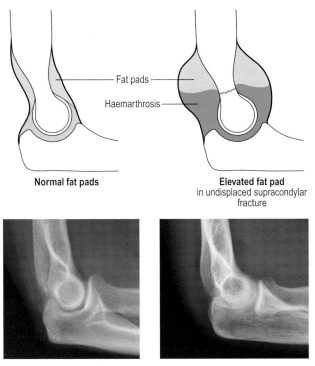

Fat pads

Haemarthrosis

**Normal fat pads**

**Elevated fat pad**
in undisplaced supracondylar
fracture

Fig. 10.7  Sail sign.

transverse component (A or C types) can also be described in relation to the fracture level as supracondylar (above the level of the condyles) or transcondylar (at the level of the condyles). Medial and lateral B-type fractures are occasionally termed condylar fractures. B3 (coronal plane) fractures are often more complex than is apparent on plain radiographs, involving the capitellum, trochlea or both.

### Bryan and Morrey classification
The Bryan and Morrey classification (**Fig. 10.9**) relates to fractures of the articular surface:

- Type I: substantial osteochondral fracture of the capitellum, also known as the Hahn–Steinthal fragment.

- Type II: thin, shell-like, fracture of the articular surface, also referred to as a Kocher–Lorenz fragment.

- Type III: comminuted fracture of the capitellum.

- Type IV: coronal shear of the capitellum with extension into the lateral portion of the trochlea, similar to an AO B3 pattern. On a lateral radiographic view, this fracture is indicated by the presence of a double arc (see Fig. 10.11); one contour is formed by the capitellum while the second is formed by part of the trochlea.

## Emergency Department management

### Clinical features
- A full examination of the elbow should be completed (p. 182).

- There is likely to be some deformity and swelling at the elbow, but bruising may not appear until a few hours after injury.

- It is important to establish whether the inverted equilateral triangle has been disrupted.

- Disruption of the brachial artery is most commonly indicated by the presence of an expanding haematoma rather than as an acutely dysvascular limb, as there is a rich collateral circulation around the elbow.

- A careful neurological examination should be performed of the three main nerves at the hand: median, ulnar and radial. Function of the AIN should also be confirmed by establishing the patient's ability to form the OK sign.

### Radiological features

- *AP and lateral elbow radiographs*: Assess the anterior humeral and radiocapitellar lines (see Fig. 10.6). Distal humeral fractures commonly fall into flexion or exten-

sion, and the entire outline of the capitellum may lie in front of, or behind, the anterior humeral line.

- *CT*: A CT scan may be helpful where there is complex intra-articular displacement, and three-dimensional reconstruction can be particularly useful.

### Reduction, immobilization and reassessment

Deformed limbs should be realigned. An above-elbow backslab (mid-humerus to metacarpal necks) will provide comfort and limit painful forearm rotation (see Fig. 4.9). Reassess the neurovascular status and obtain repeat radiographs.

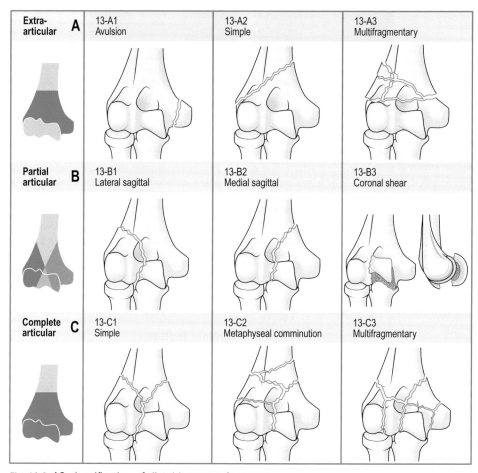

| Extra-articular | A | 13-A1 Avulsion | 13-A2 Simple | 13-A3 Multifragmentary |
| Partial articular | B | 13-B1 Lateral sagittal | 13-B2 Medial sagittal | 13-B3 Coronal shear |
| Complete articular | C | 13-C1 Simple | 13-C2 Metaphyseal comminution | 13-C3 Multifragmentary |

Fig. 10.8 AO classification of distal humerus fractures.

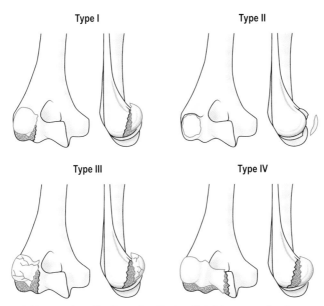

Type I    Type II

Type III    Type IV

Fig. 10.9 Bryan and Morrey classification of articular distal humerus fractures.

## Outpatient follow-up
- Undisplaced or minimally displaced fractures should be seen at the fracture clinic.

## Inpatient referral
- Intra-articular or displaced fractures.
- Neurovascular compromise.
- Open fractures.

## Orthopaedic management
### Non-operative
- *Minimally displaced fractures*: These can be treated non-operatively in a cast or splint for 6 weeks, with regular radiographic review to ensure that no displacement occurs.
- *Displaced fractures in the elderly*: In patients with poor bone quality or those too frail for surgery, displaced fractures may be managed non-operatively. Acceptance of the displacement, with early mobilization, aims to create a painless pseudoarthrosis (false joint) at the fracture site. This is frequently termed the 'bag of bones' treatment and often both starts and results in a functionally poor bag of bones. Fixation or arthroplasty is preferred, if at all possible.

### Operative
Almost all displaced distal humerus fractures are managed surgically. There are three options:

- *Fragment excision*: Small fragments such as the Kocher–Lorenz (Bryan and Morrey II) fracture may be too small to allow fixation and are generally removed to avoid restriction in range of movement.
- *Open reduction and internal fixation*: Most displaced fractures are fixed to restore normal anatomy and optimize limb function (see Fig. 10.12).
- *Elbow arthroplasty* (**Fig. 10.10**): Low transcondylar fractures in elderly, osteoporotic or rheumatoid patients may defy reconstruction and are best treated with a primary elbow arthroplasty.

### Surgical techniques
#### A-type fractures – extra-articular
Extra-articular supracondylar fractures are most common in children (p. 569). In adults, they are often minimally displaced and therefore treated non-operatively in a cast or splint. Significant displacement is defined as more than 20° of angulation in flexion or extension, varus or valgus. Displaced fractures are treated with plating (p. 189).

### B-type fractures – partial articular

- Displaced B1 (lateral condyle) and B2 (medial condyle) fractures are addressed with lag screws or buttress plating.

- B3 (coronal split) fractures are challenging injuries. Large fragments can be reduced under direct vision via a Kocher's approach (see Figs 10.18–10.19) and fixed with compact 1.5-mm or 2-mm screws, or with headless screws (**Fig. 10.11**).

### C-type fractures – complete articular

The medial and lateral columns, and the articular 'tie arch' between them, must be reduced anatomically, compressed, and fixed with absolute stability (**Fig. 10.12**). The distal humerus is approached from the posterior aspect. The overlying triceps muscle is circumvented in one of three ways:

- *Olecranon osteotomy*: The olecranon fragment and the entire triceps muscle can be elevated proximally to provide a wide articular exposure. The osteotomy is fixed at the end of the procedure with a tension band wire construct, olecranon plate or single large intramedullary screw (see below).

- *Triceps-splitting approach*: This is performed by dividing the triceps tendon in the midline and then dissecting the tendon sharply from either side of the olecranon, creating medial and lateral myotendinous sleeves. This leaves the olecranon intact, avoiding the potential problems of non-union and metalwork prominence, but partially restricts the view of the articular surface. At the conclusion of the case, the split is repaired by suturing the two sleeves together. A transosseous suture, placed through a drill hole at the tip of the olecranon, improves the strength of this repair.

- *'Triceps-sparing' approach*: It is possible to leave the extensor mechanism intact and work under the triceps muscle, retracting it alternately from side to side. This approach provides only a restricted view of the articular surface and is most commonly used for A-type extra-articular fractures.

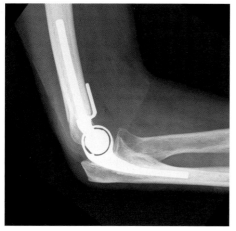

Fig. 10.10 Total elbow replacement.

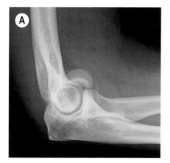 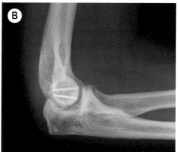 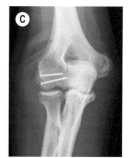

Fig. 10.11 Capitellar fracture fixation. **A**, Coronal shear fracture, Bryan and Morrey type IV. Note the 'double arc' sign of the displaced fragment. **B**, lateral radiograph after open reduction and fixation with 2-mm lag screws. **C**, AP radiograph.

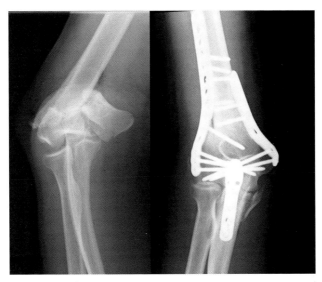

Fig. 10.12 Distal humerus plating.

## SURGICAL TECHNIQUE: Distal humerus plating – trans-olecranon approach

### Surgical set-up
The patient is placed in the lateral decubitus position, with the arm over a bolster, and the forearm hanging free and vertically downwards. A tourniquet is used. AP and lateral fluoroscopic views are taken preoperatively to ensure that the image intensifier can achieve satisfactory access (see Fig. 9.20).

### Orthopaedic equipment
- Small fragment set
- 1.6-mm k-wires
- Standard fragment reduction clamps
- Pre-contoured, region-specific plates, or a combination of pelvic reconstruction and 3.5-mm dynamic compression plates

### Incision
A longitudinal posterior incision is made through skin, fat and fascia to the triceps muscle, extending from the mid-portion of the humerus, curving around the point of the elbow and extending 10 cm along the subcutaneous border of the ulna (see Fig. 9.21).

### Approach (Fig. 10.13)
Internervous plane: There is no internervous plane, as the approach involves elevating triceps.

The approach begins with identification of the ulnar nerve as it passes around the medial epicondyle. The nerve, along with its thin investing film of vascular fatty tissue, is exposed, mobilized, marked with a vascular loop and protected throughout the case. An olecranon

*Continued*

osteotomy is made, such that it enters the articular surface in the 'bare area'– a point midway between the tip of the olecranon and the coronoid process that is not covered by articular cartilage (see Fig. 10.16). A chevron (V-shaped) osteotomy, with the tip pointing distally, is used, as this will provide maximal stability after fixation. If the plan is to fix this with a large intramedullary screw at the conclusion of the case, the pilot hole for this screw is pre-drilled at this point, before the osteotomy. The olecranon fragment is then grasped and the triceps progressively dissected proximally to expose the fracture (**Fig. 10.13B**).

### Open reduction (Fig. 10.14)

There are usually more articular fragments than have been demonstrated on preoperative imaging. These will be small and care is required to identify, disimpact and clear them without dropping them! The distal fragments of the medial and lateral columns are often shortened and rotated anteriorly (away from the surgeon) and towards each other. These are reduced with a clamp to provide compression and temporarily fixed with k-wires. Small buried screws or threaded wires may be used to secure small articular fragments.

### Internal fixation – absolute stability (Fig. 10.15)

1. *Plates*: Absolute stability must be achieved with the use of two plates, one on each column. Two equally satisfactory options are:
    a. Parallel plates: Pre-contoured locking plates may still require fine adjustments to shape before application.
    b. Orthogonal '90/90' plating: The medial column plate is placed medially and the lateral column plate is placed posteriorly. If region-specific plates are not available, a 3.5-mm pelvic reconstruction plate can be placed on the medial side while a 3.5-cm dynamic compression plate is placed posteriorly.
    Once applied, the plates can be held with clamps and temporary k-wires.
2. *Distal screws*: The distal screws should aim to pass through a plate, cross the entire width of the metaphysis, and engage with a fragment in the opposite column. By using multiple long, interdigitating screws from each side, an arch is recreated under the articular surface.
3. *Proximal screws*: Careful reduction of the reconstructed articular block to the shaft is required to re-establish stability and orientation. Where there is inadequate cortical contact owing to comminution, some shortening at the supracondylar region is required in order to allow compression.

### Closure (Fig. 10.16)

An olecranon osteotomy is repaired with an intramedullary screw or olecranon plate, or by using a tension band technique.

### Post procedure

A backslab may be applied for postoperative comfort.

### Postoperative restrictions

Movement: Early gentle active movement may be permitted. Excessive, forceful movement at this stage is painful and may encourage the development of heterotopic ossification (see 'Complications' below).

Weight-bearing: The patient should lift nothing heavier than a glass of water until union.

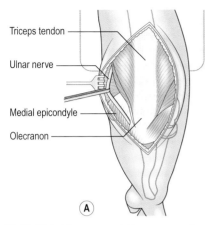
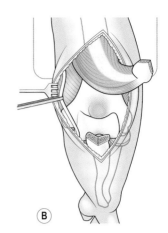

Triceps tendon

Ulnar nerve

Medial epicondyle

Olecranon

Fig. 10.13 Distal humerus plating: approach.

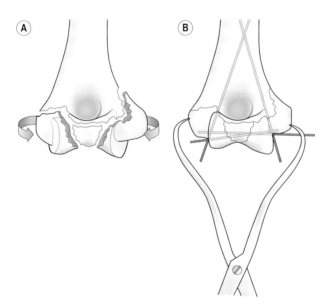

Fig. 10.14 Fracture of the distal humerus: reduction. **A**, The condyles usually displace in rotation anteriorly and are reduced by de-rotating them posteriorly. **B**, The reduction is temporarily held with k-wires (placed under the articular surface and along both columns) and clamps.

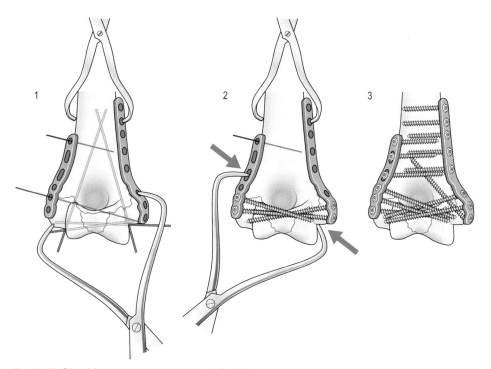

Fig. 10.15 Distal humerus plating: internal fixation.

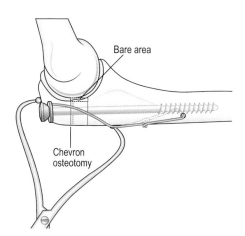

Fig. 10.16 Repair of olecranon osteotomy.

## Outpatient management

| Outpatient management summary | | | |
| --- | --- | --- | --- |
| Week | Examination | Radiographs | Additional notes |
| 1 | Neurovascular status<br>Wound check | AP and<br>lateral elbow | Begin active range of movement<br>exercises for the elbow |
| 6 | Assessment of<br>range of movement | AP and<br>lateral elbow | Continue physiotherapy |
| 12 | Confirmation of<br>clinical union | AP and<br>lateral elbow | If there is radiographic and clinical<br>union, lift restrictions on activity<br>and discharge to physiotherapy |

Further assessments at 4-week intervals if required for delayed union

Average time to union = 8 weeks

## COMPLICATIONS

### Early

Local    Ulnar nerve injury: The ulnar nerve is within the operative field and is at risk of iatrogenic injury

Loss of reduction: Poor implant selection can predispose to early construct failure. In adults, k-wires and 1/3 tubular plates are insufficiently robust to maintain fracture reduction during rehabilitation. Similarly, use of pelvic reconstruction plates for both medial and lateral columns has been shown to have insufficient strength to maintain the reduction

Infection: This may involve the elbow joint itself and can be very challenging to treat

### Late

Local    Stiffness: Loss of motion, particularly terminal extension, is common after distal humerus fracture. The minimum functional arc of elbow movement is 30–130°. An extensive capsular release and removal of metalwork are indicated if this is lost

Implant irritation: The metalwork on the medial aspect of the distal humerus and at the olecranon can be particularly irksome and may require removal

Heterotopic ossification (HO): HO is classically associated with severe elbow injuries and may compromise final range of movement and function. It is more common after recurrent manipulations or surgeries, and with overly aggressive rehabilitation. Excision of mature HO may be required, along with a capsular release and removal of metalwork as a late procedure

## RADIAL HEAD AND NECK FRACTURES

Elbow pain due to radial head fracture is a common presentation to the Emergency Department. *Most injuries are isolated, minimally displaced and stable*, and require only symptomatic treatment. However, there are unstable variants that must be actively sought and excluded:

- *Essex–Lopresti injury*: The combination of a radial head fracture and an injury to the distal radio-ulnar joint (see Fig. 11.3) can result in progressive forearm displacement and usually requires surgical treatment.

- *Monteggia fracture dislocation*: The combination of a radial head dislocation (with or without a radial head fracture) and ulnar fracture (see Fig. 11.3) is highly unstable.

- *'Terrible triad' injury*: The combination of a radial head fracture with an elbow dislocation suggests the potential for an unstable elbow (see Fig. 10.31).

## Classification

### Mason classification (Fig. 10.17)

This describes displacement and comminution:

- type I: minimally displaced fractures.

- type II: simple fractures with some displacement or angulation

- type III: comminuted or displaced fractures

- type IV: associated elbow dislocation (later addition to the classification).

## Emergency Department management

### Clinical features

- Confirm that there was no sensation of elbow dislocation at the time of injury. Exclude tenderness of the ulna shaft and any suggestion of pain or tenderness at the wrist.

- Gently assess the range of movement at the elbow in flexion/extension, as well as pronation/supination.

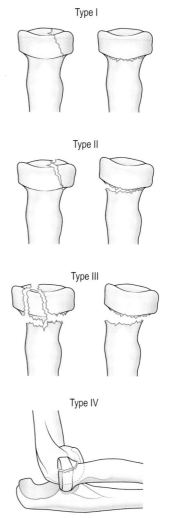

Type I

Type II

Type III

Type IV

Fig. 10.17 Mason classification of radial head and neck fractures.

### Radiological features

- *AP and lateral elbow radiographs*: There may be a clear abnormality of the radial head or neck. However, occult undisplaced fractures are common and the only abnormality may be a positive 'sail sign' (see Fig. 10.7).

- *AP and lateral views of the forearm or wrist*: These are indicated if clinical examination indicates a distal injury.

**Key point**

Always perform a careful examination of a patient's wrist if a radial head fracture has been sustained. Pain at the distal radio-ulnar joint is suggestive of an Essex–Lopresti fracture dislocation, which is a more severe injury (see p. 214).

### Inpatient referral
- Essex–Lopresti injury.
- Monteggia fracture/dislocation.
- Associated elbow dislocation.
- Neurovascular compromise.
- Open injuries.

### Outpatient follow-up
- Occult radial head fracture (sail sign only).
- Mason types 1–3.

### Patient instructions
Patients are advised to move the arm freely within the limits of comfort to prevent stiffness. They should be reminded that movement, although uncomfortable, will not lead to harm.

## Orthopaedic management

### Non-operative
- Mason type I and II fractures: These are treated conservatively with advice, reassur-ance and simple exercises. The patient should be warned that, although a gradual recovery is likely, there may ultimately be some slight loss of the last 5–10° of elbow extension.

### Operative
Indications for surgery include:

- Mason II or III fractures with persistent loss of pronation/supination
- persistent radiocapitellar crepitus or pain.

### Surgical techniques
Radial head injuries can be addressed with radial head excision, open reduction and fixa-tion, or a prosthetic replacement. Radial head excision is appropriate for most isolated, dis-placed head fractures. Caution is required with more complex acute injuries; excision of the radial head in the presence of an Essex–Lopresti lesion or a Monteggia fracture disloca-tion results in secondary wrist or elbow problems. In the presence of other injuries or where there is a suspicion of elbow instability, fixation or replacement may be indicated. Frac-tures with two substantial head fragments may be suitable for reduction and fixation, but more comminuted fractures are best treated with a prosthetic replacement of the radial head.

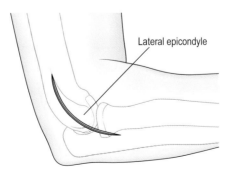

Lateral epicondyle

Fig. 10.18 Kocher's incision.

## SURGICAL TECHNIQUE: Radial head fixation/replacement – Kocher's approach

### Surgical set-up

The patient is placed supine, with the arm on a hand table. A tourniquet is used. Rehearse obtaining adequate AP and lateral fluoroscopic images before preparing and draping the patient.

### Incision (Fig. 10.18)

A lateral oblique incision is made, starting 5 cm proximal to the lateral epicondyle and extending over the epicondyle to curve over the radiocapitellar joint.

### Approach (Fig. 10.19)

Internervous plane: The plane is between anconeus (radial nerve) and extensor carpi ulnaris (PIN).

Kocher's interval is identified as a fine white stripe, best visualized away from the epicondyle. This interval is opened to expose the joint capsule (with its condensations: the lateral collateral ligament and annular ligaments) (**Fig. 10.19A**). At this point, the forearm is pronated; this has the effect of pulling the PIN away from the operative field (**Fig. 10.20**). The lateral collateral ligament is incised longitudinally through its mid-axial point; more posterior dissection may damage the lateral ulnar collateral ligament, resulting in later posterolateral instability (**Fig. 10.19B**). Proximal extension is afforded by incising along the supracondylar ridge and dissecting the anterior half of the common extensor origin and capsule anteriorly.

### Radial head fixation

A fracture with only two or three articular fragments, and no metaphyseal comminution, can be reduced and fixed. This is achieved with 1.5-mm or 2-mm interfragmentary compression screws, which are often stabilized with a small T-plate. To avoid this blocking the radio-ulnar articulation at the radial fossa, it is placed in the 90° 'safe zone' that is demarcated by the positions of the radial styloid and Lister's tubercle (**Fig. 10.21**).

### Radial head replacement (Fig. 10.22)

More comminuted fractures are treated by replacement. The radial neck is exposed carefully, then cut transversely with a small oscillating saw, and the head is excised. The head of the metal prosthesis is sized using the diameter and height of the excised radial head as a template. The stem is sized to fit the patient's radial canal. The prosthesis is impacted into the radius to sit at the correct height; this must be judged carefully, as 'overstuffing' the joint results in excessive capitellar contact pressure, chondrolysis and pain. The correct position can be judged visually at the time of surgery; the prosthetic articulating surface should align perfectly with the adjacent articular surface of the radial fossa of the ulna (**Fig. 10.23A**). Radiographically, the ulnohumeral joint space must be parallel; diverging joint lines suggest overstuffing (**Fig. 10.23B**).

### Postoperative restrictions

Movement: Early active movement should be encouraged.

Weight-bearing: The patient is instructed not to lift anything heavier than a glass of water until fracture union.

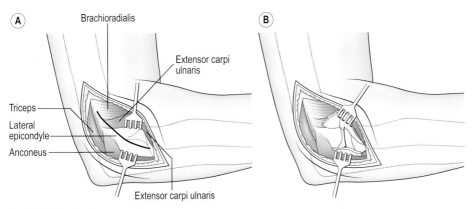

Fig. 10.19 Kocher's approach.

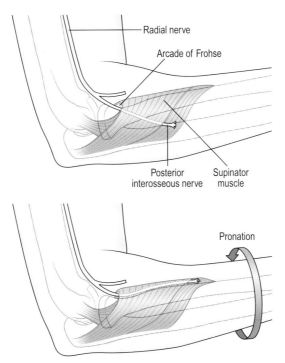

Fig. 10.20 Pronation to protect the PIN during the lateral approach to the radial head.

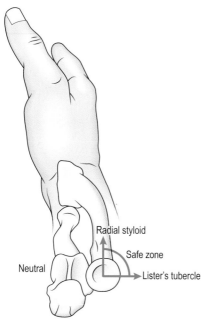

Fig. 10.21 Radial neck safe zone.

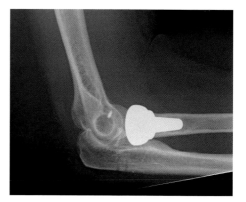

Fig. 10.22 Radial head replacement.

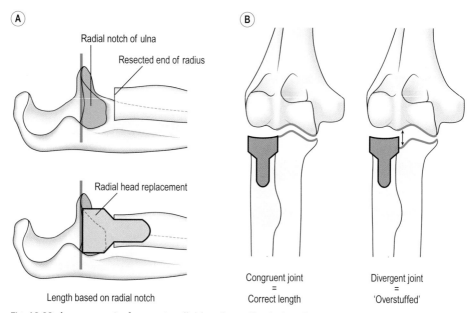

Fig. 10.23 Assessment of correct radial head prosthesis length.

## Outpatient management

| Outpatient management summary | | | |
|---|---|---|---|
| **Week** | **Examination** | **Radiographs** | **Additional notes** |
| 1 | Wound check<br>Neurovascular status | AP and lateral elbow | Allow gentle active elbow movement |
| 6 | Assessment of range of movement | AP and lateral elbow | With a radial head prosthesis, allow unrestricted movements. After fixation, lift restrictions once the fracture has united |

Further assessments at 12 weeks if required for delayed union

Average time to union=8weeks

## COMPLICATIONS

### *Early*

| Local | Stiffness: Loss of motion, particularly the last 5–10° of terminal extension, is common |
|---|---|

### *Late*

| Local | Post-traumatic arthritis: Although some incongruity remains permanently, symptomatic arthritis is rarely a problem. Where there is pain or restricted movement, however, a radial head excision is usually effective |
|---|---|

## OLECRANON FRACTURES

Olecranon fractures are common injuries, resulting from a direct fall on to the elbow. The proximal fragment is often displaced proximally by the triceps muscle.

## Classification

### Mayo classification (Fig. 10.24)

- Type 1: undisplaced. There may be some articular impaction (type 1B).
- Type 2: displaced but stable elbow joint. Type 2A fractures have a simple articular fracture and are amenable to compression fixation (often a tension band wire), whilst type 2B fractures have articular comminu- tion and may require plate fixation.
- Type 3: displaced with unstable elbow joint – a fracture dislocation of the elbow.

## Emergency Department management

### Clinical features

- Inspect any wounds for a breach in the dermis, particularly over the subcutaneous border of the ulna.
- You may be able to palpate a displaced fragment and a defect.

### Radiological features

- *AP and lateral elbow radiographs* (**Fig. 10.25**): Pay close attention to the position of the distal fragment of the olecranon. The

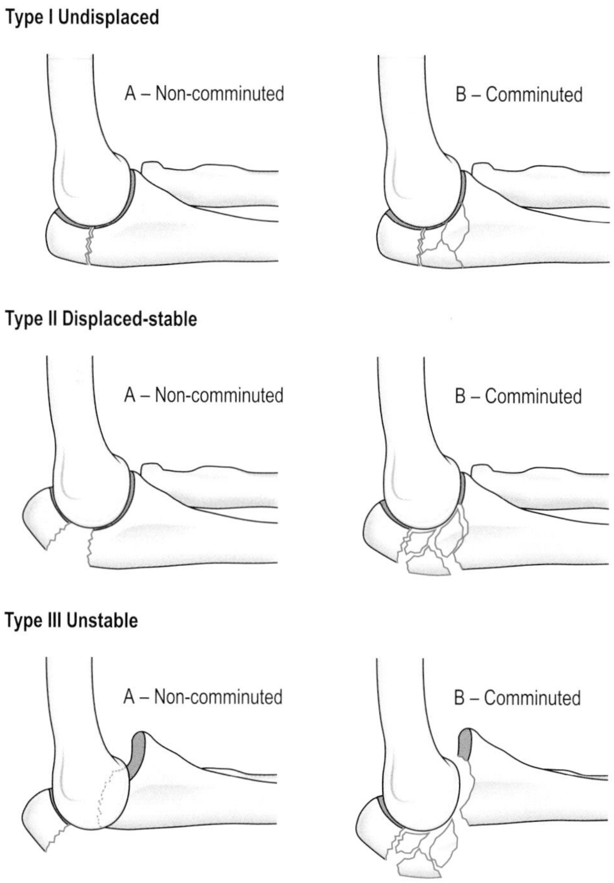

**Type I Undisplaced**

A – Non-comminuted

B – Comminuted

**Type II Displaced-stable**

A – Non-comminuted

B – Comminuted

**Type III Unstable**

A – Non-comminuted

B – Comminuted

Fig. 10.24 Mayo classification of olecranon fractures.

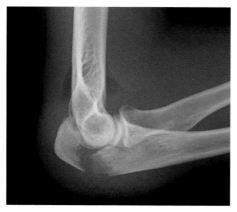

Fig. 10.25 Mayo type 2A fracture.

proximal fragment is displaced proximally by triceps but the distal piece should remain congruent with the trochlea.

### Reduction
This is only indicated in the case of a type 3 injury (fracture-dislocation) and aims to reduce the residual articular surface with the trochlea. Anatomical reduction of the proximal olecranon fragment is not feasible.

### Immobilization and reassessment
- An above elbow backslab and collar and cuff should be provided for type 1 and type 2 injuries.

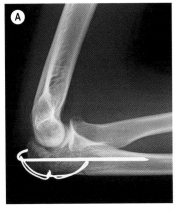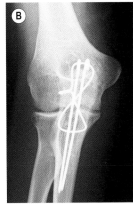

Fig. 10.26 Olecranon fracture fixed with a tension band wire. **A**, Mayo type 2A fracture, lateral. **B**, AP view.

- Type 3 injuries with elbow dislocation may be more comfortably supported with a backslab.

### Outpatient follow-up
- Type 1 injuries.

### Inpatient referral
- Type 2 and 3 injuries (displaced fractures).
- Open fractures.
- Neurovascular compromise.

## Orthopaedic management
### Non-operative
- Mayo type 1 (undisplaced) fractures: Patients are allowed a free active range of gentle movement from the outset, with a collar-and-cuff for rest.
- Mayo type 2 fractures in the elderly (>70s): These patients have surprisingly good functional outcomes with non-operative management despite complete displacement of the fracture. The slight loss of elbow extension power is more than offset by the avoidance of surgical complications. A splint may be required for comfort for the first 2 weeks.

### Operative
- Mayo type 2 fractures (displaced and/or comminuted) in patients ≤70 years old.
- Mayo type 3 (fracture-dislocation).

## Surgical techniques
### Tension band wire – Mayo type 2A
Type 2A fractures are amenable to tension band wiring (**Fig. 10.26–10.27**). This surgical technique converts distraction at the fracture site to compression of the articular surface around the fulcrum of the trochlea (p. 95). It cannot be used in fractures with articular comminution, as the joint surface will collapse.

### Olecranon plating – Mayo types 2B and 3
Where there is articular comminution, the compression effect of a tension band wire at the articular surface will often cause shortening and loss of articular congruence, and a *plating technique* is therefore preferred. Surgical set-up and exposure are as for tension band wiring. Careful articular elevation and reduction are followed by plate application. Given that the fragments are often small and osteoporotic, and that the plate is prominent in this subcutaneous position, a low-profile plate is often preferred (**Fig. 10.28**).

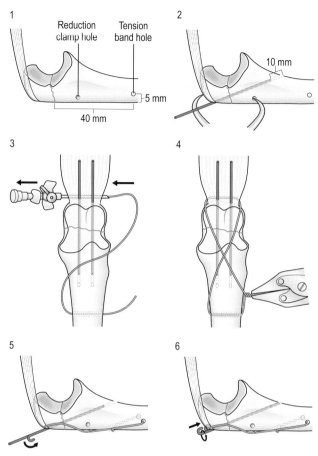

Fig. 10.27 Olecranon tension band wire.

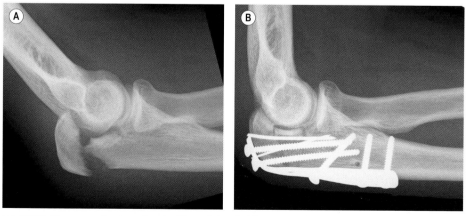

Fig. 10.28 Olecranon fracture fixed with a plate. **A**, Mayo type 2B fracture. **B**, Fracture reduced and fixed with wires, plate and screws.

## SURGICAL TECHNIQUE: Olecranon fracture fixation – tension band wiring or plating

### Surgical set-up
The patient is placed either supine, with the arm flexed over the chest, or in the lateral decubitus position, with the arm over a support. A tourniquet is used. Rehearse obtaining adequate AP and lateral fluoroscopic images before prepping and draping.

### Incision
The incision begins 2 cm proximal to the tip of the olecranon, and extends distally along the subcutaneous border of the ulna for 12 cm.

### Approach
Internervous plane: There is no internervous plane as the olecranon is subcutaneous.

Be mindful of the proximity of the ulnar nerve, as it lies around the medial epicondyle; no attempt is made to expose it in this procedure. The fracture margin is defined by dissecting the periosteum back 1–2 mm, and the fracture haematoma is removed. The muscle is dissected back from the subcutaneous edge of the ulna; posteriorly, these are the extensor compartment muscles, whereas, on the volar aspect, these are the flexors. The articular surface is examined for comminution.

### Open reduction
For a simple two-part fracture, the fragments are reduced together by extending the elbow slightly and manœuvring the olecranon fragment distally. The reduction is held with a reduction clamp; one tine is placed on the centre of the fragment, while the other is placed through a drill hole in the ulna shaft.

### Internal fixation – tension band wire (Fig. 10.27)
1. Drilling a hole: A 2.5-mm transverse hole is drilled in the shaft of the ulna for placement of the 1.2-mm flexible wire. The hole is placed around 40 mm from the fracture, and 5 mm back from the ulnar border to prevent later cutout.
2. Positioning the K-wire: Two parallel 1.6-mm k-wires are then passed across the fracture site. The start points are through the triceps tendon, one-third and two-thirds across the width of the olecranon. The wires should just penetrate the volar cortex of the ulna to improve hold. The wire positioning is checked fluoroscopically in both AP and lateral planes. The wires are now withdrawn by 10 mm to allow for later impaction.
3. Inserting the tension band wire: The tension band wire is passed through the distal hole, and then brought across the ulnar border to pass through the triceps tendon. It is important for the wire to pass deep to the tendon and sit on both the bone and the k-wires, to prevent the construct being levered out of place by the tendon during later elbow extension. This is achieved by passing a large-bore intravenous cannula through the tendon and using this to guide the passage of the flexible wire; the flexible wire tip is introduced into the bevelled end of the needle with the aim of pushing the needle back out. The needle is used to guide the wire and is gently withdrawn. Finally, the wire ends are brought together and twisted.
4. Tensioning the wire: Tension is applied by pulling and then twisting the wires (see Fig. 5.21) using pliers. When the shiny wire surface starts to look dull, the wire is reaching its tensile limit. The ends of the tension band wire are cut to leave three full twists and bent towards the bone to avoid irritation.
5. Preparing the k-wires: The exposed ends of the k-wires are bent through 180° and cut obliquely to leave pointed ends. Pliers are used to hold and bend the wire under careful control to avoid displacing the construct or loosening the grip of the wires.

*Continued*

6. Burying the k-wires: The bent ends are then rotated such that the bent tips are proximal. Small, longitudinal incisions are then made in the triceps tendon down to bone, and the bent wires are hammered down through these slits to capture the loop of flexible wire.

**Postoperative restrictions**

Movement: Early active movement is then begun immediately.

Weight-bearing: The patient is instructed not to lift anything heavier than a glass of water until fracture union.

## Outpatient management

| Outpatient management summary | | | |
|---|---|---|---|
| **Week** | **Examination** | **Radiographs** | **Additional notes** |
| 1 | Wound check if surgery performed | AP and lateral elbow | Ensure elbow joint remains congruent<br><br>Commence early range of movement |
| 6 | Assessment of range of movement and stability | AP and lateral elbow | If radiological and clinical examinations are satisfactory, discharge<br><br>Commence physiotherapy if there is a restricted range of movement |
| Further assessment at 10 weeks if required for delayed union | | | |
| Average time to union = 6 weeks | | | |

## Complications

Complications following olecranon fracture are similar to, but less frequent, than those seen in distal humerus fractures (p. 193). The most common issue is metalwork irritation at the subcutaneous border of the olecranon.

## ELBOW DISLOCATION

An elbow dislocation is typically a sporting or high-energy injury in a young adult patient. It is relatively uncommon in children, in whom a supracondylar fracture should be considered. The radius and ulna are displaced posterior to the humerus in 90% of cases. In 50% of elbow dislocations, there is disruption of the medial and lateral collateral ligaments, but no bony injury. In the other 50%, there is an additional bony injury, most commonly to the radial head or the coronoid process of the ulna. These two structures represent the static restraints to anterior movement of the humerus, and the coronoid is also the site of anterior capsular attachment. The 'terrible triad' injury consists of combined:

- elbow dislocation
- radial head fracture
- coronoid process fracture.

 **Key point**

Simple elbow dislocations are relatively benign injuries with a good prognosis after closed reduction, and have low rates of recurrence. They should be distinguished from fracture dislocations and, in particular, the 'terrible triad' injury, which is highly unstable and usually requires surgery.

## Box 10.1    Elbow stabilizers

| | |
|---|---|
| **Primary stabilizers** | Humero-ulnar joint |
| | Medial collateral ligament |
| | Lateral collateral ligament |
| **Secondary stabilizers** | Radiocapitellar joint |
| | Joint capsule – in particular the anterior aspect |
| | Origins of the common flexor and extensor tendons |

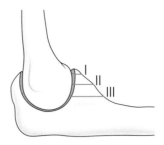

Fig. 10.29 Regan and Morrey classification of coronoid fractures.

## Pathoanatomy

The elbow is inherently stable due to the congruence of the bony anatomy, the collateral ligaments and the surrounding joint capsule. Stability is maintained by the primary stabilizers of the elbow (**Box 10.1**) and is reinforced by the secondary stabilizers. If both primary and secondary stabilizers are lost, the elbow becomes inherently unstable. For example, a dislocation resulting in rupture of the medial collateral ligament (in particular, the anterior bundle) will diminish the elbow's ability to resist valgus strain, although an intact radiocapitellar joint will limit this valgus movement of the elbow. If, however, the radial head is also injured, the elbow becomes highly unstable.

## Classification

A simple descriptive classification indicating the position of the forearm in relation to the arm is used. Some 90% of dislocations are posterior. Those without an associated fracture are referred to as 'simple', while those with fractures are 'complex'.

### Regan and Morrey classification

The Regan and Morrey classification is used for the description of any coronoid process fracture. It is based on the size of the detached fragment (**Fig. 10.29**):

I.   a small avulsion fragment from the tip of the coronoid

II.  a fragment <50% coronoid

III. a fragment >50% coronoid.

# Emergency Department management

## Clinical features

- Establish the mechanism of injury and the presence of any associated injuries or neurovascular symptoms.

- The elbow will be deformed and is usually held in near-extension. The patient will support the arm and will be unwilling to move it.

- The equilateral triangle of the elbow is disrupted in a dislocation but is preserved in a supracondylar fracture (which has a similar initial presentation).

- Neurapraxia, especially affecting the ulnar nerve, is relatively common.

- A critical appraisal of the radial pulse with a comparison to the uninjured side is required. A critically ischaemic limb will clearly need urgent surgical review and possible reconstruction (p. 58); however, more subtle degrees of impairment with an absent pulse but good capillary refill may still signify an important vascular injury disguised by the rich collateral circulation around the elbow.

## Radiological features

- *AP and lateral elbow radiographs* (**Fig. 10.30**): Examine the congruence of the radiocapitellar joint and the ulnotrochlear joint. A line through the centre of the radial neck should pass through the centre of the capitellum on any view (see Fig. 10.6). Look carefully at the radial head and at the

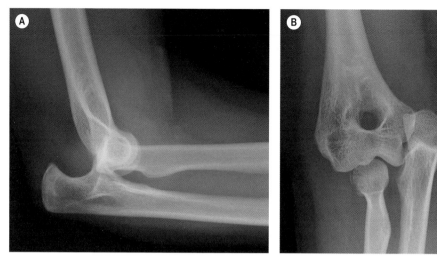

Fig. 10.30 Simple elbow dislocation. **A,** Lateral view. **B,** AP view.

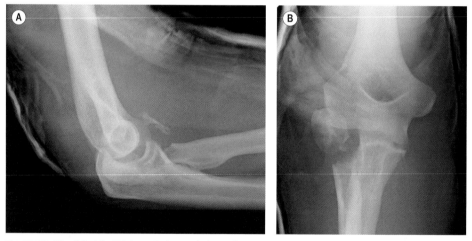

Fig. 10.31 'Terrible triad' injury. **A,** Lateral view after closed reduction of the dislocation. Note that the coronoid is blunted and there is a bone fragment anterior to the humerus. Note also that the radius remains subluxed. **B,** AP view, showing the radial head and neck fracture clearly.

coronoid in particular. Any triangular fragment of bone of any size seen anterior to the elbow should be strongly suspected of being a coronoid fracture. Radiographs of the 'terrible triad' are shown in **Figure 10.31**.

### Closed reduction

The patient is most conveniently treated supine on the examination trolley. Procedural sedation and analgesia are usually required. In a muscular individual, considerable force may be necessary (**Fig. 10.32**).

1. Ask an assistant to provide counter-traction (**Fig. 10.32A**).
2. Grasp the patient's wrist with one hand.
3. Cradle the underside of the dislocated elbow with the other hand to assess and then reduce any medial/lateral displacement,

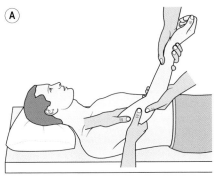

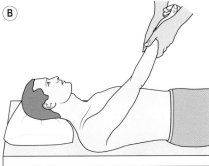

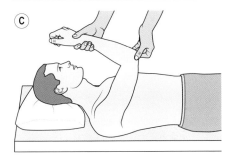

Fig. 10.32 Closed reduction: technique 1.

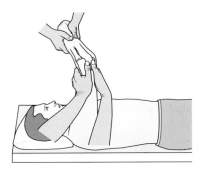

Fig. 10.33 Closed reduction: technique 2.

and medially using your thumbs, while an assistant applies traction and some flexion to the elbow (**Fig. 10.33**).

## Immobilization and reassessment

- An above-elbow backslab is applied with the elbow at 90° of flexion, extending from the wrist to the upper humerus (see Fig. 4.9).

- Acquire *repeat radiographs* of the elbow and take the opportunity to scrutinize the radial head and coronoid carefully. Any triangular fragment anterior to the elbow is likely to represent a fracture of the coronoid process. The elbow joint must be congruent with no incarcerated loose bodies.

- Repeat the neurovascular assessment paying particular attention to the ulnar nerve.

## Outpatient follow-up

- Simple (no fracture) elbow dislocations.

## Inpatient referral

- Complex (fracture) dislocations.
- Neurovascular compromise.
- Open injury.

aiming to centre the olecranon between the humeral epicondyles.

4. Apply in-line traction, using both hands. Successful reduction is accompanied by a satisfying clunk (**Fig. 10.32B**).

5. Flex the arm to a position of 90°. Reassess the equilateral triangle and the patient's ability to flex, extend and rotate the elbow (**Fig. 10.32C**).

An alternative strategy is to grasp the upper arm and push the olecranon distally, anteriorly

## Orthopaedic management

### Non-operative

- Simple elbow dislocations (those with a congruent joint post reduction and no fracture): These can be treated non-operatively with 2 weeks of backslab immobilization, followed by early rehabilitation.

## Operative

- Elbows that redisplace after reduction.
- Complex elbow dislocation: in particular, 'terrible triad' injuries.

## Surgical techniques

Elbows that re-displace after reduction, and 'terrible triad' injuries, usually require surgical stabilization. The principles of treatment are:

1. Radial head fracture fixation or replacement: Fixation is possible where there are two or three large fragments. More commonly, the fracture is comminuted and a radial head prosthesis (which acts as a spacer) is required. Simple excision of the radial head is *not* recommended, as it is likely to result in a very unstable elbow.

2. Coronoid process fracture stabilization: Small fragments are secured with transosseous sutures; large type III fractures may be fixed with a screw.

3. Lateral collateral ligament repair.

4. Medial collateral ligament repair: This may also occasionally be required where the elbow remains unstable after steps 1–3.

## SURGICAL TECHNIQUE: 'Terrible triad' stabilization – elbow utility incision

### Surgical set-up

The patient is placed supine with the upper limb on an arm-board. A tourniquet is used. Rehearse obtaining adequate AP and lateral fluoroscopic images before prepping and draping.

### Incision

The 'elbow utility incision' allows access to the posterior, the lateral and, if necessary, the medial aspects of the elbow and is commonly favoured. This is a longitudinal posterior incision through skin, fat and fascia down to, but not including, muscle. The fasciocutaneous flaps can be raised, exposing both sides of the elbow as required. Unlike the situation in the lower limb, the viability of flaps around the elbow is very rarely a concern.

### Kocher's approach

Internervous plane: The plane is between anconeus (radial nerve) and extensor carpi ulnaris (PIN).

Kocher's interval is identified as a fine white stripe between these muscles, best visualized some distance away from the epicondyle. This interval is opened to expose the joint capsule (with its condensations, the lateral collateral ligament and annular ligament). The lateral collateral ligament will often have been avulsed from the lateral epicondyle, leaving a bare area of bone exposed. The capsulotomy is formalized proximally by releasing the remaining capsule from the anterior aspect of the supracondylar ridge. Distally, exposure is completed by pronating the forearm (to take the PIN away from the operative field, Fig. 10.20) and incising the annular ligament.

### Assessment of injury

The fracture haematoma is removed with gentle irrigation and loose fragments of bone are identified. The decision whether to fix or replace the radial head is based on the number of fragments and extent of bone loss. If the radial head is to be replaced, the neck cut is made next, as this allows better exposure of the anterior elbow joint and coronoid. The PIN is at risk during resection but is least vulnerable with the forearm in full pronation. The coronoid process is then assessed for size and integrity.

### Internal fixation – absolute stability

The coronoid (**Fig. 10.34**) can be fixed with screws or a transosseous suture. A large piece can be fixed with a lag screw directed from the ulnar border. A small fragment is more securely grasped with a non-absorbable suture, the two ends of which are then drawn through separate bony tunnels drilled through the ulna, to be tightened and then tied together at the ulnar border. The radial head is then addressed by reconstruction or replacement. Fixation is achieved with the use of 1.5-mm or 2-mm screws. The lateral collateral ligament complex (**Fig. 10.35**) is then reattached by placing suture anchors in the 'bare area' of the lateral epicondyle, and passing these through lateral collateral ligament and common extensor origin as the joint is closed.

The elbow is assessed clinically and fluoroscopically for stability and congruity. If it is unstable, the medial collateral ligament should be explored and repaired with suture anchors. If it remains unstable after this repair, an external fixator is used to span the joint for 2 or 3 weeks.

### Medial approach

If still required after lateral-sided surgery, the medial skin flap of the utility incision is raised to expose the medial aspect of the elbow. The ulnar nerve is palpated in the groove behind the medial epicondyle and must be protected. The medial collateral ligament rupture is located and repaired with sutures or bone anchors.

### Postoperative restrictions

Movement: The elbow is rested in a backslab for 2 weeks. Early active movement is then begun.

Weight-bearing: The patient is instructed not to lift anything heavier than a glass of water.

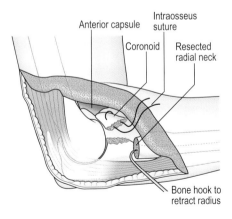
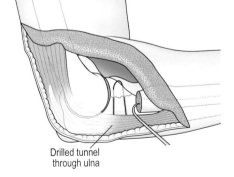

Fig. 10.34 Coronoid fixation.

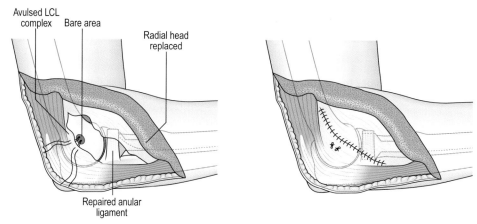

Fig. 10.35 Repair of the lateral collateral ligament (LCL) complex.

## Outpatient management

| Outpatient management summary | | | |
|---|---|---|---|
| **Week** | **Examination** | **Radiographs** | **Additional notes** |
| 1 | Neurovascular status<br><br>Wound check if treated surgically | AP and lateral elbow | Ensure elbow remains in joint |
| 2 | Removal of backslab<br><br>Assessment of range of movement and stability | AP and lateral elbow | Commence active range of movement physiotherapy without resistance |
| 6 | Assessment of range of movement and stability | AP and lateral elbow | If radiological and clinical examinations are satisfactory, discharge to physiotherapy |

## COMPLICATIONS

### Early

Local    Loss of reduction: This indicates failure of the repair, or a more unstable injury than originally appreciated. Revision of the fixation is required

PIN injury: The PIN must be protected during Kocher's approach to avoid iatrogenic injury

Infection: This may involve the elbow joint itself and can be very challenging to treat

Compartment syndrome

# COMPLICATIONS... cont'd

## *Late*

Local    Stiffness: Loss of motion, particularly terminal extension, is common after distal humerus fracture. The minimum functional arc of elbow movement is 30–130°. An extensive capsular release and removal of metalwork are indicated if this is lost

Heterotopic ossification: HO is classically associated with severe elbow injuries and may compromise final range of movement and function. It is more common after recurrent manipulations or surgeries, and with overly aggressive rehabilitation. Excision of mature HO may be required, along with a capsular release and removal of metalwork as a late procedure

## GENERAL PRINCIPLES

Forearm fractures commonly result from high-energy falls or collisions. The subcutaneous position of the ulna, in particular, leads to a relatively high incidence of open fractures. There is a modest incidence of compartment syndrome and appropriate monitoring is required where there is any suspicion of excessive swelling or neurovascular compromise.

## Anatomy

The forearm is notable in that it not only articulates at hinge joints both proximally (at the elbow) and distally (at the wrist), but also rotates (in pronation and supination) at both joints. These components are linked at the proximal radio-ulnar joint by the annular ligament, at the distal radio-ulnar joint (DRUJ) by the triangular fibrocartilage complex (TFCC), and in the mid-forearm by the interosseous membrane (**Fig. 11.1**). The axis of rotation runs from the base of the ulnar styloid to the centre of the radial head (**Fig. 11.2**). The fibres of the interosseous membrane are orientated obliquely to allow compression forces through the distal radius to be transmitted to the ulna. The ulna is straight whereas the radius has a bowed shape; loss of the normal shape of either bone prevents normal rotation and results in restricted pronation and supination. The flexor and extensor muscles of the forearm are contained within separate indistensible fascial envelopes, and high-energy fractures can be associated with compartment syndrome.

## Clinical assessment of the injured forearm

### Injury pattern
The history and examination should be performed in the knowledge that the radius and ulna are mechanically linked. Although an injury to either bone can occur in isolation, there is more commonly an associated second injury at another level. Several injury patterns should be specifically considered and excluded in the course of the assessment (**Fig. 11.3**).

● **radial fractures:**
— isolated radial shaft fracture
— Galeazzi fracture-dislocation – radial shaft fracture with DRUJ injury
— Essex–Lopresti injury – radial head and neck fracture with DRUJ injury

● **ulnar fractures:**
— isolated ulnar ('night stick') fracture
— Monteggia fracture dislocation – ulnar shaft fracture with radial head dislocation

● **both-bones forearm fracture.**

### History
Define the reason for presentation: has there been an acute definable injury, or is this an atraumatic or recurrent complaint? A high-energy mechanism of injury, such as a motor vehicle collision or fall from a height, suggests the possibility of other associated injuries and the requirement to assess and manage these first (Ch. 2).

A localized forearm injury often follows a fall on to an outstretched hand or arm, or a sporting collision. An isolated ulnar 'night stick' fracture is classically a defensive injury, sustained in the course of warding off a direct blow. However, forearm fractures are not uncommonly high-energy injuries and the possibility of swelling and a compartment syndrome must be considered. Enquire about previous injuries, operations or problems with the affected limb and obtain a medical history.

### Examination
*Look*
The patient will be in pain and will support the injured arm, which may be deformed. Carefully inspect any abrasions or lacerations to identify an open fracture.

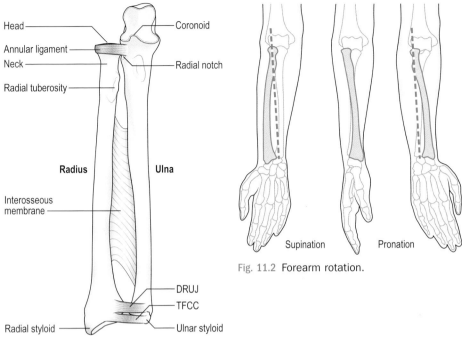

Head
Annular ligament
Neck
Radial tuberosity

Coronoid
Radial notch

**Radius**    **Ulna**

Interosseous
membrane

DRUJ
TFCC
Radial styloid
Ulnar styloid

Fig. 11.1 Osseoligamentous anatomy of the forearm. DRUJ, distal radio-ulnar joint (DRUJ); TFCC, triangular fibrocartilage complex.

Supination    Pronation

Fig. 11.2 Forearm rotation.

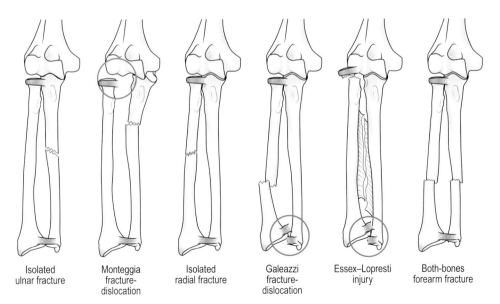

Isolated
ulnar fracture

Monteggia
fracture-
dislocation

Isolated
radial fracture

Galeazzi
fracture-
dislocation

Essex–Lopresti
injury

Both-bones
forearm fracture

Fig. 11.3 Forearm injuries.

*Feel*

Carefully assess for deformity and tenderness along the entire length of the forearm, including the elbow and wrist, paying careful attention to the radial head and the DRUJ.

*Move*

There will be pain and limitation in both active and passive movement. Crepitus may be felt when realigning a deformed limb. Active movements of the elbow and wrist will be limited by pain.

*Neurovascular assessment*

Assess the sensory and motor function of each of the radial, median and ulnar nerves at the hand (see Figs 3.17–3.19). Carefully palpate the radial pulse and check capillary refill to the fingers. Consider, and specifically exclude, a compartment syndrome (p. 226).

# Radiological assessment of the injured forearm

## Radiographs

- *AP and lateral views of the forearm* (**Fig. 11.4**): These must include both the elbow

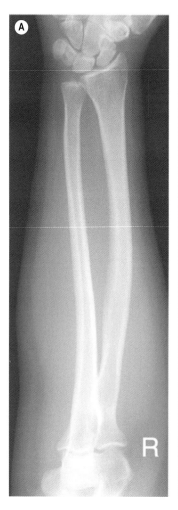
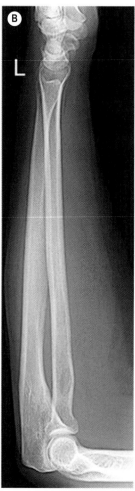

Fig. 11.4 Radiographs of the forearm. **A**, AP view. **B**, Lateral view. (From Bontrager KL, Lampignano JP: Bontrager's Handbook of Radiographic Positioning and Techniques 7th ed (Mosby 2010) with permission.)

and wrist joint. If only one joint appears on the initial radiograph, and there is clinical suspicion of an associated injury, do not hesitate to order additional views of the remainder of the forearm.

- *Additional high-quality views centred on the relevant joint*: These may be required to diagnose subtle displacement (Fig. 11.6A).

## RADIAL SHAFT FRACTURES

### Isolated fractures of the radial shaft
Isolated fractures of the radial shaft are relatively uncommon. They generally follow a direct blow and, if undisplaced, can be managed non-operatively with careful monitoring. However, a very careful assessment of the DRUJ is mandatory to ensure there is no associated injury.

### Galeazzi fracture-dislocation
This is classically a fracture of the middle and distal thirds of the radius with disruption of the DRUJ. Note that a DRUJ injury can occur with a radial fracture at any level, or indeed in both-bones forearm fractures (**Fig. 11.5**).

### Essex–Lopresti injury
This is a radial head or neck fracture with disruption of the interosseous membrane, resulting in radial shortening and DRUJ dislocation (**Fig. 11.6**). It is important to distinguish this injury from the more common and benign isolated radial head fracture.

## Emergency Department management

### Clinical features
- Enquire about pain at the wrist, which suggests a DRUJ injury.
- Carefully assess for deformity and tenderness along the entire length of the forearm, including the elbow and wrist, paying careful attention to the radial head and the DRUJ.

### Radiological features
- *Forearm series*: On the AP view, inspect the ulnar styloid for fracture and the width of the DRUJ; on the lateral view, exclude dorsal subluxation of the ulna.
- *Wrist series*: If there is any suspicion of a DRUJ injury that is not confirmed on the

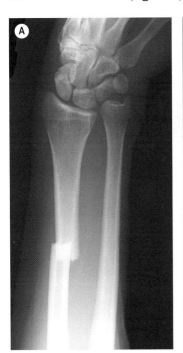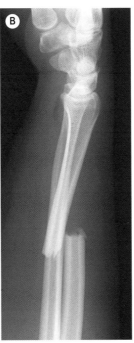

Fig. 11.5 Galeazzi fracture-dislocation. **A**, AP view, note the radial shaft fracture and DRUJ dislocation. **B**, Lateral view.

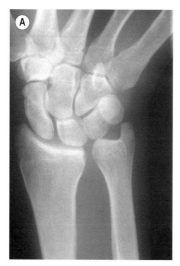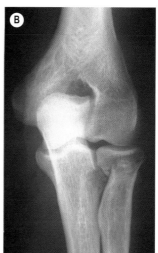

Fig. 11.6 Essex–Lopresti injury. **A**, The DRUJ has been disrupted and the ulna appears too long. **B**, The cause is an impacted radial neck fracture.

full-length forearm views, consider additional views centred on the wrist (Fig. 11.6A).

### Closed reduction

A grossly angulated and deformed forearm should be gently realigned under procedural sedation before application of a backslab.

### Immobilization and reassessment

An above-elbow backslab (see Fig. 4.9) extending from the metacarpal heads to the upper arm is required to support the fracture and prevent forearm rotation. Support the wrist with a collar-and-cuff. Carefully reassess the *neurovascular* supply to the hand after realignment and plaster application, then acquire repeat radiographs.

### Outpatient follow-up

- Undisplaced isolated radial shaft fractures.

### Inpatient referral

- Displaced radial shaft fractures.
- Galeazzi fracture-dislocations.
- Essex–Lopresti injuries.

## Orthopaedic management

### Non-operative

Undisplaced, isolated fractures of the radial shaft can be treated without surgery. Careful radiographic surveillance is required until union to ensure there is no displacement.

### Operative

#### *Galeazzi fracture-dislocations*

These are treated operatively. The radial shaft fracture is exposed via the Henry approach (see 'Surgical technique: Radial shaft plating' below), reduced anatomically and fixed with a compression plate. Particular attention is given to restoration of the radial bow. After fixation of the radius, the DRUJ is assessed clinically and fluoroscopically, and managed according to its degree of stability:

- *The DRUJ is congruent and stable, and the forearm has a full range of pronation and supination*: No further surgery is required.

- *The DRUJ is incongruent with the distal ulna displaced dorsally. The ulna can be reduced closed with gentle pressure but re-displaces when pressure is removed*: The DRUJ requires surgical stabilization. If there is an ulnar styloid fracture, this can be exposed, reduced and then stabilized with a k-wire, small screw or transosseous suture. If the TFCC remains intact, this will result in restoration of stability (**Fig. 11.7**). If this is not possible or effective, the DRUJ is reduced closed, and the distal radius and ulna are transfixed with 2-mm k-wires or a small

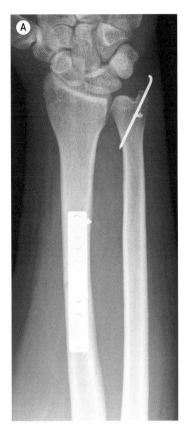

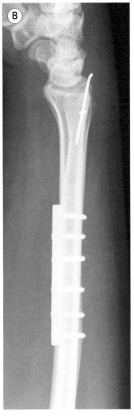

Fig. 11.7 A Galeazzi fracture-dislocation with ulnar styloid fixation. In this variant, the ulnar styloid was avulsed and has been fixed with a k-wire and suture anchor, stabilizing the DRUJ. The radius has been fixed with a plate. **A**, AP view. **B**, Lateral view.

fragment screw (**Fig. 11.8**). Postoperatively, the limb is immobilized in a cast extending from the metacarpal heads to the upper arm (to prevent attempted pronation or supination), and the wires or screw are removed at 6 weeks.

- *The DRUJ is incongruent and irreducible*: There is likely to be soft tissue interposition, often the extensor carpi ulnaris tendon. The DRUJ must be exposed through a small dorsal longitudinal incision (with care to avoid the dorsal branch of the ulnar nerve), reduced open, and then stabilized as above.

### Essex–Lopresti injury

The radial head is treated with fixation or replacement (p. 196). The distal ulna is then assessed and stabilized as above. Radial head excision alone is contraindicated, as this results in inexorable radial shortening and DRUJ dysfunction.

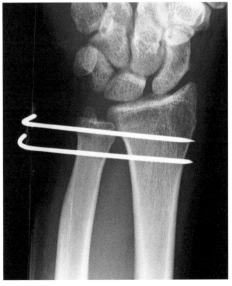

Fig. 11.8 A Galeazzi fracture-dislocation with DRUJ stabilization.

## ULNAR SHAFT FRACTURES

### Isolated 'night stick' fracture of the ulna

A night stick fracture results from a direct blow to the ulna, either from a fall directly on to the forearm, or as a defensive injury in the course of warding off a blow from a heavy blunt implement – hence its name. Unlike in the other forearm injuries, the proximal and distal radio-ulnar joints are intact, but on initial assessment the fracture should be assumed to be a Monteggia injury until proved otherwise by careful examination of the radial head.

### SURGICAL TECHNIQUE: Radial shaft plating – Henry approach

#### Surgical set-up

The patient is placed supine on the operating table, with the arm on an arm table. A tourniquet is applied.

#### Orthopaedic equipment

• Small fragment set

• 1.6-mm k-wires

• 3.5-mm dynamic compression plates

#### Incision (Fig. 11.9)

The incision is 15 cm in length, placed along a line extending from the biceps tendon to the radial styloid, and centred on the fracture.

#### Approach

This, the classic Henry's approach, allows access to the entire length of the forearm, although only a section of the approach is usually required to expose the fracture.

Internervous plane: Distally, the plane lies between brachioradialis (radial nerve) and flexor carpi radialis (median nerve). More proximally, it lies between brachioradialis and pronator teres (median nerve).

In the superficial layer, after sharply dissecting through a thin layer of fat, the fascia overlying the flexor muscles is exposed. The mobile wad of three (brachioradialis, extensor carpi radialis longus and brevis) can be palpated; retracting these muscles laterally assists in defining the plane between brachioradialis and flexor carpi radialis. The fascia is incised on the medial side of brachioradialis, in line with the skin wound. A plane is then developed with blunt dissection between brachioradialis (laterally) and pronator teres/flexor carpi radialis (medially) to reveal the radial artery. This is clearly identifiable by its two venae comitantes, which run parallel to it. The radial artery is gently retracted medially, and at the proximal end of the approach, division of recurrent branches of this artery (the leash of Henry) releases the brachioradialis muscle and allows it to be mobilized laterally (**Fig. 11.10**). The superficial radial nerve runs on the underside of brachioradialis and is retracted laterally with the muscle.

Depending on the level of the fracture, the approach to the deep layer is then continued down to the radius, in three distinct sections:

1. In the proximal third (**Fig. 11.11**), dissection of the forearm is an exercise in preserving the posterior interosseous nerve as it passes through the body of supinator. The forearm is supinated completely to move the body of supinator, and therefore the nerve, away from the operative field. Follow the biceps tendon down to its lateral border, where a small bursa is encountered, then incised, to reveal the proximal radius. The medial edge of supinator is identified, and is elevated in a subperiosteal fashion from its

insertion; do not dissect through the muscle. Caution is required during dissection and in the positioning of clamps, as the nerve is close to, or indeed touching, bone along its course.

2. In the middle third (**Fig. 11.12**) of the forearm, the plane runs between brachioradialis (laterally) and pronator teres (medially). The edge of the latter muscle is exposed by pronating the forearm fully, and then both pronator teres and flexor digitorum superficialis are progressively mobilized medially. As the radius is exposed distally, subperiosteal elevation of the flexor pollicis longus origin is performed as necessary.

3. In the distal third (**Fig. 11.13**), the forearm is supinated to reveal pronator quadratus, and the radius is exposed by incising along the lateral edge of this muscle and elevating it medially.

**Open reduction**

Each end of the fracture is delivered into the wound in turn and cleared of clot and bone fragments. The periosteum is stripped back by only a millimetre or two to expose the fractured ends. Reduction is achieved by grasping each side of the fracture with bone-holding clamps, exaggerating the fracture deformity by gently bringing the ends up into the wound, confirming rotational reduction, and then allowing the posterior cortices to come together. The fracture will now reduce as the bone ends are allowed to relax back into alignment. Ensure that the lateral bow of the radius has been restored.

**Internal fixation – absolute stability**

The fracture is most commonly transverse and can be held temporarily with an oblique k-wire. The anterior (volar) surface of the radius is, helpfully, flat and a 3.5-mm dynamic compression plate is pre-contoured (see Fig. 5.11) and used to achieve compression. Take note that the radius is bowed and the dynamic compression plate is straight. Therefore, each end of the plate will often sit towards the radial side, while the middle of the plate will sit towards the ulnar side.

**Postoperative restrictions**

Movement: The patient is allowed an unrestricted range of active movement of the elbow, wrist and forearm immediately.

Weight-bearing: The patient is instructed not to lift anything heavier than a glass of water until fracture union.

## Monteggia fracture-dislocation

The Monteggia injury is a fracture of the proximal ulna associated with a radial head dislocation (**Fig. 11.14**).

## Classification

The *Bado classification* describes the direction of displacement (**Fig. 11.15**):

1. anterior dislocation of the radial head with anterior angulation of the fracture

2. posterior dislocation of the radial head with posterior angulation of the fracture

3. lateral dislocation of the radial head, with a metaphyseal ulnar fracture

4. anterior dislocation of the radial head with fractures of both radius and ulna.

## Emergency Department management

### Clinical features

- Carefully assess for deformity and tenderness along the entire length of the forearm including the elbow and wrist, paying careful attention to the radial head.

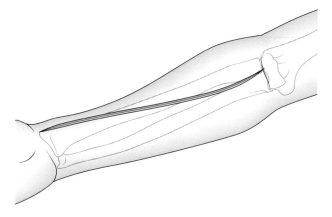

Fig. 11.9 Henry's approach: incision.

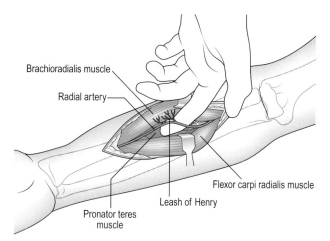

Fig. 11.10 Henry's approach: superficial dissection.

Brachioradialis muscle

Radial artery

Flexor carpi radialis muscle

Leash of Henry

Pronator teres muscle

## Radiological features

- *Forearm series*.

- *Elbow series*: Specific elbow views are indicated if the forearm radiographs do not allow confident assessment of the radio-capitellar joint. A line through the centre of the radial neck should bisect the capitellum on every view (see Fig. 10.6).

## Closed reduction

A grossly angulated and deformed fracture of the ulna should be gently realigned under procedural sedation before application of a backslab.

## Immobilization and reassessment

An above-elbow backslab extending from the metacarpal heads to the upper arm is required to support the fracture and prevent forearm rotation (see Fig. 4.9). Support the wrist with a collar-and-cuff. Carefully reassess the *neurovascular* supply to the hand after realignment and plaster application. Acquire repeat *radiographs*.

## Inpatient referral

- Monteggia fractures.

## Outpatient follow-up

- Undisplaced night stick fractures of the ulna should be referred to fracture clinic.

## Orthopaedic management

### Non-operative

Undisplaced fractures are treated with a cast or functional brace.

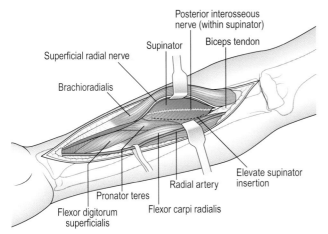

Fig. 11.11 Henry's approach: proximal third.

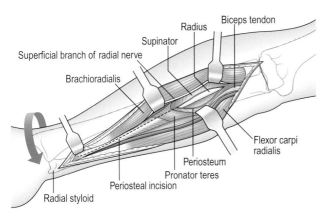

Fig. 11.12 Henry's approach: middle third.

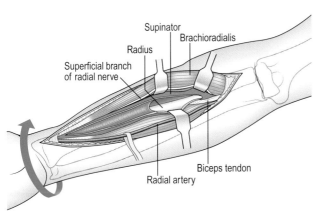

Fig. 11.13 Henry's approach: distal third.

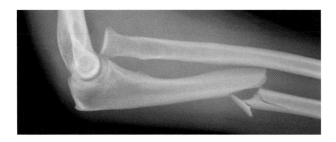

Fig. 11.14 Monteggia fracture-dislocation.

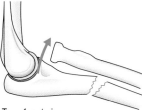

Type 1: anterior

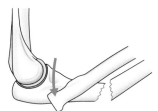

Type 2: posterior

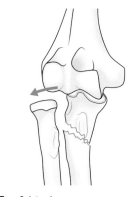

Type 3: lateral

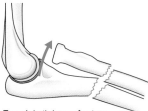

Type 4: both-bones fracture

Fig. 11.15 The Bado classification of Monteggia fracture dislocations.

## Operative

### Angulated 'night stick' fractures

Angulated or translated fractures are usually treated with compression plating to prevent further displacement and impairment of forearm rotation (see 'Surgical techniques' below).

### Monteggia fracture-dislocations

These require operative management with anatomical reduction and compression plating of the ulna (see 'Surgical techniques' below). The radial head is then assessed fluoroscopically and clinically. A number of scenarios are possible:

- *The radial head reduces closed with ulnar fracture reduction and remains stable with a full range of elbow flexion and extension, and forearm pronation and supination (the majority of cases)*: No further surgery is required.

- *The radial head remains displaced*: Most commonly, this is caused by failure to achieve anatomical reduction of the ulna. This should be scrutinized critically both visually and fluoroscopically, and revised where necessary.

- *The radial head remains displaced despite an anatomical reduction of the ulna (rare)*: This usually results from interposition of the annular ligament or other soft tissue, and an open exploration of the radiocapitellar articulation through a Kocher approach (Figs 10.18 and 10.19) is required. Once the elbow joint has been exposed, the annular ligament is usually retrieved and repaired over the radial head.

- *The radial head or neck is fractured and the elbow is unstable*: The radial head is reconstructed or, more usually, replaced (see p. 196)

---

### SURGICAL TECHNIQUE: Ulnar shaft plating – subcutaneous approach

#### Surgical set-up

The patient is placed supine on the operating table, with the arm on an arm table and the elbow flexed. A tourniquet is applied.

#### Orthopaedic equipment

- Small fragment set
- 3.5-mm dynamic compression plates

#### Incision

The incision is 15 cm in length and is centred over the fracture, along the subcutaneous border of the ulna, in a line between the tip of the olecranon and the ulnar styloid.

#### Approach

Internervous plane: The bone is subcutaneous and is exposed between the extensor carpi ulnaris (radial nerve) and the flexor carpi ulnaris (ulnar nerve).

Dissect down between the flexor and extensor compartments of the arm to expose the fracture.

#### Open reduction

Each end of the fracture is delivered into the wound in turn and cleared of clot and bone fragments. The periosteum is stripped back by only a millimetre or two to expose the fractured ends. Reduction is achieved by grasping each side of the fracture with bone-holding clamps, exaggerating the fracture deformity by gently bringing the ends up into the wound, confirming rotational reduction, and then allowing the posterior cortices to come together. The fracture will now reduce as the bone ends are allowed to relax back into alignment.

*Continued*

### Internal fixation – absolute stability

The fracture is most commonly transverse. The bone is roughly triangular in cross-section and the pre-bent compression plate is placed on the most convenient surface.

### Postoperative restrictions

Movement: The patient is allowed an unrestricted range of active movement of the elbow, wrist and forearm immediately.

Weight-bearing: The patient is instructed not to lift anything heavier than a glass of water until fracture union.

## Outpatient management

| Outpatient management summary | | | |
|---|---|---|---|
| **Week** | **Examination** | **Radiographs** | **Additional notes** |
| 1 | Wound check if treated surgically<br><br>Neurovascular status | AP and lateral forearm<br><br>Specific elbow or wrist views as appropriate | Commence early mobilization with a physiotherapist if the construct is stable |
| 6 | Assessment of range of movement at wrist, elbow and forearm<br><br>Check for tenderness at fracture site | AP and lateral forearm<br><br>Specific elbow or wrist views as appropriate | Galeazzi fractures – plan for removal of the transfixion wire, if used<br><br>Both-bones and night stick fractures – if the patient is pain-free, then discharge to ongoing rehabilitation; if not, review at 8 weeks |
| 8 | Assessment of range of movement | AP and lateral forearm<br><br>Specific elbow or wrist views as appropriate | |
| Further assessments at 4-week intervals if required for delayed union | | | |
| Average time to union = 6 weeks | | | |

## BOTH-BONES FRACTURE OF THE FOREARM

The radial and ulnar shafts are both fractured, usually at a similar level (see Fig. 11.3). The proximal and distal articulations are usually unaffected but should still be assessed for concurrent injury.

## Emergency Department management

### Clinical features

- There may be a history of a high-energy mechanism and other injuries must be excluded.
- The forearm is often deformed.

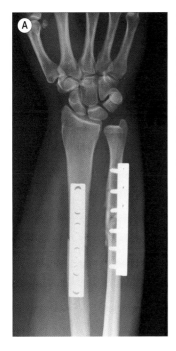

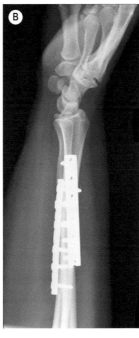

Fig. 11.16 Both-bones open reduction and internal fixation. Both radius and ulna have been reduced and fixed with dynamic compression plates. **A**, AP view. **B**, Lateral view.

- Carefully inspect any abrasions or lacerations to identify an open fracture, particularly over the subcutaneous border of the ulna.
- Compartment syndrome should be considered, as this is often a high-energy injury.

### Radiological features

- *Forearm series*: The diagnosis is usually clear. Make a careful assessment of the joints above and below the fracture.

### Closed reduction

A grossly angulated and deformed forearm should be gently realigned under procedural sedation before application of a backslab. An anatomical reduction is generally not possible. The fracture is most commonly off-ended; aim to reduce angular deformity but note that restoring normal length is not necessary at this stage.

### Immobilization and reassessment

An above-elbow backslab extending from the metacarpal heads to the upper arm is required to support the fracture and prevent forearm rotation (see Fig. 4.9). Support the wrist with a collar-and-cuff (see Fig. 4.20). Carefully reassess the neurovascular supply to the hand after realignment and plaster application. New or evolving paraesthesia, or disproportionate pain, may suggest a compartment syndrome. Split the backslab. If there are ongoing symptoms, the patient may require urgent surgery (see below).

### Inpatient referral

- All both-bones forearm injuries.

## Orthopaedic management

### Non-operative

As the forearm is a joint, allowing pronation and supination, the final position must be anatomical. Only completely undisplaced fractures are managed non-operatively.

### Operative

#### Displaced fractures

Displaced fractures require surgery (**Fig. 11.16**). The radial bow must be restored to allow normal pronation and supination. The steps of fixation are as follows:

1. The radius is approached first, anatomically reduced and fixed with compression plating (see 'Surgical techniques: Radial shaft plating' above)

2. The ulna is then addressed through a separate incision with anatomical reduction and compression (see 'Surgical techniques: Ulnar shaft plating' above).

3. The range of pronation/supination, and the fluoroscopic appearances, are assessed carefully. Restricted range of rotation suggests inadequate reduction, and revision is required. For a minor malreduction, all that may be needed is a loosening of the screws, perfection of the alignment, and retightening.

## COMPARTMENT SYNDROME OF THE FOREARM

Compartment syndrome of the forearm is not as common as that affecting the lower leg, but can accompany high-energy fractures of the radius and ulna. It is a surgical emergency. The pathophysiology, clinical features, diagnosis, Emergency Department management and principles of surgery are all described in Chapter 3.

## Orthopaedic management

Emergency fasciotomy is required; the fracture is usually stabilized at the same time. The anterior compartment is exposed through a longitudinal incision, as for the Henry approach. The deep fascia, and the fascial envelopes investing flexor digitorum superficialis and flexor carpi ulnaris, are opened. Consideration should also be given to release of the bicipital aponeurosis and the carpal tunnel. A separate decompression of the posterior compartment is then performed, opening the deep fascia widely to allow muscle inspection.

## COMPLICATIONS

### *Early*

| Local | Neurovascular injury: This may result from a high-energy mechanism or may be an iatrogenic injury, particularly to the posterior interosseous nerve, during surgery |
| --- | --- |
| | Compartment syndrome: High-energy or crush injuries to the forearm are at risk of compartment syndrome |

### *Late*

| Local | Malunion: Inadequate reduction, typically loss of radial bow, results in a reduction in pronation/supination |
| --- | --- |
| | Synostosis: This is a bony bridge between the radius and the ulna, which prevents forearm rotation. It can result from crush injuries, significant soft tissue stripping, or an attempt to fix both bones through one approach |
| | Delayed-union or non-union. This is relatively rare |

## GENERAL PRINCIPLES

Injuries around the wrist are amongst the most common injuries presenting to the Emergency Department. Injury type is highly dependent on the age of the patient and the mechanism of injury. Children commonly suffer torus fractures of the wrist after simple falls; young adults suffer complete fractures but also are prone to high-energy injuries resulting in complex distal radial fractures and fracture-dislocations of the carpus; and an ever-increasing number of elderly, osteoporotic patients present after low-energy falls with Colles' fractures. Fractures and dislocations must be distinguished from simple (ligamentous) wrist sprains and tendinous injuries.

## Anatomy

### Distal radius

The wrist is a complex joint formed by the distal radius and ulna, the eight carpal bones and their associated ligaments (**Fig. 12.1**). The radial shaft widens into the distal metaphysis and terminates at the radiocarpal joint, which has a volar tilt and ulnar inclination (see Fig. 12.7). The articular surface is irregular, having two shallow fossae for articulation with the lunate and scaphoid. The distal prominences of both the radius and the ulna are termed the styloids. The radius has a sigmoid notch, which articulates with the ulna at the distal radio-ulnar joint (DRUJ). Here it is stabilized by the triangular fibrocartilaginous complex (TFCC; see Fig. 11.1), which spans between the base of the ulnar styloid and the distal radius. The radius is longer than the ulna, but radial shortening after fracture will make the ulna appear long; this is described as positive ulnar variance. These landmarks are clearly seen in plain radiographs of the wrist (see Fig. 12.7).

### Carpus

The bones of the carpus are recalled by remembering the mnemonic 'Scottish Lads Take Presents To The Caledonian Hotel' (**Fig. 12.1**). Four bones make up the *proximal row*:

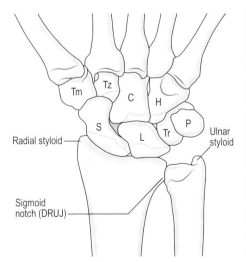
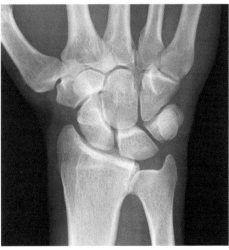

Fig. 12.1 Wrist and carpus osteology. S, scaphoid; L, lunate; Tr, triquetrum; P, pisiform; Tm, trapezium; Tz, trapezoid; C, capitate; H, hamate; DRUJ, distal radio-ulnar joint.

1. The *scaphoid* (Greek and Latin: 'boat-shaped') is considered to have proximal and distal poles connected by a waist. It is remarkable in that it has a distally based blood supply; a fracture through the waist may result in avascular necrosis of the proximal pole. The scaphoid is also noteworthy in that it bridges between the two rows of the carpus.

2. The *lunate* (Latin: 'moon-shaped') lies next to the scaphoid and resembles a crescent moon when viewed on lateral radiographs.

3. The *triquetrum* (Latin: 'three-cornered') is the third bone of the proximal row and lies distal to the ulna.

4. The *pisiform* (Latin: 'pea-shaped') is the last and least of the row. It is a sesamoid bone and lies within the flexor carpi ulnaris tendon.

In the *distal row* there are a further four carpal bones:

1. The *trapezium* (Greek and Latin: 'small table') sits under the th<u>um</u>b.

2. The *trapezoid* (Greek: 'four-sided') is the smallest bone in the distal row.

3. The *capitate* (Latin: 'head-like') sits centrally within the concave surface of the lunate and this relationship is important in defining alignment of the carpus in relation to the distal radius. The radius, lunate and capitate are described as three links in a chain, ensuring carpal stability and movement. The lunate, in the centre of this longitudinal chain, has no tendon insertions and is termed the 'intercalated segment'.

4. The *hamate* (Latin: 'hooked') is the last of the distal row. The hook of the hamate is part of the insertion of the transverse carpal ligament.

Adjacent bones are stabilized by intrinsic carpal ligaments, while the carpus is stabilized with respect to the distal radius by the extrinsic carpal ligaments (**Fig. 12.2**).

The *intrinsic carpal ligaments* of the proximal row, the scapholunate and lunotriquetral ligaments, are of particular importance, allowing dynamic flexion and extension of the row during

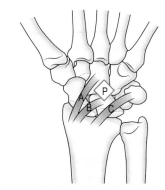

Fig. 12.2 Wrist ligaments.

wrist movement. Structurally, these two ligaments have three components: the palmar, interosseous and dorsal ligaments. The dorsal component of the scapholunate ligament is the most important, while the palmar component of the lunotriquetral ligament is most important.

The *extrinsic carpal ligaments* run from the radius to the carpus on both its volar and its dorsal aspects. The volar ligaments are stronger and more important: of these, the radioscaphocapitate (**A** on **Fig. 12.2**), radioscapholunate (**B**) and radiolunotriquetral (**C**) are most significant. An area in the capitolunate space has no ligamentous stabilizers, and this space of Poirier (**P**) is an area of potential weakness that is revealed in perilunate dissociation.

## Extensor compartments (Table 12.1)

The extensor tendons cross the wrist in six dorsal compartments under the extensor retinaculum (**Fig. 12.3**). The first four compartments (starting radially) lie over the radius, the fifth in line with the DRUJ, and the sixth over the ulna. In the *first* dorsal compartment are extensor pollicis brevis and abductor pollicis longus. These tendons can become inflamed after injury, causing de Quervain's tenosynovitis (see p. 261). In the *second* compartment are extensor carpi radialis longus and brevis. In the *third* is extensor pollicis longus (EPL), which executes a dog-leg turn in the compartment around Lister's tubercle. EPL is relatively avascular at this point and is liable to hypoxic and attritional rupture after a distal radial fracture. This risk is higher if screw tips from a volar plate are allowed to protrude dorsally, causing tendon attrition. The tendons of the first and third compartments run past the radial styloid over the scaphoid, and the sulcus between them is termed the *anatomical snuff-box* (Fig. 12.5). The *fourth* dorsal compartment is occupied by the tendons of extensor digitorum communis and extensor indicis proprius, and is the surgical route taken to expose the dorsal surface of the radius. The *fifth* compartment is occupied by extensor digiti minimi, and the *sixth* by extensor carpi ulnaris, which may become displaced in a DRUJ injury and prevent closed reduction.

## Carpal tunnel

On the volar aspect of the hand is the rectangular-shaped transverse carpal ligament. Its corners are marked by palpable carpal bones: the trapezium, the scaphoid, the pisiform and the hook of the hamate (**Fig. 12.3**). Under this ligament lies the carpal tunnel and its contents: the flexor tendons and the median nerve. Anatomically separate is Guyon's canal, which encloses the ulnar nerve.

# Clinical assessment of the painful wrist

## History

A painful wrist is an extremely common Emergency Department and fracture clinic presentation. Define the reason for presentation: has there been an acute definable injury, or is this an atraumatic or recurrent complaint? A high-energy mechanism of injury, such as a motor vehicle collision or fall from a height, suggests the possibility of other associated injuries and

| Table 12.1 The extensor compartments | |
|---|---|
| Compartment | Contents |
| I | Abductor pollicis longus |
| | Extensor pollicis brevis |
| II | Extensor carpi radialis longus |
| | Extensor carpi radialis brevis |
| III | Extensor pollicis longus |
| IV | Extensor digitorum communis |
| | Extensor indicis proprius |
| V | Extensor digiti minimi |
| VI | Extensor carpi ulnaris |

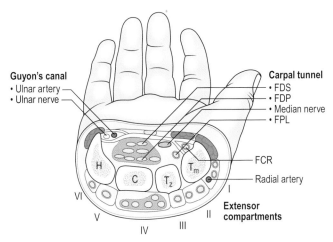

Fig. 12.3 Wrist cross-section. C, capitate; H, hamate; Tm, trapezium; Tz, trapezoid. Numbers indicate the extensor compartments.

the requirement to assess and manage these first (Ch. 2).

A localized wrist injury most commonly follows a simple fall on to an outstretched hand. Differential diagnoses for an injured wrist include a wrist sprain (p. 262), wrist fracture (p. 234), a scaphoid fracture (p. 248) or other carpal fracture (p. 253), a perilunate injury (p. 254) or De Quervain's tenosynovitis (p. 261). Patients with an *atraumatic presentation* should be assessed for an acute monoarthritis (p. 103). Features of systemic upset with fever and malaise may indicate a septic arthritis. Enquire about previous injuries, operations or problems with the affected wrist; a previous wrist fracture can make the radiographs difficult to interpret. Obtain a medical history.

### Examination

Examination of the wrist begins at the elbow and progresses in an orderly fashion to the fingertips.

#### *Look*

Inspect for the stigmata of pre-existing disease, including psoriatic skin patches, the characteristic joint deformities of inflammatory arthropathy (symmetrical small joint swelling, ulnar deviation of the fingers, swan-neck deformities) or degenerative arthropathy (Heberden's and Bouchard's nodes). Look for signs of injury, including deformity, swelling, bruising, abrasions and lacerations. A Colles' fracture has a typical 'dinner-fork' deformity (**Fig. 12.4**).

#### *Feel*

Plan to leave palpation of the injured area until last. For a distal radial injury, palpate the elbow and forearm briefly, and then palpate carefully around the distal ulna and DRUJ, the carpus, metacarpals and fingers (and their joints), and then the thumb and base of thumb, before progressing to palpate the dorsal and radial aspects of the distal radius, and the wrist joint margin. The anatomical snuff-box is the confluence of several anatomical structures; when there is tenderness here, it is important to attempt to determine which of these various structures is tender (**Fig. 12.5**):

a.  The base of the thumb metacarpal can be fractured (see p. 265).

b.  In the elderly, particularly, arthritis in the trapeziometacarpal joint (TMJ) is common (Fig. 12.42).

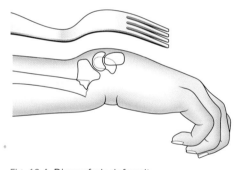

Fig. 12.4 Dinner-fork deformity.

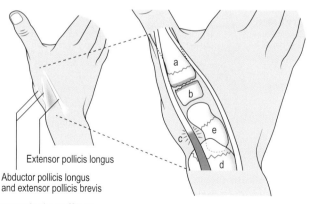

Extensor pollicis longus

Abductor pollicis longus
and extensor pollicis brevis

Fig. 12.5 Feel: anatomical snuff-box.

c. Tenderness over the first dorsal compartment (and its tendons) suggests de Quervain's tenosynovitis – inflammation within first dorsal extensor compartment (p. 261).

d. Tenderness of the radial styloid suggests a distal radial fracture.

e. Tenderness at the base of the anatomical snuff-box (ASB) itself is classically held to indicate a scaphoid fracture, but actually it is difficult to separate this from other anatomical structures and 'ASB tenderness' is a poor clinical sign. Tenderness of the scaphoid is more accurately demonstrated by placing the examining index finger and thumb on either pole and compressing it axially (see Fig. 12.29).

### Move

Assess *active* and then *passive* range of movement at the wrist, in flexion and extension, pronation and supination, and both radial and ulnar deviation (**Fig. 12.6**). Patients with a *fracture* will have restricted movement owing to pain, whilst those with an acute septic arthritis will experience exquisite pain with any attempted passive movement. Patients with pain over the first dorsal compartment suggestive of a *de Quervain's tenosynovitis* should undergo Finkelstein's test (see Fig. 12.41); the diagnosis is confirmed if pain is exaggerated on ulnar deviation of the wrist with the thumb held in the fist.

### Neurovascular assessment

Assess the sensation in each of the radial, median and ulnar nerve distributions (see Figs 3.17–3.19), and the motor power of the intrinsic muscles of the hand (median and ulnar nerves). Check the radial and ulnar pulses, and capillary return in the nailbeds.

## Radiological assessment of the painful wrist

Bony tenderness in the wrist or carpus with a history of recent trauma warrants radiographic evaluation.

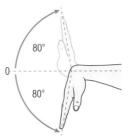

Flexion/extension

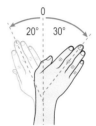

Radial/ulnar deviation

Pronation/supination

Fig. 12.6 Examination: move.

## Wrist radiographs

- The *PA view of the wrist* is taken with the hand palm down on the X-ray plate (**Fig. 12.7A**).

- The *lateral view of the wrist* is taken with the hand placed with the ulnar aspect of the wrist resting on the plate (**Fig. 12.7B**).

The radiographs should include the distal quarter of the forearm, the entire carpus and all of the metacarpals.

Assess the orientation of the articular surface of the radius, which has a normal volar tilt of 11° and a radial inclination of 22°. Beware: radiographic measurements of angles of displacement are highly dependent on rotation; two radiographs of the same fracture taken at slightly different rotations will result in markedly different measured angles. More helpful in determining displacement is the *radiocarpal alignment* (see below). Assess the relative lengths of the radius and ulna (*ulnar variance*); the radius should be a few millimetres longer than the ulna.

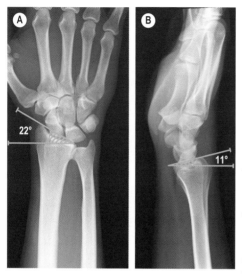

Fig. 12.7 Radiographs of the wrist. **A**, PA view showing the normal radial inclination of 22°. **B**, Lateral view showing the normal volar tilt of 11°.

### Radiocarpal alignment on the lateral radiograph

Scrutinize the lateral radiograph. Identify the scaphoid, lunate and capitate. Two curved cortices are seen adjacent to the radius, representing the overlapping scaphoid and lunate. Assess the relationship between the elements of the longitudinal anatomical chain of the wrist and carpus; this is often likened to an egg (capitate), sitting in an eggcup (lunate) resting on a table (distal radius). Lines drawn through the centre of the radius and the centre of the capitate should intersect in the carpus; if they do not, a wrist fracture should be considered displaced (**Fig. 12.8**).

### Carpal alignment on the PA radiograph

Name each of the carpal bones, assessing their bony contours, and then appraise the joint spaces in between the bones: they should be equal. In particular, an increased gap between the scaphoid and the lunate suggests scapholunate ligament disruption (see Fig. 12.34). Finally, appraise the three important anatomical Gilula's lines, which indicate a normal relationship within the carpus (**Fig. 12.9**):

- line I: a line drawn along the proximal convex curvature of the scaphoid, lunate and triquetrum

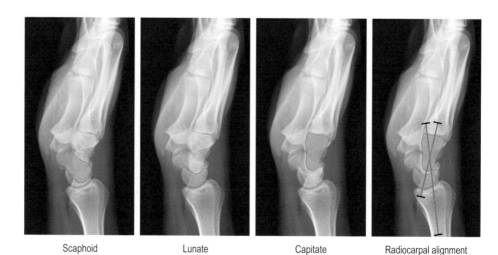

Scaphoid          Lunate          Capitate          Radiocarpal alignment

Fig. 12.8 Radiocarpal alignment.

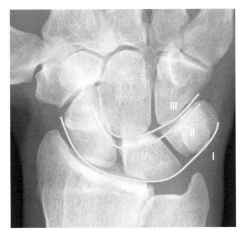

Fig. 12.9 Gilula's lines.

- line II: a line drawn along the distal concave curvature of the scaphoid, lunate and triquetrum
- line III: a line drawn along the proximal convex curvature of the capitate and hamate.

### Scaphoid series of radiographs (Fig. 12.10)

Due to the oblique position of the scaphoid, plain wrist views alone do not allow an adequate radiographic evaluation, and a series of four specific scaphoid views are required:

- *PA wrist in ulnar deviation*: The wrist is held in ulnar deviation, causing the scaphoid to extend. In this position, it looks longer (or

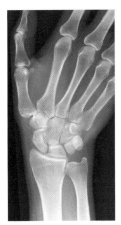

PA wrist in ulnar deviation

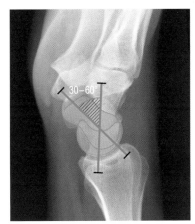

Lateral wrist: scapholunate angle

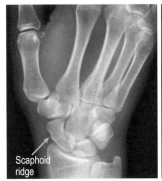

Oblique: 30° supinated

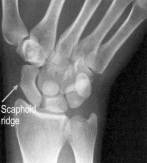

Scaphoid view

Fig. 12.10 Radiographic views of the scaphoid (the "scaphoid series").

less foreshortened) than on the PA projection, and waist fractures in particular are clearer. In the Emergency Department setting, there may be other injuries – for example, to the distal radius or metacarpals – and so this is taken like an Emergency Department wrist view, to include the distal forearm and metacarpophalangeal joints.

- *Lateral wrist.*

- *Oblique wrist*: The hand is supinated by 30°.

- *Scaphoid view*: A PA projection with the tube tilted 30° distally provides an *en face* view of the scaphoid, displaying its full length.

### Scapholunate angle

Identify the scaphoid; lines drawn through the centre of the lunate and scaphoid should intersect at a scapholunate angle of between 30 and 60°. After a scapholunate ligament injury, the angle between the scaphoid and the lunate may be abnormal (see Fig. 12.35), or the lunate may have been expelled completely (see Fig. 12.33).

### CT

CT is commonly employed to evaluate patients with complex distal radial fractures or traumatic carpal instability.

### MRI

MRI allows assessment of the intrinsic and extrinsic carpal ligaments, and is often used to exclude an occult scaphoid fracture.

---

### DISTAL RADIAL FRACTURES

## Classification

Distal radial (wrist) fractures are most commonly described eponymously or according to recognized patterns, although a number of classification systems are also used. Of these, the AO and Frykman classification systems are most widely quoted (see below).

### Specific fracture patterns (Fig. 12.11)

#### Colles' fracture (Fig. 12.12)

This is one of the most common of all fractures, and is usually sustained by an elderly patient after a fall on to an outstretched hand. It was first described by Abraham Colles, Professor of Surgery at the Royal College of Surgeons in Dublin, before the discovery of X-rays. The original description is of a fracture in the distal inch and a half of the radius with dorsal displacement. Colles also described the natural history, which is of gradual return of normal function despite persisting deformity.

#### Smith's fracture (Fig. 12.13)

Smith was Colles' successor in Dublin and performed his postmortem. He described this oblique extra-articular fracture with volar displacement. It is an inherently unstable fracture and is treated surgically.

#### Barton's fracture (Fig. 12.14)

This fracture, named after an American surgeon, is an intra-articular fracture of the distal radius with volar displacement. An equivalent injury with dorsal displacement is often termed a dorsal (or reverse) Barton's fracture.

#### Chauffeur (radial styloid) fracture (Fig. 12.15)

This is an isolated fracture of the radial styloid, caused by forced loading of the scaphoid against the radius. Classically, this resulted from the starting handle of a car kicking back against the chauffeur's hand; the same type of mechanism may result in a scaphoid fracture.

#### Lunate fossa

The volar aspect of the lunate fossa, in particular, is important because of the attachment of the extrinsic carpal ligaments (see Fig. 12.2); displacement of this fragment may result in subluxation of the entire carpus.

#### Die-punch fragments

Intra-articular fractures can represent a particular challenge. Displacement may take the form of a step, a gap or a 'die-punch' fragment: a section of articular surface impacted below the level of the adjacent cartilage. These fractures may require delicate manipulation and fixation with levers and wires.

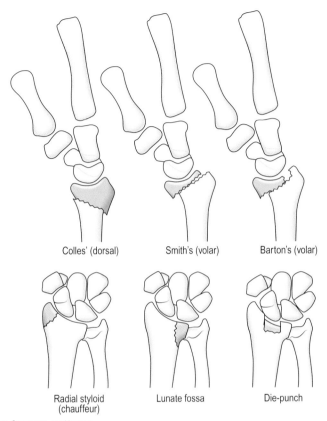

Colles' (dorsal)    Smith's (volar)    Barton's (volar)

Radial styloid
(chauffeur)    Lunate fossa    Die-punch

Fig. 12.11 Wrist fracture patterns.

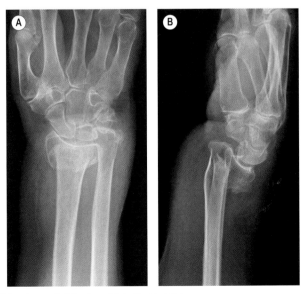

Fig. 12.12 Colles' fracture. **A**, PA view. **B**, Lateral view.

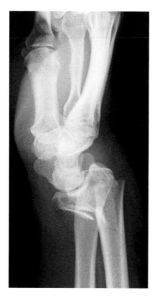

Fig. 12.13 Smith's fracture.

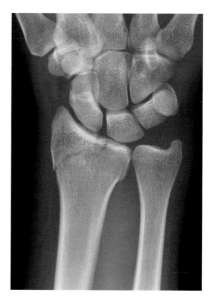

Fig. 12.15 Radial styloid fracture.

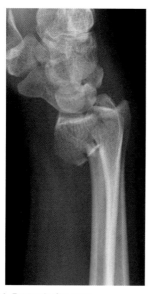

Fig. 12.14 Barton's fracture.

## AO classification

The AO classification of wrist fractures follows the universal system of separating extra-articular, partial articular and complete articular fracture types, with subsequent identification of groups and subgroups (see Fig. 1.21).

## Frykman classification

The Frykman classification assesses articular involvement and identifies injuries to the ulnar styloid. There are eight types in four pairs. The odd numbers represent differing degrees of intra-articular involvement of the two joints at the wrist: the radiocarpal joint and the DRUJ. The even numbers represent the preceding fracture with the additional involvement of an ulnar styloid fracture.

1. extra-articular fractures (type 2 is this injury plus an ulnar styloid fracture)

3. intra-articular fractures involving the radio-carpal joint (type 4 is this injury plus an ulnar styloid fracture)

5. intra-articular fractures involving the DRUJ (type 6 is this injury plus an ulnar styloid fracture)

7. intra-articular fractures involving both the radiocarpal joint and DRUJ (type 8 is this injury plus an ulnar styloid fracture).

## Classification according to stability and displacement

Pragmatically, fractures are usually described in terms of stability and displacement. Stability may be interpreted from the fracture morphology and the age of the patient. Smith's and Barton's fractures are inherently unstable, and are therefore usually treated operatively. Colles' fractures with dorsal comminution, particularly in osteoporotic patients, are also often unstable and are usually manipulated or treated operatively if displaced. There is no consensus as to what should be considered significant displacement. The clinical assessment will include an appreciation of the age, occupation, hand dominance and functional requirements of an individual patient. Radiographic assessment will include evaluation of the dorsal tilt, loss of radial inclination, ulnar variance and radiocarpal alignment. As a guide, displacement is commonly considered significant where there is:

- loss of radiocarpal alignment
- >10° of dorsal tilt (i.e. >20° from the normal position of volar tilt)
- >5 mm positive ulnar variance
- >2 mm articular step.

## Emergency Department management

### Clinical features

- The patient will usually have suffered a fall on to an outstretched hand.
- The wrist may be held protectively to the chest and supported with the contralateral hand.
- There may be clear deformity and swelling of the wrist. A 'dinner-fork' deformity (see Fig. 12.4) is typical of a Colles' fracture, indicating substantial dorsal displacement.
- Assess any abrasions or lacerations for potential communication with a fracture or joint.
- Establish carefully the location of any tenderness or deformity.
- Exclude injury to the joint above (elbow) and below (fingers).

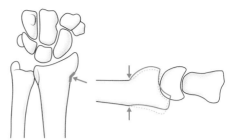

Fig. 12.16 Subtle signs of wrist fracture.

- A median nerve palsy suggests an acute carpal tunnel syndrome, which may require urgent intervention (p. 259).
- In high-energy injuries, a forearm compartment syndrome (p. 226) may develop. This is a surgical emergency.

### Radiological features

- *PA and lateral wrist radiographs*: Orientate the radiographs, recalling that on the lateral projection, the thumb metacarpal projects to the volar side of the carpus. Scrutinize the cortex of the radius, and the ulnar styloid, and assess the radiocarpal alignment, volar tilt and radial inclination. Assess the disposition and spacing of the carpal bones and reconstruct Gilula's lines. In a minimally displaced fracture, the radiographic appearances may be subtle (**Fig. 12.16**):

  an increase in the dorsal concavity, often with kinking

  an accompanying break in the smooth curve of the anterior cortex

  an irregularity on the lateral aspect of the radius.

  Where there is uncertainty regarding the significance of a radiographic appearance, re-examine the patient for local tenderness. This correlation of clinical signs with radiographic assessment is most important.

- *Scaphoid series*: These are required where there is suspicion of a scaphoid fracture or a significant ligamentous injury in the carpus.

- *CT*: This is indicated in highly comminuted and displaced fractures for preoperative planning.
- *MRI*: This is helpful for occult carpal fractures, diagnosis of ligamentous injuries and assessment of the TFCC (see Fig. 11.1), but is not required for acute wrist fractures.

## Closed reduction and immobilization

- Undisplaced (or minimally displaced) fractures do not require reduction and can be managed with a removable splint (see Fig. 4.27).
- Most displaced Colles' fractures have neither neurovascular impairment nor compromised skin, and can be reduced under Bier's block (p. 35) or a haematoma block (see Fig. 2.7) in a planned manner. The sequence of manœuvres required to reduce a Colles' fracture and apply a backslab is detailed on page 62.
- Uncommonly, the fracture is complicated by acute neurovascular impairment or potential skin compromise, and an urgent reduction under conscious sedation is required.
- Very comminuted and unstable patterns, and those with significant articular displacement, may not be suitable for attempted closed reduction and may be considered for primary surgical fixation.
- Smith's and Barton's fractures are inherently unstable and are usually not amenable to closed reduction. A Colles' backslab is

applied to the limb for comfort whilst awaiting surgery.

## Reassessment

- Neurovascular status should be reassessed after backslab application, before obtaining repeat radiographs to demonstrate adequate fracture position.
- Cast appraisal is important because poor application can restrict the patient's movement or cause skin abrasion. The edges of the plaster should not extend beyond the palmar crease (**A** on **Fig. 12.17**), restrict movement of the thumb metacarpal or dig in to the first web space (**B**). Trim excess material to allow free movement. An exaggerated position of wrist flexion (the Cotton–Loader position, **C**) risks the development of an acute carpal tunnel syndrome (p. 259) and should be avoided.

## Inpatient referral

- Open fractures.
- Grossly displaced and comminuted fractures.
- Failed closed reduction.
- Neurovascular compromise.

## Outpatient follow-up

Patients with undisplaced (or minimally displaced) fractures, or those adequately reduced by closed manipulation, should be reviewed in the fracture clinic with radiographs after a week.

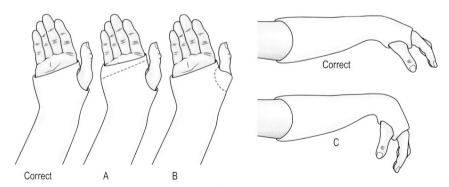

Fig. 12.17 Cast appraisal. **A**, **B**, The cast should be trimmed where it obstructs finger or thumb movement. **C**, The "Cotton-Loader" position of excessive flexion must be avoided.

## Orthopaedic management of Colles' fractures

### Non-operative

Conservative management is applicable in the majority of Colles' wrist fractures and is appropriate for:

- minimally displaced fractures treated with splint immobilization
- displaced fractures, which have been successfully reduced with closed manipulation; these are managed with cast immobilization and subsequent radiographic review to ensure that there is no deterioration in position
- displaced fractures in patients with cognitive impairment, significant illness, or low functional demands.

### Operative

Fractures that are inherently unstable, grossly displaced or irreducible, and those that subsequently displace in cast, should be considered for surgical fixation.

### Surgical techniques

A number of surgical procedures have been described for the treatment of Colles' fractures. There is no objective evidence of clear superiority of any one technique.

#### Kirschner wires (Fig. 12.18)

This relatively simple and inexpensive technique involves closed reduction of the fracture and percutaneous stabilization with 1.6-mm k-wires; it is particularly applicable to fractures with no intra-articular extension or displacement. Two common wire positions are preferred. The first is placed in the coronal plane, through the radial styloid, and passed medially to engage with the medial cortex of the radial shaft. The second is placed in the sagittal plane, through the dorsal cortex in the region of Lister's tubercle, passing forwards and out through the volar cortex. Reduction may also be achieved by means of the Kapandji technique, which is performed by placing the k-wire into the fracture and using it to lever the dorsal segment forwards into a reduction, before driving the wire forwards into the intact volar cortex. The wire then acts as a buttress against dorsal re-displacement. K-wire fixation may be prone to wire loosening, particularly in comminuted, osteoporotic bone, and may be augmented by external fixation.

#### Volar locked plates (Fig. 12.19)

Plating has become extremely popular with the development of locking plate technology, as, in order to resist collapse back into dorsal tilt, a volar plate applied to a Colles'-type fracture must be locked. Note that this is different from the buttress plating principle used for management of Smith's and Barton's fractures. Various surgical techniques may be employed to achieve reduction:

- The fracture may be reduced and stabilized temporarily with k-wires, before application of the locking plate.

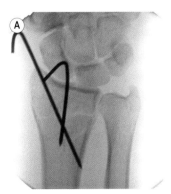
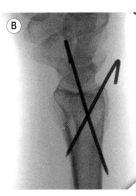

Fig. 12.18 K-wires. **A**, PA view. **B**, Lateral view.

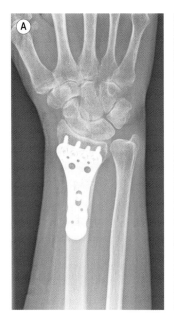

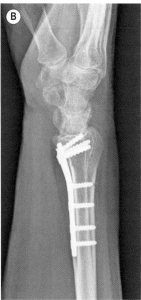

Fig. 12.19 Volar plate. **A**, PA view. **B**, Lateral view.

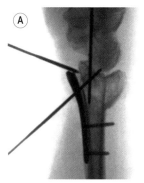

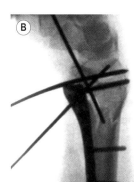

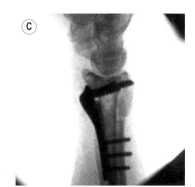

Fig. 12.20 K-wire joystick technique. **A**, The fracture has been partially reduced and a volar plate and two temporary k-wires have been inserted. The joystick k-wire is placed immediately distal to, and touching, the volar plate. **B**, The joystick wire is levered proximally to lift the distal fragment back into a position of volar tilt. **C**, Locking screws provide definitive fixation.

- The plate may be applied to the shaft of the radius, and the wrist is then flexed maximally to bring the distal fragment into reduction assisted by the surgeon applying firm digital pressure over the dorsal surface of the distal fragment. It is held either by an assistant, or by the surgeon with one hand, whilst the distal locking screws are inserted.

- The plate may be applied to the shaft of the radius, and the metaphyseal fragment then levered into position with an elevator or k-wire passed over the plate, or through a separate dorsal incision (**Fig. 12.20**).

- The plate may be applied to the distal fragment first, with the shaft of the plate angled away from the radius. When the plate is

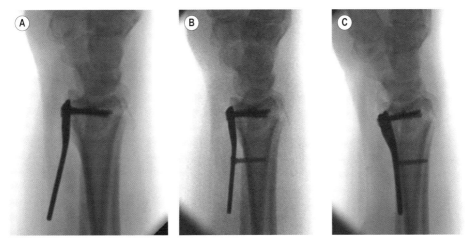

Fig. 12.21 Lift technique. **A**, The plate is applied to the distal fragment first, with subarticular locking screws. The shaft of the plate is angled away from the radius. The angle here is the same as the angle of correction desired. **B**, A non-locking screw is inserted. **C**, As this is tightened, the distal articular surface is elevated into a reduced position.

then brought down to the cortex of the radial shaft, the distal fragment is levered up into a reduction (**Fig. 12.21**).

More complex fracture patterns may require additional reduction manoeuvres, and augmentation with k-wires or additional plates placed dorsally, or laterally against the styloid.

### Dorsal plates

A dorsally based plate is well positioned mechanically to resist fracture displacement, but plates placed over the dorsal surface of the radius have a tendency to cause attritional damage to the extensor tendons. The technique is not, therefore, commonly used for primary fixation of simple Colles'-type fractures. However, a dorsal plate is useful for augmenting volar fixation where there is a complex intra-articular fracture, with small dorsal fragments that are insufficiently controlled by the volar plate.

### Non-bridging external fixation (Fig. 12.22)

An external fixator has the advantages of being applied percutaneously, being dorsal (and therefore well sited mechanically to resist the tendency to dorsal collapse) and easily removable. However, there is an incidence of pin-track infection requiring antibiotic treatment. A non-bridging fixator is sited in the distal fragment and allows some wrist movement. The technique involves placing two 10-mm longitudinal incisions over the distal metaphysis, and blunt dissection to bone. Self-drilling, self-tapping external fixator pins are implanted as far as the volar cortex. Two pins are then placed in the radial shaft. The pins are used to reduce the joint surface and are then secured with an external bar. All of the hardware is removed in the outpatient clinic after union at 6 weeks.

### Bridging external fixation (Fig. 12.23)

Fractures with intra-articular displacement are not amenable to non-bridging fixation, and in this situation the distal pins are placed in the second metacarpal to bridge the wrist joint. This technique is particularly useful for spanning irreducible, highly comminuted fractures that are not amenable to plate fixation. Bridging external fixators cannot address dorsal tilt. The volar wrist joint capsule is tighter than the dorsal capsule and with ligamentotaxis there is inevitable dorsal tilt; supplemental k-wire fixation is required.

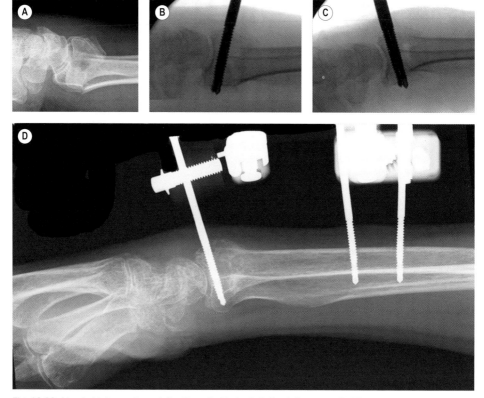

Fig. 12.22 Non-bridging external fixation. **A**, Typical Colles' fracture. **B**, The distal pins are inserted percutaneously parallel with the joint surface. **C**, The pins are levered distally to correct the orientation of the joint. **D**, The fixation is maintained by the proximal pins and bar.

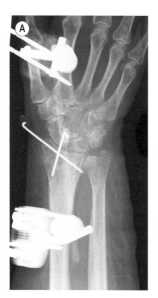 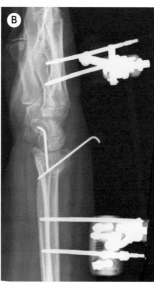

Fig. 12.23 Bridging external fixation. **A**, AP view. **B**, Lateral view. Note that, despite the supplemental k-wires, bridging external fixation does not reliably restore volar tilt.

# Orthopaedic management of Smith's and Barton's fractures

Both Smith's and Barton's fractures are shear fractures and surgery to reduce and stabilize these uses a buttress (anti-glide) plating technique (Fig. 12.25). Unless the dorsal cortex is also fractured, there is no additional advantage to using a locking plate. It is advisable to place cancellous screws in the distal segment to resist the displacement forces that can occur during wrist flexion and extension, and forearm rotation, while healing takes place. The concept that no distal screws are required because this is a buttress plate would only apply if the patient were strictly limited to axial loading of the construct during healing!

## SURGICAL TECHNIQUE: Volar plating of the distal radius – modified Henry approach

### Surgical set-up

The patient is positioned supine with an arm tourniquet, and the arm on a hand table.

Ensure adequate fluoroscopic images are obtained before beginning surgery. In complex fractures, traction views can help to identify the fracture pattern more clearly. Lateral images taken with the arm held at 20° to the table (so that the inclined articular surface is aligned with the fluoroscopic beam) will allow a clearer view of the orientation and displacement of the distal radial articular surface (see Fig. 12.27).

### Orthopaedic equipment

- 1.6-mm k-wires
- T-plate (not locking): Smith's or Barton's fracture
- Volar locking plate: comminuted or Colles' fracture

### Incision

The incision is placed directly over the palpable flexor carpi radialis tendon and extends from the wrist skin crease proximally.

### Approach (Fig. 12.24)

This is a modification of the true Henry approach (p. 218), in that the radial artery and nerve are taken laterally rather than medially. The flexor carpi radialis tendon is retracted medially and the fascial bed of that tendon is incised to reveal the flexor tendons; these are then retracted medially too to protect the median nerve. The transverse fibres of pronator quadratus, which covers the distal radius, are now revealed (A). These are incised at their radial edge, and the whole muscle is elevated towards the ulna to expose the volar aspect of the distal radius. The exposure can be improved in several ways. An additional transverse periosteal incision can be made at the margin of the wrist joint to release the pronator muscle more completely. A Hohmann retractor can then be placed under the muscle, its tip engaging with the DRUJ to expose the ulnar corner of the distal radius (B). At the radial edge of the field, the radial styloid can be released from the deforming force of brachioradialis by sharp dissection of the fibres of that muscle at its insertion.

### Open reduction

An anatomical reduction of the volar cortex is performed. A small, rolled drape placed under the wrist may assist in positioning the hand. For simple Smith's and volar Barton's fractures, the reduction is often achieved as the plate is compressed against the radial shaft (**Fig. 12.25**).

*Continued*

### Internal fixation – absolute stability

The selection and position of the plate will depend on the type of fracture being treated:

● A Smith's or Barton's fracture requires a simple T-plate for buttressing the fracture.

● A Colles'-type fracture demands a locked plate.

● Highly comminuted fractures may require specialized plates with multiple screw options.

● Fractures with a volar fragment bearing the lunate fossa are particularly vulnerable to poor plate placement. The fragment must be carefully reduced, and may be compressed and held initially with wires or a bone clamp (**Fig. 12.26**). The plate must then be placed over the fragment and should extend to the border of the DRUJ, with a screw inserted through the fragment to prevent later displacement of that fragment around the edge of the plate. Failure to do so can result in volar carpal subluxation.

### Post procedure

Casting is only required where there is concern over the stability of fixation achieved. Otherwise, a soft dressing will suffice.

### Postoperative restrictions

Movement: Gentle movements of the wrist are permitted immediately.

Weight-bearing: The patient should lift nothing heavier than a glass of water until union is confirmed.

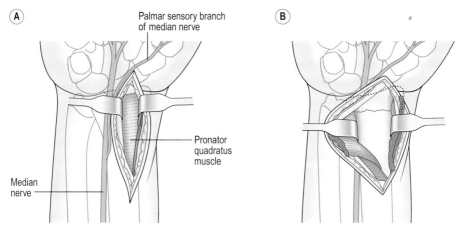

Fig. 12.24 Volar plating: modified Henry's approach.

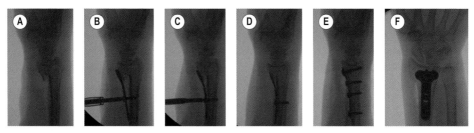

Fig. 12.25 Plate reduction of Smith's and Barton's fractures. **A**, Volar displacement. **B**, A buttress (antiglide) plate is applied to the volar cortex. **C**, As the screw is tightened, the fracture is reduced and compressed. **D**, Reduced position. **E**, Distal screws are required to resist rotational and radial/ulnar movements. **F**, AP view.

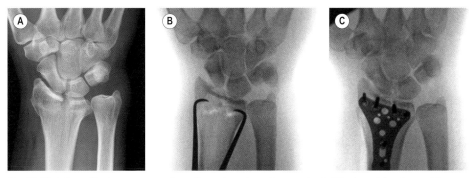

Fig. 12.26 Intra-articular compression of a volar ulnar fragment. **A**, Displaced fracture with intra-articular split. **B**, Joint reduction achieved with a pointed clamp. **C**, fixation with a volar locking plate. (See technique box on p. 243).

## ✓ Technical tip

Assessment of both the reduction of volar tilt and screw placement can be difficult on the lateral view; with the forearm flat on the table, an oblique view of the distal radius may suggest penetration (**Fig. 12.27A**). Raise the wrist so that the beam is in line with the distal radial articular surface (i.e. allowing for the 20° radial inclination; **Fig. 12.27B**).

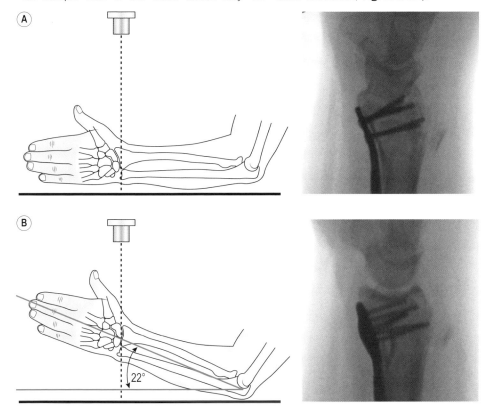

Fig. 12.27 Volar plate screw assessment.

## Orthopaedic management of a chauffeur (isolated radial styloid) fracture

Displaced chauffeur fractures are often reduced open and stabilized with a lag screw.

## Orthopaedic management of die-punch fragments

Die-punch fragments may require careful elevation with a lever, and stabilization with a k-wire or fine screws, before plate fixation. Numerous specialist plate sets, incorporating site-specific volar, dorsal and lateral plates, are available for plating complex fractures.

## Orthopaedic management of lunate fossa fractures

Lunate fossa fragments may not be adequately appreciated in the initial assessment of the injury and have a particular propensity to displacement, with subsequent volar carpal subluxation. The volar plate must be aligned with the ulnar side of the radius at the DRUJ, and at least one screw must pass through the fragment.

## Outpatient management

### Colles' fracture: non-operative management

| Outpatient management summary | | | |
|---|---|---|---|
| **Week** | **Examination** | **Radiographs** | **Additional notes** |
| 1 | If the fracture has not required manipulation: application of a light-weight cast and review at 6 weeks<br><br>If manipulation was required: simple reinforcement of the backslab and review at 2 weeks | PA and lateral wrist in new or reinforced cast | Check fracture/reduction position. If unsatisfactory, consider operative management |
| 2 | For those patients who have had a manipulation: conversion to a full cast at this stage | PA and lateral wrist in new cast | Check fracture/reduction position. If unsatisfactory, or there is evidence of progressive movement, consider operative management. If there is no change in fracture position from the initial (or post-reduction) Emergency Department films, the fracture is likely to be stable and can be reviewed at 6 weeks |
| 6 | Removal of cast<br><br>Check for absence of tenderness at fracture site<br><br>Assessment of range of movement | PA and lateral wrist if clinical signs of union are equivocal | If the patient is pain-free, discharge with exercise instructions |

Average time to union = 6 weeks

## Distal radius plating

| Outpatient management summary | | | |
| --- | --- | --- | --- |
| **Week** | **Examination** | **Radiographs** | **Additional notes** |
| 1 post surgery | Wound check<br><br>Neurovascular status | PA and lateral wrist | Commence early mobilization with a physiotherapist if the construct is stable |
| 6 | Assessment of range of movement<br><br>Check for tenderness at fracture site | PA and lateral wrist | If the patient is pain-free, discharge to physiotherapy or home exercises |

Further assessments at 2-week intervals if required for delayed union
Average time to union = 6 weeks

## COMPLICATIONS

### Early

Local    Median nerve injury: This is at risk during injury, cast application and surgery. Paraesthesia is usually relieved by fracture reduction. Progressive symptoms mandate cast release and consideration of acute carpal tunnel decompression (p. 259)

Infection: Surgical wounds, particularly around external fixation pins, may become infected and require prompt attention

Loss of reduction: Early loss of position after both non-operative and operative treatment may occur. Before 3 weeks, this is often amenable to (revision) fixation. Beyond this time point, it may be preferable to allow the fracture to unite fully and then address any pain or loss of function with a planned osteotomy

### Late

Local    Malunion: Modest malunion is common after Colles' fractures but is rarely accompanied by significant functional loss. Malunion resulting in a restricted range of movement or weakness may be amenable to corrective osteotomy or DRUJ excision hemiarthroplasty (Bower's procedure)

Extensor pollicis longus rupture: The EPL is at risk as it passes around Lister's tubercle, where the tendon is relatively avascular. EPL rupture can occur after undisplaced fractures, but is more common where there is attrition from prominent screw tips or after dorsal plating. Diagnosis is confirmed by an inability to lift the thumb from the table when the hand is placed flat, palm down. An extensor indicis transfer will restore function

*Continued*

Complex regional pain syndrome: This condition can arise after either operative or non-operative treatment. It is said to be more common following excessively tight plaster immobilization. Management is with analgesia and vigorous supervised physiotherapy (p. 120)

Stiffness: Loss of range of movement is common, particularly after prolonged immobilization. Simple instructions regarding mobilization are usually sufficient for return of function but recalcitrant cases may require supervised physiotherapy rehabilitation

## DISTAL ULNAR FRACTURES

Fractures of the ulnar styloid usually occur in conjunction with distal radius fractures. These are avulsions with varying displacement, the importance of which remains unclear. Usually, reduction of the displaced distal radius fracture will also result in the reduction of the ulnar styloid component, which is not itself usually exposed or fixed. Isolated ulnar styloid fractures are rare and can be treated with a wrist splint for comfort and early, unrestricted range of movement.

Fractures of the distal ulnar shaft may occur in isolation and are similar to ulnar shaft 'night stick' injuries (p. 218). If the ulnar shaft is fractured in conjunction with the distal radius, it is usually fixed at the time of radial fixation.

## SCAPHOID FRACTURES

Scaphoid fractures are of particular concern for two reasons:

1. Acute fractures are not always visible on initial radiographs.
2. A scaphoid waist fracture can interrupt the tenuous retrograde blood supply, resulting in avascular necrosis of the proximal pole.

This potential to miss and neglect an acute fracture, with the subsequent potential complications of non-union and avascular necrosis, leads to a great deal of anxiety when managing these patients initially. There is a substantial group of patients with clinical features that are possibly suggestive of a scaphoid fracture whose initial radiographs are normal (the so-called 'clinical scaphoid'), and these often require further clinical and radiographic review.

## Classification

### Herbert classification

The Herbert classification is shown in **Figure 12.28**.

## Emergency Department management

### Clinical features

- A scaphoid fracture is rare in the absence of a specific history of significant injury, which would typically involve a sporting injury or high-energy fall on to the out-stretched hand.

- There is a significant male predominance.

- An isolated scaphoid fracture will not usually cause any discernible deformity, although deformity may be seen when associated with a dislocation of the carpus: for example, trans-scaphoid perilu-nate fracture-dislocation.

- Begin by palpating away from the most painful area, ensuring there is no tender-ness over the metacarpals or the distal radius and ulna. Then palpate the anatomi-cal snuff-box (see Fig. 12.5) and the scaphoid tubercle, and perform the scaphoid compression test (see Fig. 12.29).

The anatomical snuff-box lies between the first extensor compartment (abductor pollicis longus and extensor pollicis brevis)

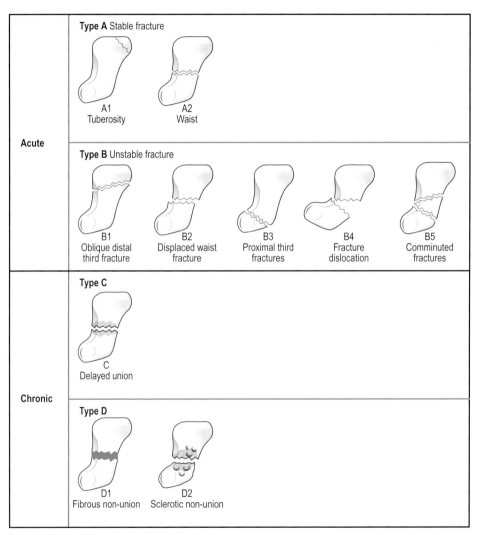

Fig. 12.28 Herbert classification of scaphoid fractures.

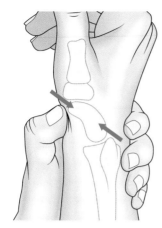

Fig. 12.29 Scaphoid compression test.

 **Key point**

None of the features in the history or examination is absolutely diagnostic of a scaphoid fracture, but the likelihood of a fracture increases with the number of features present. A scaphoid fracture is most likely in a male patient who has suffered a high-energy fall or sporting accident, and who has a positive scaphoid compression test and ASB pain on ulnar deviation of the wrist. With fewer of these features, the likelihood of there being a fracture recedes sharply. However, in order not to miss scaphoid fractures, further review and, occasionally, investigations are usually warranted where suspicion of an occult fracture remains.

and third extensor compartment (extensor pollicis longus). Tenderness in this area may indicate a number of different pathologies and it is important to locate the precise point of discomfort (see Fig. 12.5).

The scaphoid tubercle is identified by running a thumb along the flexor carpi radialis tendon. Just distal to the distal palmar wrist crease, a bony prominence will be felt a little to the radial side of the tendon.

The scaphoid axial compression test is performed with a thumb over the tubercle and the index finger of the same hand on the proximal pole of the scaphoid, on the dorsal aspect of the wrist (**Fig. 12.29**).

- Pain on ulnar deviation of the wrist is highly suggestive of scaphoid fracture. Conversely, lack of ASB pain on ulnar deviation is highly indicative of the *absence* of a fracture.

### Radiological features

- *Scaphoid series*: Scrutinize the four views for any subtle cortical abnormalities. The scaphoid ridge is visible on the lateral aspect of the scaphoid in the PA, oblique and scaphoid views, and should not be mis-construed as cortical abnormality (see Fig. 12.10).

- *MRI*: This is highly sensitive for detecting a scaphoid fracture but will also demonstrate bone bruising/oedema and other soft tissue pathologies. It is expensive and may not be readily available for acute assessment in the Emergency Department.

- *CT*: This is also sensitive for detecting a fracture and is a suitable alternative to MRI. However, the risks associated with radiation must be considered and CT will not identify associated potentially significant soft tissue injuries around the carpus, such as a scapholunate ligament disruption.

### Closed reduction

No reduction manœuvre is effective for a displaced scaphoid fracture.

### Immobilization and reassessment

Patients are provided with a wrist splint or below-elbow backslab for comfort. More extensive immobilization (e.g. the traditional scaphoid cast enclosing the thumb) is an encumbrance for the patient and has not been proven to influence outcome.

## Outpatient follow-up

- Confirmed scaphoid fractures are reviewed in the fracture clinic within 1 week for assessment of displacement/instability and to determine the definitive treatment.

- Suspected scaphoid fractures should be seen at the fracture clinic 2 weeks after the initial injury for repeat clinical assessment and radiographs. Bone resorption at the fracture site may make this clearer to discern.

## Patient instructions

Patients with a suspected scaphoid fracture but normal radiographs should be advised that only a small possibility of fracture remains; ultimately, only approximately 10% will be found to have a true scaphoid fracture.

# Orthopaedic management

## Non-operative

Suspected occult fractures and confirmed undisplaced scaphoid fractures (**Fig. 12.30**) are usually treated non-operatively with immobilization in a Colles' cast. Various more complex casts are described but offer no additional advantage.

## Operative

Indications for surgery include:

- Displaced fractures, particularly with a 'hump-backed' deformity.

- Undisplaced fractures – some surgeons advocate early surgery of undisplaced fractures with percutaneous screw fixation to expedite return to normal activity. The relevance of this is clearly influenced by the patient's age, occupation and hand dominance.

- Proximal pole injuries – owing to the tenuous blood supply to the proximal pole.

- Associated perilunate dissociation.

## Surgical techniques

Undisplaced scaphoid fractures are most commonly treated with percutaneous buried variable-pitch compression screws, which may be placed antegrade or retrograde (**Fig. 12.31**). Displaced or collapsed fractures routinely require open reduction and internal fixation with or without bone grafting.

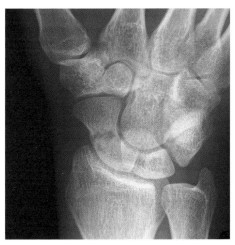

Fig. 12.30 Undisplaced scaphoid waist.

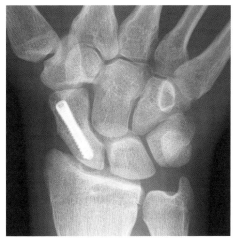

Fig. 12.31 Scaphoid screw fixation.

## Outpatient management

### Suspected and undisplaced scaphoid waist fractures

| Outpatient management summary | | | |
|---|---|---|---|
| **Week** | **Examination** | **Radiographs** | **Additional notes** |
| 1 | Review of confirmed scaphoid fractures for discussion of early surgery in young or active patients | Scaphoid series – repeat to assess for displacement | Apply a full Colles' cast |
| 2 | Review of suspected scaphoid fractures for reassessment | Scaphoid series – repeat if still tender | If clinical signs have resolved, discharge<br><br>If radiographs confirm fracture, offer definitive management. If still uncertain, consider MRI |
| 6 (distal pole)<br><br>8 (scaphoid waist)<br><br>12 (proximal pole) | Clinical assessment should be repeated | Scaphoid series | If the patient is pain-free and the fracture is united, discharge<br><br>If there is delayed or non-union, consider MRI or CT assessment and possible surgery |

Time to union and percentage of united fractures are shown in **Table 12.2**.

### COMPLICATIONS

#### *Late*

Local    Delayed union: Prolonged times to union are common, and investigation with CT may ultimately be required to confirm union

Non-union: Fractures that fail to unite are treated with screw fixation, usually with bone graft. Long-standing scaphoid non-union advanced collapse (SNAC) has three stages:

- stage 1 – radioscaphoid arthritis
- stage 2 – scaphocapitate arthritis
- stage 3 – lunocapitate arthritis

SNAC is an end-stage condition, and often requires salvage surgery in the form of a proximal row carpectomy or a wrist fusion

Avascular necrosis of the proximal pole also results in a degenerative wrist

# OTHER CARPAL FRACTURES

Fractures of the carpal bones other than the scaphoid are rare, and diagnosis can be difficult because they are usually small avulsion or impaction fractures that are not easily appreciated on plain radiographs. Many are detected on further investigation for a suspected scaphoid fracture. The most important feature is well-localized tenderness over the carpus. Oblique radiographs or CT may be required to characterize these adequately. Large fragments are occasionally amenable to fixation; however, these fractures are generally too small to be surgically fixable and are treated empirically as for a soft tissue injury with immobilization for comfort. Three common injuries are dorsal rim shear fractures of the hamate,

avulsion flake fractures and hook of hamate fractures.

## Dorsal rim shear fracture of the hamate

This occurs with dorsal displacement of the bases of the fourth and fifth metacarpals (**Fig. 12.32**). The mechanism is that of an axial load to the affected metacarpals, usually in the course of throwing a punch. If significantly displaced, this type of fracture is treated with closed reduction and k-wire transfixion of the metacarpal bases for 4 weeks.

## Avulsion flake fractures

A severe hand sprain results in tearing of the extrinsic carpal ligaments but no carpal instability. On occasion, the ligament may avulse a small flake of bone from the dorsum of the carpus. The injury may be seen on a lateral or oblique hand radiograph. The origin of the flake is often the triquetrum but this is usually difficult to establish. Treatment is as for a soft tissue injury with early mobilization.

## Hook of hamate fractures

The hamate hook may be fractured by direct impact: for example, from falling or catching a hard ball. Clinical examination reveals local tenderness over the volar aspect of the hamate.

### Table 12.2  Scaphoid fractures: time to union and rate of union

| Fracture position | Time to union (weeks) | Union (%) |
|---|---|---|
| Distal third and tuberosity | 6 | 100 |
| Waist | 8 | 85 |
| Proximal pole | 12 | 70 |

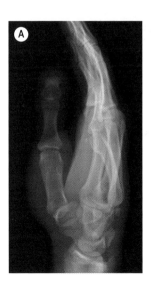
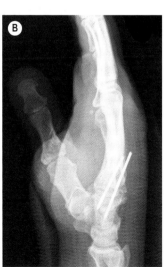

Fig. 12.32 Dorsal rim shear fracture of hamate. **A**, The bases of the fourth and fifth metacarpals are displaced dorsally, attached to a small dorsal rim fragment from the hamate. **B**, Reduced position stabilized with two k-wires through the metacarpal bases and into the hamate.

The proximity of Guyon's canal often results in a partial ulnar nerve neurapraxia. A CT scan is usually required to confirm the diagnosis. Treatment is symptomatic with splintage until union. Occasionally, a painful non-union may necessitate excision of the un-united fragment.

## CARPAL INSTABILITY

Carpal instability is a term that encompasses a spectrum of injuries within or around the carpus, resulting in loss of congruity or abnormal loading between the carpal bones. An appreciation of the osseoligamentous anatomy of the carpus helps in understanding this condition (see Figs 12.1–12.2). Commonly used terms include:

- *Dissociation*: loss of the normal ligamentous attachment between bones. This implies rupture of the intervening ligament. The bones may maintain a normal position, may be subluxed or may be dislocated. Do not confuse this with a similar word, 'dissociative', which has a specific meaning in the context of carpal injuries (see below).

- *Subluxation*: partial loss of articular congruity.

- *Dislocation*: complete loss of articular congruity.

- *Instability*: the functional effect of dissociation. An unstable joint may be subluxed or dislocated at rest (static instability) or may behave abnormally only during use or movement (dynamic instability).

### Carpal biomechanics

The lunate is the 'keystone' of the carpus and is essential to understanding carpal instability. It lies at the centre of the proximal carpal row (linking the scaphoid and the triquetrum), and also at the centre of the longitudinal chain (linking the radius with the capitate); it is therefore sometimes termed the *intercalated segment*. In the proximal row, the scaphoid has an inherent tendency to flex, while the triquetrum has an inherent tendency to extend. The lunate, placed between the two, is in dynamic equilibrium and maintains the alignment of the proximal row.

## Classification

A rather complex-sounding terminology is employed to describe the location of the carpal instability:

- *Carpal instability – dissociative (CID;* instability within a single carpal row): This usually affects the proximal row, comprising either a scapholunate or a lunotriquetral injury (see below). Isolated injury to the distal carpal row is rare.

- *Carpal instability – non-dissociative (CIND;* instability between intact carpal rows): This results from rupture of the extrinsic carpal ligaments and can occur between the proximal and distal carpal rows (intercarpal), or the proximal row and radius (wrist dislocation) (**Fig. 12.33**).

- *Carpal instability – combined (CIC;* instability within *and* between the carpal rows): This is a complex carpal injury.

- *Carpal instability – adaptive (CIA;* abnormal carpal alignment that is secondary to a more proximal abnormality): This is a chronic condition, often arising from a malunion of a distal radial fracture.

### Scapholunate dissociation

This is the most common dissociative carpal injury (CID). Rupture of the scapholunate ligament disconnects the scaphoid and lunate, widening the interval between them. The scaphoid flexes while the lunate (which is still connected to the triquetrum) extends. Three typical radiographic features result:

1. *Terry Thomas sign* (**Fig. 12.34**): There is excessive gapping between the scaphoid and lunate on the PA view. The name refers to a British actor from the 1950s, who had a striking gap between his front teeth.

2. *Ring sign*. Also on the PA film, the abnormally flexed scaphoid is seen end-on, giving a foreshortened appearance and producing a 'ring' of cortex.

3. *Dorsal intercalated segment instability (DISI)*: This overly complex term is used to describe the excessive dorsal tilt of the lunate (the intercalated segment) seen on the lateral

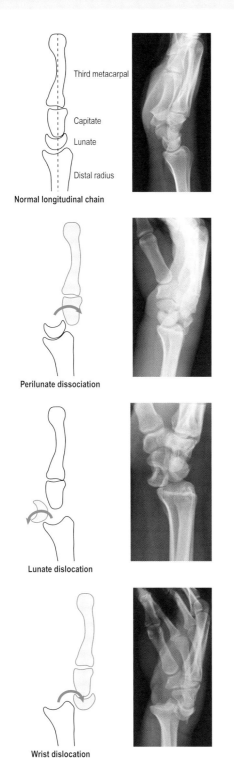

Normal longitudinal chain

Perilunate dissociation

Lunate dislocation

Wrist dislocation

Fig. 12.33 Perilunate injuries.

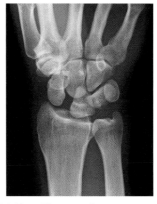

Fig. 12.34 Terry Thomas sign.

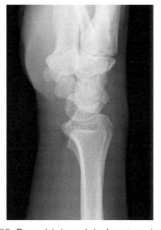

Fig. 12.35 Dorsal intercalated segment instability.

wrist radiograph (**Fig. 12.35**; see also Fig. 12.10). The scaphoid is also seen in abnormal flexion, resulting in an *increased* scapholunate angle of >70° (see Fig. 12.10).

## Lunotriquetral dissociation

This is also a proximal row CID. Rupture of the lunotriquetral ligament results in the lunate being pulled into flexion by the scaphoid, while the triquetrum falls into excessive extension. With the lunate tilted in a volar direction, there is a *reduced* scapholunate angle of <30° (see Fig. 12.10), which is described as a *volar intercalated segment instability* (*VISI*) deformity.

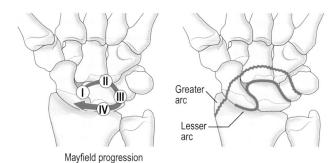

Mayfield progression

Fig. 12.36 Mayfield progression and the greater and lesser arcs.

## Perilunate injuries (Fig. 12.33)

These make up a collection of high-energy injuries sustained in a fall on to a hyperextended wrist. The pattern of injury follows a predictable sequence termed the *Mayfield progression* (**Fig. 12.36**):

- *Stage I*: The *scapholunate ligament* is disrupted first, causing the scaphoid and lunate to separate. Therefore a *scapholunate dissociation* is actually the first stage of the Mayfield progression.

- *Stage II*: The *capitolunate ligament* is disrupted at the space of Poirier and the capitate dislocates dorsally, leaving the lunate within its fossa. This is termed a *perilunate dislocation*.

- *Stage III*: The *lunotriquetral ligament* is disrupted and the triquetrum follows the capitate and dislocates dorsally. Again, the lunate remains in its fossa. As with stage II, this can also be described as a *perilunate dislocation*.

- *Stage IV*: The dorsal radiolunate ligament is disrupted and the lunate is extruded in a volar direction into the carpal tunnel. The capitate falls into the space vacated by the lunate, but remains correctly aligned with the radius on the lateral radiograph. This is termed a *lunate dislocation*.

Perilunate injuries may be purely ligamentous and include both CID (Mayfield stage I) and CIC (Mayfield stages II–IV) types. However, perilunate injuries are often complicated by fractures

(osseoligamentous injury), reflecting a different location of force dissipation:

- *Lesser arc* injuries are those that involve purely ligamentous disruption around the lunate.

- *Greater arc* injury occurs when the force is dissipated in fractures of the radial styloid, the scaphoid, the capitate or the triquetrum. A common variant is the trans-scaphoid perilunate fracture-dislocation.

## Emergency Department management

### Clinical features

- Patients report severe pain in the wrist and hand.

- There may be paraesthesia due to compromise of the median nerve.

- While an isolated scapholunate dissociation may not result in any visible abnormality, a wrist dislocation leads to a severe deformity; volar displacement is common, while dorsal displacement results in a characteristic 'dinner-fork' deformity like a Colles' fracture.

- Patients with a lunate dislocation may have blanched, compromised skin in the palmar aspect of the hand, just distal to the wrist crease, where the lunate has been extruded.

- Gently localize the site of maximal tenderness. In subtler Mayfield grade I injuries to the scapholunate ligament, tenderness will typically be elicited dorsally, just distal to Lister's tubercle.

## Radiological features

- *PA and lateral wrist radiographs ± scaphoid series*: The two standard wrist views are usually sufficient to make the diagnosis of a dislocation but may be complemented by scaphoid views, if required, for more subtle injuries. On the PA view, assess each carpal bone, the joint spaces and Gilula's arcs, and check for the presence of the 'Terry Thomas' or scaphoid 'ring' sign. On the lateral view, identify the scaphoid, lunate and capitate, and assess alignment and the scapholunate angle.

## Closed reduction of perilunate and lunate dislocations

### Tavernier's manœuvre

Procedural sedation is required. Reduction is most easily accomplished by applying both thumbs to the lunate while grasping the patient's wrist (*a* on **Fig. 12.37**), and using an assistant to apply the traction and wrist movement (*b*). The manœuvre consists of three steps (**Fig. 12.38**):

1. *Thumb pressure and traction*: Direct pressure over the lunate stabilizes and extends it, and, if it is dislocated, induces it to reduce dorsally. Simultaneously, firm traction is applied to the fingers (to create a gap for the lunate).

2. *Extension*: The wrist is extended (to bring the base of the capitate forwards to key in to the curvature of the lunate).

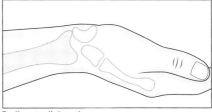
Perilunate dislocation

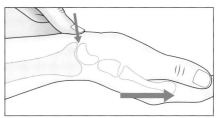
1 Traction and thumb pressure

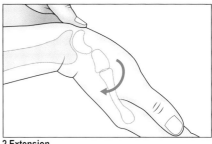
2 Extension

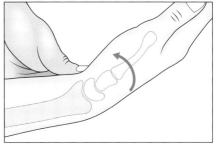
3 Flexion

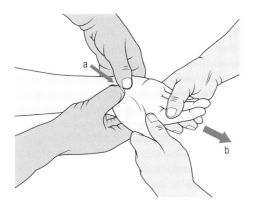

Fig. 12.37 Perilunate reduction: hand position.

Fig. 12.38 Tavernier's manœuvre.

3. *Flexion*: Finally, the wrist is flexed (to reduce the base of the capitate and restore carpal alignment).

A closed reduction may not be possible, in which case an open surgical reduction is required. This is urgent in the presence of an acute median nerve palsy.

### Wrist dislocation

Reduction is performed under procedural sedation and mirrors the principles and movements of distal radial fracture reduction (see Figs 4.2 and 4.4): longitudinal traction is followed by wrist extension, with the thumbs acting as a fulcrum at the level of the dislocation, followed by flexion.

### Immobilization and reassessment

A below-elbow backslab is applied in a neutral wrist position (see Fig. 4.11). Reassess the neurovascular status of the hand. Failure of an acute nerve palsy to resolve, or the development of a new palsy after manipulation, requires urgent surgical assessment. Repeat radiographs confirm reduction.

### Inpatient referral

- Perilunate or lunate dislocations.
- Wrist dislocation.
- Displaced greater arc fractures.
- High-energy injuries.
- Neurovascular compromise.
- Open injury.

### Outpatient follow-up

- Isolated scapholunate dissociation (Mayfield stage I injury).
- Undisplaced greater arc fractures.

## Orthopaedic management

### Non-operative

Undisplaced ligament injuries or fractures are initially treated as wrist sprains with temporary immobilization for comfort.

### Operative

Injuries with displacement or dislocation usually require surgery.

Persistent functional pain or clicking after an undisplaced carpal injury may indicate subtle dynamic instability. This can be assessed clinically with the Watson provocation test for scapholunate dissociation. The test is performed with the thumb over the scaphoid tubercle (as shown in Fig. 12.29), pushing the scaphoid dorsally into extension. Movement of the wrist in radial and ulnar deviation will produce a painful click or clunk. The nature of the injury can be clarified further with an MRI scan of the carpal ligaments. Local ligament reconstruction or limited carpal fusion may be required.

### Surgical techniques

The repair of acute scapholunate dissociation (Mayfield stage I) and lunate dislocations (Mayfield IV) is conceptually similar.

Perilunate dislocations are approached via both volar and dorsal incisions. From the volar incision, the carpal tunnel is decompressed (p. 260); caution is required, as the median nerve is displaced by the presence of the lunate. This allows access to the lunate and the volar extrinsic ligaments. The strongest component of the scapholunate articulation is, however, the dorsal ligament, and this is assessed and repaired through a dorsal approach centred over the scapholunate interval. The injury is often found to be an avulsion of the intact ligament from either the scaphoid or the lunate, leaving a small cancellous bare area. With traction and the occasional use of k-wire joysticks, the lunate can be reduced back under the capitate, via both incisions. The excessive extension of the lunate can be reduced by flexing the wrist and engaging the dorsal surface of the lunate with a k-wire (**Fig. 12.39A**) before allowing the wrist to return to a neutral position (**Fig. 12.39B**). The reduction can then be perfected and stabilized with transfixion k-wires (**Fig. 12.39C,D**). Finally, the scapholunate ligament is repaired or reattached with suture anchors. The k-wires are usually removed at 10 weeks.

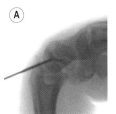 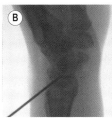 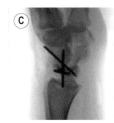 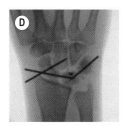

Fig. 12.39 Scapholunate dissociation: operative steps. See text for details.

## COMPLICATIONS

### Early

Local   Median nerve palsy: The displacement of the lunate into the carpal tunnel commonly results in an acute carpal tunnel syndrome (see below)

### Late

Local   Persistent instability: Some persistent or recurrent displacement may occur after initial repair or present after non-operative treatment. This often progresses to secondary post-traumatic arthritis of the wrist and carpus with pain and instability. This is termed a scapholunate advanced collapse (SLAC) wrist. Arthritic degeneration proceeds in a predictable sequence, according to the Watson classification, between:

- stage 1 – the scaphoid and the radial styloid
- stage 2 – the entire radioscaphoid articulation
- stage 3 – the lunocapitate joint.

Salvage surgery in the form of intercarpal fusion, proximal row carpectomy or wrist fusion may be required.

## CARPAL TUNNEL SYNDROME

Acute carpal tunnel syndrome may develop after injuries or infection of the distal forearm or wrist. The aetiology is usually tissue oedema in the carpal tunnel, but occasionally, direct pressure on the median nerve can result from an extruded lunate, or from tenting of the nerve over a dorsally tilted or displaced wrist fracture (Fig. 3.11). Chronic carpal tunnel syndrome is a related condition, developing either primarily or in association with a condition such as pregnancy or inflammatory joint disease.

## Emergency Department management

### Clinical features

- The patient will have an injury or infection in the region of the hand or wrist, and may complain of swelling, pain, paraesthesia and numbness in the wrist and hand.

- Clinical examination will reveal reduced or absent sensation in the median nerve distribution (see Fig. 3.17), with preserved sensation in the ulnar and radial distributions.

- The patient will have weakness of thumb opposition and abduction (median nerve), but a normal 'OK' sign (anterior interosseous nerve), as well as finger abduction/adduction (ulnar nerve).
- Two confirmatory features commonly assessed in the context of chronic carpal tunnel syndrome – Tinel's sign (paraesthesia in the distribution of the median nerve, elicited by tapping over the transverse carpal ligament) and Phalen's test (symptoms provoked by maximal flexion of the wrist) – are usually uncomfortable and impractical in the emergency setting.

## Radiological features
- *PA and lateral wrist radiographs*: Radiographs of the wrist are required to exclude a bony abnormality.

## Closed reduction
A displaced fracture or dislocation of the wrist or carpus, complicated by a dense or progressive median nerve palsy, must be reduced urgently under procedural sedation.

### Immobilization and reassessment
If there is already a bandage or cast in place, this should be split along its whole length, down to skin, to relieve any circumferential constriction. The wrist should be splinted for comfort, taking care not to recreate any constriction. The limb should be elevated in a high-elevation arm sling or Bradford sling (see Figs 4.22 and 4.23). Repeat neurovascular examination is required to ensure symptoms are improving.

### Inpatient referral
- All patients with neurovascular complications – refer to Orthopaedics.

## Orthopaedic management
### Non-operative
Patients who are clearly improving, particularly where the cause of the palsy has been addressed by the reduction of a fracture or dislocation, can be kept in high elevation and observed closely.

### Operative
Patients who have a persistent or worsening acute carpal tunnel syndrome usually require surgical decompression.

### SURGICAL TECHNIQUE: Carpal tunnel decompression

#### Surgical set-up
The patient is positioned supine with an arm tourniquet, and the arm on a hand table.

#### Incision (Fig. 12.40)
The incision is 2–4 cm long, in line with the ulnar border of the tip of the flexed ring finger, starting just proximal to Kaplan's cardinal line (the location of the deep palmar arterial arch, see Fig. 2.9) and extending proximally towards the distal transverse wrist skin crease. Where an additional (modified) Henry approach to the distal radius is needed for wrist plating, either an S-shaped incision or two separate incisions can be used. If a single incision is used, it is important to dissect bluntly and carefully around the palmar cutaneous branch of the median nerve (which lies superficial to the retinaculum) to avoid injury to this structure.

#### Procedure
Four layers are opened separately in turn, under direct vision:

1. Skin: This is divided sharply with a knife.
2. Subcutaneous fat: This layer can be split and retracted.
3. Palmar fascia: This is divided sharply with a knife.
4. Transverse carpal ligament: This is divided with a knife after clearing the surface of the ligament and checking visually for the presence of the recurrent motor branch of

the median nerve, which may overlie or even penetrate the ligament. It is safest to make a small incision and then place a small dissector, such as a MacDonald's, through this opening to protect the contents of the canal; reverse the knife to cut upwards whilst completing the division.

The completeness of the release is checked both proximally and distally. The contents of the canal, particularly the median nerve, are inspected and confirmed to be intact. The skin only is closed with mattress sutures.

### Post procedure

The hand is lightly bandaged in absorbent gauze and elevated postoperatively.

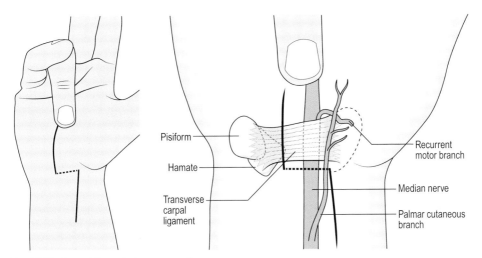

Fig. 12.40 Carpal tunnel decompression.

## DIFFERENTIAL DIAGNOSES FOR ACUTE WRIST PAIN

### De Quervain's tenosynovitis

This is one of the most common differential diagnoses for wrist pain. The tendons of the first dorsal compartment (extensor pollicis brevis and abductor pollicis longus) become inflamed following a direct blow or a wrist sprain, or injury may be related to overuse or inflammatory joint disease.

### Clinical features

- There is tenderness, and sometimes crepitus, on palpation of the first dorsal compartment over the distal radius, and of the associated tendons. These structures can be identified by asking the patient to demonstrate a 'thumbs up' position.

- Finkelstein's test stretches the tendons and exacerbates the pain. Ask the patient to form a fist, enclosing the thumb. Ulnar deviation of the wrist produces a characteristic severe pain at the first dorsal compartment (**Fig. 12.41**).

- This is a clinical diagnosis and no investigation is specifically indicated.

### Management

Management is principally with splintage to protect the wrist during activity (provide a wrist splint with thumb extension), accompanied by progressive mobilization and stretching. An injection of local anaesthetic and steroid into the first dorsal compartment can be helpful to confirm the diagnosis and to alleviate symptoms (**Fig. 12.41**). Occasionally, surgical release of the compartment is required after

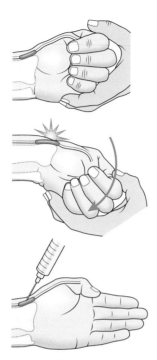

Fig. 12.41 Finkelstein's test and injection.

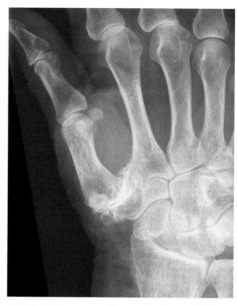

Fig. 12.42 Trapeziometacarpal osteoarthritis.

failure of non-operative treatment. An incision is made directly over the compartment; blunt dissection through fat is necessary in order to avoid injury to the dorsal branch of the radial nerve. The compartment is opened and then carefully inspected; there are often septa within it around one or other of the tendons, and these septa must also be divided.

## Wrist sprain

This is a diagnosis of exclusion, based on a history of injury, the presence of localized tenderness but not deformity, and the absence of radiographic abnormality. Tenderness is maximal at the radiocarpal joint, usually dor-sally, rather than over the bones of the distal radius or carpus.

Treatment is with advice regarding RICE: *r*est, application of *i*ce, *c*ompression or the provision of a stockingette bandage or a splint, and *e*levation.

## Trapeziometacarpal arthritis

This is a very common site of degenerative arthritis, which may have been relatively asymptomatic prior to a minor injury. Patients will present with a localized exacerbation of pain and tenderness, and radiographic evidence of established arthritis (**Fig. 12.42**). Treatment is symptomatic, with reassurance, splintage, analgesia and advice regarding gradual mobilization. Recalcitrant cases may respond to an intra-articular injection or, ultimately, a trapeziectomy.

## GENERAL PRINCIPLES

Injuries to the metacarpals and fingers are the most common orthopaedic presentation to Emergency Departments and fracture clinics. Many injuries can be successfully managed non-operatively with splintage and active rehabilitation. Some problems, however, such as the presence of a rotational deformity, require early recognition and intervention.

## Anatomy

The normal hand has five *rays*, with a metacarpal subtending each digit (**Fig. 13.1**). Although the rays and metacarpals are commonly numbered from one to five, starting from the radial side, this can cause confusion when describing the fingers and so these must always be named: thumb, index, middle, ring and little. The bones of the hand are described as having a metaphyseal base and a shaft. The metacarpals terminate in a neck and head, while the proximal and intermediate phalanges have a distal metaphysis with medial and lateral condyles, and the distal phalanges have a terminal tuft. The metacarpophalangeal joints (MCPJs) and interphalangeal joints (IPJs) are stabilized by radial and ulnar collateral ligaments. The *metacarpal head* is not circular but cam-shaped, such that the collateral ligaments are longest at 90° of MCPJ flexion but are able to shorten in extension (**Fig. 13.2**). In contrast, the collateral ligaments of the IPJs are longer in extension and will shorten in flexion. When these joints are immobilized, it is essential to do so in the 'position of safety', where these ligaments are at their longest (Fig. 13.11). Immobilization in any other position risks contracture of the collateral ligaments, which can result in permanent disability. The metacarpals articulate with the carpus at the carpometacarpal joints (CMCJs). The thumb metacarpal articulation with the trapezium (trapeziometacarpal joint, TMJ) is considered separately because of its high degree of mobility and vulnerability to injury.

### Volar plate

The volar plate is a fibrocartilaginous reinforcement of the joint capsule of the MCPJs and IPJs. The volar plates contribute greatly to finger joint stability, as they merge not only with the volar joint capsule, but also with the sagittal bands of the extensor tendons, and with the transverse metacarpal ligament that connects all of the metacarpal heads. In finger dislocations, a small fragment of bone is often seen at the volar base of the phalanx, representing an avulsion injury to the volar plate. The plate can occasionally fall into the joint, blocking reduction (see Fig. 13.33).

### Extensor tendons

The extensor tendon to each finger broadens out into a flat extensor hood as it reaches the MCPJ (**Fig. 13.3**). This blends with the joint capsule and reinforces it before dividing into central and lateral slips. The central slip attaches to the proximal phalanx and volar plate (via sagittal bands) before terminating on the intermediate (middle) phalanx. The lateral bands are joined by the lumbricals before reuniting to insert into the base of the distal phalanx. This arrangement is the basis by which a boutonnière deformity occurs (p. 283).

### Flexor tendons

The flexor tendons travel through a sheath on the volar aspect of each digit (**Fig. 13.3**). The sheath has a number of thickenings termed the annular and cruciate pulleys, which are numbered. The flexor digitorum superficialis (FDS) tendon in each digit divides to form Camper's chiasm and then inserts into the intermediate phalanx. The flexor digitorum profundus (FDP) tendon passes through this chiasm to insert into the base of the terminal phalanx. The FDP

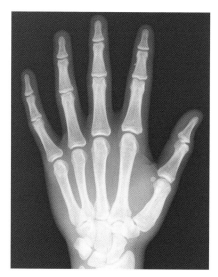

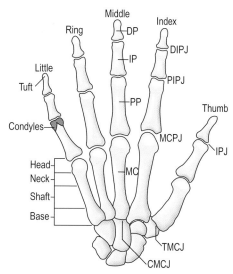

Fig. 13.1 Hand osteology. CMCJ, carpometacarpal joint; DIPJ, distal interphalangeal joint; DP, distal phalanx; IP, intermediate phalanx; IPJ, interphalangeal joint; MC, metacarpal; MCPJ, metacarpophalangeal joint; PIPJ, proximal interphalangeal joint; PP, proximal phalanx; TMCJ, trapeziometacarpal joint.

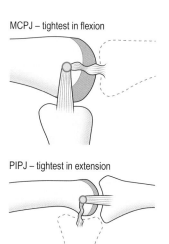

Fig. 13.2 Finger collateral ligaments. MCPJ, metacarpophalangeal joint; PIPJ, proximal interphalangeal joint.

has a single common muscle belly and flexes all of the digits simultaneously (to form a power grip). The FDS has separate muscle bellies for each digit, allowing each to be flexed separately (such as when playing the piano).

## Thumb

The thumb is highly independently mobile, allowing the useful movement of thumb opposition, enabling grip and fine prehensile manipulation. It is extended by extensor pollicis longus (EPL) and brevis (EPB). The tendon of EPL passes through the third dorsal extensor compartment and around Lister's tubercle of the radius before inserting into the base of the distal phalanx. EPB passes through the first dorsal compartment and inserts into the proximal phalanx. The thumb is flexed by flexor pollicis longus (inserting at the base of the distal phalanx) and flexor pollicis brevis (inserting into the proximal phalanx).

## Clinical assessment of the painful hand

Given the multiplicity of activities for which the hand is used, it is not surprising that injuries and infection are common. As for many conditions, the history not only provides the context, but also often gives a clear indication of the diagnosis.

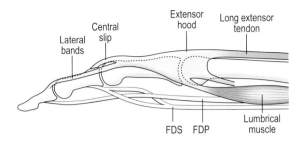

Fig. 13.3 Flexor and extensor tendons. FDP, flexor digitorum profundus; FDS, flexor digitorum superficialis.

## History

Enquire about the patient and the nature of the injury. Is the patient left or right hand-dominant? Ask about occupation, sports and hobbies. Previous injuries and operations should be noted, as they may complicate the clinical picture. Ask about conditions that commonly affect hand form and function, most notably rheumatoid arthritis, psoriatic arthritis and gout. Several common injuries affect the hand:

- *Crush injuries* often occur to the fingertips and may cause a tuft fracture, subungual haematoma or nailbed injury.

- *Penetrating injuries* may breach joints or the flexor sheath. How clean was the environment and the sharp implement involved? Wounds caused by broken glass are noteworthy, as the skin wound may look benign but the underlying soft tissue injury can be significant. The only structure that will stop the penetration of glass is bone.

- A *'fight bite'* injury occurs when the patient's closed fist strikes another individual's teeth. The resulting wound over the MCPJ can look innocuous, and may appear to be a superficial skin laceration when the hand is held straight. However, when the fingers are flexed to form a fist, the penetrating injury to the extensor hood and MCPJ is usually revealed.

- *Twisting and pulling* injuries may cause avulsions at the insertions of tendons (mallet finger and rugger jersey finger), the collateral ligaments or the volar plate, or may lead to spiral fractures.

- *Axial loading* injuries (e.g. from being struck by a ball on the fingertip) may cause joint dislocations or articular fractures.

- Deep *infection* of the joints or a flexor tendon sheath often presents with worsening pain, swelling and loss of function.

## Examination

### Look

Inspect the hand for bruising, swelling, wounds and deformity. In particular, rotational deformity may not be apparent on initial inspection or on subsequent radiographs (see below for assessment of rotation). Note the *cascade* of the hand: the normal, partially flexed positions of the fingers when the hand is at rest (**Fig. 13.4A**). With passive wrist extension, this cascade becomes more obvious as the fingers flex (**Fig. 13.4B**). Where there is a flexor tendon injury, this cascade is disturbed and the injured finger will be straight (see ***arrow*** on Fig. 13.4). With passive wrist flexion, the fingers extend and any deformity may be less apparent (**Fig. 13.4C**). Infections of the skin (cellulitis or paronychia) should be distinguished from infections of the joints (septic arthritis) and of the flexor tendon sheath (see Kanavel's signs, Fig. 13.42). Pre-existing conditions may cause confusion. Inflammatory joint disease, in particular, causes deforming small-joint polyarthropathy. Osteoarthritis may present with osteophytes of the distal IPJs (Heberden's nodes) or proximal IPJs (Bouchard's nodes).

### Feel

Palpate the bones and joints carefully to identify any site of tenderness, swelling or crepitus.

### Move

- *Screening movements*: Ask the patient to flex and extend each of the digits fully. Lack of active movement may indicate division of a tendon or pain inhibition from an injured or infected joint.

Flexor tendon injury

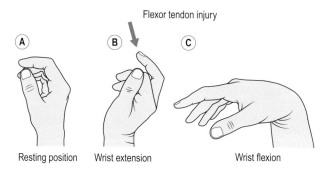

(A) Resting position   (B) Wrist extension   (C) Wrist flexion

Fig. 13.4 The hand cascade. Division of the flexor tendons in the finger is revealed when the wrist is extended (arrow).

Flexor digitorum profundus

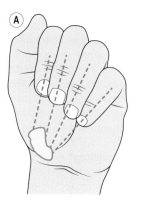

Flexor digitorum superficialis

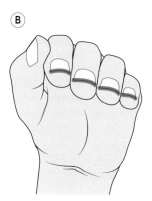

Fig. 13.5 Flexor tendon assessment.

Fig. 13.6 Rotational assessment.

- *Extensor tendons*: Confirm that patients can demonstrate active joint extension of all joints in all digits by asking them to hold their hand with the palm down and all the fingers straight out.
- *Flexor tendons*: Where there is suspected injury to the flexor tendons, the FDS and FDP tendons must be examined separately. For each digit, check that the patient has active flexion at the distal IPJ (only FDP can do this; **Fig. 13.5A**). Then check that the patient has active flexion of that digit at the proximal IPJ when the tips of the adjacent digits are held in extension (only FDS can do this; **Fig. 13.5B**).
- *Rotational assessment*: When the fingers are flexed, each finger should point towards the scaphoid (**Fig. 13.6A**). If the patient cannot flex their fingers, look at the orientation of the fingernails in the position of safety (**Fig. 13.6B**).

- *Joint stability*: Where there is a question of instability (e.g. ulnar collateral ligament injury to the thumb), gently but firmly stress the joint and compare it to the contralateral joint (see Fig. 13.31).

### Neurovascular assessment

The sensory supply to the hand is described on page 32. For the purposes of examination (and surgical repair), only the larger volar digital nerves are considered; check for sensation along the radial and ulnar borders of each digit. Assess capillary refill at the nailbed. If there is a laceration, carefully inspect the capillary refill of any distal skin flap.

## Radiological assessment of the painful hand

### Hand series of radiographs

The hand series includes three radiographs:

- *PA view* (**Fig. 13.7A**): This is taken with the hand laid flat, palm down. It includes the carpus, metacarpals and all phalanges.

- *Oblique view* (**Fig. 13.7B**): A view in mid-pronation provides additional information and can allow subtle fractures to be identified.

- *Lateral view* (**Fig. 13.7C**): The hand rests against the plate, ulnar side down.

### Finger radiographs

Patients with suspected phalangeal injury should have specific finger views taken, including a PA (**Fig. 13.8A**) and a lateral (**Fig. 13.8B**).

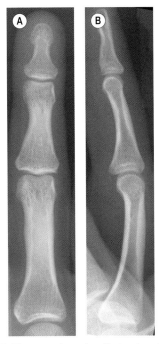

Fig. 13.8 Finger series of radiographs. **A**, PA view. **B**, Lateral view.

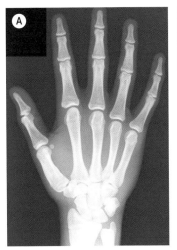
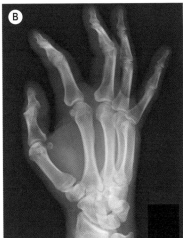
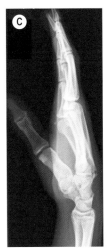

Fig. 13.7 Hands series of radiographs. **A**, PA view. **B**, Oblique view. **C**, Lateral view.

## IMMOBILIZATION OF HAND INJURIES

The majority of hand injuries are managed non-operatively with simple splintage.

### Mallet splint

A mallet splint is used primarily to maintain DIPJ extension in the treatment of a mallet finger (p. 279), but can also be used to protect tuft fractures and other painful conditions of the fingertip. Correct sizing is important to ensure that the finger is not constricted (too small) or is allowed to flex (too large). The splint is secured with tape. When a mallet splint is used to treat mallet injuries, the patient must be given explicit instructions on how to remove and re-apply it; poor technique will result in temporary loss of extension and will disrupt the healing tissue. Two important instructions should be given to patients:

1. During tape change, the fingertip should rest on a surface to maintain distal IPJ extension while allowing access to the tape (**Fig. 13.9A**).

2. When the splint is removed/applied for cleaning, the whole finger should rest on a flat surface (**Fig. 13.9B**).

## Buddy strapping

Simple, stable fractures and IPJ dislocations can be treated effectively with buddy (neighbour) strapping. Before application, prepare a gauze swab (cut to the length of the affected finger and folded, but not left bulky such that it forces the fingers apart); several strips of zinc oxide tape (less adhesive tapes such as micropore are not suitable), cut to the correct length, will also be needed. Place the gauze swab pad between the injured finger and an adjacent finger (**Fig. 13.10A**). Use the tape above and below the IPJs to splint the two together (**Fig. 13.10B**). Ensure that the tape is snug but does not constrict the circulation.

## Hand splintage

Potentially unstable phalangeal fractures, or fractures of the metacarpals, are most comfortably immobilized with a hand splint in the *position of safety*.

This position is maintained using either:

- a *padded malleable splint* commonly referred to as a 'Zimmer splint'; this is a metal strip padded with foam
- a *plaster slab*
- a *thermoplastic splint* supported with straps.

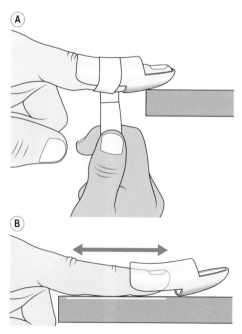

Fig. 13.9 Mallet splint.

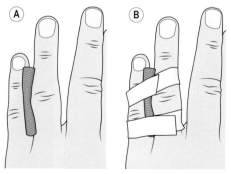

Fig. 13.10 Buddy strapping.

##  Key point

The position of safety is 90° of flexion at the MCPJs and full extension of the IPJs, with slight extension of the wrist (**Fig. 13.11**). This minimizes the risk of stiffness and contractures (p. 263 and Fig. 13.2).

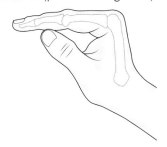

Fig. 13.11 Position of safety.

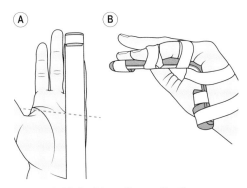

Fig. 13.12 Malleable splint application.

## Application of malleable splintage

This splint supports the fingers and metacarpals, and has the advantages of being light and leaving the wrist free. Application of the splint is as follows:

1. Size and shape the splint against the uninjured side (**Fig. 13.12A**). The right-angled bend in the splint lies at the level of the transverse palmar crease. If it is placed any further distally, the MCPJs will be held in a certain degree of extension.

2. Buddy-strap the affected fingers first before placing them on the splint.

3. Apply the splint to the palm of the hand and flex the fingers down on to it.

4. Secure the splint around the fingers with two strips of tape and use two more strips around the hand (**Fig. 13.12B**).

## Application of a volar hand slab (Fig. 13.13)

1. *Prepare the equipment*:
   - 8–10-cm width plaster slab, eight layers thick.
   - Soft wool roll.
   - 8-cm diameter bandage.
   - Bucket of tepid water.
   - Ring removal from the patient's fingers.

The slab should extend from the tip of the middle finger to the mid-forearm. Wrap the slab in wool or stockingette before immersing it in water to prevent the plaster material from coming into contact with the patient's skin. Wrapping the wool or stockingette around the slab rather than around the patient's hand allows for easier moulding and girdering (see below), and subsequent removal.

2. *Wet the slab*: Keep hold of both ends of the slab and concertina it between your hands. Immerse it completely for 4 seconds in tepid water. Squeeze firmly to remove water – the plaster material will be retained by the wool bandage.

3. *Add a girder (ridge) to the slab*: After immersing it in water but before applying it to the injured hand, lay the slab on a flat surface and pinch up a girder. This increases the strength of the slab enormously.

4. *Apply the slab*: Apply the girdered slab to the palmar aspect of the hand, with the bend level with the distal palmar crease. Take care to ensure that the MCPJs are flexed to 90°, the fingers are straight, the thumb is free and the wrist is slightly extended.

5. *Bandage*: Secure the slab with a bandage. The tips of the fingers should be visible.

6. *Appraise the cast*: The whole length of all of the fingers should be supported. Rubbing is

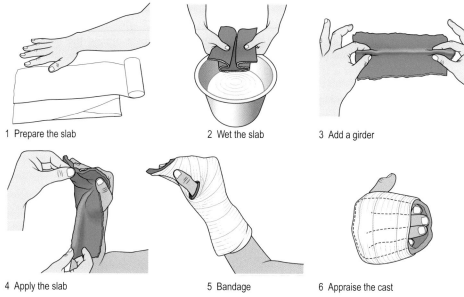

1 Prepare the slab     2 Wet the slab     3 Add a girder

4 Apply the slab     5 Bandage     6 Appraise the cast

Fig. 13.13 Hand volar slab application.

common in the first web space between the thumb and index finger – trim or pad as necessary. Reassess the rotational alignment, capillary refill and sensation to the fingers.

An *ulnar slab* is a modification that is useful for injuries to the little finger or metacarpal. It uses a narrower strip of plaster slab applied to the ulnar aspect of the hand; this splints the little and ring fingers, leaving the middle and index fingers free.

## Thumb immobilization

The thumb can be immobilized by a simple plaster slab (**Fig. 13.14**).

### Application of a thumb slab
1. *Prepare the equipment*:
   - 8–10-cm width plaster slab, eight layers thick.
   - Stockingette.
   - Finger stockingette.
   - Soft wool roll.
   - 8-cm diameter bandage.
   - Bucket of tepid water.
   - Ring removal from the patient's fingers.

The slab should extend from the base of the thumbnail to mid-forearm, immobilizing the wrist in order to afford additional strength. The hand is positioned as though holding a glass, with the wrist in slight extension.

2. *Apply stockingette*: Begin by placing a small piece of the finger stockingette over the thumb, cutting a small slit at the base to cover the first web space. Then apply the stockingette over the wrist as for a normal wrist backslab, cutting a small hole to allow the passage of the thumb.

3. *Apply soft wool*: Run a double layer of wool from the mid-forearm up to the tip of the thumb.

4. *Wet the slab*: Keep hold of both ends of the slab and concertina it between your hands. Immerse it completely for 4 seconds in tepid water. Squeeze to remove water.

5. *Apply the slab*: Apply the slab from the base of the thumbnail over the radial aspect of the thumb and wrist.

6. *Bandage*: Fold back the stockingette and wool, and apply a damp crepe bandage to secure the slab. This should be firm enough to prevent the slab from moving but should not constrict the soft tissues.

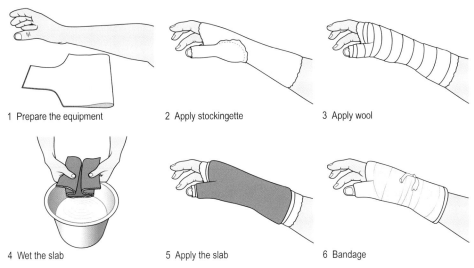

1  Prepare the equipment    2  Apply stockingette    3  Apply wool

4  Wet the slab    5  Apply the slab    6  Bandage

Fig. 13.14 Application of a thumb slab.

### Full casts for thumb injuries

Certain thumb injuries (such as 'gamekeeper's thumb'; p. 280) are treated definitively in a full cast. The Brunner cast encloses the palm, and the thumb up to the distal IPJ, but does not include the wrist. The thumb is held in a neutral position, as if the patient were holding a glass.

## Elevation

Patients should be instructed to keep the injured hand elevated, with regular active movements of the shoulder and elbow. This may simply involve them holding the injured hand on the contralateral shoulder. However, provision of a high-elevation arm sling may be more comfortable (see Fig. 4.22).

Avoid the use of a broad arm sling or collar-and-cuff for hand injuries; these allow the hand to hang down in a dependent position and cause constriction at the wrist, exacerbating the development of swelling. Inpatients with swelling should be provided with a Bradford sling (see Fig. 4.23).

## METACARPAL FRACTURES

Metacarpal fractures are extremely common following sporting and recreational activity.

Many are stable and minimally displaced, and require only symptomatic treatment. However, some metacarpal fractures will require reduction, or are unstable and may require fixation.

## METACARPAL HEAD FRACTURES

Fracture of the metacarpal head often occurs after a direct blow, with a resulting small osteochondral chip.

## Emergency Department management

No reduction is required and patients are managed initially with buddy strapping (see Fig. 13.10) and a high-elevation arm sling (see Fig. 4.22). Open fractures and grossly displaced or comminuted fractures should be referred to the orthopaedic service. All other fractures are referred to the fracture clinic.

## Orthopaedic management

### Non-operative

Simple fractures can be reviewed at 1 week in the fracture clinic and treated with buddy strapping for comfort and early mobilization.

### Operative

Displaced fractures may require reduction and fixation with wires, screws or sutures to maintain the stability and orientation of the MCPJ. Small fragments may simply require excision.

## METACARPAL NECK FRACTURES

These are usually the result of a direct impact to (or, more often, by) the fist, and have a dorsal angulation with variable volar comminution. The term 'boxer's fracture' describes a fracture to the fifth metacarpal neck (**Fig. 13.15**).

## Emergency Department management

In the *index and middle* metacarpals, up to 20° of angulation can be accepted without any effect on MCPJ function. In the *ring and little* metacarpals, up to 45° of angulation can be accepted. Angulation greater than this can be

corrected under metacarpal block (see p. 33) by a simple reduction manœuvre (**Fig. 13.16**). With one finger over the apex of the fracture, flex the MCPJ and use the patient's finger to provide a posteriorly directed force to the metacarpal head. The position is secured with a malleable splint or plaster slab (see Figs 13.12 and 13.13) in the position of safety. The patient is given a high-elevation arm sling (see Fig. 4.22) and referred to the fracture clinic.

## Orthopaedic management

### Non-operative

Fractures within acceptable degrees of angulation can be reviewed at 1 week and managed with early mobilization, along with buddy strapping for comfort if required. If a reduction manœuvre has been necessary, immobilize the fracture for 3 weeks using a malleable splint before commencing mobilization (see Fig. 13.12).

### Operative

These fractures only rarely require surgery but where there is marked angulation, or instability with displacement in a splint, fixation with k-wires or small blade plates is effective.

## METACARPAL SHAFT FRACTURES

Like metacarpal neck fractures, these are typically angulated dorsally but may also

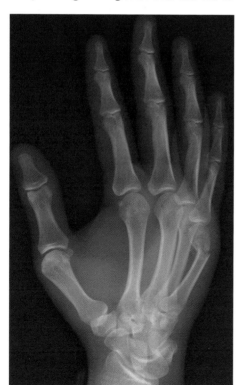

Fig. 13.15 Boxer's fracture.

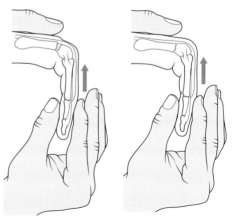

Fig. 13.16 Metacarpal neck and shaft reduction manœuvre.

be rotated. Fractures are usually transverse (**Fig. 13.17A**) or spiral (**Fig. 13.17B**) in morphology. Spiral fractures commonly follow twisting injuries and should be treated with particular suspicion, as they are more liable to shortening and rotation. In particular, the index and little finger metacarpals are prone to rotation, whereas the middle and ring fingers are supported on both sides by the transverse metacarpal ligaments.

## Emergency Department management

Up to 20° of dorsal angulation can be accepted. These fractures can be immobilized with buddy strapping (or if the patient is very uncomfortable, a plaster slab; see Fig. 13.13) and a high-elevation sling (see Fig. 4.22). Greater degrees of angulation can usually be corrected under a metacarpal block (as for a metacarpal neck fracture; see above), followed by slab immobilization and elevation sling (see Fig. 4.22). Where there is residual deformity of more than 20° or an evident rotational deformity, an orthopaedic review is required. Patients should otherwise be referred to the fracture clinic.

## Orthopaedic management

### Non-operative
Simple fractures within the acceptable parameters described above can be mobilized as pain allows. Formal immobilization is not required but buddy strapping may be supplied for comfort. Fractures requiring closed reduction are rested in cast for 3 weeks before mobilization is commenced.

### Operative
Fractures that have a residual deformity of more than 20° angulation should be considered for surgical intervention. Similarly, a rotational deformity that is clearly evident or prevents the formation of a fist usually requires reduction and operative stabilization. Metacarpal shaft fractures may be treated using a number of operative techniques:

- *Transverse k-wires*: The fracture is reduced closed, with longitudinal traction, rotation and angulation as required. K-wires are then driven from the border of the hand, aiming to splint the fractured metacarpal to an adjacent ray. The surgeon grasps each metacarpal in turn between thumb and index finger, and this palpation of the volar and dorsal surfaces allows the wire to be advanced in the correct trajectory (**Fig. 13.18**). Two wires are usually required in the distal fragment to control angulation, and a third wire just proximal to the fracture provides additional stability (**Fig. 13.19**).

- *Intramedullary k-wires*: (**Fig. 13.20**) Longitudinal wires act powerfully to maintain angular stability. A large-diameter (2-mm) wire or a drill bit is used to breach the metacarpal base dorsally, and a smaller-diameter (1.6-mm) wire is then introduced and passed across the fracture. A small bend at

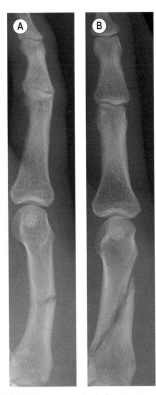

Fig. 13.17 Metacarpal shaft fracture morphology. **A**, Transverse. **B**, Spiral.

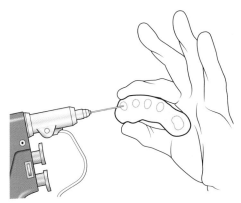

Fig. 13.18 Transverse k-wire technique.

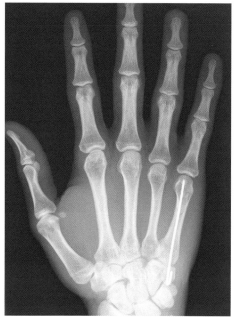

Fig. 13.20 Metacarpal longitudinal k-wire.

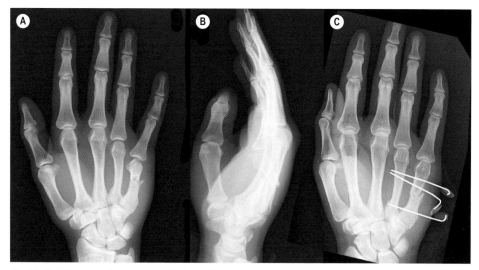

Fig. 13.19 Metacarpal transverse k-wires. **A,B,** The fifth metacarpal is shortened and angulated. AP and lateral views. **C,** The reduced fracture is stabilized with transverse k-wires, which splint it to the fourth metacarpal.

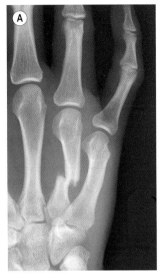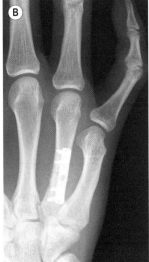

Fig. 13.21 Metacarpal plating.
**A**, Displaced fracture of the fourth metacarpal.
**B**, Fracture fixed with a dorsal compact hand set plate.

the tip of the wire helps its introduction into the medullary canal.

- *Open reduction and internal fixation*: (**Fig. 13.21**) Where a closed reduction cannot be obtained or maintained, a formal open reduction is required with the application of a mini-fragment plate. The metacarpal is exposed via a longitudinal incision, which is placed to one side of the extensor tendon. Two adjacent metacarpals can be addressed through one incision placed midway between them. There is an incidence of extensor tendon adhesion to the plate.

## FINGER METACARPAL BASE FRACTURES

These are common, caused by axial loading injuries such as a punch. They most commonly affect the fourth and fifth rays. Fractures to the base of the thumb metacarpal are considered separately.

## Emergency Department management

Simple undisplaced fractures are treated with a wrist splint or volar slab for comfort, with fracture clinic follow-up. Displaced metacarpal base fractures are usually dorsal shear frac-tures or CMCJ dislocations that require ortho-paedic review.

## Orthopaedic management

### Non-operative

The majority of injuries are treated with removable splintage for comfort and early mobilization.

### Operative

Displaced fractures and dislocations are treated by closed reduction and k-wire fixation (see Fig. 12.32).

## THUMB METACARPAL BASE FRACTURES

### Extra-articular fractures

These are commonly transverse or short-oblique in orientation and are therefore rela-tively stable. Modest angulation is very common and does not require reduction, as this is easily compensated for by the TMJ. Surgery is reserved for very displaced fractures.

### Intra-articular fractures

- *Bennett's fracture* (**Fig. 13.22**): This partial articular fracture is very common. A small volar lip fragment of the metacarpal base

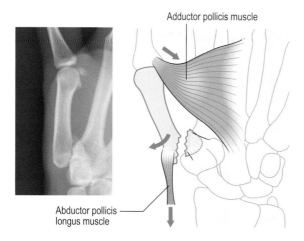

Adductor pollicis muscle

Abductor pollicis longus muscle

Fig. 13.22 Bennett's fracture.

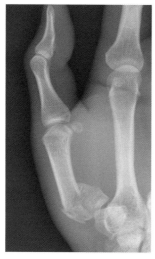

Fig. 13.23 Rolando fracture.

remains in an anatomical and stable position attached to the trapezium. The remainder of the metacarpal and the thumb, however, are displaced proximally (by abductor pollicis longus) and into adduction and supination (by adductor pollicis).

- *Rolando fracture* (**Fig. 13.23**): This is a complete articular fracture and is usually highly unstable.

## Emergency Department management

Minimally displaced Bennett's fractures can be immobilized in a thumb slab (see Fig. 13.14) or a removable splint with thumb extension. A high-elevation sling (see Fig. 4.22) is provided for comfort and the patient referred for fracture clinic follow-up. Where there is marked displacement, refer to the orthopaedic service.

## Orthopaedic management
### Non-operative
Minimally displaced Bennett's fractures are treated in a Bennett's cast or removable splint for 6 weeks.

### Operative
In displaced extra-articular or intra-articular (Bennett's and Rolando) fractures, reduction is usually simple, but is very difficult to maintain in cast. Operative closed reduction and k-wire fixation are usually required. Reduction is achieved with longitudinal traction and direct pressure over the metacarpal base (**Fig. 13.24**). This position can be maintained by passing one or two k-wires transversely from the thumb metacarpal into the second metacarpal. Alternatively, a Bennett's fracture can be fixed by directing the wire into the trapezium, either as a 'blocking' wire, or through the thumb metacarpal base as a transfixion wire. **Figure 13.25** shows both a transverse and a transfixion wire, although one of these is generally sufficient. Postoperatively, the thumb is immobilized for 3 weeks. Wires are then removed in clinic before commencing mobilization.

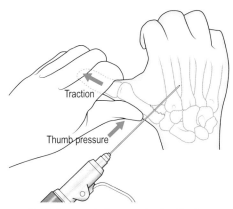

Fig. 13.24 Bennett's fracture k-wire fixation technique.

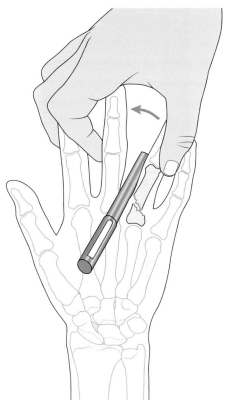

Fig. 13.26 Proximal phalanx reduction manœuvre.

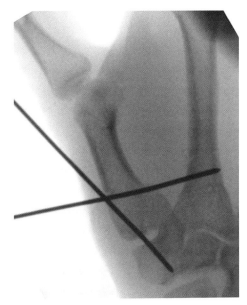

Fig. 13.25 Bennett's fracture k-wire fixation.

# PHALANGEAL FRACTURES

## PROXIMAL AND INTERMEDIATE PHALANGES: EXTRA-ARTICULAR FRACTURES

### Emergency Department management

Fractures of the phalangeal shafts are often minimally displaced and stable, and can be managed non-operatively with buddy strapping.

Minor degrees of angulation can be corrected with manipulation under a metacarpal or ring block. Place a pen in the web space to act as a fulcrum and gently apply a corrective force to the finger (**Fig. 13.26**). Buddy-strap the same two fingers together (in the illustration above, the middle and ring fingers) to maintain this force vector.

## Orthopaedic management
### Non-operative
Undisplaced fractures are treated with buddy strapping for 3 weeks before commencing early mobilization.

### Operative
Persistent angulation, and particularly rotational displacement, may require operative reduction and stabilization with wires, screws or small plates (**Fig. 13.27**).

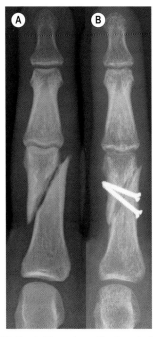

Fig. 13.27 Unstable extra-articular phalangeal fracture with screw fixation. **A,** Oblique fracture with shortening. **B,** After lag screw fixation.

## PROXIMAL AND INTERMEDIATE PHALANGES: INTRA-ARTICULAR FRACTURES

Intra-articular (condylar) fractures of either the proximal or the distal metaphysis may result in joint instability and displacement.

## Emergency Department management

Splint the injured digit with buddy strapping. Where there is minimal displacement, refer to the fracture clinic. Where these fractures are displaced, they generally require surgery; refer to Orthopaedics.

## Orthopaedic management

### Non-operative

Minimally displaced fractures are splinted in buddy strapping for 3 or 4 weeks.

### Operative

Displaced intra-articular fractures are fixed with wires, screws or mini T-plates. Severely comminuted 'pilon' fractures (with impaction of the articular surface) may not be amenable to fixation and can be spanned with mini-external fixation devices (**Fig. 13.28**).

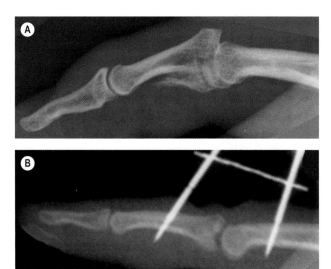

Fig. 13.28 Intra-articular phalangeal fracture. **A,** Comminuted 'pilon' fracture. **B,** After treatment with spanning external fixation.

## DISTAL PHALANX: MALLET FINGER INJURY

This is an avulsion of the extensor tendon insertion into the base of the distal phalanx, with or without a bony fragment (**Fig. 13.29**). Injury results in a typical flexion deformity, or 'droop' to the DIPJ. Bony avulsions may be large, and specific attention should be paid to the congruence of the DIPJ, as in more severe injuries the joint can sublux.

## Emergency Department management

Provided the joint is congruent, both types of mallet injury can be treated in a mallet splint (see Fig. 13.9). For bony injuries, a repeat radiograph should be taken in the splint to confirm reduction of the bony fragment. The position of full extension must be maintained throughout treatment, even when removing the splint for cleaning, and patients should be warned to keep their hand flat on a table during this manœuvre.

## Orthopaedic management

### Non-operative

Provided that the DIPJ remains congruent, these injuries are treated with continuous extension splintage for 6 weeks, and then nocturnal and sporting splintage for a further 2 weeks, followed by active mobilization. After healing, a minor extensor lag (droop) at the DIPJ is not uncommon but does not result in any functional deficit.

### Operative

Subluxation of the distal IPJ may occur if a bony fragment is large. This is treated with a dorsal blocking wire, with or without a transfixion wire, for 4 weeks. The wire is then removed in clinic before physiotherapy is commenced.

## DISTAL PHALANX: RUGGER JERSEY FINGER

This is an avulsion of the insertion of the FDP tendon at the base of the distal phalanx (**Fig. 13.30**). The fragment is usually obvious at the base of the distal phalanx, but occasionally a bony fragment can retract proximally before being caught on the A1 flexor sheath

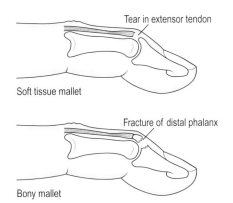

Tear in extensor tendon

Soft tissue mallet

Fracture of distal phalanx

Bony mallet

Fig. 13.29 Mallet finger injuries.

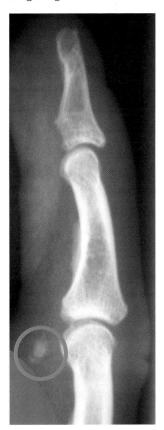

Fig. 13.30 Retracted fragment in rugger jersey finger.

pulley, or can occasionally displace into the palm; inspect the lateral radiograph carefully.

## Emergency Department management

The cascade of the hand may be abnormal (see Fig. 13.4). Importantly, the patient will be unable to flex the affected DIPJ actively (see Fig. 13.5). Assess the location of any tenderness and take radiographs of the finger or hand as appropriate. Refer to the orthopaedic service.

## Orthopaedic management

### Operative

These injuries are treated operatively. The bony fragment is reduced and then held with mini-fragment screws, plates, or transosseous sutures either secured with a suture anchor or passed through the distal phalanx and then tied over a button on the dorsum of the fingertip.

### DISTAL PHALANX: CLOSED TUFT FRACTURES

Crush injuries to the fingertips may result in a tuft fracture of the distal phalanx.

## Emergency Department management

These fractures require symptomatic treatment only, with a mallet splint to protect the injured tip. A subungual haematoma can be trephined if very painful. More complex nailbed injuries may need further assessment and treatment (p. 285).

## DISLOCATIONS

### CARPOMETACARPAL JOINT DISLOCATIONS

CMCJ dislocations may include a fracture to the base of the metacarpal or a dorsal rim fracture of the carpus, most commonly the hamate. Displaced fracture dislocations are unstable and are usually treated with k-wire stabilization

(Fig. 12.32). Thumb metacarpal base injuries (Bennett's and Rolando fractures) are described above.

### THUMB METACARPOPHALANGEAL JOINT INSTABILITY: ULNAR COLLATERAL LIGAMENT RUPTURE OR 'GAMEKEEPER'S THUMB'

The thumb is commonly injured in isolation because of a fall in which the thumb is forcibly abducted, such as when skiing, resulting in rupture of the ulnar collateral ligament (UCL). The term 'gamekeeper's thumb' refers to an attrition rupture of the same ligament from repetitive wringing of animals' necks! The injury leads to instability of the thumb, weakness, and inability to form a pinch grip.

## Emergency Department management

The injury is diagnosed on the basis of local pain over the UCL and clinical instability. Start by examining the uninjured side, as there is often a surprising degree of freedom in normal lateral movement. Stabilize the metacarpal with one hand and apply a radial force to the thumb with the other, gently stressing the UCL; there may be some movement but there should be a firm end point. Now examine the injured side (**Fig. 13.31**). If this is abnormal, obtain

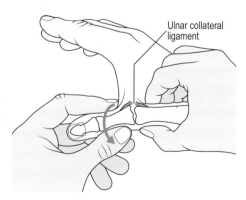

Fig. 13.31 Testing of the ulnar collateral ligament.

plain radiographs of the thumb and look for the presence of an avulsed fragment or joint subluxation. Where there is no fracture and a firm end point, the injury can be treated as a sprain. Where there is a displaced fragment, subluxation or clinical laxity, refer to Orthopaedics.

## Orthopaedic management

### Non-operative
A Brunner cast is applied for 3 weeks and the ligament is then reassessed. If stability has returned, early rehabilitation is commenced.

### Operative
Where there is a large bone fragment, or persistence of complete instability after initial cast management, surgical repair (with a suture anchor, wire or screw as appropriate) should be considered. The *Stenner lesion* is a UCL disruption in which the torn end of the ligament, with or without a small bony fragment, becomes displaced in a position superficial to the adductor pollicis aponeurosis, and is thus prevented from healing down anatomically (**Fig. 13.32**). The true incidence of Stenner lesions is unknown but they should be suspected where there is a grossly displaced bony fragment on the initial radiographs, or where there is persisting instability after cast treatment.

## METACARPOPHALANGEAL JOINT DISLOCATIONS

Most MCPJ dislocations occur as a result of hyperextension of the joint (**Fig. 13.33**).

## Emergency Department management

Confirm the injury radiographically. The dislocation can usually be reduced easily under a metacarpal block (see Fig. 2.9). Apply gentle traction, flexion of the wrist and finger, and pressure over the metacarpal base, allowing it to slide back into position (**Fig. 13.33B**). Obtain a post-reduction radiograph to confirm congruence. The injured finger is

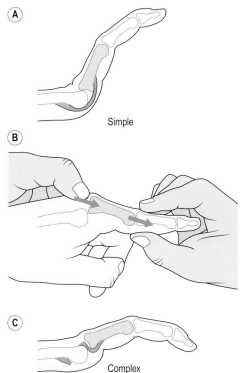

Fig. 13.33 Metacarpophalangeal joint dislocation and reduction. See text for details.

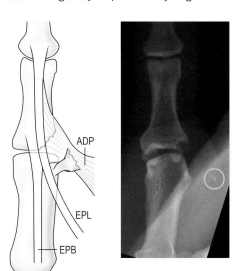

Fig. 13.32 Stenner lesion. ADP, adductor pollicis; EPB, extensor pollicis brevis; EPL, extensor pollicis longus.

then immobilized with buddy strapping and the patient is referred to the fracture clinic. Irreducible dislocations should be referred to Orthopaedics.

## Orthopaedic management

### Non-operative

Reduced dislocations with a congruent joint on post-reduction radiographs and normal movement are managed with buddy strapping for comfort for 2 weeks, and then active mobilization.

### Operative

Failure to reduce the dislocation may result from interposition of an avulsed volar plate within the joint (**Fig. 13.33C**), or 'button-holing' of the metacarpal head between the flexor tendons and lumbricals. The incarcerated plate may result in a visible dimple of the skin over the volar aspect of the joint, and the joint will remain incongruent radiographically. An operative open reduction is required. The joint is exposed dorsally and the volar plate is pushed out, allowing joint reduction. The volar plate itself may have to be incised in order to achieve enough mobility for reduction. Alternatively, the joint can be exposed from a volar approach, by dividing the A1 pulley.

## PROXIMAL INTERPHALANGEAL JOINT DISLOCATIONS

These are extremely common injuries and often present after a spontaneous reduction as a 'finger sprain'. The intermediate phalanx can dislocate in any direction but dorsal is the most common (**Fig. 13.34**).

## Emergency Department management

Dislocated PIPJs joints require reduction under a ring block (p. 32). Dorsally dislocated joints are reduced with longitudinal traction and flexion, with pressure over the phalangeal base (**Fig. 13.35**). Volar dislocations are treated by the application of traction, flexion and then pushing the phalanx base dorsally. Following successful reduction, assess the joint for stability and exclude a central slip injury (see below).

Post-reduction radiographs usually show a congruent reduction, occasionally with a small avulsion fracture related to either a collateral ligament or a volar plate. The joint is usually stable, and treatment is with buddy strapping and fracture clinic follow-up. Check radiographs may, however, reveal persisting incongruity or subluxation. This requires a referral to Orthopaedics for open reduction.

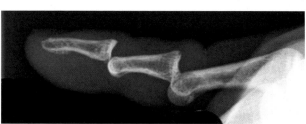

Fig. 13.34 "Stepladder finger". Dislocations of the distal and proximal interphalangeal joints.

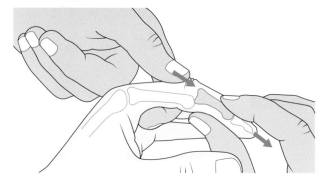

Fig. 13.35 Proximal interphalangeal joint reduction manœuvre.

## Orthopaedic management

### Non-operative

Congruent and stable reductions are treated with buddy strapping for 2 weeks and subsequent active mobilization. Persistent dorsal subluxation in extension can be treated non-operatively with dorsal blocking splintage (to prevent extension) for 6 weeks.

### Operative

Persistently incongruent joints are usually caused by a phalangeal base fracture. Reduction may entail the operative placement of a dorsal blocking k-wire, particularly where more than 40% of the volar lip is fractured. A very large volar lip fragment may require open reduction and fixation.

### Extensor central slip injury

PIPJ dislocations and extensor tendon injuries may cause disruption of the extensor central slip (see Fig. 13.3). Classically, this results in a *boutonnière deformity* (French: 'buttonhole'), reflecting the fact that with loss of the central slip, the lateral bands sublux in a volar direction around each side of the phalangeal head 'button', causing the PIPJ to flex while the DIPJ extends. This deformity develops within days or weeks of injury. This injury may only be revealed by flexing the injured PIPJ to 90° and noting weakness on attempted active extension. A central slip injury is treated acutely with 6 weeks of splintage, holding the PIPJ in extension while leaving the DIPJ free. Active DIPJ flexion should be encouraged during healing; this helps to pull the lateral bands back into their normal posterior location. The opposite injury to the volar aspect of the joint, causing stretching of the volar plate, may allow late hyperextension of the PIPJ and a compensatory *swan-neck* flexion deformity at the DIPJ.

## DISTAL INTERPHALANGEAL JOINT DISLOCATIONS

## Emergency Department management

Isolated distal IPJ dislocations (**Fig. 13.36**) without a bony avulsion fracture are rare but are treated with closed reduction under digital block. This simple relocation is achieved by traction and pushing the phalanx base back into position. Immobilize with a mallet splint for 3 weeks.

## Orthopaedic management

Instability after reduction may necessitate operative splintage with a dorsal blocking wire or a longitudinal transfixion k-wire through the tip of the finger into the intermediate phalanx.

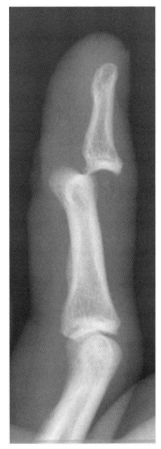

Fig. 13.36 Distal interphalangeal joint dislocation.

# SOFT TISSUE INJURIES OF THE HAND

## EXTENSOR TENDON INJURY

Extensor tendon injuries in the hand are extremely common. It is important to distinguish those that:

- have >50% tendon division
- penetrate a joint
- involve the central slip (boutonnière deformity, see above under PIPJ dislocations).

### Emergency Department management

Establish the mechanism of injury. What type of implement caused the wound? Was it dirty or contaminated? Was it a human tooth ('fight bite')? These should be considered highly contaminated. What position was the hand in at the time of injury? Examine the hand in the position of injury so that the skin wound and any extensor tendon injury line up together. Ensure that the affected digit retains active extension against resistance and has no neurovascular injury.

- *Injuries that involve <50% of the extensor tendon and do not overlie joint*: The tendon injury requires no specific treatment. The skin wound should be thoroughly cleaned, and then sutured under local anaesthetic. No modification of activity is necessary.
- *Injuries with >50% disruption or joint penetration*: Refer to Orthopaedics.

### Orthopaedic management

#### Operative

Injuries with >50% disruption or joint penetration should undergo formal exploration under local, regional or general anaesthesia. The wound should be extended both proximally and distally, usually producing an S-shaped outline. Identify the tendon edges. If the joint has been penetrated, expose it further, enough to allow thorough irrigation. This is easiest using a 10-mL syringe and a 16G (green) needle bevel (with the needle itself snapped off) to create a jet of saline. Inspect the articular surface and remove any loose fragments. Repair the

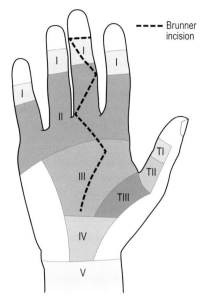

Fig. 13.37 Flexor tendon injury zones and Brunner incision.

extensor tendon with a fine, non-absorbable suture (e.g. 5/0 prolene). Close the skin wound with interrupted nylon and apply a bulky dressing. The digit should be splinted in extension with malleable splintage or a plaster strip (see Figs 13.12 and 13.13) for 4 weeks, followed by active mobilization.

## FLEXOR TENDON INJURY

Flexor tendon injuries are common, usually arising from contact with a sharp implement. The complexity of the injury and the outcome are dictated by the anatomical site, described in terms of *zones of injury* (**Fig. 13.37**).

### Emergency Department management

Assess the site of the wounds and the natural cascade of the fingers (see Fig. 13.4). Ask what position the hand was in at the time of injury. Examine the hand in the position of injury so that the skin wound and any flexor tendon injury line up together. Assess flexion power of the FDP and FDS to each digit (see Fig. 13.5). Assess the neurovascular supply; associated digital nerve and artery injury is common. Where there is a nerve injury, division of a flexor tendon or any uncertainty, refer to Orthopaedics or to the local hand surgery service.

## Orthopaedic management

### Operative

Flexor tendon divisions are repaired surgically. Zone II injuries are of particular concern, as there may be coexisting FDP and FDS division within a tight flexor sheath, with a risk of failed repair and finger stiffness. Repair here is a demanding technical exercise and may be undertaken within a local orthoplastic hand surgery unit.

### Skin incisions

Incisions must not cross flexor creases directly, as scar shortening will result in a flexion contracture of the joint. A *Brunner incision* consists of multiple limbs that cross the flexor creases at an angle (**Fig. 13.37**).

### Tendon repair

The strength of the repair is related principally to the number of strands of core suture material that cross the injury, and to secure knot tying. Many core sutures have been described; the Adelaide suture is a good example of a four-core suture with locking loops that is strong enough to allow immediate finger movement (**Fig. 13.38**). A 3/0 core suture is used and, in zone II particularly, is usually reinforced by a 5/0 epitendinous suture that improves tendon gliding, and decreases the formation of gaps at the repair site.

### Rehabilitation

The principal complications of tendon repair are re-rupture and tendon adhesion. Risk of these complications can be minimized by the adoption of an intensive supervised rehabilitation protocol that encourages early movement while protecting the repair with dorsal splintage that limits extension.

## FINGERTIP INJURIES

The *fingernail* (**Fig. 13.39**) is a specialized region consisting of the nail plate (the hard nail itself), the nailbed (the skin underlying it) and the germinal matrix (the specialized region of soft tissue in the proximal nailbed from which

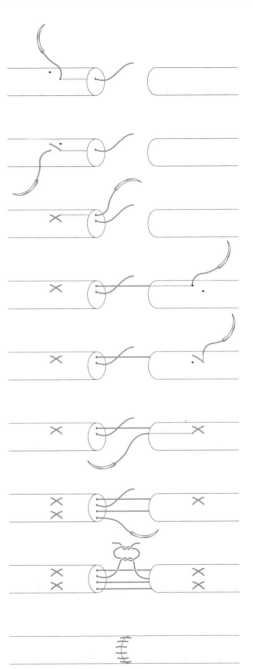

Fig. 13.38 Tendon repair: Adelaide suture.

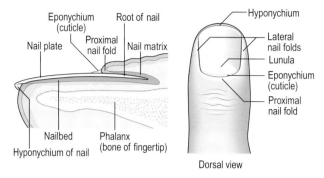

Fig. 13.39 Nail-tip anatomy.

the new nail is formed). The matrix can be seen through the nail as a whitish, semicircular region termed the lunula. The root of the nail is the deepest part, concealed under the proximal nail fold. The nailbed is sealed off under free edge of the nail by the eponychium or 'cuticle', and at the tip of the finger by the hyponychium or 'quick'.

Fingertip injuries present after a crushing or flexion injury to the distal phalanx. The patient will present with a swollen, bruised fingertip that may demonstrate:

- a subungual haematoma: a collection of blood under the nail
- a nailbed laceration: a laceration to the nailbed or germinal matrix
- nail root avulsion: dislodging of the nail root from under the eponychium and proximal nail fold
- a tuft fracture
- a combination of the above; a nailbed injury with a tuft fracture is considered an open fracture.

## Emergency Department management

Differentiate between a simple subungual haematoma and the more complex nailbed laceration. A subungual haematoma has a normal overall appearance to the fingertip with dark blood pooling under part or all of the nail. A significant nailbed laceration, which might require surgical exploration, is often associated with an avulsion of the nail root or a displaced

fracture. Obtain radiographs of the affected digit.

- *Subungual haematoma*: This is treated with a trephine for symptomatic relief. Prepare the affected digit with iodine or chlorhexidine. A ring block is not required, as the nail is insensate. A hole in the nail directly over the haematoma is produced with a hot trephine, a heated paper clip or a large-bore needle using a rotating motion. The release of blood under pressure is accompanied by relief of pain. Apply a dressing.

- *Nailbed laceration:* Refer to Orthopaedics or a local orthoplastic hand surgery unit.

## Orthopaedic management
### Operative
More complex nailbed injuries are treated surgically. Under a ring block and finger tourniquet, the following sequence of steps is performed (**Fig. 13.40**):

1. *Nail removal*: This is performed by pushing a small artery clip under the nail as far as the lunula, and then twisting to rotate the nail root out from under the proximal nail fold. Clean and preserve the nail for use later.

2. *Fracture fixation*: Minimally displaced or stable fractures do not require stabilization but should be exposed through the nailbed injury to allow thorough lavage with sterile saline. If there is persistent angulation of the fracture, it will require stabilization. After lavage, pass a fine double-ended k-wire in an anterograde direction through the distal

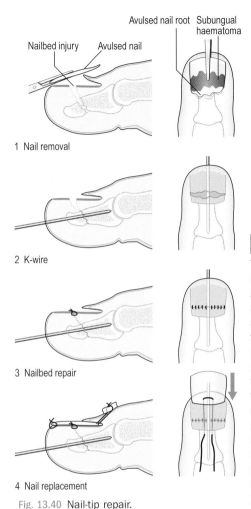

1 Nail removal

2 K-wire

3 Nailbed repair

4 Nail replacement

Fig. 13.40 Nail-tip repair.

and distally. Proximally, a suture is passed through the proximal nail fold, avoiding the germinal matrix, through the nail as a horizontal mattress, then back through the nail fold. The knot is tied over a small piece of padding to avoid skin pressure. Distally, a simple interrupted suture though the nail and underlying soft tissue secures the nail plate in place. A piece of the aluminium foil packaging of a suture can be used as a substitute if the nail is lost or damaged. The old nail can be discarded after around 4 weeks once the new nail has begun to grow.

## TRIGGER FINGER

This is a swelling of the flexor tendon that becomes hitched up as it passes beneath the A1 pulley. Although it does not usually arise as a result of acute trauma, it may present acutely and be attributed to injury. The cardinal features are a finger that remains flexed when the patient attempts to extend, but which then releases suddenly (like a trigger) and painfully with further exertion or with passive manipulation of the finger. There is often a palpable swelling of the flexor tendon at the level of the A1 pulley, which can be felt moving to and fro as the finger is moved passively. Patients should be referred non-urgently to the hand clinic, where they may undergo an injection of steroid into the flexor sheath or be offered A1 pulley release surgery.

## HAND INFECTIONS

### FINGERTIP INFECTIONS

A *paronychia* (Greek: *para*, 'around', and *onyx*, 'nail') is an infection in the fold of tissue at the base or sides of a nail. It may follow minor trauma, such as picking or biting at the nail or surrounding skin, a minor penetrating wound, or waterlogging of the skin after immersion.

A *felon* is an infection of the fingertip pulp and often follows a direct penetration such as a needlestick injury.

fragment, reduce the fracture, and then pass the wire in a retrograde fashion into the proximal fragment. Bend and cut the wire.

3. *Nailbed repair*: The nailbed is carefully approximated and repaired with a 6/0 absorbable suture. Special care must be taken to avoid inverting or everting the wound edges in order to prevent permanent nail deformity.

4. *Nail plate replacement*: The cleaned nail is then replaced under the proximal nail fold as a dressing and spacer. It is held in place with non-absorbable 5/0 sutures, proximally

## Emergency Department management

● *Simple infections without a collection of pus*: These can be treated with a course of oral antibiotics.

● *Paronychia* (**Fig. 13.41A**): A collection of pus is usually very superficial and can be drained simply in the Emergency Department under ring block. An incision directly over the abscess with an 11 blade releases the abscess cavity. The finger is then dressed and the patient is provided with a short course of oral antibiotics.

● *Felon* (**Fig. 13.41B**): Under ring block, a small incision is made over the area of swelling at the pulp of the finger, 5mm distal to the distal IPJ crease. Fibrous septa within the abscess cavity are broken down with a small artery clip to ensure complete drainage. The finger is then dressed and the patient is provided with a short course of oral antibiotics.

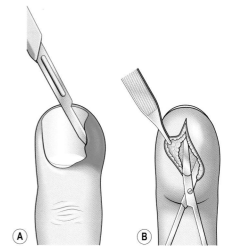

Fig. 13.41 Treatment of fingertip infections. **A**, Paronychia. **B**, Felon.

### FLEXOR SHEATH INFECTION

This is an important diagnosis because flexor sheath infections usually require urgent surgical drainage, and neglected infections are complicated by severe tendon adhesions and permanent finger stiffness.

## Emergency Department management

The patient will display Kanavel's cardinal signs (**Fig. 13.42**):

1. fusiform (spindle-shaped) swelling of the digit

2. tenderness on palpation of the flexor tendon sheath, not only from the volar side of the finger but also when the sides of the finger are gently squeezed

3. a flexed posture of the finger

4. severe pain in the finger, which is exacerbated by attempted passive extension.

Patients with suspected flexor sheath infections should be referred urgently to Orthopaedics or the local orthoplastic hand surgery service. Do not start empirical antibiotics, as a bacteriology swab will be taken in theatre.

## Orthopaedic management

### Operative

Flexor sheath infection is an orthopaedic emergency and surgery should not be delayed. Drain the flexor sheath surgically under general anaesthesia (**Fig. 13.43**). Make a transverse or Brunner incision over the volar aspect of the distal IPJ to expose the distal end of the sheath. Alternatively, use a *mid-axial incision*. The line of this incision is drawn between the flexion creases of the proximal and distal IPJs. Use blunt dissection to expose the sheath and to avoid dividing the distal ends of the digital nerves. Make a second transverse incision within the transverse palmar crease. Again, blunt dissection is used to expose the proximal end of the sheath at the A1 pulley. Incise the sheath at both ends and send a sample of pus for microbiological investigations. Then insert a size 20 cannula into the proximal or distal end of the sheath and use it to irrigate through and through with sterile saline until it runs clear. Leave the wounds open and dress them with absorbent gauze. Begin empirical intravenous antibiotics immediately after this lavage, rationalizing them later according to the results of culture and sensitivity analysis.

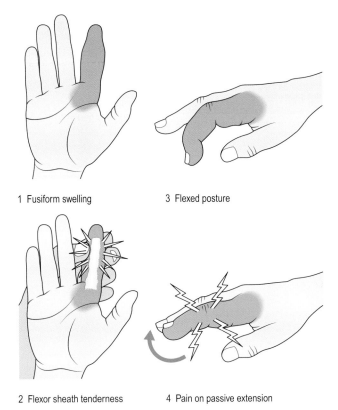

1 Fusiform swelling

3 Flexed posture

2 Flexor sheath tenderness

4 Pain on passive extension

Fig. 13.42 Kanavel's signs.

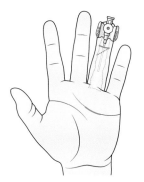

Fig. 13.43 Flexor sheath drainage.

## SEPTIC ARTHRITIS

### Emergency Department management

Septic arthritis of the wrist or fingers presents with severe pain at the joint, localized swelling, and exquisite pain on attempted passive movement. The investigation and treatment of septic arthritis are described in Chapter 6 on page 108. The wrist can be aspirated (see Fig. 6.5) but the smaller joints of the hand cannot. Do not start empirical antibiotics, as a bacteriology swab will be taken in theatre.

### Orthopaedic management

Arthrotomy and surgical lavage are indicated for most cases, including patients presenting late with contaminated wounds. A longitudinal, para-midline, dorsal incision is made over the affected joint to avoid dividing the extensor tendon. Less severe infections of small interphalangeal joints may be managed non-operatively with elevation and systemic anti-biotics. Chondral damage is common and a later joint fusion may be required.

# 14 Spine

*Alexander DL Baker*

## GENERAL PRINCIPLES

Injuries affecting the spinal column range from the common and frequently innocuous 'wedge compression fracture' to the potentially life-changing fracture-dislocation with associated spinal cord injury. Few injuries are as potentially devastating. Spinal fractures tend to occur at zones of mechanical transition in the spine; the thoracolumbar junction (T12–L2) is the most commonly fractured region, followed by the craniocervical and cervicothoracic junctions.

## Anatomy

### Vertebrae

The vertebral column consists of 33 vertebrae: 7 cervical, 12 thoracic, 5 lumbar, 5 sacral and 4 coccygeal. When viewed in the coronal plane, the spine appears straight, while in the sagittal plane the spine is curved with a cervical lordosis, thoracic kyphosis and lumbar lordosis.

Vertebral shape varies according to location. However, all vertebrae have certain features in common (**Fig. 14.1**):

- *Body*: The cortical circumference of the body is termed the *wall*, while the superior and inferior aspects that articulate with the intervertebral discs are the *endplates*. The interior is comprised of cancellous bone.

- *Vertebral arch*: These arches, together with the posterior wall of the vertebral body, create a longitudinal tube termed the *vertebral canal*. The components of the vertebral arch comprise:

  *Pedicles*: These cylindrical projections connect the body to the vertebral arch.

  *Laminae*: These sheets of bone are attached to the pedicles and coalesce at the base of the spinous process to complete the vertebral canal.

*Pars interarticularis*: These are the regions of the laminae that lie between the superior and inferior facets.

*Superior facets*: These bilateral projections extend superiorly from each pedicle and articulate with the inferior facet of the vertebra above to form bilateral *facet joints*.

*Inferior facets*: These projections extend inferiorly from the laminae and articulate with the superior facet of the vertebra below, at the facet joint.

*Transverse processes*: These lateral projections form the sites of attachment of muscles and ligaments bilaterally.

*Spinous processes*: These project posteriorly in the midline and form the bony prominences that are palpable subcutaneously.

The vertebral canal contains the spinal cord, which ends in the cauda equina (Latin: 'horse's tail'). The cord is bathed in cerebrospinal fluid (CSF) and is covered by the meninges. Nerve roots exit from either side of the spine between the pedicles of adjacent vertebrae, through a space known as the *neural foramen*.

### Intervertebral disc

The intervertebral disc (see Fig. 14.33) consists of the:

- *annulus fibrosus*: the tough outer layer of the disc, formed from around 20 concentric rings of lamellar fibrocartilage
- *nucleus pulposus*: a highly hydrated, aggrecan-containing gel in the centre of the disc.

The normal appearances of the disc change with age, the nucleus pulposus becoming progressively more dehydrated. Degradation or tears of the annulus may result in disc herniation (see Fig. 14.33).

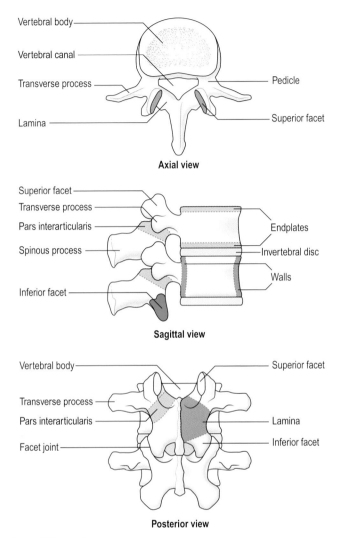

Fig. 14.1  Osteology of the vertebrae.

## Ligaments of the spine

The spinal column is supported by a number of strong ligaments (**Fig. 14.2**) that maintain alignment during loading and movement:

- the anterior longitudinal ligament
- the posterior longitudinal ligament
- the *posterior ligamentous complex*, comprising the:

  facet joint capsule

  ligamentum flavum

  interspinous ligament

  supraspinous ligament.

## Posterior elements

The posterior ligamentous complex and the intervening vertebral arches, considered together, are termed the posterior elements (an osseoligamentous structure).

## Columns of the spine

The spine may be thought of as consisting of three columns (**Fig. 14.2**):

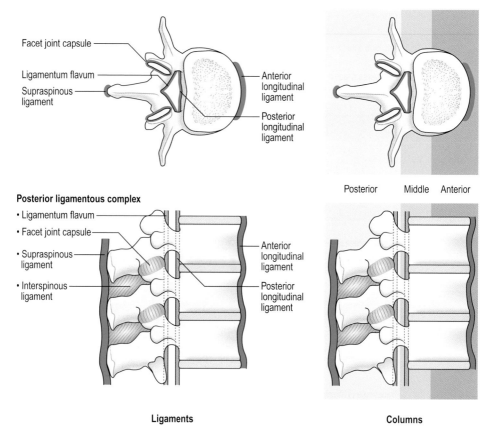

Facet joint capsule

Ligamentum flavum

Supraspinous ligament

Anterior longitudinal ligament

Posterior longitudinal ligament

Posterior     Middle     Anterior

**Posterior ligamentous complex**
• Ligamentum flavum
• Facet joint capsule
• Supraspinous ligament
• Interspinous ligament

Anterior longitudinal ligament

Posterior longitudinal ligament

Ligaments

Columns

Fig. 14.2 Ligaments and columns of the spine.

- *The anterior column* comprises the anterior longitudinal ligament and the anterior half of the vertebral body and disc.
- *The middle column* comprises the posterior half of the vertebral body and disc, and the posterior longitudinal ligament.
- *The posterior column* comprises the posterior elements.

## Cervical spine

The first two cervical vertebrae are significantly different in shape from the remaining five.

### C1

The *atlas* (named after the Greek titan who held aloft the celestial spheres) does not have a vertebral body but rather anterior and posterior arches that connect the two *lateral masses* (Fig. 14.3). The articulation between the skull (the occipital condyles) and the cervical spine is termed the *atlanto-occipital joint*.

### C2

The *axis* has a peg-like process (referred to as the odontoid peg, or dens) that projects superiorly into the ring of the atlas, forming the *atlanto-axial joint* (**Fig. 14.3**). The odontoid peg is held in place by two ligamentous structures: the alar ligaments, which emanate from the occipital condyles and insert into the tip of the peg; and the transverse ligament, which lies behind the posterior aspect of the peg and spans the anterior arch of the atlas. Approximately half of all cervical rotation happens at the atlanto-axial joint.

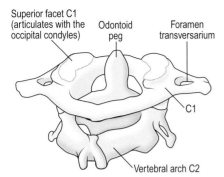

Superior facet C1
(articulates with the
occipital condyles)
Odontoid peg
Foramen transversarium
C1
Vertebral arch C2

**Posterior view without ligaments**

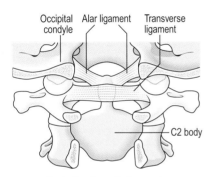

Occipital condyle
Alar ligament
Transverse ligament
C2 body

**Posterior view with ligaments
(vertebral arches removed)**

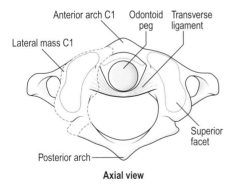

Anterior arch C1
Odontoid peg
Transverse ligament
Lateral mass C1
Superior facet
Posterior arch

**Axial view**

Fig. 14.3 Atlanto-axial joint.

The *subaxial cervical spine* (C3–C7) consists of the remaining five cervical vertebrae.

## Spinal cord

The spinal cord is made up of peripheral white matter and central grey matter. The grey matter contains the cell bodies and synapses of the cord, while the white matter consists of the ascending and descending tracts that transmit sensory and motor information (the long tracts). Knowledge of the anatomy of the long tracts helps in understanding and identifying patterns of spinal cord injury.

Information is transmitted via four main tracts (**Fig. 14.4**):

- The *dorsal columns* transmit proprioceptive and vibration sense. These tracts ascend the cord and do not decussate (cross to the contralateral side) until they reach the brain.

- The *spinothalamic tracts* transmit the sensation of pain (pin-prick test) and temperature. They decussate at the level of entry into the cord before ascending.

  Sensory examination of both pain and proprioception is quite specific to these two tracts: an abnormality in one or other sensation will locate the cross-sectional position of an incomplete spinal cord lesion, giving useful prognostic information. Beware when assessing light touch sensation – it is unreliable for locating an incomplete spinal cord injury. This is because light touch sensation ascends in both the ipsilateral posterior dorsal column and the contralateral anterior spinothalamic tract (i.e. it ascends on both sides and in both the anterior and posterior sections of the spinal cord).

- The *spinocerebellar tract* transmits unconscious proprioception that allows the coordination of movement.

- The *corticospinal tract* transmits efferent motor signals from the brain to the peripheral musculature.

The cell bodies of the preganglionic nerves of the *autonomic nervous system* are located in the spinal cord grey matter. Injuries to the spinal cord above the mid-thoracic level may affect autonomic nervous system function, resulting in loss of 'sympathetic tone'. This leads to peripheral vasodilatation and hypotension (neurogenic shock).

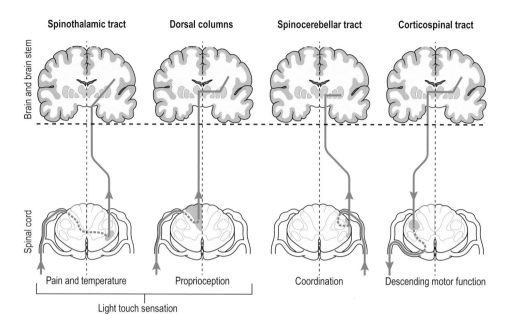

Fig. 14.4 Long tracts of the spinal cord.

## Biomechanics of vertebral column injury

Vertebral column injury results from excessive force being applied to the spine. The magnitude, location and trajectory of this force can result in displacement with six degrees of freedom:

1. compression/distraction
2. anteroposterior translation/shear
3. lateral translation/shear
4. axial rotation
5. lateral bending (coronal rotation)
6. flexion and extension (sagittal rotation).

### Spinal tension bands

In *flexion injuries*, the posterior elements act as a tension band. As the spine flexes, these structures come under tension. If they remain intact, the vertebral bodies will fail in compression (resulting in wedge and burst fractures). Alternatively, the posterior elements may fail in tension (distraction), through either the bone or the ligaments, resulting in a far more unstable fracture. In *extension injuries*, the anterior longitudinal ligament acts as the tension band (see Fig. 14.24).

## PRINCIPLES OF MANAGEMENT OF MAJOR SPINAL TRAUMA

A seriously injured patient should initially be assumed to have an unstable spinal injury. Movement at the level of an unstable fracture can cause further neurological deficit, and so patients suspected of having a spinal injury should be handled with the minimum amount of force and movement applied to the spine. At the scene of injury, the patient is immobilized with a spinal board, a rigid cervical collar, neck blocks and straps.

## Emergency Department management

Patients suspected of having a spinal injury should arrive in the Emergency Department already immobilized as described above; if this is not the case, the cervical spine should be immobilized as soon as a spinal injury is suspected.

### Primary survey

This follows the ABCDE sequence described on page 21. Some additional considerations apply in the context of spinal injury.

### Airway

A compromised airway is protected with simple measures and the use of adjuncts (p. 21), while maintaining stabilization of the cervical spine. Progressive airway compromise may be caused by the development of a retropharyngeal haematoma (see Fig. 14.8).

### Breathing

Thoracic breathing movements may be abolished or impaired after a cervical or thoracic spine injury, and diaphragmatic breathing may also be impaired in a high cervical injury (phrenic nerve, C3,4,5). Thoracic injury may affect the chest wall, lungs or heart and should be assessed during the primary survey.

### Circulation

*Neurogenic shock* is defined as vascular hypotension that occurs as the result of *spinal cord injury*, and is characterized by low blood pressure with warm peripheries and a bradycardia (p. 293). Do not assume, however, that hypotension after trauma is solely due to a cord injury; patients with spinal cord injuries are also unable to respond in a normal way to the hypovolaemia caused by haemorrhage. Neurogenic shock may be the only indication of spinal cord injury in an unconscious patient. Neurogenic shock should be distinguished from *spinal shock* (a syndrome of cord dysfunction; p. 317).

### Disability – the neurological examination

A rapid assessment of *central* neurological function is made using AVPU and the Glasgow Coma Scale (p. 23). If a spinal injury or neurological deficit is identified, a detailed *peripheral* neurological examination is required. The American Spinal Injuries Association (ASIA) chart (**Fig. 14.5**) guides examination and allows an accurate and reproducible record to be made. Neurological assessment in the conscious patient (see also Figs 3.14–3.16) includes:

- sensory function in all dermatomes (light touch and pin prick)

- muscle power using the MRC grading scale (see Table 3.4)

- reflexes in the upper and lower limbs

- rectal examination, including perianal and perineal sensation bilaterally, and anal tone and anal sphincter contraction.

### Exposure

- Patients should be completely exposed to allow examination. This involves cutting their clothing free whilst preserving warmth and dignity.

- Log-roll the patient to allow inspection of the back and to remove debris and clothing (**Box 14.1**).

## Secondary survey

Once immediately life-threatening injuries have been identified and addressed, a secondary survey is carried out (p. 23) and, depending on the clinical context, radiographic and other investigations are undertaken. During this phase, a clinical examination of the neck and back is performed. Where there is no evidence of spinal injury, the spine is 'cleared' (**Box 14.2**) and spinal precautions are lifted.

## Additional considerations in children

### Positioning

The Emergency Department management of childhood spinal injuries follows the same principles as for adults. A correctly sized cervical collar, with a spinal board, sandbags and tape, is required. Under the age of 7 years, children have a relatively large occiput, which will cause flexion of the neck on conventional spinal boards. This should be accommodated with a 'double mattress' pad placed under the trunk, or a modified board.

### Spinal cord injury without radiological abnormality (SCIWORA)

This syndrome occurs primarily in children and can range in severity from minor cord contusion to complete cord disruption. Neurological dysfunction can be delayed or progressive in the first few days. MRI will often show cord or surrounding soft tissue contusion. A child who has presented with signs of any cord dysfunction following trauma should have spinal instability excluded and, once fit for discharge, be advised to avoid contact sports for 3 months.

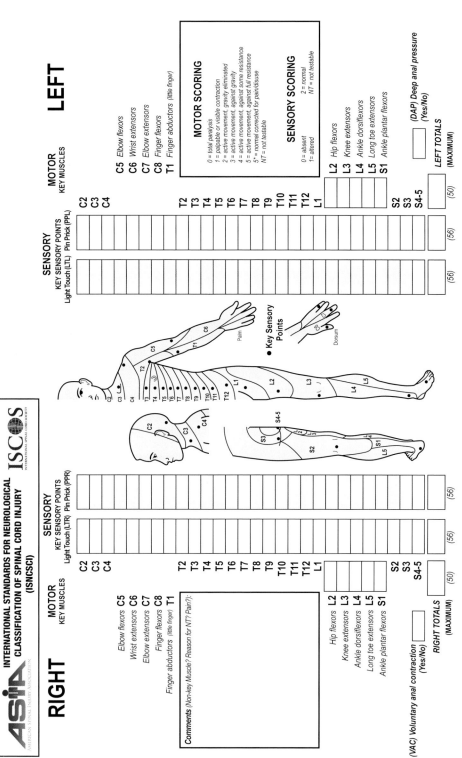

Fig. 14.5 ASIA chart. (From American Spinal Injury Association: International Standards for Neurological Classification of Spinal Cord Injury, revised 2013; Atlanta, GA. Reprinted 2013. With permission.)

## Box 14.1 Log roll

A 'log roll' (Fig. 14.6) is the safe, coordinated turning of the patient to allow inspection and palpation of the back, and a rectal examination.

The cervical collar is taken off to allow examination of the neck and occiput, and the removal of clothing, debris and jewellery.

A minimum of five people should be involved. One person controls the head, neck and airway, providing manual in-line stabilization of the cervical spine and directing the manoeuvre. Three people stand on the side towards which the patient is to be turned. Their six hands are positioned as follows:

1. shoulder
2. chest
3. pelvis
4. thigh
5. calf
6. ankle.

Additional coordination is achieved if these personnel cross hands, as shown in **Figure 14.6**. The fifth member of the team carries out the examination.

Clear instructions from the person immobilizing the cervical spine and coordinating the log roll should be given both to the patient and to the team:

To the patient: 'We are going to roll you on to your side. You do not need to do anything to help; we will hold you carefully. Lie as still as you can. This doctor will feel your back and ask whether you are sore, and will then examine your back passage and ask you to squeeze his finger. Is that OK?'

To the team: 'We are going to log-roll this patient. I am going to count to three and then say roll, and we will move on the command "roll". One, two, three, *roll*.'

At this point, the spinal board is usually removed. The fifth member of the team performs a complete examination, checking for:

- signs of injury and abrasions
- bruising
- boggy swelling
- palpable steps in the arrangement of the spinous processes, including uneven spacing between processes, or loss of longitudinal alignment in either the coronal or the sagittal plane
- tenderness of the spinous processes – ask the patient to respond 'yes' or 'no' at each point of palpation
- tone, voluntary power and sensation, as assessed by a rectal examination.

Once the examination is completed, the patient and the team are given instructions as above and the patient is thus returned to the supine position. Immobilization is reinstated with sandbags and straps or tape.

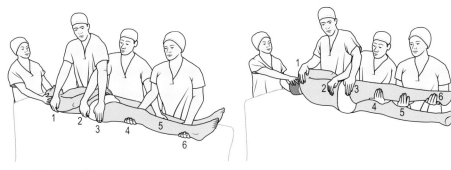

Fig. 14.6 Log roll.

## Box 14.2 Clearing the cervical spine in the conscious patient

### Principles

- All patients should be immobilized until their spine is fully assessed and cleared.

- Immobilization with full spinal precautions for prolonged periods is associated with pressure sores and pulmonary complications, and restrictions should be lifted as soon as it is possible to 'clear the spine'.

- A clinical examination of the whole spine, *including neurological status*, must be made in all at-risk patients; any sign of spinal cord injury mandates urgent scanning.

### Examination

The spine can only be cleared clinically in the following circumstances:

- The patient must be fully alert and orientated.

- There should be no associated head injury.

- There should be no impairment from sedative drugs or alcohol.

- There should be no other 'distracting' injury (such as a long bone fracture).

- A complete neurological examination should be normal and clearly documented.

Under these circumstances, the cervical collar can be removed and the neck examined. A supine patient is most easily assessed if the examiner stands at the head of the trolley, loosens the collar and then slides the examining hand round behind the patient's neck. An ambulant patient who has not been immobilized is most conveniently examined sitting in a chair, with the examiner standing behind. Assess for:

- swelling
- deformity
- bony tenderness in the midline.

If there is *no* midline tenderness, the examination proceeds with assessment of:

- movement: ask the patient to rotate the head to place the chin on each shoulder in turn, and then flex the neck to touch the chin to the chest.

If there is no pain on movement, the supine patient can safely be allowed to sit up gradually and the examination is then repeated, starting with a visual inspection of the back of the neck.

If this examination is normal, the cervical spine can be considered clear and radiographic studies are not required.

### Cervical spine imaging

If there are clinical abnormalities on examination, particularly midline pain or tenderness, cervical spine radiographs are required (see Figs 14.7–14.13). If radiographs are normal but the patient continues to have moderate to severe spine pain or tenderness, then the immobilization is left in place. Review by a senior doctor is often helpful and the patient may require further imaging with CT or MRI.

### Clearing the spine in the unconscious patient

Clearing the spine in unconscious patients remains controversial and local protocols should be consulted. If it is anticipated that a patient will remain unconscious, or be unable to cooperate with clinical examination, for more than 48 hours, radiological clearance of the spine may be undertaken.

## Radiological assessment of the injured spine

### Cervical spine series

Three radiographs are commonly performed:

1. lateral cervical spine (with the addition of a 'swimmer's view' if necessary; see below)
2. open mouth (odontoid peg) view
3. AP cervical spine.

*Lateral view of the cervical spine*

The entire cervical spine from the occiput to T1 must be shown. Assessment of the lateral cervical spine radiograph is described in **Box 14.3**.

---

### Box 14.3 Assessment of the lateral cervical spine radiograph

**Adequacy**

Ensure that the radiograph includes the entire cervical spine from the occiput to the C7/T1 junction.

**Five lines of alignment (Fig. 14.7)**

Begin with an assessment of the five key longitudinal lines:

1. Anterior soft tissue shadow: The prevertebral soft tissues lie between the pharynx and trachea (which appear lucent) and the vertebral bodies. Swelling suggests significant injury.
   a. C1–C4: The soft tissue should be no more than 50% of the width of the corresponding body (**Fig. 14.8**).
   b. C5–C7: The soft tissue should be no more than 100% of the width of the corresponding body.
2. Anterior vertebral body line: This line is most easily assessed, and any step or break in it is indicative of an unstable injury.
3. Posterior vertebral body line (anterior border of the spinal canal).
4. Base of spinous process line (the 'spinolaminar' line): This represents the posterior border of spinal canal.
5. Tip of spinous process line: Review the tips of the processes for avulsion fractures. Note that the line passes through the C2 spinous process, which is longer than the processes above and below.

**C1 vertebra (atlas) (Fig. 14.9)**

Identify and assess the atlas. This is a thin bone but the anterior arch can be seen clearly as a bean-shaped, opaque ring lying anterior to the odontoid peg of C2. Once

this is identified, trace the rest of C1, looking for any fracture lines.

**Atlanto-axial joint (C1/C2) (Fig. 14.9)**

Identify the odontoid peg, which protrudes superiorly from the vertebral body of C2 into the ring of C1. There are two corresponding measurements that indicate the positioning of C1 on C2. The atlanto-dens interval anteriorly should be <3 mm in an adult and <5 mm in a child. A larger interval suggests anterior subluxation of C1. The space available for the cord posteriorly should be >14 mm.

**C2 vertebra (axis) (Fig. 14.9)**

Assess the remainder of the axis by following the anterior margin of the peg distally, ensuring it is in line with the anterior aspect of the C2 body. Repeat this process on the posterior aspect of the peg and body. Finish by assessing the posterior elements of the vertebra.

**C3–C7 vertebrae**

The subaxial vertebrae should be assessed sequentially, tracing out the contour of each and checking the relationship of the joints above and below.

**C7/T1 junction**

The normal relationship of the cervical vertebrae should continue into the thoracic spine, and this cervicothoracic relationship must be imaged in all suspected injuries.

**Facets (Fig. 14.10)**

Examine each facet joint. These are best appreciated by visualizing a rhomboid shape at each level. Loss of alignment of these rhomboids suggests a facet joint dislocation (p. 300).

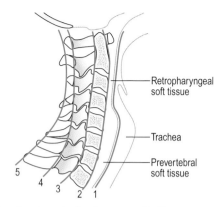 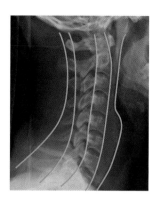

Fig. 14.7 Lateral cervical spine: overall alignment.

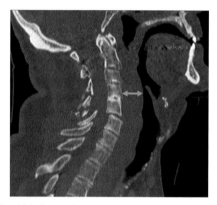

Fig. 14.8 Retropharyngeal swelling. Increased soft tissue width is evident following cervical spine fracture with traumatic C5/6 spondylolisthesis, in this case a retrolisthesis, and formation of a retropharyngeal haematoma. The patient developed critical airway obstruction.

If an adequate view is not achieved initially, there are three possibilities:

1. *Gentle traction* to the arms: The lower cervical vertebrae are often obscured by the shoulders, which can be lowered by gentle traction on the arms.

2. *Swimmer's view*: One of the arms is abducted (as if the patient were doing the back stroke) to reduce overlap over the

lower cervical spine. Identify the cervical level by assessing the shape of the spinous processes, and match these with the existing lateral view in order to identify and count the vertebrae (**Fig. 14.11**).

3. *CT*: Where adequate plain radiographic views are not possible, a CT of the cervical spine is required.

### Open mouth (odontoid peg) view (Fig. 14.12)

This view allows assessment of the odontoid peg and the relationship between the peg and the lateral masses of C1:

- Trace the contour of the *odontoid peg* and look for lucent lines or tilting of the peg. Intervening structures, including soft tissues or the teeth, can cause spurious 'Mach lines', which make interpretation difficult.

- Assess the alignment of the corners of the *lateral masses* of C1 and C2, and the space between the odontoid peg and the lateral masses of C1 (**Fig. 14.12**). If the C1 lateral masses are displaced laterally, a C1 fracture is present.

### AP view of the cervical spine (Fig. 14.13)

Assess the alignment of the spinous processes; deviation may indicate facet joint dislocation or other rotational injury.

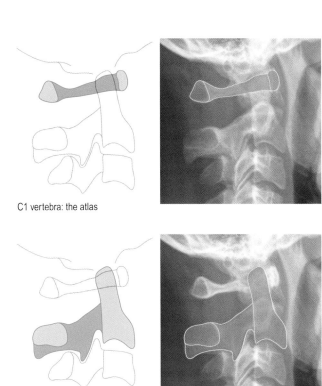

C1 vertebra: the atlas

C2 vertebra: the axis

Atlanto-axial joint: ADI and SAC

Fig. 14.9 Lateral cervical spine: atlas and axis. ADI, atlanto-dens interval; SAC, space available for the cord. Compare with Figure 14.20.

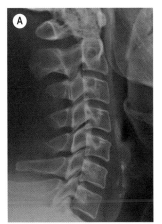
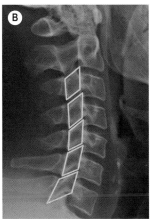

Fig. 14.10 Lateral cervical spine: facet joint alignment. **A**, Lateral view. **B**, The same radiograph with the facet joints highlighted; note the regular distribution and normal alignment.

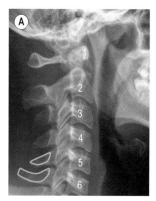
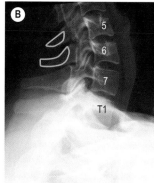

Fig. 14.11 Swimmer's view. **A**, This lateral cervical spine radiograph is inadequate on its own, as it fails to demonstrate C7 and the cervicothoracic junction. **B**, This swimmer's view shows the remaining cervical spine and junction clearly. Accurate identification of the spinal level is possible by comparing the shape and size of the spinous processes.

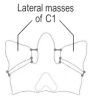

Lateral masses of C1

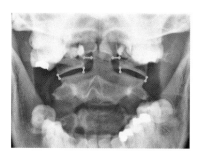

Fig. 14.12 Open mouth odontoid peg view.

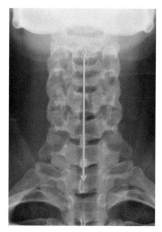

Fig. 14.13 AP view of the cervical spine.

### ✓ Key points

- Ten per cent of spinal fractures occur with a second spinal fracture at another vertebral level. If one spinal fracture is identified, careful consideration should be given to imaging the whole spine.

- Head injuries and cervical spine injuries commonly occur together. Patients with multiple injuries will usually undergo a full trauma scan, but when ordering a CT view of the head in a patient with head injuries, add a CT of the cervical spine as well, and vice versa.

- Adequate imaging of the cervicothoracic junction (C7/T1) is vital after neck injury. CT may offer higher sensitivity than standard radiographs.

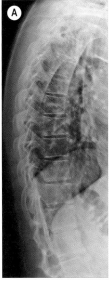
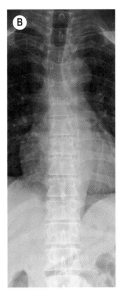

Fig. 14.14 Radiographs of the normal thoracic spine. **A**, Lateral view. **B**, AP view.

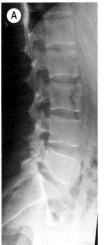
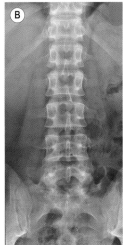

Fig. 14.15 Radiographs of the normal lumbar spine. **A**, Lateral view. **B**, AP view.

## Thoracic and lumbar spine series (Figs 14.14–14.15)

Two orthogonal views (AP and lateral), including the thoracolumbar junction, are required. Also assess the thoracic cage. An additional sternal fracture or multiple rib fractures (as opposed to a solitary spinal fracture) increase the likelihood of spinal instability.

### Lateral thoracic/lumbar spine

- Assess *overall alignment* by tracing the anterior and posterior margins of the vertebrae and of the spinous processes.
- For each *vertebral body*, trace the outline, paying particular attention to the anterior and posterior height. Compare the height of the vertebral body to that of the vertebrae above and below. Loss of anterior height produces a kyphosis and suggests a wedge fracture. Loss of height of the posterior wall of the vertebral body indicates the presence of a burst fracture.
- Assess the *posterior bony elements* for uneven spacing (separation) or a fracture, indicative of a posterior element injury.

### AP thoracic/lumbar spine

Look for widening or displacement of the pedicles, which is indicative of a burst fracture (see Fig. 14.27), on the AP radiograph. The alignment of the spinous processes should be assessed as for the cervical spine.

## CT

CT is invaluable for the assessment of spinal fractures, both in the diagnosis of occult injuries and for the characterization of fractures that are only partially appreciated on plain radiographs (such as burst fractures with retropulsion). In unstable injuries, CT is usually required to allow preoperative planning.

## MRI

MRI is used to assess soft tissue anatomy, including the intervertebral discs, spinal cord, nerve roots and posterior ligamentous complex (see Fig. 14.34). MRI is also helpful in identifying inflammatory pathology such as discitis, osteomyelitis or malignancy.

## Orthopaedic management of spinal injuries

### Non-operative

#### Cervical spine

Non-operative management is appropriate for stable injuries, defined as those that will not displace under normal physiological load, or injuries in patients for whom surgical management poses an unacceptable risk (**Fig. 14.16**).

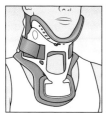 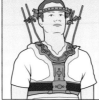 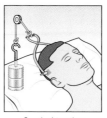

Cervical hard collar         Cervical halo         Cervical traction

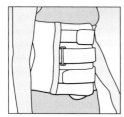 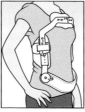

Lumbar corset     Jewitt extension brace

Fig. 14.16 Non-operative management of spinal injuries.

Rigid collars are used for immobilization of the cervical spine during extrication and initial assessment. Various collars with greater padding, such as the Philadelphia collar, provide definitive support for stable cervical spine fractures.

Halo vests are used when more rigid support is needed, and are favoured for the non-operative treatment of unstable cervical spine fractures. Pins are placed in the outer table of the skull under local anaesthesia, and these are connected to a halo device, which is mounted on a padded thoracic brace. Halo vests provide stability at the craniocervical junction, where cervical collars may allow pivoting.

Traction is used for definitive treatment when operative treatment is contraindicated (e.g. in extremes of age) and may be the treatment of choice in some cases (e.g. reduction of a facet joint dislocation).

### Thoracolumbar spine

Extension bracing may provide some support to the spine but is unlikely to prevent progressive deformity in an unstable fracture. Removable orthoses, such as lumbar corsets and extension braces that aim to resist progressive kyphosis (such as the Jewitt brace or custom-moulded thermoplastic braces), are used to provide comfort and assist mobility in stable thoracolumbar injuries, in the same way that removable orthoses are used in stable limb injuries.

### Operative

Unstable fractures are usually treated operatively by fusing across the injured segment of the spine to the uninjured segments above and below, with or without decompression of the vertebral canal. Stabilization is most commonly performed via a posterior approach with the patient lying prone. Fixation is achieved using pedicle screws and rods (see Fig. 14.28). Alternatively, stabilization is attained via an anterior approach. In the cervical spine, this is achieved by dissecting between the sternocleidomastoid muscle and carotid artery laterally, and trachea and strap muscles medially (see Fig. 14.23). In the thoracic spine, a thoracotomy is required; in the lumbar spine, either an extraperitoneal or a transperitoneal dissection is performed.

## MAJOR SPINAL INJURIES

### ATLANTO-OCCIPITAL INJURIES

Occipital condyle fractures arise from compression and are associated with C1 fractures. They are usually stable and treated in a rigid collar, although the rare condylar avulsion fracture may be unstable.

Atlanto-occipital dislocations are usually fatal. Rare survivors may have injuries to the spinal cord or to cranial nerves VII–X. Power's ratio is used to determine the relationship between the skull base and the cervical spine. The ratio is calculated by dividing the distance between the basion and the posterior C1 arch by the distance between the opisthion and the anterior C1 arch on CT scan. A ratio of either greater or less than 1 is suggestive of an atlanto-occipital dislocation. Treatment is with halo vest immobilization. Traction should be avoided, as there is a risk of over-distraction and subsequent neurological injury. An occiput to upper cervical fusion may be considered to prevent late displacement.

## ATLANTO-AXIAL FRACTURES AND INSTABILITY

These include fractures of C1 or C2, or rupture of the transverse ligament (**Fig. 14.17**). Where one injury is diagnosed, there is a high incidence of other associated fractures.

## Classification

### C1 (atlas) fracture classification (Levine)

1. *Isolated apophyseal fracture*: This is usually stable.

2. *Isolated posterior arch fracture*: This accounts for two-thirds of atlas fractures and is often stable.

3. *Isolated anterior arch fracture*: This is less common and is unstable.

4. *Lateral mass*: This is less common and is unstable.

5. *Burst fracture* involving both posterior and anterior arches, separating the lateral masses: This type is referred to as a *Jefferson fracture* (**Fig. 14.17**). They are usually unstable and account for one-third of atlas fractures.

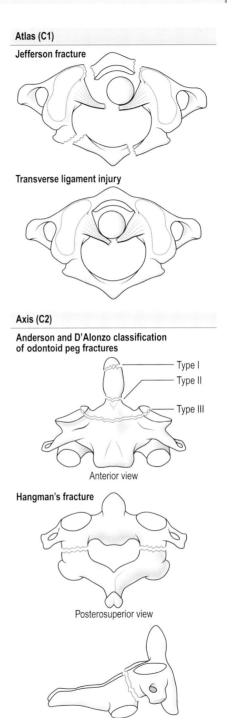

**Atlas (C1)**

Jefferson fracture

Transverse ligament injury

**Axis (C2)**

Anderson and D'Alonzo classification of odontoid peg fractures

Type I
Type II
Type III

Anterior view

Hangman's fracture

Posterosuperior view

Lateral view

Fig. 14.17 Injuries to the atlas and axis.

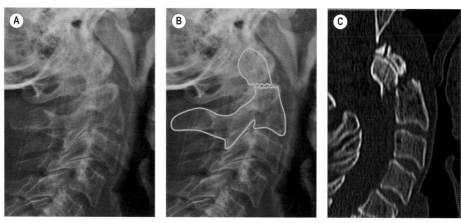

Fig. 14.18 Type II odontoid peg fracture. **A**, Abnormal radiograph of the upper cervical spine. **B**, The same radiograph with the abnormality highlighted. Note the step in the anterior border of C2, which breaks the anterior vertebral body line (see Fig. 14.07). **C**, The fracture is clearly demonstrated on the subsequent CT scan.

## C2 odontoid peg fracture classification (Anderson and D'Alonzo; Fig. 14.17)

- Type I: Fracture of the tip caused by avulsion of the alar ligaments (which connect the dens to the occiput). This type is rare but often stable.

- Type II: Fracture of the middle of the odontoid peg (**Fig. 14.18**).

- Type III: Fracture through the vertebral body of C2. The majority of these are stable.

## C2 hangman's fracture classification (Effendi; Fig. 14.19)

- Type I: Minimally displaced with no angulation.

- Type II: Angulated and displaced.

- Type III: Anterior translation with unilateral or bilateral facet dislocation at C2/3.

## Radiological features

- *Plain radiography or CT* will usually confirm a fracture (see Fig. 14.17). Rupture of the transverse ligament is diagnosed directly on MRI, or can be surmised from an abnormally large atlanto-dens interval of >3 mm on the lateral view (see Fig. 14.9) or a combined lateral mass displacement of >7 mm from

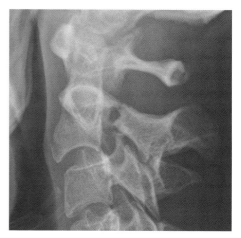

Fig. 14.19 Hangman's fracture.

their anatomical positions on the AP view (see Fig. 4.12).

- *Flexion/extension views* are specialist investigations that should *not* be ordered in the Emergency Department setting. For limited indications (such as confirming that a fracture has healed) and in expert hands, these may reveal dynamic instability of the cervical spine (**Fig. 14.20**).

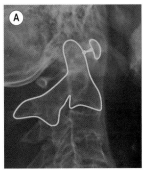 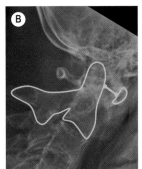 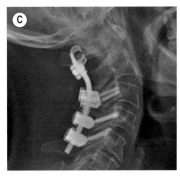

Fig. 14.20 Dynamic atlanto-axial instability. **A, B**, Flexion/extension views demonstrate an increase in the atlanto-dens interval in flexion due to failure of the transverse ligament. **C**, This was managed with posterior fusion.

## Emergency Department management

See Principles of management of Major Spinal Trauma (p. 294).

## Orthopaedic management

### Non-operative

Non-operative management for 12 weeks is appropriate for stable fracture types and for most elderly patients. A rigid cervical collar is more comfortable but a halo vest may be required for greater stability but is often poorly tolerated by elderly patients. A rigid cervical collar is more comfortable but provides less stability. Some unstable or displaced C1 fractures may require an initial period of traction for 3 weeks, or until reduction of the lateral masses is achieved.

### Operative

Operative fixation is required for unstable injuries or those with impaired healing ability, or as a later procedure for those with chronic instability or pain.

- *C1 (atlas) fractures*: Occipito-cervical fusion may be required for unstable injuries.
- *Transverse and alar ligaments*: A mid-substance tear will not usually heal and a C1/C2 fusion (with resultant loss in cervical rotation) is indicated (**Fig. 14.20**).

- *Peg fractures*: Type II fractures with displacement of >5 mm are associated with instability and non-union. They are managed with either posterior stabilization and a C1/C2 fusion, or odontoid lag-screw fixation. In patients over 50, management frequently depends on comorbidities.
- *Hangman's fractures*: Type II and III fractures with a significant disc or facet joint injury may require C2/C3 fusion.

## SUBAXIAL CERVICAL FRACTURES C3–C7

Fractures at the remaining levels of the cervical spine are considered together, as the vertebral morphology is relatively uniform and injury biomechanics follows a more consistent pattern at these levels.

## Emergency Department management

See Principles of management of Major Spinal Trauma (p. 294).

## Orthopaedic management

Orthopaedic management is guided by the *Allen and Fergusson classification*. Six mechanisms of injury are described:

1. *Flexion–compression injuries*: This mechanism causes failure of the anterior column

in flexion (**Fig. 14.21**). Minimally displaced injuries may be managed conservatively in a cervical collar or halo vest, but higher-grade injuries may require surgery.

2. *Flexion–distraction injuries* (facet joint dislocations): This mechanism typically causes failure of the posterior tension band, and subluxation and dislocation of the facet joints. These injuries are frequently missed. Lateral radiographs may show anterior subluxation of the vertebra and soft tissue

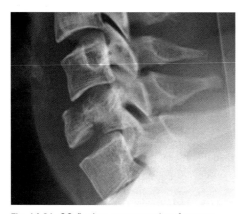

Fig. 14.21 C6 flexion–compression fracture. (From Raby N et al: Accident and Emergency Radiology: A Survival Guide 3rd ed (Saunders 2014) with permission.)

swelling, and the articular processes may overlap more (**Fig. 14.22**). On an AP radiograph, the spinous process may be deviated to the affected side. Facet joint dislocations require reduction with traction (up to one-third body weight) and subsequent stabilization.

3. *Vertical compression injuries*: Fractures resulting in compression of the vertebral endplate are usually managed conservatively with a cervical collar or halo vest; a fracture with displacement or fragmentation may require surgery (**Fig. 14.23**).

4. *Extension–compression injuries*: These injuries cause failure of the posterior column in compression. A laminar fracture can be treated with immobilization in a cervical collar or halo vest. Bilateral displaced fractures or severely displaced fractures are treated with posterior cervical fusion.

5. *Extension–distraction injuries*: Failure of the anterior longitudinal ligament with a vertebral body fracture is treated with halo vest immobilization, while an injury to the posterior column requires surgical stabilization.

6. *Lateral flexion injuries*: An undisplaced unilateral fracture can be treated with immobilization in a cervical collar; a displaced fracture with a contralateral ligamentous injury requires surgical stabilization.

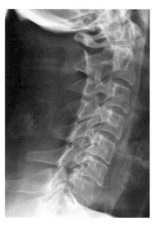
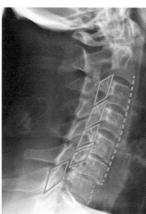

Fig. 14.22 C6/C7 facet joint dislocation. **A**, Abnormal lateral radiograph. **B**, The same radiograph with superimposed lines to highlight the loss of alignment of the facet joints (see Fig. 14.10) and anterior vertebral body line (see Fig. 14.07).

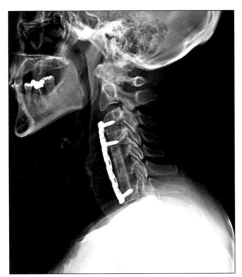

Fig. 14.23 Anterior fusion of the cervical spine. (From Angeles CF, Park J: Anterior Cervical Corpectomy and Fusion, in Jandial R, McCormick PC, Black PM: Core Techniques in Operative Neurosurgery 1st ed (Elsevier 2011) with permission.)

## FRACTURES OF THE THORACIC AND LUMBAR (THORACOLUMBAR) SPINE

Amongst young patients, thoracolumbar fractures are usually the result of high-energy trauma, while many fractures in the elderly are due to bony insufficiency. Those with rheumatoid arthritis, osteoporosis or a history of long-term steroid use are at particular risk of such fractures. The thoracic vertebrae are splinted by the ribs and sternum anteriorly, providing the region with mechanical support. In contrast, the thoracolumbar transitional zone is particularly vulnerable, with 40–60% of all spinal fractures involving T12, L1 and L2.

## Classification

### AO thoracolumbar injury classification
This morphological classification of thoracolumbar fractures is based on the familiar AO system of three groups divided into subgroups (**Fig. 14.24**). A diagnostic algorithm for this classification is most easily approached *in reverse order* by exclusion of the most severe injuries.

### C-type: displacement or dislocation injuries
- These are rare and represent severe spinal disruption with dissociation between cranial and caudal spinal segments (**Fig. 14.25**). Cord injury is common.

### B-type: tension band injuries
- Anterior tension band failure in extension:

  *B3 Hyperextension*: In these injuries, the anterior tension band fails under tension.

- Posterior tension band failure in flexion:

  *B2 Osseoligamentous disruption*: These injuries are important, as they are often unstable, and the extent of the injury may not be apparent initially on plain radiographs.

  *B1 Osseous disruption (Chance fractures)*: These are characterized by failure of the posterior bony elements (spinous process, lamina) in tension (**Fig. 14.26**).

### A-type: compression injuries
In these injuries, the anterior structures fail under compression:

- *A4 Burst fractures*: These occur when the entire vertebral body fails under compression. The radiological features of burst fractures include loss of vertebral height and loss of cortical integrity of the posterior vertebral body on the lateral radiograph, and widened pedicles on the AP view (**Fig. 14.27**). On CT scan, retropulsion of fragments into the vertebral canal will be appreciated (**Fig. 14.28**). This may result in spinal cord injury.
- *A3 Incomplete burst fractures*: These fractures involve the posterior bony wall but only one endplate.
- *A2 Pincer fractures*: In these fractures, both endplates fail but both the posterior and anterior walls of the vertebral body remain intact.
- *A1 Simple wedge compression fractures*: These are the most commonly encountered

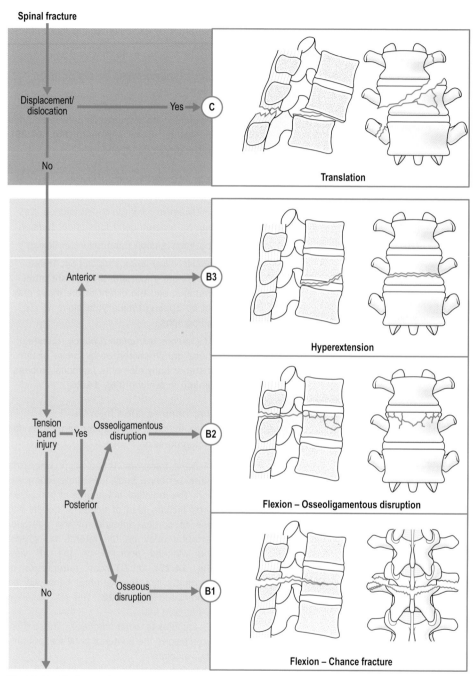

Fig. 14.24 AO thoracolumbar spine fracture classification. (From Vaccaro AL et al: AO Spine thoracolumbar spine injury classification system: fracture description, neurological status, and key modifiers. Spine (Phila Pa 1976). 2013 Nov 1;38(23): with permission.)

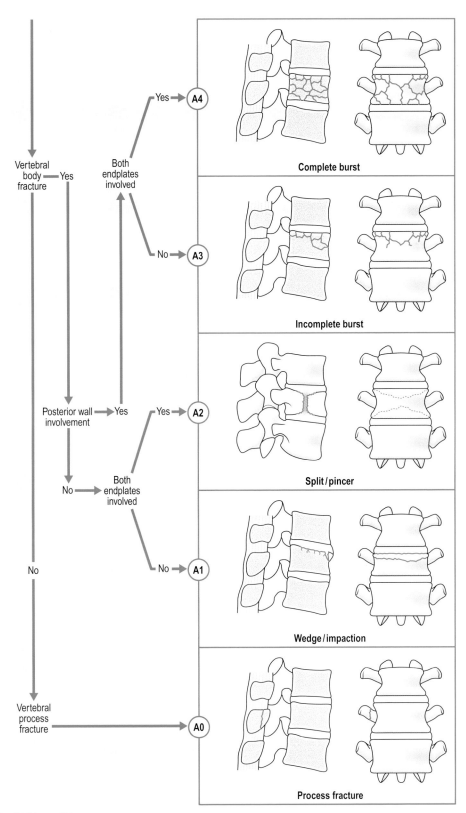

Fig. 14.24 cont'd.

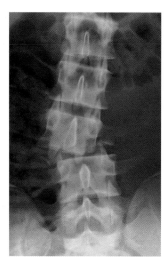

Fig. 14.25 AO type C: dislocation.

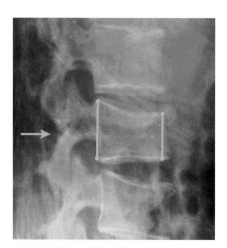

Fig. 14.26 AO type B1. Although the lines show only a 15% loss of height of the anterior wall of the vertebral body, the distraction (Chance) fracture through the vertebral arch (arrow) renders this fracture unstable.

spinal fractures. The posterior elements are intact but the anterior vertebral body fails in flexion and compression. Spinal cord injury is uncommon.

- *AO Minor fractures (non-structural)*: These are fractures that in themselves are minor

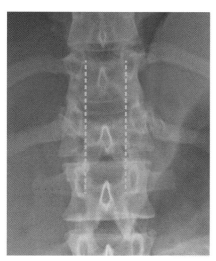

Fig. 14.27 AO type A4: complete burst. This AP radiograph shows pedicular widening.

and not associated with instability (e.g. transverse process). Note that these fractures may be markers of other injuries, such as unstable pelvic fractures or renal injuries.

### AO neurological score

Neurological injury is recorded in addition to the morphological classification above:

- N0: neurologically intact
- N1: transient neurological deficit, which is no longer present
- N2: radicular symptoms
- N3: incomplete spinal cord injury or any degree of cauda equina injury
- N4: complete spinal cord injury
- NX: neurological status unknown due to sedation or head injury.

## Assessing stability

### Fracture morphology

Wedge fractures are often thought to be unstable injuries when there is a kyphosis of >30° or loss of vertebral body height of >50% (see **Figs 14.29** and **14.30**). However, this is largely empirical and the TLICS score (below) is more helpful.

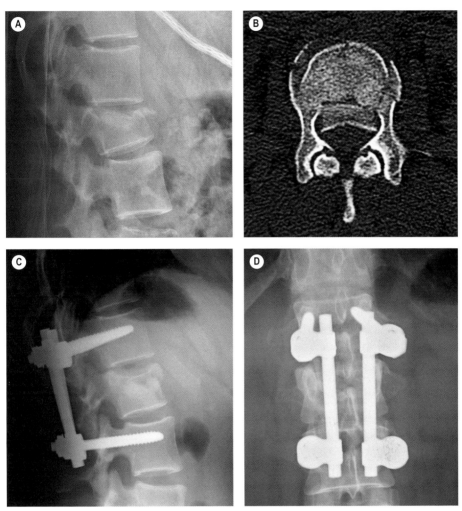

Fig. 14.28 AO type A4: complete burst fracture. **A, B,** Plain lateral radiograph and axial reformat CT showing retropulsion of the posterior wall. **C, D,** This fracture was unstable and required posterior reduction and fixation.

## Denis three-column theory of spinal stability

The Denis three-column theory of spinal stability (see Fig. 14.2) deserves mention, as it is commonly (and unhelpfully) quoted. The key concept of the classification relates to complete burst fractures in which both the middle and anterior columns are disrupted. These 'two-column injuries' are unstable, according to the strict application of Denis's theory. However, the assumptions underpinning this classification are no longer considered robust, and it is widely accepted that many 'two-column' burst fractures are mechanically stable and are well managed non-operatively.

## Thoracolumbar Injury Classification and Severity (TLICS) Score (Box 14.4)

In the absence of high quality prospective outcome data to guide the treatment of spinal fractures Alexander Vaccaro's TLICS system

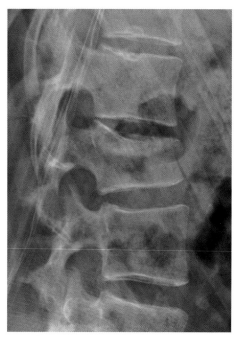

Fig. 14.29 AO type A1: wedge.

**Box 14.4** Thoracolumbar Injury Classification and Severity (TLICS) score

| Morphology | |
|---|---|
| Compression | 1 |
| Burst | 2 |
| Translation/rotation | 3 |
| Distraction | 4 |
| **Neurological status** | |
| Intact | 0 |
| Nerve root | 2 |
| Complete cord injury | 2 |
| Incomplete cord injury | 3 |
| Cauda equina injury | 3 |
| **Integrity of posterior elements** | |
| Intact | 0 |
| Indeterminate | 2 |
| Injured | 3 |

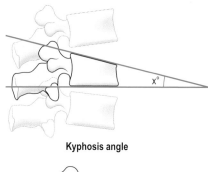

**Kyphosis angle**

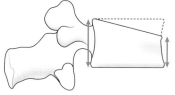

**Loss of anterior vertebral body height**

Fig. 14.30 A kyphosis angle of >30° or >50% loss of anterior wall vertebral body height are radiological markers that might indicate an increased risk of instability.

provides a pragmatic and logical approach to decision-making based on expert opinion. The TLICS scoring system indicates the likelihood of instability and the requirement for surgery. It is based on a combined analysis of injury morphology, the neurological status of the patient, and the integrity of the posterior elements (posterior tension band). Posterior element injury may be revealed on clinical examination, or on radiological examination as spinal process splaying. Each of these three components is scored, producing a total score out of 10. A higher score reflects increasing fracture instability and a greater potential benefit from neurological decompression. Although the score is not absolutely prescriptive, injuries that score 5 or more are usually treated surgically and those that score 3 or less are usually treated conservatively. Note that a lower neurological status score is awarded for a complete cord injury (where surgery is unlikely to be successful in restoring function) than for an incomplete cord injury or cauda equina syndrome (where intervention may restore function or at least protect against deterioration).

## Emergency Department management

See Principles of management of Major Spinal Trauma (p. 294).

### Radiological features

If one fracture is detected, the whole spine should be carefully examined. In most cases, the remaining spine should be imaged in its entirety.

- *AP and lateral radiographs*:

  The *AP view* may reveal coronal deformity or widening of the pedicles, indicating middle column disruption.

  The *lateral view* may reveal loss of normal vertebral shape or loss of sagittal alignment (such as a kyphotic deformity).

- *CT*: This is indicated if there is a significant fracture on the plain film, a neurological deficit clinically or inadequate plain films. Axial imaging provides a particularly good indication of whether there is retropulsion of bone into the canal.

- *MRI*: This is most useful for evaluating the spinal cord and soft tissues for signs of injury. High signal on T2 weighted scans may also indicate posterior ligament complex injury.

### Outpatient follow-up

- Patients with stable fractures, and who have no neurological abnormality, can be treated with analgesia and mobilization in Emergency Department. They may be referred to physiotherapy, or to the fracture or spinal clinic, depending on local protocols. Such injuries comprise:

  A0 fractures

  A1 fractures: simple, single-level wedge fractures with <50% loss of body height anteriorly and <30° kyphosis (see Fig. 14.30).

### Inpatient referral

- All other spinal fractures should be considered potentially unstable, and these, as well as any spinal fracture with neurological deficit, should be discussed with a senior colleague and/or referred for orthopaedic review.

---

 **Key point**

While there is consensus regarding the treatment of spinal injuries at both the innocuous and severe extremes of the spectrum, there is disagreement between experts regarding some aspects of spinal trauma. Areas of ongoing uncertainty include whether (and to what degree) certain types of spinal fracture are unstable, when surgical intervention is required (and what form this should take), and indeed the degree to which an intervention will improve the patient's long-term functional outcome. Similarly, the relative risks and benefits of surgery for influencing recovery after spinal cord injury are unclear. It is vital to consult senior colleagues and local protocols where there is any uncertainty in individual cases.

---

## Orthopaedic management

### Non-operative

*Stable fractures*

Stable fractures are usually managed non-operatively. For those patients admitted to the ward, the aim is to provide analgesia and bed rest initially, then progressive mobilization once *trunk control* returns. Patients are said to have trunk control once they can comfortably roll themselves around the bed, are able to tense their abdominal musculature and feel as if they can sit up. This is used as a clinical indicator of mechanical stability. However, this sign is not reliable in the early post-injury period and should not be used in the Emergency Department to clear the spine; neither is it used when the patient is intoxicated or delirious, or has a head injury.

Bracing (see Fig. 14.16) may help early mobilization, provide pain relief and prevent some fractures from deteriorating. However, when patients are comfortable, neurologically intact and mechanically stable, bracing may not be required.

*Outpatient follow-up* with imaging is required to ensure there is no deterioration in position. Follow-up is usually at 6 weeks and 3 months with radiographs, and subsequent follow-up is guided by pain. While 50% of fractures will have healed by 3 months, 20% of patients still complain of pain after 1 year.

### Operative

For unstable fractures, operative treatment usually takes the form of posterior surgical decompression and instrumented spinal fusion (see Fig. 14.28). Intraoperative ligamentotaxis (tension on the posterior longitudinal ligament; see Fig. 14.2) may be used intraoperatively to restore height and sagittal alignment, and in some cases to reduce retropulsed fragments. Decompression with laminectomy alone should be avoided, as it will further destabilize the spine by compromising the posterior supporting structures. Posterior fusion alone (no decompression) may be undertaken where there are no signs of neurological compromise. Anterior decompression and stabilization may also be considered and has the potential advantage of providing direct visualization of fracture fragments and therefore better canal clearance and better anterior column support.

## SACRAL FRACTURES

Sacral fractures are frequently missed, and potentially unstable, fractures associated with pelvic ring injuries and are described on page 332.

## SPINAL CORD INJURIES

## Classification

Spinal cord injuries can be classified as complete or incomplete:

- *Complete cord injury*: This is defined as complete loss of motor and sensory function below the level of a spinal cord injury.

- *Incomplete cord injury*: This is defined as partial preservation of sensory or motor function below the level of a spinal cord injury with sensory or motor function in the lowest sacral segment.

The ASIA grading system (based on Frankel) is a refinement of this and comprises:

A. complete paralysis

B. sensory incomplete – sensory function but no motor function below the level of injury

C. motor incomplete – useless motor function below the level of injury (more than half of key muscles have power of MRC grade 2 or less)

D. motor incomplete – useful motor function below the level of injury (more than half of key muscles have power of MRC grade 3 or more)

E. **normal function.**

As a 'rule of thumb', incomplete injuries have a greater potential for recovery than complete injuries. Different patterns of incomplete injury have been identified.

### Incomplete spinal cord syndromes

*Brown-Séquard syndrome*

This represents an injury to one side of the spinal cord. It will result in loss of ipsilateral motor function, conscious proprioception and contralateral pain and temperature sensation with decreased sensation to light touch (see Fig. 14.4). The prognosis is relatively good, with 90% of patients regaining bowel and bladder function and independent ambulatory capacity.

*Anterior cord syndrome*

In this syndrome, light touch and proprioception are preserved in dorsal columns with loss of motor function, pain and temperature sensation. The prognosis is more guarded, with recovery only if symptoms resolve within a short period (24 hours).

*Central cord syndrome*

This is the most common incomplete spinal cord injury and frequently results from an extension injury in a spine with pre-existing degenerative change. The upper limbs are more affected than the lower limbs. Upper limb flaccid paralysis occurs with lower limb hypertonic paralysis or preservation of function. The prognosis is fair, with 50–60% of patients regaining lower limb function; however, damage to the central synapses and cell bodies (in the spinal cord grey matter) frequently result in poor hand function.

### Spinal shock

This is defined as spinal cord dysfunction due to physiological rather than anatomical disruption. It is the result of swelling, oedema and inflammation, and it typically resolves over the first few days following spinal cord injury. Reflex arcs below the level of injury return to normal with the resolution of spinal shock.

## Management of spinal cord injuries

Patients with spinal cord injuries are at risk of a number of complications and careful consideration is required regarding:

- *Positioning*: Patients should be nursed flat, as sitting up may reduce the perfusion of a critically ischaemic spinal cord.

- *Skin*: Careful log-rolling is required to turn the patient every 2 hours in order to avoid decubitus (Latin: 'to lie down') ulceration. The spinal board should be removed as soon as possible after admission.

- *Gastrointestinal system*:

  *Stress ulceration* is common and ranitidine or proton pump inhibitors are given prophylactically.

  *Paralytic ileus* is also common and is treated with nasogastric tube insertion and intravenous fluids.

  *Bowel function* is frequently abnormal and faecal impaction requires suppositories or manual evacuation.

- *Genitourinary system*: Early catheterization is required.

- *Autonomic dysreflexia*: This is a potentially life-threatening condition that is commonly caused by a blocked urinary catheter or bowel obstruction, resulting in severe (paradoxical) hypertension and bradycardia. Treatment is by removal of the initiating stimulus and pharmacological treatment with antihypertensives and vasopressors.

- *Deep vein thrombosis*: This is a substantial risk in immobile patients. Prophylaxis should be considered for all patients, balancing the benefits of anticoagulants against the risk of epidural haematoma.

- *Joint contracture*: Joint contracture as a result of loss of voluntary movement occurs rapidly unless regular passive range of movement exercise of all affected joints is undertaken regularly. Resting splints should be provided overnight.

## MINOR SPINAL INJURIES

### SPINOUS PROCESS FRACTURES (Fig. 14.31)

A 'clay-shoveller's fracture' is an isolated avulsion fracture of the tip of the spinous process of C6 or C7; it is caused by sudden

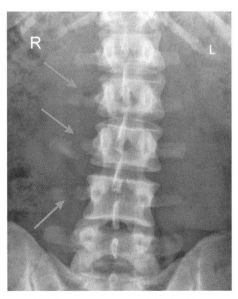

Fig. 14.31 Transverse process fractures (arrows).

contractions of trapezius, associated with sporting activities such as rock climbing. Analgesia and a hard collar are usually provided until the pain settles over 2–3 weeks. If a painful non-union occurs, excision of the avulsed fragment may be considered.

---

 **Key point**

A spinous process fracture occurring with an anterior injury indicates disruption of the posterior tension band and the likelihood of an unstable fracture pattern.

---

## COCCYX FRACTURES

Coccygeal fractures present with localized pain following a fall or a direct blow (such as a kick during sport). Clinical examination confirms tenderness on palpation over the dorsal surface of the coccyx externally, and on the anterior surface of the coccyx on rectal examination. Although extremely painful, coccygeal fractures do not require radiological investigation, as they are not normally visible on plain radiographs. Similarly, there is no form of surgical management that is of benefit in the acute stage. Patients should be reassured, and discharged with analgesia. Rarely, prolonged intractable symptoms are treated on an elective basis with local injections or coccygectomy.

## OTHER SPINAL PATHOLOGY

### THE AMBULANT PATIENT WITH BACK PAIN

This group of patients includes a wide range of different conditions. Assessment is based on applying *Waddell's diagnostic triage*, which assigns patients to one of three groups:

1. *Mechanical low back pain*: This type of back pain is not related to any specific disease or new injury, although it is often related to degeneration, and frequently presents following an incident where the patient has slipped, fallen, twisted or attempted to lift something. It is usually worse with movement and eased by rest. It is almost ubiquitous and up to 90% of the population will suffer from it at some point in their life. Occasionally, the pain can be severe, leading to attendance at Emergency Departments.

2. *Radiculopathy*: Radiculopathy (nerve root pain) is characterized by pain, paraesthesia and numbness in a dermatomal distribution affecting the upper or lower limbs (see below). The pain is often described as electric, shooting or burning in nature. The term *sciatica* indicates pain in the distribution of the sciatic nerve with symptoms below the knee; it is frequently used imprecisely and should generally be avoided.

3. *Major spinal pathology*: Patients with major spinal pathology, such as fractures (p. 304), infections (p. 324), tumours or cauda equina syndrome (p. 323), need prompt attention and frequently require admission for investigation and treatment.

## Clinical assessment of the ambulant patient with back pain

### History

History-taking in the patient presenting with back pain is an exercise in the exclusion of major spinal pathology. The 'red flags' are symptoms that are used to identify patients who are likely to require further investigation (**Box 14.5**).

### Examination

*Look*

- Observe the patient, their use of walking aids and how they stand and walk.

- Inspect for swelling, bruising or deformity of the neck and back.

- Assess the skin for localized abnormalities. *Erythema ab igne* (Latin: 'redness from fire') is a common marking caused by persistent and excessive use of heat therapy (water bottle or heat pads).

- Appraise the normal sagittal curvatures of the cervical, thoracic and lumbar regions,

## Box 14.5 Back pain: red flags

- History of trauma
- Age <20 or >55 years
- Thoracic or abdominal pain
- Nocturnal pain
- Pain that is constant, progressive or non-mechanical in nature
- Constitutional symptoms (fever, night sweats, weight loss)
- History of malignancy, steroid use, drug abuse or human immunodeficiency virus (HIV) infection
- Persisting severe restriction of lumbar spine flexion
- Structural spinal deformity
- Widespread neurological abnormality
- Saddle anaesthesia, urinary or bowel symptoms

and the normally straight spine in the coronal plane. Patients with a disc herniation will frequently present with a 'list', with the shoulders (and therefore centre of mass) displaced to one side in order to offload a disc herniation and ease nerve root irritation.

### Feel

- Palpate the spine for deformity, warmth, swelling and tenderness.
- Patients with mechanical back pain will indicate generalized tenderness of the paraspinal muscles, as opposed to the midline (bony) tenderness that is suggestive of spinal trauma or other major pathology.

### Move

- *Range of movement of the spine*: Most patients presenting to the Emergency Department will have a limited range of movement as a result of pain. *Persistent* restriction in range of movement of the spine over many weeks is a 'red flag' (see Box 14.5).
- *Gait*: This allows a global assessment of neurological function, as well as assessment of

power and coordination (cerebellar function) in the lower limbs. Tiptoe walking (S1/2) and heel-walking (L4/5) will identify weakness in their respective myotomes: for example, a 'foot drop'.

### Neurovascular assessment

- Perform a neurological examination, including:

  *Sensation* of light touch in each dermatome (see Fig. 14.5). Where there is an abnormality, also test for pin-prick sensation and proprioception.

  *Tone*: Test tone by gently moving (uninjured) joints.

  *Power*: Test power in the major muscle groups (see Figs 14.5, 3.14 and 3.15).

  *Reflexes* (see Figs 3.14 and 3.15).

- Examine the peripheral pulses (popliteal, posterior tibial and dorsalis pedis) to exclude vascular claudication. Assess for an aortic aneurysm as the cause of thoracolumbar pain.

### Special tests

- *Nerve root tension signs* (**Fig. 14.32**): These tests apply tension to the nerve roots as they exit the neural foramina and, if positive, demonstrate nerve root irritation (radiculopathy):

  *Straight-leg raise* (Lasègue's sign, SLR): The patient is placed supine. Raise the patient's lower limb by flexing the hip with the knee in full extension (*a* on **Fig. 14.32A**). A positive sign is achieved when this movement is limited by radicular pain. Note the angle achieved on each side (normal is 90°). A positive SLR can be confirmed by additionally dorsiflexing the foot (*b* on **Fig. 14.32B**; which applies increased tension on the sciatic nerve and exacerbates the pain), and then by flexing the knee (which eases the tension on the nerve and reduces the pain). Limited movement due to hamstring tightness and discomfort in the posterior thigh is not a positive SLR test.

  *Femoral nerve stretch test* (for radiculopathy at levels L2–4): The patient

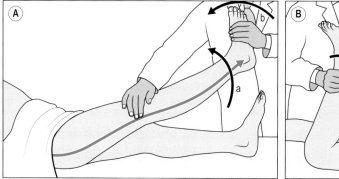
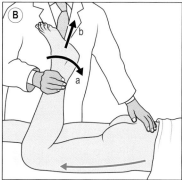

Sciatic nerve stretch test – Lasègue's sign          Femoral nerve stretch test

Fig. 14.32 Nerve root tension signs.

is positioned prone and tension is applied to the femoral nerve by first flexing the knee (*a* on **Fig. 14.32A**) and then extending the hip (*b* on **Fig. 14.32B**).

- *Plantar reflex*: The lateral side of the sole of the foot is firmly stroked with a blunt instrument. Flexion of the toes is normal. Extension of the toes indicates an abnormality of the brain or spinal cord (an upper motor neurone lesion, Babinski's sign). Extension is a normal finding in infants (0–1 years).

- *Rectal examination*: Rectal, perianal and perineal sensation, as well as tone, must be recorded.

- *Other systemic examinations*: Other examinations may be required as directed by the history. For example, thyroid, breast and respiratory examinations may be needed if there is a significant history of weight loss or systemic upset (looking for signs of malignancy).

## Investigations

Investigations for the ambulatory patient with back pain should be kept to a minimum, except in the context of red flags:

- *Inflammatory indices* (full blood count, erythrocyte sedimentation rate, C-reactive protein) may be required to exclude infection in the context of raised temperature or symptoms of systemic upset.

- *Plain radiographs* are seldom indicated, unless there is a history of trauma.

- *MRI of the spine* is required urgently for suspected cauda equina syndrome, but is performed in the outpatient setting for nerve root assessment.

## Emergency Department management

The management of mechanical low back pain in the Emergency Department may be problematic. Patients may present unable to cope with their pain, frequently anticipating serious pathology and expecting urgent investigation and admission. The majority of patients do not require either. The diagnosis is one of exclusion and is reached after a thorough clinical assessment – something that the patient will find reassuring in itself. Management consists of:

- *Counselling*: A sympathetic approach is required. Reassure the patient that the condition will improve spontaneously over the course of a few days or weeks.

- *Analgesia*: Patients should be provided with sufficient analgesia. Taking into consideration allergies and contraindications, a multimodal analgesic approach is usually more effective than a single agent. Consider paracetamol, a non-steroidal anti-inflammatory drug (NSAID) and a weak opioid.

- *Activity and physiotherapy*: The patient should be warned that protracted periods of recumbency will worsen their symptoms. On discharge, the patient should be advised against sitting or lying (expect during sleep) for longer than 30 minutes at a time. Once the exacerbation has abated, outpatient physiotherapy may be helpful.

- *Adjuncts*: In those patients with difficulty mobilizing despite analgesia, provision of elbow crutches can be helpful. Back braces are not recommended, as they can result in loss of lumbar muscle tone.

## THE AMBULANT PATIENT WITH NECK PAIN

## Clinical assessment of the ambulant patient with neck pain

### History

Mechanical neck pain is another common cause of presentation to the Emergency Department and commonly takes two forms:

- *Torticollis*: This is spasm of the sternocleidomastoid muscles, presenting with rotation and flexion of the neck; it is most often related to a new or repetitive activity that has commonly been performed the preceding day.

- *Whiplash-type injuries*: Classically, patients present following a low-speed motor vehicle collision, in which they have been the restrained occupant of a stationary car that has been struck from behind by another vehicle. There is considerable controversy regarding the pathophysiology of this condition. At the moment of collision, the head is thrown back, causing abnormal motion of the cervical spine. The recoil of the seat then throws the individual forwards and, as the torso is restrained by the seatbelt, the cervical spine flexes. Patients will usually present complaining of the gradual development of neck pain, which may be associated with head or shoulder pain, nausea, dizziness or paraesthesia in the upper limbs.

Spasm and a reduced range of movement commonly develop over several hours after injury.

### Examination

The procedure for clearing the spine in the conscious patient is followed (see Box 14.2). Provided there is no abnormality in this clinical examination, the patient can be reassured and discharged with advice and analgesia.

### Radiological assessment of the painful neck

An abnormal clinical examination requires cervical spine radiographs.

## Emergency Department management

Early return to normal function is key. The principles of management of back pain are followed, with appropriate counselling, analgesia, activity and physiotherapy. Soft neck collars do not assist in early return to mobility and should be avoided.

## LUMBAR RADICULOPATHY

This term implies dysfunction of a lumbar nerve root, presenting with pain, paraesthesia and numbness in a dermatomal distribution. The key elements are that sensory symptoms are felt *below the knee*, and that pain in the leg is worse than that in the back. The term 'sciatica' is often used imprecisely and is best avoided. Sensory symptoms felt in the loin, buttock or posterior thigh are considered to be radiating mechanical back pain (often colloquially termed 'lumbago') and not radiculopathy. Motor weakness (such as a 'foot drop') may also occur.

The most common cause of lumbar radiculopathy is a herniation of the intervertebral disc, which typically affects those between 20 and 50 years. An acute presentation may be prompted after a bending, lifting or jarring movement. The natural history of most lumbar disc herniations is one of spontaneous resolution with time. Other causes of radiculopathy include degenerative stenosis, spondylolisthesis (p. 324) and facet joint cysts.

## Nomenclature of disc herniation

The terms 'prolapse', 'rupture' and 'slipped disc' are often used synonymously, but are imprecise and should be avoided. Accepted terms used to describe disc pathology include:

- *Degeneration*: Most disc abnormalities are thought to arise as a result of pre-existing degeneration of the disc.

- *Herniation*: This applies to displacement of disc material beyond the normal limits of the intervertebral disc space (**Fig. 14.33**):

  *Protrusion*: The displaced material has a broad base that is wider than the area of displaced disc material (**Fig. 14.34**).

  *Extrusion*: The displaced material has a narrow base that is not as wide as the area of displaced material.

  *Sequestration*: The disc material has lost continuity with the disc from which it herniated.

- *Location of the herniation*:

  A '*central*' disc herniation is one that is located posteriorly, in the midline.

  Other locations include *para-central*, *foraminal* and *far-lateral* disc herniation.

## Emergency Department management

### Clinical features

Radiculopathy usually predominates over back pain and is often described as burning in nature, and associated with paraesthesia and numbness. Exclude any 'red flags' (see Box 14.5).

---

### ✅ Key point

Beware of the patient with bilateral lower limb radiculopathy: this, along with urinary and bowel symptoms, is a cardinal feature of cauda equina syndrome (see below). The patient should be instructed to return urgently should these symptoms develop.

---

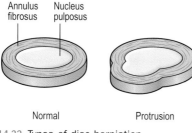
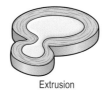
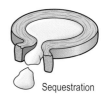

Annulus fibrosus  Nucleus pulposus

Normal          Protrusion          Extrusion          Sequestration

Fig. 14.33 Types of disc herniation.

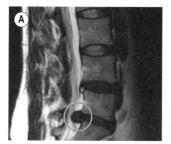
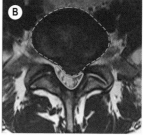

Fig. 14.34 Lumbar disc herniation. **A**, Note that in this case the extent of the herniation is appreciated better on the sagittal image than the axial image. **B**, The axial image shows the disc herniation (dotted line) encroaching into the vertebral canal. CSF surrounds the cauda equina (solid line), which is not compressed.

A detailed neurological examination of the lower limbs should be undertaken including tone, power, sensation, reflexes, and a rectal examination.

Examination may reveal positive nerve root tension signs (see Fig. 14.32), altered sensation in the affected dermatome, and decreased motor power and reflexes in the affected nerve root myotome (see Figs 3.14 and 3.15).

### Radiological features

Radiological investigations are not usually warranted in the Emergency Department in the absence of 'red flag' symptoms. Where there is specific concern, consideration should be given to MRI (e.g. for a suspected cauda equina syndrome).

### Treatment

Initial treatment is non-operative. This involves the provision of analgesia, including NSAIDs if not contraindicated. Consideration should be given to the short-term use of antispasmodics (a benzodiazepine). The use of neuropathic analgesics may be considered.

### Outpatient follow-up

Most patients with new-onset radiculopathy and no 'red flags' do not need to be seen in a spinal clinic and can be discharged to their GP with advice. However, if leg pain has not resolved after 6–12 weeks of conservative management, a referral to a spinal clinic is appropriate, as decompressive surgery may be considered.

### Inpatient referral

Patients experiencing severe pain frequently expect urgent investigation and admission. The majority of patients do not require either.

## Orthopaedic management

### Operative

Decompression surgery for radiculopathy is indicated as an elective procedure for persistent intractable pain or for motor weakness.

## CAUDA EQUINA SYNDROME

Cauda equina syndrome (CES) is a compressive injury to the lumbosacral nerve roots from a central lumbar disc herniation, resulting in impairment of bladder, bowel or sexual function, and perianal or 'saddle area' numbness. Bilateral radiculopathy is also a cardinal feature. CES is a surgical emergency, which, left untreated, can lead to devastating long-term complications such as incontinence of bladder or bowel, loss of lower limb function and sexual dysfunction. Surgical decompression within 48 hours of the onset of symptoms is considered to result in an improved outcome.

CES can progress rapidly over a matter of hours, or more slowly over days or weeks, and patients present at various points along this process. The most important distinction relates to urinary function:

- *CES-incomplete* (CES-I): There are subtle urinary difficulties, including altered sensation, loss of the desire to void, poor urinary stream, stress incontinence or difficulty in initiating micturition. Saddle area sensory change may be subtle, unilateral or partial. Trigone (catheter-tug) sensation should be present.

- *CES-retention* (CES-R): This is characterized by complete loss of bladder sensation. Painless urinary retention results, with overflow incontinence. There is extensive loss of sensation in the saddle area with absent trigone sensation.

The outcome of surgery for patients with CES-I is generally more favourable; surgery aims to prevent progression to CES-R.

## Emergency Department management

A detailed neurological examination should be undertaken, including a rectal examination. In the presence of a history of bilateral radiculopathy, or altered bladder or bowel function, or in the presence of physical findings on examination (altered sensation, tone or power), an urgent MRI scan should be arranged, with referral to a spinal surgeon if the diagnosis is confirmed.

## Orthopaedic management
### Operative

In most cases, surgery will be undertaken as soon as possible, within a matter of hours. A wide decompressive laminectomy, followed by microdiscectomy, is indicated in order to decompress the nerve roots and maximize the chances of recovery.

The long-term outcome for patients presenting with CES, particularly when the presentation is delayed or after neurological dysfunction has become established, may be poor, despite adequate management.

## SPINAL INFECTION

Spinal infections can affect the disc (discitis), the vertebrae (osteomyelitis), the spinal canal (epidural abscess), or the soft tissues surrounding the spine (e.g., psoas abscess). Symptoms can be severe and prolonged, and there is a risk of neurological injury. The diagnosis is often delayed, as pain may be vague and poorly localized. Risk factors include intravenous drug use and immunocompromised states. Most infections are caused by *Staphylococcus aureus* or *Streptococcus* species, but tuberculosis (TB, Pott's disease of the spine) is increasing in incidence.

## Emergency Department management
### Clinical features

- Assess for evidence of primary sources of infection (chest, urinary tract infection) that could have spread to the spine.
- A detailed neurological examination should be undertaken, including a rectal examination.
- Send blood for culture as well as testing for inflammatory markers.

### Radiological features

- *AP and lateral radiographs*: These may reveal a loss of disc space, although this may not be apparent for several weeks after infection.
- *MRI*: This is the investigation of choice.

- *MRI- or CT-guided percutaneous biopsy*: This may provide tissue for culture and pathology.

### Inpatient referral

Patients with suspected spinal infection should be referred to a spinal surgeon.

## Orthopaedic management
### Non-operative

In the absence of neurological compromise, initial treatment is usually with high-dose intravenous antibiotics for 6 weeks or until the C-reactive protein normalizes; oral antibiotics should then be given until there are no signs of infection. Bracing may provide pain relief.

### Operative

Indications for surgery include:

- Localized collection of pus.
- Progressive vertebral collapse and deformity.
- Neurological abnormality.

## SPONDYLOLISTHESIS

*Spondylolisthesis* (Greek: *spondylos*, 'spine'; *listhesis*, 'to slip') is the anterior displacement of a vertebra in relation to the vertebra below. It is a normal (incidental) finding in 6% of the population, and these may be commonly misinterpreted as acute injuries. It occurs most often at L5/S1 and is most commonly caused by a *spondylolysis* (**Fig. 14.35**): a defect or fracture of the pars interarticularis (see 'Wiltze classification' below). A *spondyloptosis* is an off-ended complete slip.

## Classification
### Wiltze classification

The Wiltze classification describes the *aetiology* of a spondylolisthesis:

I.  Dysplastic: Congenital abnormalities of the sacrum or L5 allow the slip to occur.

II. Isthmic: Here the defect is in the pars interarticularis (a spondylolysis) and it is subdivided into a lytic failure, an acute fracture, or an elongated but intact pars.

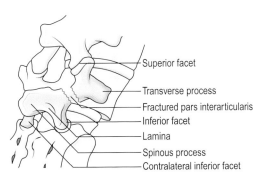

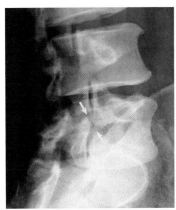

Fig. 14.35 Spondylolysis. The arrows show the fracture of the pars interarticularis (the collar of the Scottie dog). (Image from Kim, W: Plain Film Examination of Spinal Trauma, in Pretorius, ES, Solomon JA: Radiology Secrets Plus 3rd ed (Mosby 2011) with permission.)

III. Degenerative: This is due to degenerative change that produces instability (caused by changes in disc, joint capsules and facet joints).

IV. Traumatic: This is due to a fracture (but not of the pars, e.g. pedicle).

IV. Pathological: This is caused by local bone disease.

### Meyerding's grading system

Meyerding's grading system describes the *severity* of spondylolisthesis according to the proportion of vertebral body depth by which the more cranial vertebral body has slipped forwards:

- grade I: a slip of <25%
- grade II: 25–50%
- grade III: 50–75%
- grade IV: >75%

- grade V (added later): a spondyloptosis with 100% slip.

## Radiological assessment

The fracture is most commonly diagnosed on MRI or CT but may also be seen on oblique or lateral radiographs of the lumbar spine. In the oblique projection the pars interarticularis has the appearance of the neck of a *Scottie dog*, with the fracture appearing as the dog's collar (Fig. 14.35).

## Outpatient follow-up

Referral to a spinal surgical service is appropriate but patients can usually be investigated and managed on an outpatient basis. Activity modification, core stability exercises and bracing may allow healing. Operative treatment may be required for intractable symptoms.

## GENERAL PRINCIPLES

### Anatomy
#### Osseous anatomy
The pelvis is comprised of the two innominate bones (each having three components: the ilium, ischium and pubis; **Fig. 15.1**) and the sacrum.

The bones of the pelvis are joined by strong fibrocartilaginous joints, which form the *pelvic ring* (**Figs 15.2–15.3**). In pelvic ring fractures, this fails at a minimum of two points, either bony or ligamentous (**Box 15.1**).

#### Soft tissues within the pelvis
The true pelvis contains the rectum (*a* on **Fig. 15.4**), uterus (*b*) and bladder (*c*). A muscular floor (*d*) supports these structures and permits the passage of the rectum, vagina and urethra. At the back of the true pelvis, in the retroperitoneum, lie a plexus of veins, the iliac vessels (**Fig. 15.5A**) and the lumbosacral nerve roots (**Fig. 15.5B**). Disruption of the pelvis may therefore be associated with life-threatening haemorrhage, neurological deficit, urogenital trauma and bowel injury.

### Clinical assessment of pelvic injuries
#### History
Understanding the mechanism and the energy of the injury is vital. A high-energy mechanism of injury, such as a motor vehicle collision or fall from a height, suggests the possibility of other associated injuries. Airway and breathing problems will need immediate assessment and treatment first (see Ch. 2). Other associated injuries are common, and careful secondary and tertiary surveys are mandatory.

Low-energy injuries in young patients are typically avulsion fractures, reported as a sudden severe pain felt whilst performing a rapid, powerful movement, such as kicking a ball or starting to sprint. Avulsions of the anterior superior iliac spine, anterior inferior iliac spine or ischial tuberosity may occur (see Fig. 15.14), and pain may be poorly localized to the hip region. In the elderly, pelvic injuries often occur after a fall from standing height. This more commonly causes fractures of the hip and pubic rami, although more complex pelvic and acetabular fractures can occur in this group.

### Examination in low-energy pelvic injuries
*Look*
Limb lengths are usually equal. Bruising is unusual when presentation is prompt after the fall.

*Feel*
The superior pubic ramus is usually palpated easily at the groin; a fracture results in local tenderness. The inferior pubic ramus can be palpated at the ischial tuberosity; flex the hip a few degrees and palpate under the buttock crease.

*Move*
In contrast to a hip fracture, gentle passive hip rotation of the extended leg is usually tolerated well in fractures of the pubic rami.

*Neurovascular assessment*
Assess power and sensation to the tibial nerve, and the superficial and deep peroneal nerves (see Figs 3.20–3.22). Palpate the dorsalis pedis and posterior tibial pulses, and check capillary refill to the toes.

### Examination in high-energy pelvic injury
Initial management of a patient with high-energy trauma begins with a primary survey to exclude life-threatening injuries (see Ch. 2). Pelvic disruption can cause significant blood loss resulting in hypovolaemic shock, which is

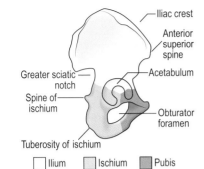

Fig. 15.1 Innominate bone.

Iliac crest
Anterior superior spine
Greater sciatic notch
Spine of ischium
Acetabulum
Obturator foramen
Tuberosity of ischium

☐ Ilium   ☐ Ischium   ■ Pubis

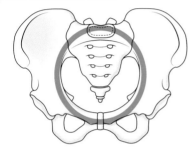

Fig. 15.2 Pelvic ring.

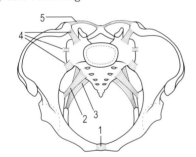

Fig. 15.3 Osseoligamentous anatomy of the pelvis. See **Box 15.1** for details.

addressed as part of *C: circulation and haemorrhage control*.

Following the primary survey, application of a pelvic binder (p. 333) and the taking of initial radiographs, a *secondary survey* is performed. This will include a full head-to-toe assessment. A number of pathologies are directly related to pelvic disruption, including:

- *Abdominal injury*: Assess the abdomen for swelling and guarding, suggesting peritonism or intraperitoneal haemorrhage. A *trauma CT or focused abdominal scan for trauma* (FAST) will often be part of this assessment.

- *Urethral injury*: Check for signs of urethral disruption (a triad of blood at the external meatus, a high-riding prostate and perineal bruising). Catheterize if there is no evidence of urogenital trauma; otherwise, obtain advice. A single, careful attempt to pass a urethral catheter is usually acceptable. A retrograde cystourethrogram will demonstrate the integrity of the bladder and urethra. A suprapubic catheter may be necessary if there is disruption, but colonization of the tract may risk deep wound infection if subsequent surgery to the anterior pelvic ring is required. A combined orthopaedic and urological plan is essential.

- *Open fracture*: Assess for signs of an open fracture (e.g. a perineal tear) or an 'internal open fracture' (e.g. blood, mucosal tear or bone fragments in the vaginal vault or rectum). A formal internal examination may be required (e.g. by speculum or sigmoidoscopy).

**Box 15.1    Ligaments of the pelvic ring (see Fig. 15.2)**

**Anterior**     1. **Pubic symphysis** – joins the pubic rami

**Posterior**   2. **Sacrospinous ligament** – originates from the lateral margin of the distal sacrum and inserts into the ischial spine
3. **Sacrotuberous ligament** – lies superficial to the sacrospinous ligament and arises from the sacrum to insert into the ischial tuberosity
4. **Sacroiliac ligaments** – comprised of three main parts: the anterior, interosseous and posterior ligaments
5. **Lumbar fascia** – arises from the transverse processes of the lumbar spine to insert into the iliac crest

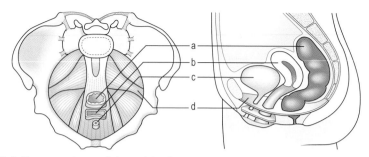

Fig. 15.4 Soft tissue anatomy of the pelvis. See text for details.

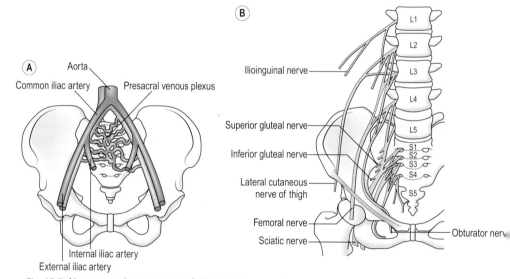

Fig. 15.5 Neurovascular anatomy of the pelvis.

● *Sacral nerve root injury*: Check for loss of anal tone or sensation, or a distal neurovascular deficit in the lower limbs.

Avoid performing a log roll or 'springing' the pelvis; the danger of dislodging the 'first clot' (p. 25) outweighs the benefits in the situation where CT scanning is easily obtainable. Rectal examination to check for internal injury should be performed in the supine position.

## Radiological assessment of pelvic injuries

### Radiographs

Three radiographs are required for full assessment of the pelvic ring:

1. *AP view of the pelvis* (**Fig. 15.6**): This should include the entire pelvis, fifth lumbar vertebra, sacrum and coccyx, and both proximal femora, including the femoral head, neck and greater trochanter.

2. *Inlet view* (**Fig. 15.7**): This is taken with the beam angled 60° caudally and shows the shape of the pelvic ring. It allows assessment of *horizontal stability*, as it shows the pubic symphysis and both anterior and posterior displacement of the sacroiliac joints clearly.

3. *Outlet view* (**Fig. 15.8**): This is taken with the beam angled 45° cephalad and shows the sacrum and sacroiliac joints *en face*. It allows assessment of *vertical stability*, as it

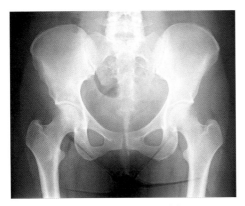

Fig. 15.6 AP radiograph of the pelvis.

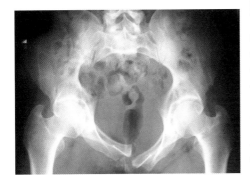

Fig. 15.7 Pelvic inlet view. Note the malreduction of the symphysis.

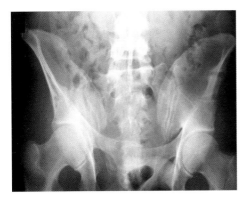

Fig. 15.8 Pelvic outlet view. Note that in this case the symphyses are overlapping or 'locked'.

shows displacement of the sacroiliac joints clearly, as well as the sacral foramina.

In practice, the AP view of the pelvis is usually complemented by CT scanning, with the inlet and outlet views obtained as reformatted images. Plain inlet and outlet views are often helpful at follow-up outpatient attendances. In the low-energy injury, an AP view of the pelvis alone is usually sufficient.

## CT

CT images of the pelvis are commonly acquired as part of the trauma scan and may replace the plain radiographic series. CT allows more detailed assessment of the injury and assists in preoperative planning.

## PELVIC RING INJURIES

## Classification

### Young and Burgess classification

The Young and Burgess classification describes the vector of the disrupting force and the resulting degree of displacement. The forces are broadly divided into three main types: anteroposterior compression (force applied from the front), lateral compression (side-on impact) and vertical shear (upwards movement of the hemipelvis in relation to the sacrum, often the result of landing from a height on to one leg). With greater violence, the fragments are displaced more widely, resulting in stepwise progression of injury.

#### Anteroposterior compression (APC) injuries (Fig. 15.9)

- APC 1: There is disruption of the pubic symphysis, resulting in an 'open book'. The diastasis (joint separation) is <2.5 cm and the posterior ligamentous elements of the pelvis are intact.

- APC 2: The pubic diastasis is >2.5 cm (**1** on **Fig. 15.9**) and the sacrotuberous (**2**), sacrospinous (**3**) and anterior sacroiliac ligaments (**4**) are disrupted, resulting in greater rotational instability. There is opening of the sacroiliac joint but, as the posterior sacroiliac ligaments remain intact, there is no vertical instability.

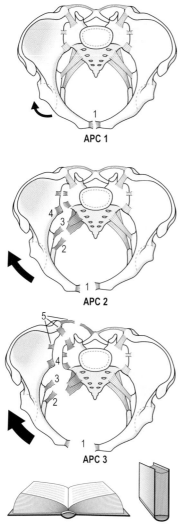

Fig. 15.9 Anteroposterior compression injuries.

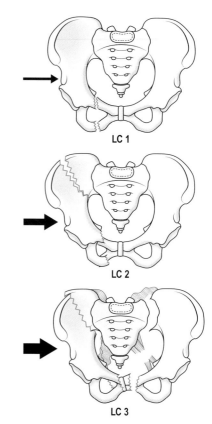

Fig. 15.10 Lateral compression injuries.

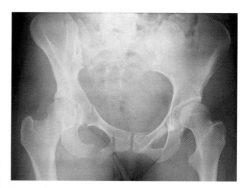

Fig. 15.11 Lateral compression injury: LC 3.

- *APC 3*: The posterior sacroiliac joint injury (**5**) is complete, resulting in vertical instability. This is indistinguishable from a vertical shear injury pattern, although the latter more commonly involves a sacral fracture.

### Lateral compression (LC) injuries (Fig. 15.10)

- *LC 1*: The pubic rami fail first with a characteristic transverse fracture, often accompanied by a crush fracture of the anterior margin of the sacrum.

- *LC 2*: The iliac blade fractures, often leaving a 'crescent fragment' attached at the sacroiliac joint (**Fig. 15.11**).

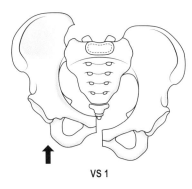

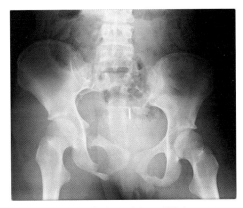

Fig. 15.13 Vertical shear injury: VS 1.

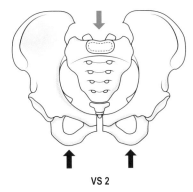

Fig. 15.12 Vertical shear injuries.

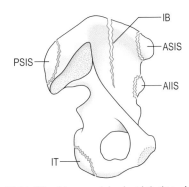

Fig. 15.14 Tile A-type pelvic ring injuries. AIIS, anterior inferior iliac spine; ASIS, anterior superior iliac spine; IB, iliac blade; IT, ischial tuberosity; PSIS, posterior superior iliac spine.

- *LC 3*: The contralateral wing opens as an open book, producing a 'windswept' pelvis.

### Vertical shear (VS) fractures
These are severe injuries resulting in complete loss of attachment between the sacrum and the lower limb (**Fig. 15.12**). The posterior pelvic ring may fail through the sacroiliac joint, sacrum or ilium.

- *VS 1*: Injury is unilateral (**Fig. 15.13**).
- *VS 2*: Injury is bilateral.

### Combined mechanism (CM) injuries
Some injuries result from a more complex force vector and involve a combination of the fractures listed above.

## Tile classification
The Tile classification is occasionally preferred, as it groups fractures based on the horizontal and vertical stability of the pelvic ring.

### A-type fractures
These have an intact pelvic ring (**Fig. 15.14**) and include:

- Avulsion fractures of the anterior superior iliac spine (*ASIS*, from sartorius), anterior inferior iliac spine (*AIIS*, from rectus femoris) and the ischial tuberosity (*IT*, from the hamstrings). Where the fragment is displaced >2 cm, open reduction and internal fixation is often performed. Fractures involving the iliac blade (*IB*) or posterior superior iliac spine (*PSIS*) in isolation are also classified as A-type.

### B-type fractures
These are horizontally unstable but vertically stable:

- *B1* is an APC (open book) injury.
- *B2* is an LC 1 or 2 injury.
- *B3* is an LC 3 injury.

### C-type fractures

These are both horizontally and vertically unstable:

- *C1* is unilateral and is an APC 3 or VS 1 injury.
- *C2* is bilateral and is a VS 2 injury.

## Other specific fracture types

Other specific fracture types of note are the tilt fracture (**Fig. 15.15**), in which a displaced segment of ramus impinges on the vaginal vault and may obstruct the birth canal, and the butterfly (or straddle) fracture (**Fig. 15.16**), arising from an anteroinferior force, such as when the perineum experiences a rapid deceleration against a motorcycle fuel tank or horse's saddle. The most common pelvic fracture of all is the *pubic rami fracture* of the

elderly following a simple fall from standing (usually classified as an LC 1 injury).

## Sacral fractures

The pelvic ring may fail through the body of the sacrum. The Denis classification relates the line of the fracture to the sacral foramina (**Fig. 15.17**).

- *Type I* fractures are lateral to the foramina.
- *Type II* fractures are transforaminal.
- *Type III* fractures are medial to the foramina.

Types 2 and 3 risk nerve root injury. A transverse component may result in an H-shaped or U-shaped fracture pattern (**Fig. 15.18**). The classic 'jumper's fracture' results from the spine 'falling through' the pelvis and typically comprises bilateral Denis type 2 fractures with a horizontal component (H-type). The sacrum may rotate into a flexed position on the lateral view. Often there is no anterior pelvic ring injury.

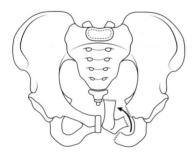

Fig. 15.15 Tilt fracture.

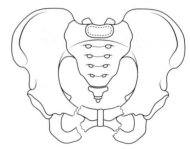

Fig. 15.16 Butterfly fracture.

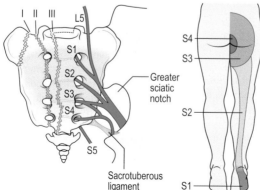

| Nerve root | Myotome |
|---|---|
| S1 | Ankle plantar flexion |
| S2 | Ankle plantar flexion |
| S3 | Bowel and bladder sphincters |
| S4 | |

Fig. 15.17 Denis classification of sacral fractures and their neurological implications.

## Emergency Department management

The initial assessment of the seriously injured patient is described in Chapter 2. The specific assessment of pelvic injuries is described above.

### Immobilization

### Key point

Trauma+haemodynamic compromise = immediate application of pelvic binder

Haemodynamic stability requires skeletal stability.

#### *Pelvic binder application*

A hypotensive patient with a history of high-energy trauma should be assumed to have a pelvic fracture until this has been excluded. An unstable pelvis will be a source of ongoing blood loss resulting from venous ooze from the low-pressure presacral plexus and the fractured bone surfaces. The binder imparts the skeletal stability required for the formation and protection of the retroperitoneal clot, which is essential for regaining haemodynamic stability. Circumferential compression is applied at the level of the trochanters (not the iliac crest) with a pelvic binder (**Fig. 15.19**) or with a simple draw sheet binder, which is applied by passing the ends of the sheet tightly around the pelvis at the level of the trochanters (**Fig. 15.20A**) and securing this with clamps (**Fig. 15.20B**). A number of proprietary binders are widely used (**Fig. 15.21A**). Alternatively, a G-clamp, if available, will provide mechanically powerful stabilization but requires technical experience in its application (**Fig. 15.21B**). For VS fractures, traction should first be applied to the displaced lower limb to correct shortening before applying the binder (**Fig. 15.22**). Although most effective for APC and VS fractures, a binder applied to an LC fracture has not been shown to cause visceral injury and is therefore considered safe; this allows one protocol to be applied to all pelvic ring fractures.

### Radiological features
#### *Low-energy injury*
● *AP view of the pelvis.*

The films will usually confirm a pubic rami fracture, although an undisplaced fracture of the posterior portion of the pelvic ring, most commonly a small sacral crush fracture, is usually present. In young patients, careful inspection

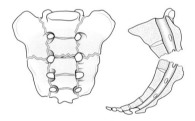

Fig. 15.18 'H' type sacral fracture.

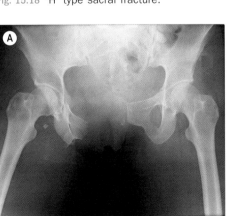

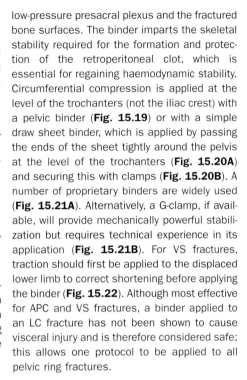

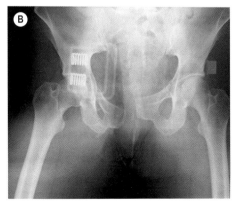

Fig. 15.19 Pelvic binder application radiographs. **A**, An APC 2 fracture with bilateral pubic rami fractures before treatment. **B**, The same fracture after application of a pelvic binder.

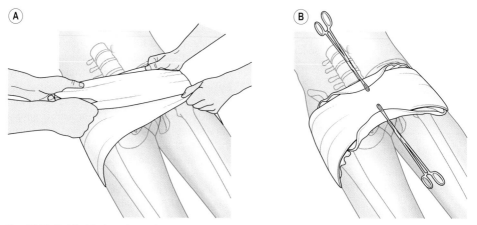

Fig. 15.20 Pelvis binder: draw sheet application.

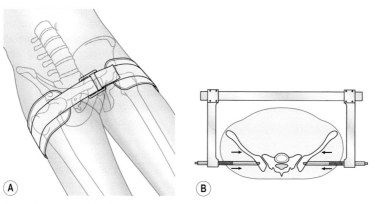

Fig. 15.21 Pelvic binders and G-clamp.

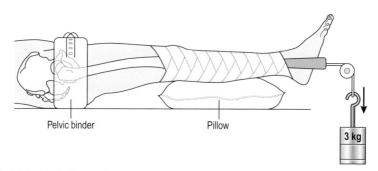

Pelvic binder

Pillow

3 kg

Fig. 15.22 Pelvic binder in vertical shear injuries.

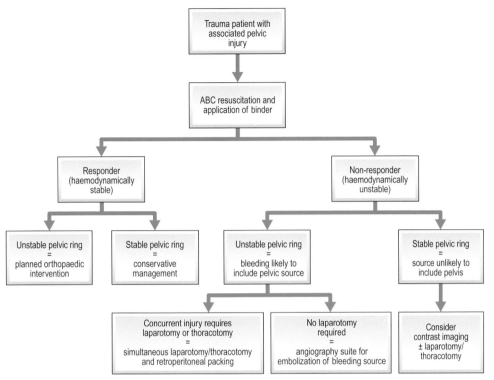

Fig. 15.23 Pelvic trauma algorithm.

of plain films may reveal a Tile A-type fracture, but the injury may be subtle and a CT may be required for diagnosis.

### High-energy injury

For high-energy injuries, radiographs should be taken after the application of a pelvic binder; application should not be delayed for radiographs.

- *Trauma series*: These include an AP view of the pelvis and AP chest radiograph.
- *Inlet and outlet pelvis radiographs*: These provide useful additional information but are not required in a patient undergoing CT of the pelvis.
- *CT*: A trauma scan may be obtained during the resuscitation phase and may negate the need for plain radiographs.

### Inpatient referral

Disposition will depend on the response to resuscitation and is defined in the algorithm shown in

**Figure 15.23**. In the haemodynamically unstable patient, haemorrhage most commonly arises from the low-pressure venous plexus at the back of the pelvis and is most effectively treated by retroperitoneal packing. Arterial bleeding from branches of the internal iliac artery may be evident on the trauma CT with contrast, and can be controlled by angiographic embolization. Whether to go to theatre for packing or the angiography suite depends on local protocols and expertise. Pragmatically, if any other emergency surgical procedure (e.g. laparotomy or thoracotomy) is required, then packing may be preferred.

## Orthopaedic management

### Non-operative

- LC 1 fractures, (including pubic rami fractures in the elderly) are treated conservatively with analgesia and mobilization. Elderly patients who are unable to walk may require admission for analgesia and physiotherapy.

- APC 1 injuries are stable and can be managed with gradual mobilization. Surgery is performed for ongoing symptoms of crepitus, movement or pain.
- Avulsion fractures (Tile A) rarely require operative intervention. Patients are encouraged to make a gradual return to activity. Operative treatment is only required where there is a large, displaced fragment.

## Operative

Indications for surgery include:

- life-threatening haemorrhage: pelvic packing
- unstable fractures
- open fractures
- urological injury.

The approach and method of stabilization are guided by the Young and Burgess classification (**Table 15.1**).

## Surgical techniques

### Pelvic packing (Fig. 15.24)

The surgical control of life-threatening haemorrhage is addressed as part of resuscitation and before surgical stabilization. A pelvic binder or clamp should be in place to prevent separation of the bony fragments. In the operating theatre, a transverse Pfannenstiel incision and a midline rectus split expose the peritoneum. The peritoneum and its contents can then be mobilized medially to expose the internal aspect of the pelvic ring and the overlying iliopsoas muscle. Work progressively towards the midline posteriorly, and then pack this space with abdominal packs in order to tamponade the venous haemorrhage.

### Table 15.1  Pelvic fracture: surgical management

| Injury | Surgical management |
|---|---|
| APC 1 | Anterior stabilization if symptomatic; otherwise, non-operative |
| APC 2 | Anterior stabilization ± posterior stabilization |
| APC 3 | Anterior and posterior stabilization |
| LC 1 | Non-operative; mobilize and permit weight-bearing as comfort allows. Deformity or ongoing pain is an indication for plate or 'in-fix' stabilization |
| LC 2 | Iliac fixation (open reduction and internal fixation, or screw ± anterior stabilization |
| LC 3 | Anterior and posterior stabilization |
| VS | Anterior and posterior stabilization |

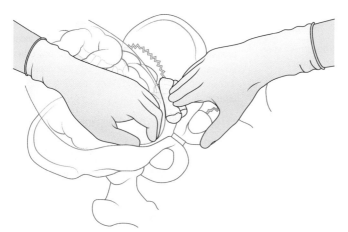

Fig. 15.24 Pelvic packing.

### Treatment of open fractures and urogenital injury

Open fractures require debridement and irrigation. Internal open fractures with bowel involvement require a loop colostomy and washout of the distal segment to prevent faecal contamination of the fracture. A partial urethral tear may be treated with the careful passage of a catheter and spontaneous healing, but a complete urethral tear or a bladder rupture requires exploration and repair.

### Anterior pelvic ring stabilization

Soft tissue symphyseal injuries (a pubic diastasis) heal slowly over 15 weeks and are usually plated (**Fig. 15.25**). Bony injuries heal more rapidly and can be successfully treated with either external or internal fixation. External fixator pins may be placed in either the iliac crest or the supra-acetabular corridor.

- *Iliac crest frame*: The subcutaneous iliac crest is easily identified. Separate incisions, orientated towards the umbilicus, are required for each pin (**Fig. 15.26A**). The trajectory can be established by passing instruments or wires down the outer and inner tables of the pelvis (**Fig. 15.26B**). After the cortex is drilled, a threaded pin is inserted by hand (**Fig. 15.26C**). The bone of the crest is relatively weak and three pins are required (**Fig. 15.26D**). The pelvic deformity is reduced using the pins, and the external fixator apparatus is assembled, without obstructing access to the abdomen.
- *Supra-acetabular frame*: A single pin via the anterior inferior iliac spine is

biomechanically stronger. However, it requires a limited Smith–Peterson approach (**Fig. 15.27A**) and is technically more challenging, requiring clear identification of the safe corridor above the acetabulum, between the AIIS and PSIS, using combined outlet/obturator oblique (**Fig. 15.27B**) and iliac oblique (**Fig. 15.27C**) views on fluoroscopy. The pins can be connected with an external fixator construct, as above. Alternatively, an all-inside construct ('in-fix'), with both pins and fixator bars tunnelled in the subcutaneous plane, can avoid pin track problems. Occasionally, anterior ring fractures (e.g. tilt fractures; see Fig. 15.15) are not amenable to closed reduction. These may require open reduction and plating, or percutaneous reduction and screw fixation.

### Posterior ring stabilization (Fig. 15.28)

Injuries to the sacrum or sacroiliac joints that can be reduced with traction are amenable to

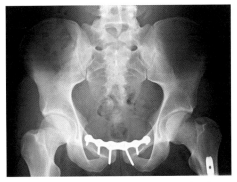

Fig. 15.25 Anterior pelvic ring open reduction and internal fixation.

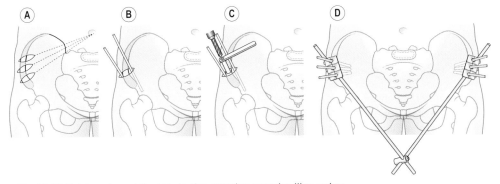

Fig. 15.26 Pelvic external fixator via the anterior superior iliac spine.

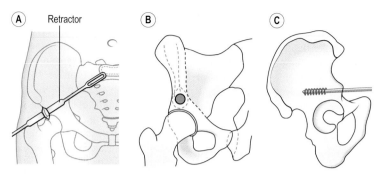

Fig. 15.27 Pelvic external fixator via the anterior inferior iliac spine. See text for details.

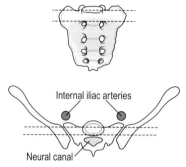

Fig. 15.28 Posterior pelvic stabilization with screws.

percutaneous fixation with the patient supine. The path of the guide wire and lag screw is a straight corridor that is navigated fluoroscopically between the L5 nerve root (which passes over the sacral ala) above, the S1 nerve root passing through its foramen below, the neural canal behind and the iliac vessels anteriorly. The screw is partially threaded to allow compression and should pass across the midline; it is maximally stable when it passes completely through the sacrum and engages the far sacroiliac cortex.

Posterior ring injuries that cannot be reduced closed require open reduction. Sacroiliac joint injuries may be approached and reduced from the front via the lateral window of the ilio-inguinal approach (see Fig. 16.10) and either fixed with sacroiliac screws or plated (**Fig. 15.29A**). Irreducible sacral fractures require open reduction in the prone position, allowing fixation with screws, a plate (**Fig. 15.29B**) or bars (**Fig. 15.29C**). The wounds should not be placed over the bony prominence of the

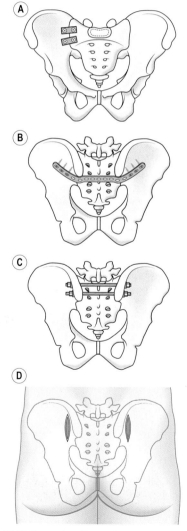

Fig. 15.29 Posterior ring stabilization with plates and bars.

posterior superior iliac spine, where they are vulnerable to dehiscence, but are placed just lateral to these prominences (**Fig. 15.29D**). The crescent fracture of an LC 2 injury is either plated or stabilized percutaneously with a screw (which lies in the same corridor as the supra-acetabular screw (see Fig. 15.27).

### Spinopelvic dissociation

Certain complex H-shaped sacral fractures (see Fig. 15.18) and lumbosacral fracture dislocations dissociate the entire pelvis from the spine (**Fig. 15.30A, B**) and cannot be fixed with sacral screws. These injuries require a formal exposure in the prone position. Spinal

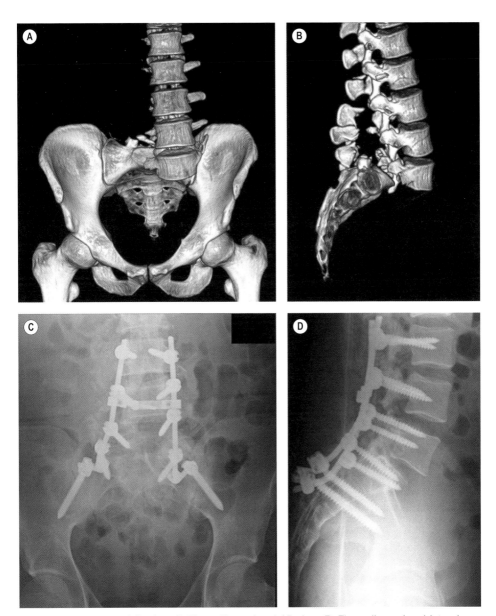

Fig. 15.30 Lumbosacral fixation. **A**, Three-dimensional AP view. **B**, Three-dimensional lateral view. **C**, AP view. **D**, Lateral view.

instrumentation is used to bridge the sacral fracture, with lumbar pedicle screws proximally and transiliac screws distally via the posterior superior iliac spines (**Fig. 15.30C, D**).

### Postoperative management

- *Deep venous thrombosis prophylaxis*: Formal anticoagulation may be required. An inferior vena caval filter should be considered in patients who cannot receive chemoprophy-laxis (e.g. those with severe head injuries).

- *Mobilization*: This will usually consist of pro-tected weight-bearing until stability returns between 6 and 15 weeks.

# Outpatient management

- Stable pubic rami fractures in the elderly do not routinely require follow-up.

- In the patient with a surgically stabilized pelvic ring fracture, protected weight-bearing on the affected side for 8 weeks is required, with regular radiographic review.

- Patients with bilateral fixed injuries (LC 3 and VS 2, as well as spinopelvic dissocia-tion injuries) are usually restricted to bed-to-wheelchair transfers for a prolonged period.

## COMPLICATIONS

### *Early*

| Local | Haemorrhagic shock: This is the principal concern. Initial management centres on rapid diagnosis and intervention with the application of a binder and surgical packing or embolization, along with concurrent resuscitation with blood and blood products |
| --- | --- |
| | Urinary tract injury: This must be excluded early by clinical and radiographic examination as appropriate. The injury can be worsened by injudicious attempts at catheterization |
| | Infection: Careful inspection is required to avoid missing an open fracture or an internal-open fracture |
| General | Multiply injured patients: These individuals are at risk of a lethal triad of hypothermia, acidosis and coagulopathy (p. 26), and aggressive resuscitation is required to reduce mortality, both acutely and later, from development of the systemic inflammatory response syndrome (SIRS) and acute respiratory distress syndrome (ARDS) |
| | Deep venous thrombosis and pulmonary embolism: These are common after pelvic fractures |

### *Late*

| Local | Long-term sequelae: The majority of patients suffer some form of long-term sequelae, including erectile dysfunction, mechanical pelvic pain and psychological disturbance |
| --- | --- |

## GENERAL PRINCIPLES

## Anatomy

The name for the hip socket derives from the Latin word for a small cup used to serve vinegar. Structurally, it is considered to have two columns:

- The anterior column extends from the anterior iliac spines and the rami to the pubis (**a** on **Fig. 16.1**).
- The posterior column extends from the sciatic notch to the ischium (**b**).

The acetabulum is bounded by a roof or *tectum* (**c**), a posterior wall (**d**) and an anterior wall (**e**), and is floored by the quadrilateral plate (**f**).

## Clinical assessment of acetabular injury

### History

An acetabular fracture usually follows a high-energy injury, such as a motor vehicle collision or fall from a height; there may be other associated injuries and it is important to assess and manage these first (see Ch. 2). In the older patient, an acetabular fracture may occur after a simple fall from a standing height; acetabular fractures at the root of the pubis behave much like pubic rami fractures.

### Examination

Acetabular fractures are different from pelvic ring fractures: although there may be internal bleeding from the cancellous bone surface of the fracture, the major, life-threatening haemorrhage that accompanies severe pelvic ring disruption is rarely present. The application of a pelvic binder worsens the deformity and is not indicated, except in the rare circumstance of a combined pelvic and acetabular fracture where there is haemodynamic instability. Associated abdominal or urethral injuries are rare, but associated hip dislocation, femoral neck fracture or sciatic nerve palsy should be excluded. Assess the condition of the skin overlying the pelvis and hip; the Morel-Lavallée lesion is a degloving injury of the skin overlying the hip that predisposes to wound dehiscence and may complicate a planned posterior surgical exposure.

## Radiological assessment of acetabular injury

### Radiographs

- *AP pelvis*: An AP radiograph of the pelvis gives an oblique view of the acetabulum and many features of this radiograph are effectively compound shadows of a number of structures. The roof can be seen (**a** on **Fig. 16.2**), along with the anterior (**b**) and posterior (**c**) walls, as well as the teardrop (**d**) that represents the acetabular floor and quadrilateral plate. The iliopectineal line (**e**) represents the anterior column, the ilio-ischial line (**f**) the posterior column.

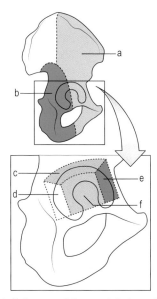

Fig. 16.1 Columns of the acetabulum. See text for details.

● *Judet views* (**Fig. 16.3**): These were classically obtained preoperatively by tilting the patient 45° in either direction, but have largely been supplanted by CT scanning. However, Judet views remain central to intraoperative fluoroscopic assessment. The c-arm is tilted 45° in either direction to give clearer views of the key pelvic structures. The iliac oblique shows the ilium *en face*, and reveals the anterior wall and posterior column. The obturator oblique shows the obturator foramen, seen *en face* as an 'O', and reveals the anterior column and posterior wall.

### CT
Commonly, a CT scan is performed to assist in preoperative planning (**Fig. 16.4**).

## ACETABULAR FRACTURES

## Classification
### Judet and Letournel classification (Fig. 16.5)
This classification system groups acetabular fractures into five elementary types and five associated types. The term 'elementary' pattern implies the involvement of one element

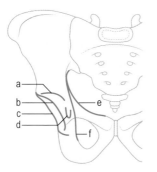

Fig. 16.2 AP view of the pelvis for assessment of the acetabulum.

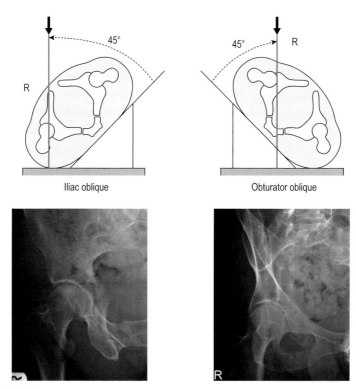

Iliac oblique

Obturator oblique

Fig. 16.3 Judet views.

of the pelvis, not that these fractures are necessarily either simple to treat or associated with a good outcome.

Note that although several injury patterns involve both columns, rather confusingly they are not all termed both-column fractures according to the Judet and Letournel classification. The *both-column fracture* pattern is unique in that no element of the joint surface remains attached to the 'constant fragment' (that part of the ilium that remains attached to the sacrum). It is sometimes referred to as the 'associated both-column' pattern for clarity. The medialized hip joint gives rise to the classical radiographic appearance of the both-column fracture: the spur sign, which is the 'constant fragment' of ilium in profile (**Fig. 16.6**).

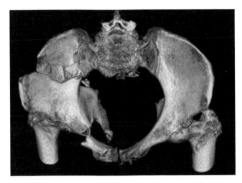

Fig. 16.4 CT scan of a both-column acetabular fracture.

## Emergency Department management

### Clinical features

- There is usually a history of a significant injury, and initial management should follow a standard primary survey and resuscitation. However, unlike pelvic ring fractures, life-threatening haemorrhage is unusual and a pelvic binder is not indicated.

- Assess the condition of the skin to exclude a Morel-Lavallée lesion or open fracture.

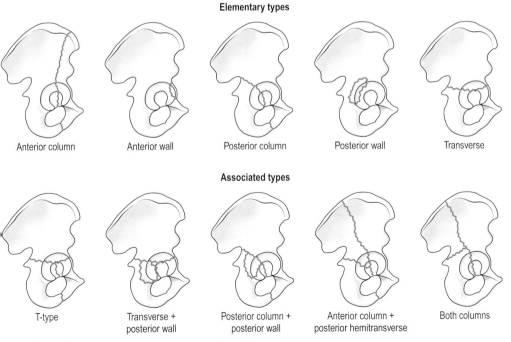

**Elementary types**

| | | | | |
|---|---|---|---|---|
| Anterior column | Anterior wall | Posterior column | Posterior wall | Transverse |

**Associated types**

| | | | | |
|---|---|---|---|---|
| T-type | Transverse + posterior wall | Posterior column + posterior wall | Anterior column + posterior hemitransverse | Both columns |

Fig. 16.5 Judet and Letournel classification of acetabular fractures.

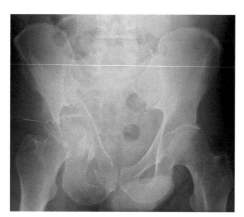

Fig. 16.6 Spur sign. This is pathognomic of a both-column acetabular fracture.

- Assess leg lengths and rotation: an acetabular fracture may be complicated by a dislocation of the hip (p. 375), which should be reduced urgently.
- A careful neurovascular examination is required.

### Radiological features
- *AP radiograph of the pelvis*: Assess the integrity of the pelvic ring itself, including the sacroiliac joints. Then carefully assess and compare the radiographic features of the acetabula on the injured and uninjured sides (see Fig. 16.2).
- *CT*: This will usually be required for complete assessment and operative planning.

### Closed reduction and immobilization
If there is significant joint incongruity, skin traction (see Fig. 18.6) should be applied to the lower limb to minimize further acetabular cartilage damage. A dislocation of the hip (p. 375), should be reduced urgently.

### Inpatient referral
All acetabular fractures should be referred to the orthopaedic service.

## Orthopaedic management
### Non-operative
- Undisplaced fractures or those with minimal displacement may be managed conservatively.

- Both-column fractures may have a surprising degree of secondary congruence, as all of the articular components may coalesce around the femoral head. In selected patients, this may allow the fracture to be treated non-operatively.

### Operative
- In young patients with displaced fractures, surgery is usually performed to restore acetabular congruence and pelvic stability.
- In elderly patients, reconstruction of severely displaced fractures may be performed as a precursor to total hip replacement, as either a single-stage or a two-stage procedure.

The choice of surgical approach is dictated by the fracture pattern. In general, fractures with most displacement at the front are addressed through an anterior approach and similarly those with most displacement at the back are addressed through a posterior approach.

### Anterior surgical approaches
#### Ilio-inguinal approach
The ilio-inguinal approach is used when the majority of the displacement is at the front of the pelvis and allows access to a wide area of the internal surface of the pelvis (**Fig. 16.7**). It uses a single crescentic incision from the iliac crest to the pubic symphysis (**Fig. 16.8**). Division of the external oblique aponeurosis (***a*** on **Fig. 16.9**) exposes the inguinal canal and the spermatic cord, which is mobilized and protected by a sling. Further dissection through the internal oblique aponeurosis (***b***), the transversus abdominis aponeurosis (***c***) (and their conjoint tendon) and the rectus abdominis insertion (with ligation of the inferior epigastric artery) exposes preperitoneal fat. The iliopsoas muscle (with the femoral nerve) (***d*** on **Fig. 16.10**) and external iliac vascular bundle (***e***) can now be isolated separately to form three 'windows'.

1. The lateral window is developed by reflecting the iliacus muscle from the inner surface of the pelvis and allows access to the iliac blade, internal aspect of the quadrilateral plate, and posterior column.

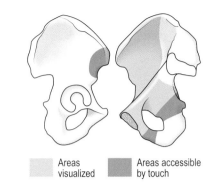

Areas visualized

Areas accessible by touch

Fig. 16.7 Ilio-inguinal approach: access.

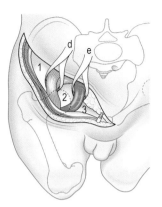

Fig. 16.10 Ilio-inguinal approach: exposure. See text for details.

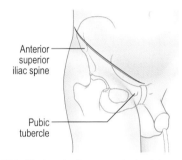

Anterior superior iliac spine

Pubic tubercle

Fig. 16.8 Ilio-inguinal approach: incision.

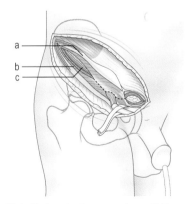

a
b
c

Fig. 16.9 Ilio-inguinal approach: soft tissue dissection. See text for details.

2. The middle window lies between the ilio-psoas muscle (and femoral nerve) and the vascular bundle, allowing access to the pubic root.

3. The medial window lies to the medial side of the femoral artery, vein and canal, and allows access to the superior pubic ramus and pubis.

### Stoppa approach

The Stoppa approach is a modification of the ilio-inguinal approach, allowing access to the internal surface of the true pelvis, the sciatic notch and the pelvic brim with minimal dissection (**Fig. 16.11**). A midline or Pfannenstiel incision is made and a rectus split is performed (**Fig. 16.12**). Blunt dissection allows mobilization of the peritoneum medially, lifting it from the internal surface of the true pelvis (**Fig. 16.13**). The corona mortis artery is identified and divided, and this allows the internal iliac artery and vein to be lifted up to expose the pelvic brim. Subperiosteal dissection exposes the fracture. The Stoppa approach can be used in combination with the lateral window of the ilio-inguinal approach to provide additional access to the iliac blade.

### Smith-Peterson approach

The Smith-Peterson (iliofemoral) approach allows limited access to the anterior column and the hip joint. It is used principally for access to the joint and femoral head and neck, and the anterior iliac spines (e.g. for placement of supra-acetabular external fixation pins). The incision lies around the iliac crest and is then extended vertically down from the anterior

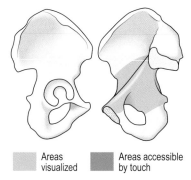

Areas visualized

Areas accessible by touch

Fig. 16.11 Stoppa approach: access.

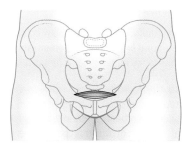

Fig. 16.12 Stoppa approach: incision.

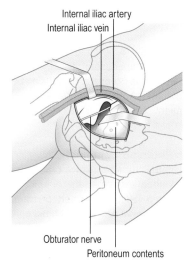

Internal iliac artery
Internal iliac vein

Obturator nerve
Peritoneum contents

Fig. 16.13 Stoppa approach: exposure.

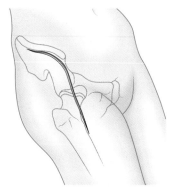

Fig. 16.14 Smith-Peterson approach: incision.

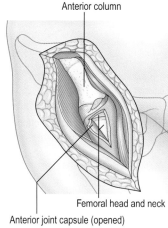

Anterior column

Femoral head and neck

Anterior joint capsule (opened)

Fig. 16.15 Smith-Peterson approach: exposure.

superior iliac spine over the anterior aspect of the thigh (**Fig. 16.14**). It exploits a superficial internervous plane between tensor fasciae latae (superior gluteal nerve) and sartorius (femoral nerve). The fascia of sartorius covers the lateral cutaneous nerve of the thigh, which can be damaged in this approach. A deep internervous plane is then developed between gluteus medius (superior gluteal nerve) and the reflected head of rectus femoris (femoral nerve), exposing the hip joint capsule and the anterior column (**Fig. 16.15**).

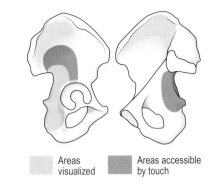

Fig. 16.16 Kocher–Langenbeck approach: access.

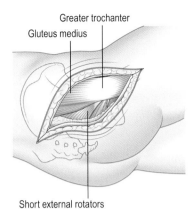

Fig. 16.18 Kocher–Langenbeck approach: soft tissue dissection.

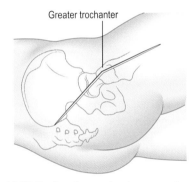

Fig. 16.17 Kocher–Langenbeck approach: incision.

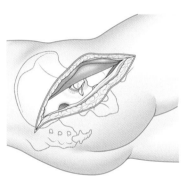

Fig. 16.19 Kocher–Langenbeck approach: exposure.

## Posterior surgical approach

### Kocher–Langenbeck approach

The Kocher–Langenbeck approach is used for access to the posterior wall and column (**Fig. 16.16**). The patient can be placed in either the lateral or the prone position. The incision runs from the posterior superior iliac spine to the greater trochanter, and then runs distally over the lateral aspect of the femur (**Fig. 16.17**). Incising the fascia lata and splitting gluteus maximus exposes the sciatic nerve and short external rotators (**Fig. 16.18**). Piriformis, obturator internus and the gemelli are divided at their femoral insertions but quadratus femoris is preserved, along with the medial circumflex femoral artery, which runs under its superior border and supplies the femoral head. The

posterior column and wall are thus exposed (**Fig. 16.19**) and a finger can be placed through the sciatic notch and on to the internal surface of the quadrilateral plate.

## Extensile approaches

The extensile approaches are only occasionally required for extensively displaced and comminuted fractures. The *triradiate* approach constitutes a Kocher–Langenbeck incision with an additional limb that passes anteriorly through the belly of tensor fasciae latae and then ascends in the Smith-Peterson interval (**Fig. 16.20**). The greater trochanter with its attached

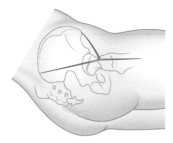

Fig. 16.20 Triradiate approach.

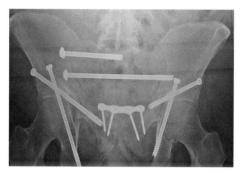

Fig. 16.21 Percutaneous acetabular fixation.

glutei is then detached with a saw and retracted proximally to give an extensive exposure of the lateral aspect of the pelvis and acetabulum. The *extended iliofemoral* approach is an extension of the Smith-Peterson approach, with detachment of the insertion of the gluteal tendons from the greater trochanter. The entire external surface of the pelvis is thus exposed, leaving the gluteal muscles dependent on the superior gluteal artery.

### Percutaneous surgery

This is demanding, and an intimate understanding of pelvic anatomy and safe corridors is essential. However, the skilful use of percutaneous screws can avoid considerable soft tissue stripping and morbidity (**Fig. 16.21**). Adjuncts to reduction, such as pelvic reduction frames, can be used in combination with percutaneous fixation.

### Surgical techniques

Surgery is challenging and is performed by a surgeon with experience and expertise in this type of injury. The operation is planned carefully, based on the preoperative radiographs and scans. A specialized radiolucent table and an experienced radiographer are invaluable, along with the use of blood autotransfusion. Surgery should usually be performed through one approach where possible, using specialist clamps, retractors and plates. Two approaches can usefully be combined in one stage, particularly the Stoppa with the lateral window of the ilio-inguinal. Rarely, a two-stage operation is required, with an initial posterior approach followed by an anterior approach, or *vice versa.* In the elderly patient, there is often extensive articular impaction and the advantages of joint reconstruction are fewer; a definitive single procedure to stabilize the major elements of the acetabulum and then implant a total hip replacement should be considered.

### Postoperative management

- *Deep venous thrombosis (DVT) prophylaxis*: Formal anticoagulation may be required. An inferior vena caval filter should be considered in patients who cannot receive chemoprophylaxis (e.g. those with severe head injuries).

- *Heterotopic ossification*: Consideration should be given to the use of an extended postoperative course of indomethicin or even elective radiotherapy.

- *Mobilization*: This will usually consist of restriction in the range of hip movement to 90° of flexion in neutral rotation for 3 weeks, and toe-touch weight-bearing and crutches for up to 12 weeks.

## Outpatient management

Patients are reviewed at 2, 6 and 12 weeks and at 6 months with AP pelvis and Judet views, and may undergo subsequent surveillance for the development of complications.

# COMPLICATIONS

## *Early*

| | |
|---|---|
| Local | Infection and wound dehiscence: These are feared complications and are more common after extensile incisions, and combined anterior and posterior approaches; in the presence of the Morel-Lavallée lesion; and following pelvic embolization |
| | Neurovascular dysfunction: This may follow injury to the sciatic, femoral or obturator nerves. There is a particular risk of thigh numbness following injury to the lateral cutaneous nerve to the thigh in the ilio-inguinal approach |
| | Heterotopic ossification: This is more common following posterior and extensile approaches |
| General | DVT: This is virtually ubiquitous following pelvic and acetabular injury |

## *Late*

| | |
|---|---|
| Local | Post-traumatic osteoarthritis: This is inevitable after this intra-articular injury with articular disruption. Incidence and severity are related to patient age, fracture pattern and accuracy of reduction. Posterior wall fractures and transverse and T-type fractures are amongst those with the worst prognosis |

## GENERAL PRINCIPLES

Hip joint injuries are extremely common. The type of injury is related to the age of the patient and the energy involved. The most common surgically treated fracture is the hip fracture, usually sustained by an elderly patient after a low-energy fall. In the same age group, there is an increasing incidence of periprosthetic fractures related to hip or knee arthroplasty. Younger patients usually present after high-energy trauma with fractures of the hip or femoral head, or with hip dislocation.

## Clinical assessment of the painful hip

### History

A description of the mechanism and energy of the injury guides the initial assessment. Those patients with a high-energy injury may have important associated injuries and require a full assessment and primary survey (see Ch. 2). Older patients who have suffered a lower-energy injury require a detailed medical assessment to elucidate the cause of the fall and to allow optimization pre-surgery (p. 35). Establish whether the patient has had any previous hip or pelvic surgery.

Atraumatic hip pain is also a common Emergency Department presentation. As with all atraumatic monoarthritides, the most important differential diagnosis to exclude is a septic arthritis (p. 103). Important symptoms include fever, rigors and an irritable hip. If the patient has a prosthetic joint, enquire about previous infection or any wound problems postoperatively.

### Examination

#### Look

Inspection of the exposed lower limbs often indicates a particular hip pathology. A shortened, externally rotated limb is a classic feature of a hip fracture (see Fig. 17.8) but may also indicate a femoral shaft fracture or anterior hip dislocation. A shortened, internally rotated limb suggests a posterior hip dislocation.

#### Feel

The hip joint itself is too deep to assess for effusion or heat but localized tenderness around the hip region can indicate important pathology. Palpate the:

- *superior pubic ramus*, felt along its length by finding the pubic symphysis then palpating along its border laterally
- *hip joint*, located just inferior to the mid-inguinal point (halfway between the pubic symphysis and the anterior superior ischial spine); firm pressure over an irritable hip will be uncomfortable
- *ischial tuberosity*, felt at the buttock crease when the hip is flexed slightly; tenderness here is indicative of an inferior pubic ramus fracture.

#### Move

Establish whether patients can perform a straight-leg raise (see Fig. 19.4). If they can, assess the active range of movement that is possible in terms of flexion and rotation. Comfortable active hip movement usually excludes a hip or acetabular fracture. Passive testing beyond gentle rotation or limited flexion before acquiring radiographs is likely to cause unnecessary discomfort, but assess:

- passive *hip rotation* with the hip extended; this is painful with a hip fracture but much less so with a ramus fracture
- *axial loading* of the hip by pressing up on the sole of the foot; patients with a hip fracture find this uncomfortable but it is often normal in those with a ramus fracture.

#### Neurovascular assessment

Integrity is confirmed by ensuring active dorsiflexion and plantar flexion of the ankle and

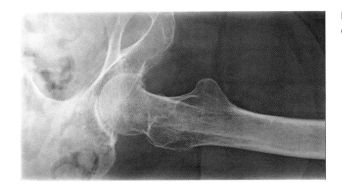

Fig. 17.1 Lateral radiograph of the hip.

checking that sensation is present over the dorsal and plantar surfaces of the foot (see Figs 3.20–3.22). Locate the dorsalis pedis and posterior tibial pulses (although these may be impalpable in peripheral vascular disease) and confirm capillary refill.

## Radiological assessment of the painful hip

### Radiographs

- *AP view of the pelvis* (see Fig. 15.6): This is required to allow full assessment of the hip and pelvic ring.

- *Lateral view of the hip* (**Fig. 17.1**): The lateral radiograph of the affected hip is taken with the contralateral hip flexed out of the path of the beam.

- *AP and lateral femur*: This additional view is needed if there is suspicion of a malignant pathology of if intramedullary fixation is planned.

On the AP pelvis, assess the integrity of Shenton's arcs (**Fig. 17.2**); a break in this line will reveal a subtle intracapsular fracture. Carefully inspect the trabecular lines, looking for discontinuity or angulation (Fig. 17.6). If the fracture line, or the extent of displacement, is not clear, a coned AP view of the affected hip is required. Often, a poor radiograph arises from the injured limb lying in external rotation, resulting in an oblique view with a prominent lesser trochanter; provide analgesia and then hold the foot in a position of internal rotation to obtain a true AP hip. In the context of an unremarkable AP radiograph (**Fig. 17.3A**), the lateral is often helpful

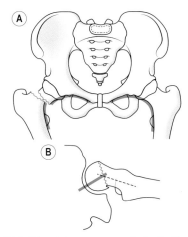

Fig. 17.2 AP pelvis assessment. **A**, On the AP view, assess Shenton's arcs (highlighted). In this illustration there is an intracapsular fracture of the right hip and this has caused a break in Shenton's arc. **B**, On the lateral view, assess for any displacement of the head, which should normally be aligned centrally on the neck (dotted black line). Here, there is a fracture with posterior tilt.

in distinguishing a displaced from an undisplaced intracapsular fracture (**Fig. 17.3B**). Assess bone quality to exclude a primary bone disease (e.g. Paget's) or a tumour (most commonly, a metastatic deposit). Malignant metastases have a predilection for the lesser trochanter (see Fig. 1.1).

### CT

CT is required in the evaluation of complex hip injury, such as a native hip dislocation or

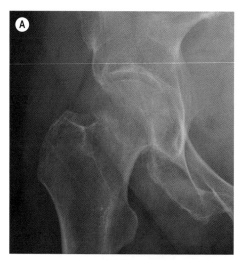

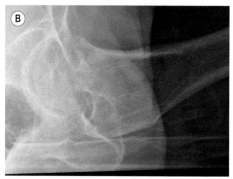

Fig. 17.3 Hip radiographs. **A**, A patient with an unremarkable AP view. **B**, The lateral view shows an intracapsular fracture. Compare with Figs 17.1 and 17.2.

femoral head fracture. It can also be used in the assessment of occult hip fracture.

### MRI

MRI is also a suitable modality for the assessment of occult hip fracture, and it will also demonstrate other soft tissue causes of hip pain, such as a psoas abscess.

### HIP FRACTURES

Hip fracture is the most common fracture requiring surgical treatment. The worldwide annual incidence is projected to rise from 1.6 million patients in 1990 to a predicted

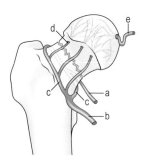

Fig. 17.4 Vascular anatomy of the femoral head.

6 million in 2050. Up to 50% of women can expect to suffer a hip fracture in their lifetime. It is a typical fragility fracture, as a consequence of osteoporosis, advancing age or chronic disease. The fracture is often indicative of a generalized decline in health, including cognitive ability, balance, muscle power and eyesight. In addition, an acute intercurrent illness, such as urinary tract infection, is often the precipitant of the fall that breaks the hip. These patients are often medically and socially vulnerable and have a high level of perioperative and postoperative mortality and dependency. Around 30% will die within a year of their fall and 25% of the remainder will never return to independent living. Prompt and effective surgical and medical care has a substantial effect on improving this prognosis.

## Anatomy and vascular supply

Classification is key to deciding on management, and is based on the vascular anatomy of the proximal femur. The vascular supply to the femoral head arises from three sources. The most important supply arises from the lateral and medial circumflex arteries (**a** and **b** on **Fig. 17.4**), which are branches of the profunda femoris artery. These form a vascular ring (**c**) within the capsule of the hip joint. From this, retinacular vessels (held down by a retinaculum) run on the surface of the femoral neck to penetrate the head (**d**). Secondly, there is small contribution from the medullary canal and, thirdly, a negligible contribution from the ligamentum teres (**e**) in adults.

The hip joint capsule inserts into the intertrochanteric line (anteriorly) and crest (posteriorly) in the region of the vascular ring.

- *Intracapsular* fractures (**Fig. 17.5**) disrupt the retinacular vessels and threaten the blood supply to the head. This can result in avascular necrosis (AVN) and subsequent bony collapse, and so, when displaced, these fractures are usually treated by removal of the femoral head and an arthroplasty in the elderly.

- *Extracapsular* fractures rarely affect this blood supply and so are usually treated with fixation.

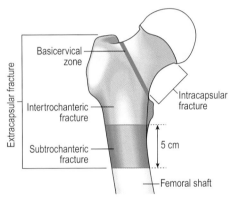

Fig. 17.5 Regions of the proximal femur.

## Classification of intracapsular fractures

### Garden classification

The Garden classification (**Fig. 17.6**) describes four patterns of intracapsular fracture, as seen on the AP radiograph:

- Garden 1: The fracture is *valgus impacted* (i.e. the apex of the fracture points medially). Classically, the medial cortical fracture is not seen on the radiograph.

- Garden 2: The fracture is complete but *undisplaced*, but the trabeculae remain aligned.

- Garden 3: The fracture is moderately displaced with disturbance of the trabecular pattern.

- Garden 4: The fracture is displaced but the trabeculae line up to indicate that the head lies in neutral rotation.

In practice, it is neither possible nor very useful to differentiate between these four types consistently or reliably. However, identifying displacement (and therefore the likelihood of retinacular vessel disruption) *is* crucial, and Garden 1 and 2 fractures are best termed '*undisplaced*' and Garden 3 and 4 '*displaced*'.

The Garden classification does not take into account the displacement, usually *posterior tilt*,

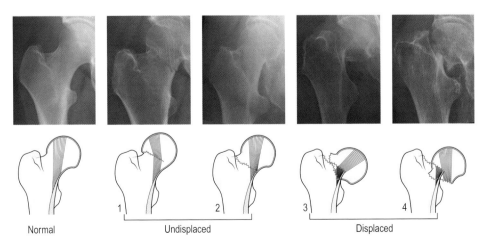

Fig. 17.6 Garden classification of intracapsular fractures.

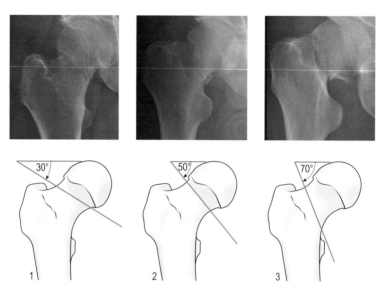

Fig. 17.7 Pauwel classification of intracapsular fractures.

that may be present on the lateral hip radio-graph. Although there is no current consensus, a hip fracture with a posterior tilt of >10° should be viewed as *displaced* (see Fig. 17.3B).

## Pauwel's classification

Pauwel's classification indicates the orientation of the fracture (**Fig. 17.7**). Most fragility frac-tures are of type 2, but young patients suffering higher-energy trauma often have a more verti-cal, Pauwel's 3, orientation. While type 1 and 2 fractures are relatively stable and can be fixed with screws, type 3 fractures are subject to shear and may be better treated with angle-stable fixation such as the use of a dynamic hip screw (DHS).

## Classification of extracapsular fractures

Extracapsular fractures include basicervical, intertrochanteric and subtrochanteric types (see Fig. 17.5):

- *Basicervical*: Basicervical fractures occur at the base of the femoral neck, but are extra-capsular and do not impair the blood supply to the femoral head.

- *Intertrochanteric*: These fractures are the most common. Both the terms *intertro-chanteric* and *pertrochanteric* are frequently used, and although they do have subtly dif-ferent meanings (the fracture line in the former passes transversely below the greater trochanter and above the lesser tro-chanter, whereas in the latter the fracture line passes obliquely from one trochanter to the other), they are often used interchangeably.

- *Subtrochanteric*: These fractures originate in the 5 cm distal to the lesser trochanter. They account for only 5% of extracapsular fractures but are considered separately because of their biomechanical character-istics. Pathological metastases have a predilection for the subtrochanteric region (see Fig. 1.1). In addition, a small propor-tion of low-energy subtrochanteric fractures are termed 'atypical fractures' (p. 383).

The method of fracture fixation is dependent on the fracture pattern and its inherent stability. There is no useful single classification system, although various modifications of a classifica-tion by Evans have been proposed and are discussed on page 364.

## Emergency Department management

The majority of hip fractures occur following a simple fall by a frail elderly patient, who will often have a number of comorbidities and intercurrent illnesses. A thorough medical assessment is crucial in order to ascertain the cause of the fall and to identify potentially remediable medical problems (p. 35). Young patients with hip fractures have often suffered high-energy trauma and should undergo a full primary and secondary survey (p. 21).

### Clinical features

- Most hip fractures in the elderly follow a simple fall from a standing position, although 5% occur whilst the patient is upright, often in the course of a stumble.
- The lower limb will be shortened and externally rotated if the fracture is displaced (**a** on **Fig. 17.8**). Bruising only appears later.
- There will be tenderness over the groin (**b**).
- There will be pain on attempted passive rotation of the limb (**c**).
- The patient will be unable to perform a straight-leg raise.

### Radiological features

- *AP view of the pelvis and lateral view of the affected hip.*
- *Coned AP view of the hip*: The hip is often seen in external rotation (with the lesser trochanter prominent) and this can obscure a fracture line. Where there is uncertainty, provide analgesia and repeat the AP radiograph of the affected hip while holding the limb in internal rotation. This gives a higher-quality 'coned view' of the proximal femur.
- *AP and lateral femur radiographs*: These should be performed when there is a suggestion of a pathological lesion, or when intramedullary nailing is planned.

### Immobilization

No formal immobilization or traction is indicated for most hip fractures and the leg is allowed to rest in as comfortable a position as possible. Occasionally, extensive subtrochanteric fractures may display significant shortening and the patient may find relief from fixed or balanced traction (Figs 18.12 and 18.13).

### Inpatient referral

Patients with compromised physiology and those who are thought to have suffered an acute cardiopulmonary or neurological event may require initial assessment and monitoring in a critical care area under an appropriate medical specialty. In all cases, appropriate pain relief is provided, comprising systemic analgesia and local anaesthetic blocks (p. 34). Local hip fracture protocols may also include the commencement of intravenous fluids in appropriate cases, inspection of pressure areas, and frailty and delirium assessments (p. 36). Hip fractures should be referred to the orthopaedic service for surgical management.

#### Occult hip fracture

Where there is no fracture on the plain radiographs and patients are ambulant, they may be discharged, with instructions to return for further assessment if symptoms persist or deteriorate. Where the patient is not ambulant due to pain, further investigation is indicated. Both MRI and CT scans have high sensitivity and specificity for occult hip fractures. MRI has the additional advantage of occasionally identifying other pathologies that are causing the hip

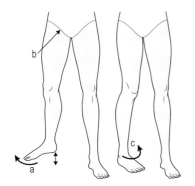

Fig. 17.8 Clinical examination of a hip fracture. See text for details.

**Box 17.1**   SUMMARY OF SURGICAL STRATEGIES FOR HIP FRACTURE

| Intracapsular | Undisplaced | | | Fixation |
|---|---|---|---|---|
| | Displaced | Young | | Urgent reduction and fixation |
| | | Elderly | High demand | Total hip replacement |
| | | | Low demand | Hemiarthroplasty |
| Extracapsular | Intertrochanteric (including basicervical) | Simple | | Dynamic hip screw |
| | | Highly comminuted | | Dynamic hip screw or nail |
| | | Reverse oblique | | Nail |
| | Subtrochanteric | | | Nail |

pain, such as a psoas abscess. Finally, radio-nucleotide scanning is occasionally helpful, although it is not sensitive in the first 3 days after fracture.

## Orthopaedic management of intracapsular fractures

Management of hip fractures is surgical, except in the rare circumstances where the patient is too physiologically compromised to undergo anaesthesia and surgery. The aim of management is to optimize the patient's physiological condition and then perform a single definitive procedure within 24–48 hours of injury that will allow immediate weight-bearing and early reha-bilitation. The surgical technique is selected according to the fracture pattern and the patient's age and physiological condition (**Box 17.1**).

### Undisplaced intracapsular fractures
Undisplaced and valgus impacted fractures are most commonly fixed in situ with either can-nulated screws or a DHS, although there may be a preference for a definitive arthroplasty. Contraindications to screw fixation exist where bone quality is abnormal (e.g. rheumatoid arthritis, renal failure, osteomalacia) or in the rare event that the hip is already affected by symptomatic osteoarthritis.

### SURGICAL TECHNIQUE: Cannulated screw fixation

**Surgical set-up**
Patient set-up is as shown in Figure 17.25.

Ensure the image intensifier can provide AP and true lateral fluoroscopic images of the hip (Fig. 17.26), and confirm that the fracture is undisplaced before proceeding.

**Closed reduction**
No reduction manœuvre is required. Care should be taken whilst positioning the patient to avoid displacing the fracture.

**Incision**
The procedure is percutaneous and only a 3-cm incision at the level of the lesser trochanter is required.

**Starting point**

The entry point for the guide wire is at the level of the lesser trochanter (Fig. 17.9). A screw placed in a more distal position causes a stress riser in the lateral cortex that can result in a comminuted subtrochanteric fracture.

**Procedure**

1. Threaded guide wires:

   The central area of the neck comprises very soft bone and the screws should rest against or near the cortex.

   The first guide wire is placed low in the neck, immediately above the calcar and into the femoral head (**1** on **Fig. 17.9**). It acts as a cantilever, maintaining reduction in the standing position.

   The second wire is placed posteriorly (**2**), to lie adjacent to the posterior cortex of the neck on the lateral view. It also acts as a cantilever, maintaining reduction while the patient is sitting or rising.

   The third wire is placed anteriorly and superiorly (**3**), well away from the first two.

2. Measurement: The measuring device is slid over each wire in turn to provide a screw length.

3. Drilling the lateral cortex: A cannulated drill is passed over each wire to widen the hole at the lateral cortex of the femur. This does not need to ream the length of the guide wire – the screws are self-cutting and self-tapping.

4. Screw insertion: All three screws are inserted before removal of the guide wires. Washers are often used, although compression at the fracture site is principally produced during mobilization rather than intraoperatively.

**Postoperative restrictions**

Movement: No restrictions are imposed.

Weight-bearing: Full weight-bearing is permitted.

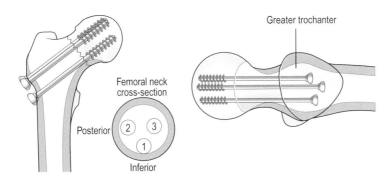

Fig. 17.9 Cannulated screws: insertion technique.

## Displaced intracapsular fractures in elderly patients

Displaced hip fractures have a much higher risk of AVN, non-union and construct failure after attempted fixation than do undisplaced frac- tures. In elderly patients, the advantages of a definitive arthroplasty outweigh any potential benefits of preserving the femoral head. A high-demand patient who is cognitively intact, inde- pendently mobile and active will benefit from a

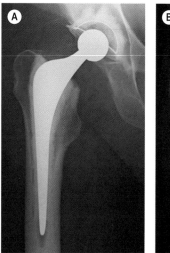
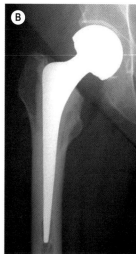
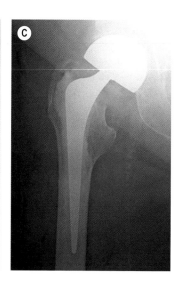

Fig. 17.10 Arthroplasty for hip fractures.

total hip replacement (THR; **Fig. 17.10A**). Those who are less active, are socially dependent and do not walk independently outside the home are more appropriately treated with a hemiarthroplasty, which is a faster, simpler (and therefore safer and more predictable) operation, with a lower rate of dislocation. The implant chosen should have satisfactory long-term joint registry survival data. The head of the hemiarthroplasty may be a single block (unipolar; **Fig. 17.10B**) or may have an independent articulation between a small head and a larger outer shell (bipolar; **Fig. 17.10C**). The latter theoretically reduces acetabular wear but this advantage has yet to be proven conclusively.

A cemented stem is preferred in this patient group. A layer of cement acts as a grout, creating an interface to distribute load between the smooth surface of the femoral stem and the irregular surface of the bone. The principal concern regarding cementation has been hypoxaemia from fat embolism; however, it is now clear that overall survival is, in fact, higher with cemented implants. Uncemented stems should be viewed with caution in patients with hip fractures. Initial stability of uncemented devices is obtained by impacting the stem into the cone of cancellous bone of the proximal femur, providing a tight 'interference' fit. However, the quality of the cancellous bone in the hip fracture patient may be inadequate, preventing satisfactory impaction and resulting in poor initial stability. Moreover, in weak, osteoporotic bone, impaction carries a risk of femoral fracture.

## SURGICAL TECHNIQUE: Hip hemiarthroplasty

### Surgical set-up (Fig. 17.11)
The patient is placed in the lateral position and the pelvis is held securely with supports placed on the sacrum and anterior superior iliac spine. A leg bag is positioned over the anterior side of the table to allow the limb to be placed in flexion and external rotation during the canal preparation stages of the procedure. The surgeon stands behind the patient, the assistant in front.

No intraoperative imaging is required but the radiographs from the Emergency Department should be scrutinized and templated preoperatively. Likely femoral stem size and offset, and head size, should be assessed. Offset is the distance between the centre of the femoral head and a line drawn down the anatomical axis of the femur. The stem size chosen should match the patient's anatomy as closely as possible.

### Incision

The longitudinal skin incision is centred on the tip of the greater trochanter and is 20 cm in length (**Fig. 17.12**). It may curve slightly posteriorly at the proximal end.

### Approach: anterolateral

Internervous plane: The approach runs between split fibres of the glutei, supplied by the inferior gluteal nerve (maximus) and superior gluteal nerve (minimus and medius). Splitting these muscles at the level of the hip spares their innervation. This approach is therefore a plane between branches of the same nerve rather than between two distinct nerves.

The subcutaneous fat is divided sharply in the line of the skin incision, revealing the fascia lata. This fibrous sheet is incised in line with the underlying femur and greater trochanter, and is curved slightly posteriorly at the proximal end of the wound, so as to split the fibres of gluteus maximus. A Charnley retractor is inserted. Any trochanteric bursa is excised to expose the greater trochanter clearly. The vastogluteal sling consists of gluteus medius, vastus lateralis and the intervening tendon attached to the greater trochanter, and is a continuous musculotendinous unit that controls hip stability. These structures are conveniently considered as one anatomical unit and must be divided longitudinally to expose the hip joint. An indentation on the anterosuperior corner of the greater trochanter, which marks the point between the anterior third and posterior two-thirds of the tendon, is a convenient position to start this incision (**Fig. 17.13**). Distal to this point, diathermy is used to develop a subperiosteal plane beneath the tendon and vastus lateralis, exposing the femur and its neck. Above this point, the femoral neck is palpated, then the gluteus medius muscle belly is split in line with its fibres. The underlying gluteus minimus and capsule are then divided as one layer as far as the acetabular margin to expose the femoral head (**Fig. 17.14**). Progressive external rotation and retraction are extremely helpful during this exposure. The femoral neck can now be brought into the wound, usually leaving the femoral head behind in the acetabulum.

### Procedure

1. Femoral neck cut (see Fig. 17.16): The limb is flexed and externally rotated, such that the foot hangs towards the floor within the leg bag. The assistant maintains this position with their knees. The femoral neck cut is dependent on the type of prosthesis. Some stems have a collar that rests on the cortical bone of the calcar, and the neck cut thereby dictates the final position of the femoral component. Special care must be taken when orientating the angle of the saw blade. In most cases, however, a collarless stem is used, and some leeway exists in the location of the cut. The neck cut is made along a line between the superior aspect of the neck and a spot 1 cm above the lesser trochanter.

2. Removal of the femoral head (**Fig. 17.15**): The femoral head is removed using a corkscrew device. Care should be taken to insert the corkscrew into the centre of the femoral head to allow sufficient grip for extraction. The neck should first be palpated with the index and middle fingers. The head is manipulated so that the neck is facing outwards; then the corkscrew is slid between the fingers and the

*Continued*

centre of the neck engaged. A hammer blow to the corkscrew can help engage it if the bone is unusually hard. Keep turning until the head spins within the socket to ensure that any remaining capsule is detached. If head removal proves difficult despite a good corkscrew grip, the capsule cut is checked to ensure it extends to the acetabular lip; then a spoon-shaped retractor is used to lever the head from the socket.

3. Measurement of the femoral head: The femoral head is measured to allow correct sizing of the prosthetic head. If the head is between sizes, opt for the smaller one, as an oversized head may not fit into the acetabulum and is at risk of dislocation.

4. Femoral canal preparation: A box chisel is used to open the top of the femoral canal and remove any remnant of neck at the greater trochanter. The chisel is seated posterolaterally, care being taken not to damage the gluteus medius insertion (**Fig. 17.16A**). A T-handled reamer is then passed down the canal, in line with the anatomical axis. It is useful to place one hand on the knee during this process, as proprioception guides the trajectory of the reamer and can avoid breaching the femoral canal, especially in osteoporotic bone. Stem-specific broaches of incremental size are then used to prepare the proximal femur. The correct size has been reached when the broach resists attempted rotational movement of the broach handle, yet still has several millimetres of cancellous bone surrounding it. The orientation of the broach will reflect the desired position of the definitive stem and so should be inserted with 10–15° of anteversion (**Fig. 17.16B**). The correct depth is achieved when the centre of the broach neck is in line with the tip of the greater trochanter (**Fig. 17.16C**). Most stems have depth markings on the side, and a corresponding mark should be made on the femur (with diathermy or small rongeur) to ensure that the definitive stem rests in the same position.

5. Trial: Because of the intrinsic stability of a large hemiarthroplasty head, a trial reduction is not always performed. However, if desired, with the last broach still in situ, attach the chosen trial head. With the assistant applying gentle traction, the leg is slowly rotated internally and the head guided into the socket. A smooth reduction confirms the correct depth of the broach. A difficult reduction usually indicates that the stem is proud and needs to be inserted deeper into the femoral canal, but may also suggest that the offset is too great or there is obstruction by soft tissue interposition. To dislocate the trial components, a bone hook or swab is placed around the broach neck to apply traction, then the leg is gently rotated externally. The broach is removed.

6. Cement restrictor insertion: A cement restrictor is then inserted to close off the distal canal. It should be inserted to a depth of 2 cm more than the stem length.

7. Lavage: The femoral canal is thoroughly cleared of fat, marrow and blood with pulsed lavage and brushing. This has the dual effect of providing a clean bone interface for cement interdigitation, and minimizing the amount of fat intravasated into the venous circulation during pressurization. The canal is then dried by packing with gauze.

8. Cement insertion: This is a stepwise process that aims to fill the canal and interstices of the cancellous bone with cement. The quality of the bone/cement interface is continually at risk from back-bleeding from the cancellous bone, and poor technique or delays will impair the final result. Once mixed, the cement is loaded into a gun, the gauze is removed and the nozzle is introduced fully into the

canal. Inform the anaesthetist that cementation is about to commence. Begin injecting the cement with rapid compressions on the cement gun and allow the gun to back up as the canal fills, keeping the tip of the nozzle below the cement surface (**Fig. 17.17A**). This retrograde filling occurs at low pressure and is performed rapidly to minimize the back-bleeding time. Once the canal is filled, the nozzle is cut short and a pressurizing collar attached. The gun is then reapplied to the femur and more cement is forced into the canal. Filling is now slow and controlled, aiming to create and maintain a high pressure – above mean arterial pressure – that will force cement into the interstices of the bone, and prevent the cement being pushed back out of the bone by blood (**Fig. 17.17B**). Pressure is maintained throughout the viscous phase of the cement, until it loses its tacky feel and begins to turn rubbery. The gun is removed. This will cause the pressure to drop again and so the stem must be introduced without delay.

9. Stem insertion: The stem is mounted on an introducer. A centralizer is attached at the tip. The tip should be placed in the posterolateral corner of the exposed cement-filled canal with 10–15° of anteversion. The stem is then implanted smoothly and firmly to the predetermined depth. This re-establishes the high canal cement pressure (**Fig. 17.17C**), which will then be maintained as the cement cures. Once the stem is at the correct depth, do not attempt to change the anteversion – this will leave large gaps between the metal and cement. The most common error is to start – or drift – too far medially, which results in implanting the stem in varus. A varus stem has a higher chance of failing early. Allow the cement to set completely before proceeding.

10. Head attachment: The trunion of the femoral stem is cleaned and the head applied. If a bipolar design is selected, apply the bipolar head.

11. Reduction: With the assistant applying gentle traction, the leg is slowly rotated internally and the head guided into the socket. Stability is assessed by placing the limb in maximal internal rotation at 90° of hip flexion, and maximal external rotation with the hip fully extended. An unstable hip requires careful assessment and consideration of greater offset neck or head components.

### Closure

Capsule: The longitudinal incisions in the capsule should be repaired with 2–3 interrupted stitches using a heavy, absorbable, braided suture. Suturing at this depth may be a challenge; the assistant should place two Langenbeck retractors into the wound.

Abductors: The vasto-gluteal sling is now repaired along the omega-shaped tendinotomy. If the tendon is of poor quality, consider driving the needle through the bone to provide a more secure repair.

Fascia lata: The fascia lata is repaired with a continuous stitch using a heavy, absorbable suture (braided or unbraided).

Subcutaneous tissue and skin: These can then be closed according to the surgeon's preference.

### Post procedure

Maintain control of the legs while the patient is moved from their side on to their back and into bed. Bring the heels together and compare the lengths of the operated and non-operated sides.

### Postoperative restrictions

Movement: Standard THR precautions only are applied.

Weight-bearing: Full weight-bearing is permitted.

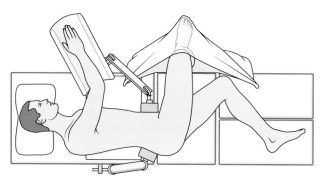

Fig. 17.11 Hip hemiarthroplasty: set-up.

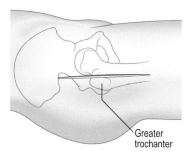

Greater trochanter

Fig. 17.12 Anterolateral approach to the hip: skin incision.

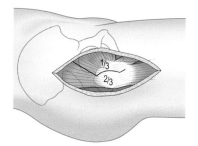

Fig. 17.13 Anterolateral approach to the hip: abductor release.

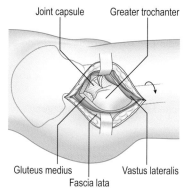

Joint capsule   Greater trochanter

Gluteus medius   Vastus lateralis
Fascia lata

Fig. 17.14 Anterolateral approach to the hip: capsular release.

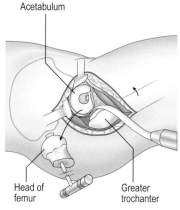

Acetabulum

Head of femur   Greater trochanter

Fig. 17.15 Anterolateral approach to the hip: femoral head removal.

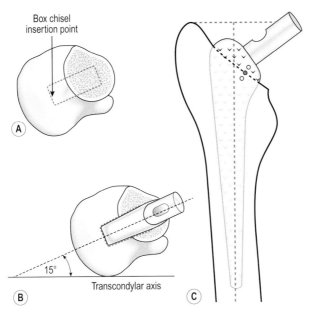

Fig. 17.16 Femoral canal preparation.

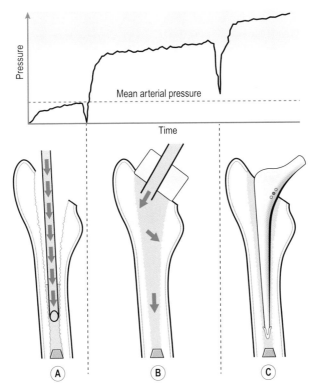

Fig. 17.17 Cement and stem insertion. The correct technique is to maintain the cement pressure (black line) above the mean arterial pressure to avoid back-bleeding into the canal. **A**, Rapid filling phase. **B**, Pressurization phase. **C**, Implant insertion and cement curing.

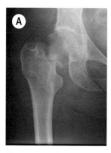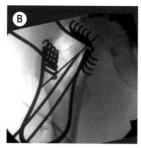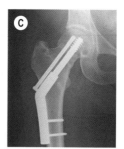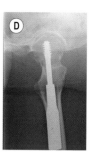

Fig. 17.18 Surgery for displaced intracapsular fractures in the young. See text for details.

## Displaced intracapsular fractures in young patients

In healthy patients under the age of 55, who have usually sustained high-energy fractures, displaced fractures are normally reduced and fixed because of the limited life-span of a hip replacement (**Fig. 17.18A**). If a perfect closed reduction cannot be achieved with closed traction, it may be necessary to perform an open reduction, which is most conveniently done on traction. Two incisions are required. Through an anterior Smith-Peterson approach, the fracture and femoral head are exposed. Two large (2-mm) guide wires are placed in the femoral head to act as joysticks, allowing reduction of the rotational and angulatory components of the displacement (**Fig. 17.18B**). Through a second, lateral, incision, a DHS with an anti-rotation screw is used to stabilize the reduced fracture. As these fractures are often vertically orientated (Pauwel's type 3) with a tendency to displace through shear, this fixed-angle construct is mechanically more stable than using cannulated screws (**Fig. 17.18C,D**). The femoral head is clearly at risk of AVN, and intuitively these patients should undergo reduction and stabilization surgery within 24 hours of injury, although there is no clear scientific evidence for this. If the fracture is fixed closed, there is a theoretical advantage in performing a joint aspiration to decompress the intracapsular haematoma, but again the benefits of this procedure have not been clearly established. The patient should be toe-touch weight-bearing for 6 weeks.

## Orthopaedic management of extracapsular hip fractures

Management of hip fractures is surgical, except in the rare circumstances where the patient is too physiologically compromised to undergo anaesthesia and surgery. The aim of management is to optimize the patient's physiological condition and then perform a single definitive procedure within 24–48 hours of injury that will allow immediate weight-bearing and early rehabilitation.

### Classification and principles of fixation
*Modified Evans Classification*
These fractures are best described according to their morphology. The Modified Evans classification serves as a guide to operative management (**Fig. 17.19**).

1. *Basicervical fractures.* See 2.

2. *Simple intertrochanteric fractures* and basicervical fractures are relatively stable after reduction and are fixed with a dynamic (or sliding) hip screw.

3. *Comminuted intertrochanteric fractures* are less stable and are prone to collapse during healing. They may involve separation of the greater or lesser trochanters, or both, or have extensions distally into the subtrochanteric region. They are generally treated with a DHS. A cephalomedullary nail is sometimes preferred to minimize shortening of the femoral neck.

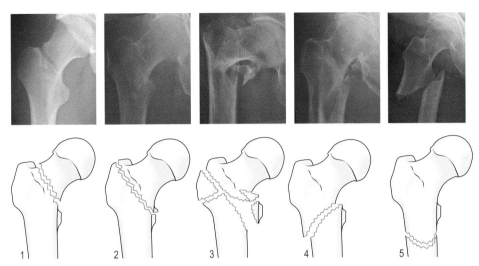

Fig. 17.19 The modified Evans classification of extracapsular fractures.

4. *Reverse oblique fractures* have a fracture orientation that is intrinsically unstable and will progressively displace following DHS fixation. They require a cephalomedullary nail.

5. *Subtrochanteric fractures* are highly unstable. Stress concentrations in the subtrochanteric region result in huge compressive forces on the medial cortex during weight-bearing. As there is often fracture comminution at this site, rotational forces tending to cause fracture collapse are common, and subtrochanteric fractures are therefore usually treated with cephalomedullary nailing.

### AO classification

The AO classification groups together:

- A1 fractures: simple intertrochanteric fractures
- A2 fractures: comminuted intertrochanteric fractures
- A3 fractures: reverse oblique and subtrochanteric fractures.

## Surgical techniques

### Dynamic hip screw

The dynamic (or sliding) hip screw (DHS) is a remarkably successful device comprising a lag

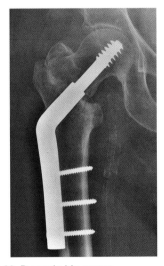

Fig. 17.20 Dynamic hip screw.

screw in the femoral head and neck, which articulates with the barrel of a side plate that is secured to the femoral shaft (**Fig. 17.20**). The screw has flat sides that correspond to the internal shape of the barrel, allowing longitudinal sliding but preventing postoperative rotation (**Fig. 17.21**). This construct allows maintenance of fixed neck-shaft angle, and linear controlled collapse and compression of the fracture, as the lag screw slides into the

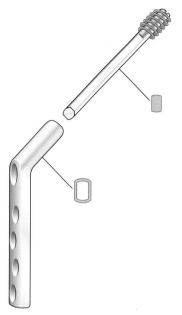

Fig. 17.21 Dynamic hip screw components.

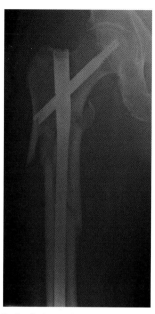

Fig. 17.23 Cephalomedullary nail.

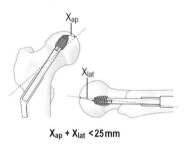

$$X_{ap} + X_{lat} < 25\,mm$$

Fig. 17.22 The tip–apex distance (TAD) of Baumgaertner.

barrel of the plate during postoperative mobilization. Importantly, the lag screw must lie in the centre of the femoral head, near the apex. The tip–apex distance (TAD) is calculated by adding the two distances X from the AP and lateral images ($X_{ap}$ and $X_{lat}$ on **Fig. 17.22**). The risk of screw cut-out and construct failure is minimized by ensuring that the sum of these two distances is <25 mm. A very slightly inferior and posterior position of the wire tip may be accepted but any superior or anterior position increases the risk of failure and should not be tolerated. An eccentric position will tend to result in the femoral head displacing through rotation during mobilization.

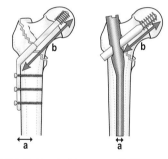

Fig. 17.24 Dynamic hip screw (left) versus intramedullary nail (right).

## Cephalomedullary nailing

The cephalomedullary nail (so called as it extends from the femoral head – Greek: *cephalus* – to the medullary canal of the shaft) is a robust device that allows the secure fixation of proximal femoral fractures (**Fig. 17.23**). It has a number of important features (**Fig. 17.24**). Like the DHS it has:

- a lag screw that is placed centrally adjacent to the apex of the head (see TAD, Fig. 17.22)
- a fixed angle between the femoral neck and shaft to allow controlled linear collapse.

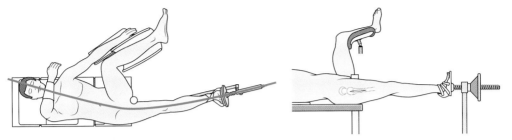

Fig. 17.25 Surgical set-up: percutaneous screws, dynamic hip screws and femoral nailing.

In contrast to the DHS, it has the advantages that it:

- has a relatively short lever arm between the device and the fracture (*a* on **Fig. 17.24**) (see also Fig. 5.2), making it more suited to comminuted fractures or those involving the subtrochanteric region

- has a reduced sliding distance of the lag screw (*b*), which minimizes the distance by which the femoral neck shortens in comminuted intertrochanteric fractures, (in theory) improving subsequent function by maintaining hip offset

- can be implanted percutaneously.

However, it has some disadvantages compared with the DHS, in that:

- there is a higher rate of implant-related fracture, principally at the distal tip of the nail, and particularly with short nails

- it is considerably more expensive

- it is a technically more difficult operation

- despite its theoretical advantages, it has not been shown conclusively that any intertrochanteric fractures (i.e. excluding reverse oblique and subtrochanteric patterns) have a better clinical outcome with a nail than with a DHS.

### Surgical set-up: percutaneous screws, dynamic hip screw, and cephalomedullary and femoral nailing

The set-up for cannulated screw fixation, DHS fixation and femoral nailing is very similar (**Fig. 17.25**). The patient is placed on a radiolucent traction table with the foot in a traction boot. The uninjured limb must be placed out of the way of the image intensifier, most commonly by flexing the hip and knee into the lithotomy position and resting the leg in a leg-holder. Alternatively, both hip and knee can be extended to drop the leg below the level of the injured leg. When setting up for cannulated screws, remember that no reduction is required, and care must be taken not to displace the fracture by excessive movement or traction. For extracapsular injuries, the fracture is reduced first by longitudinal traction, and then by internal rotation of the foot. For nailing procedures, access to the starting point is greatly improved by orientating the patient's trunk away from the hip into the 'banana position'.

Ensure the fluoroscopic images are optimal. Firstly, the lateral image should be rotated on the screen to show the groin post vertically to allow you to orientate yourself (**Fig. 17.26A**). However, with the c-arm in a horizontal position, an oblique view of the hip will often be shown because of anteversion of the femoral neck and external rotation of the distal fragment. This makes interpretation of the image more difficult, particularly when identifying the start point. The c-arm should now be orientated to show a true lateral projection of the hip with the greater trochanter superimposed on the femoral neck (**Fig. 17.26B**). This usually involves rotating the c-arm such that the end nearest the surgeon is lowered and the other end raised.

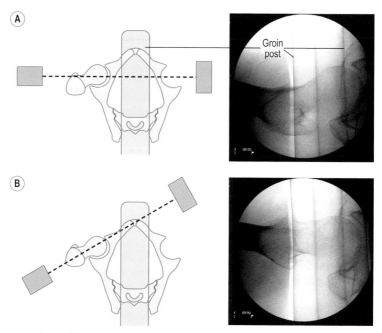

Fig. 17.26 Image intensifier positioning.

## SURGICAL TECHNIQUE: Dynamic hip screw insertion

### Patient set-up
See Figure 17.25.

### Closed reduction
Longitudinal traction and internal rotation of the foot until the patella points directly up will give a satisfactory reduction in the majority of cases. Rarely, in comminuted fractures, adequate reduction is not possible with traction alone. Typically, the fracture 'sags' backwards and an assistant is required to lift the proximal femur anteriorly during fixation.

Preoperative fluoroscopy: Check the AP and true lateral fluoroscopic images carefully and make fine adjustments where necessary to the amount of traction and rotation.

### Incision
The incision starts just below the greater trochanter and proceeds distally in line with the femur. A more precise start point for the proximal end of the incision can be gauged by placing a guide wire over the front of the patient's hip in the planned orientation of the lag screw, confirming the position with fluoroscopy, and locating the point where this would pierce the skin. The length of the incision is dependent on the size of the patient and the plate to be used.

### Approach: direct proximal femoral
Internervous plane: There is no internervous plane, as this technique employs a muscle-splitting technique.

The subcutaneous tissue is sharply dissected to reveal the fascia lata. This is incised in line with the skin incision to reveal the vastus lateralis. The muscle is pulled anteriorly and its aponeurosis incised longitudinally 2 cm from its insertion into the intermuscular septum. A Bristow elevator is then used to elevate the muscle belly anteriorly from the septum and the lateral aspect of the femur. A large self-retaining retractor is useful.

### Procedure (Fig. 17.27)

1. Guide wire placement: A jig is placed on the lateral femoral shaft; the starting position is central on the femoral shaft and can be gauged by direct vision, feel and use of the lateral projection on the fluoroscopic image. Selecting the starting point on the AP fluoroscopic image is more challenging and requires a visual assessment of where the wire tip will end up once driven into the femoral head. The wire tip must sit as close as possible to the apex of the femoral head (**a** on **Fig. 17.27**; see also Fig. 17.22). In an unstable or basicervical fracture, there is a risk of proximal fragment rotation and displacement during drilling and screw insertion, and a second 'anti-rotation' wire and/or screw can be placed well out of the way above the first wire at this point (**b**). When used, the anti-rotation screw is inserted and tightened to provide maximal compression and stability <u>before</u> the DHS wire is overdrilled.

2. Measurement: The measuring device, which slides over the guide wire and must sit on the lateral femoral cortex, is then used to select the correct length of lag screw.

3. Drilling: The guide wire is over-drilled with the composite drill, which cuts a channel to accommodate the lag screw and barrel. A tap may be used in young bone but is not usually necessary in the elderly.

4. Lag screw insertion: The lag screw (**c**) is then inserted with a handle (**d**), ensuring that the final position of the flat sides of the screw will accommodate the plate barrel correctly.

5. Plate application: The plate barrel then slides over the screw to lie against the femur. Occasionally, light taps with an impactor will help to seat the plate but be cautious: injudicious hammering can displace the lag screw forwards into the hip joint or even into the pelvis in weak bone. Finally, the plate is secured to the shaft with position screws. Placing the most distal screw first will ensure that the whole plate lies centrally against the femur. Fracture compression usually occurs with postoperative patient ambulation, but can be generated intraoperatively using a compression screw if desired.

### Postoperative restrictions

Movement: No restrictions are imposed.

Weight-bearing: Full weight-bearing is permitted.

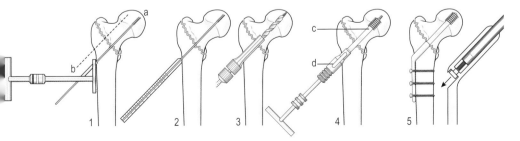

Fig. 17.27 Dynamic hip screw insertion technique.

## SURGICAL TECHNIQUE: Cephalomedullary nail insertion

**Patient set-up**

See Figure 17.25.

**Closed reduction**

Traction and internal rotation are usually sufficient to overcome the deforming forces. However, the combined muscular forces of the glutei producing abduction (*a* on **Fig. 17.28**), the iliopsoas producing flexion and external rotation (*b*), and the adductors, quadriceps and hamstrings producing medial translation and shortening of the shaft (*c*) may necessitate an open reduction and application of a reduction clamp or a cerclage wire.

Preoperative fluoroscopy: Check the reduction with AP and true lateral fluoroscopic images of the hip (see Fig. 17.26).

**Incision**

A stab incision is placed 10 cm proximal to the tip of the greater trochanter in line with the anatomical axis of the femur (see Fig. 18.16). No further dissection is necessary – the guide wire is placed directly through this skin incision.

**Start point**

As with all nailing procedures, selection of the correct start point is crucial. Different nails are designed to exploit different start points: lateral to the tip of the greater trochanter (*a* on **Fig. 17.29**), the tip of the trochanter (*b*; most cephalomedullary nails), or the piriformis fossa (for straight femoral nails; *c*). For trochanteric start-point nails, be aware that the process of sequential broaching and reaming will gradually move the entry point laterally as the instruments lever against the soft tissues. An entry point that is too lateral will result in a varus fracture malalignment, a high screw position in the head and a risk of construct failure (**Fig. 17.30**). Similarly, the start point on the lateral image is important. For example, placing the guide wire into a proximal fracture extension may result in the nail missing the proximal fragment (**Fig. 17.31**).

**Procedure (Fig. 17.32)**

1. Guide wire placement: A threaded guide wire is passed to rest on the start point (see Fig. 18.16). The position is checked on AP and true lateral fluoroscopic images and the wire is then advanced into the proximal femur. This is then over-drilled before the wire is withdrawn.

2. Ball-tipped guide wire: The longer flexible guide wire is inserted and passed into the distal segment. A reduction spoon is often very helpful in directing the wire, particularly in preventing the wire from escaping through the medial fracture line (see Fig. 18.18). The length is then measured before the distal segment is reamed.

3. Nail insertion: The nail, mounted on a jig, is then introduced over the wire; how far it is inserted is determined by the location of the lag screw holes, which must allow the lag screw to be positioned in the centre of the head on the AP view. The screw head placement on the lateral view is controlled by rotating the nail and jig. A radiolucent targeting arm will help to determine this position. As with the DHS, the tip-apex distance (TAD) should be <2.5 cm (see Fig. 17.22). Check that the nail is seated distally within the bone and at the correct length before proceeding.

4. Lag screw guide wire: Once the nail is seated, a sleeve is introduced through a second small incision and guide wire positioned.

5. Lag screw insertion: The guide wire is measured and reamed, and the lag screw is then inserted. As for the DHS, fracture compression most commonly occurs postoperatively by weight-bearing mobilization, but some nails incorporate techniques of allowing compression to be applied intraoperatively if desired.

6. Some nails incorporate a set-screw designed to control the movement of the lag screw within the nail postoperatively to allow sliding but not rotation (like a DHS), or to lock the screw rigidly (preventing any compression or shortening, converting the nail into a rigid fixed-angle device).

7. Distal locking screw placement (see Fig. 18.20). Finally, a distal locking screw is placed free-hand using the 'perfect circles' technique to prevent shortening or rotation of the nail within the distal fragment.

**Postoperative restrictions**

Range of movement: No restrictions are imposed.

Weight-bearing: In the elderly, it is rarely practicable to restrict weight-bearing. In younger patients with highly comminuted fractures, particularly where the construct has been 'locked' to prevent controlled collapse, restricted weight-bearing for 8 weeks may be appropriate, until there is radiographic callus.

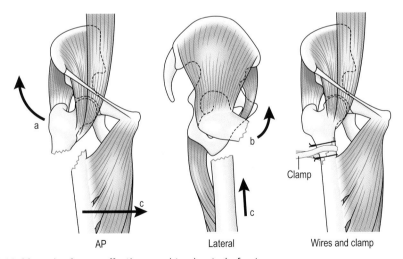

Fig. 17.28 Muscular forces affecting a subtrochanteric fracture.

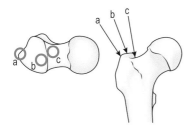

Fig. 17.29 Cephalomedullary nail: starting point.

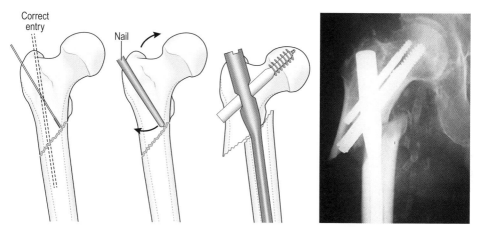

Fig. 17.30 Varus malalignment.

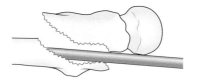

Fig. 17.31 Posterior starting point.

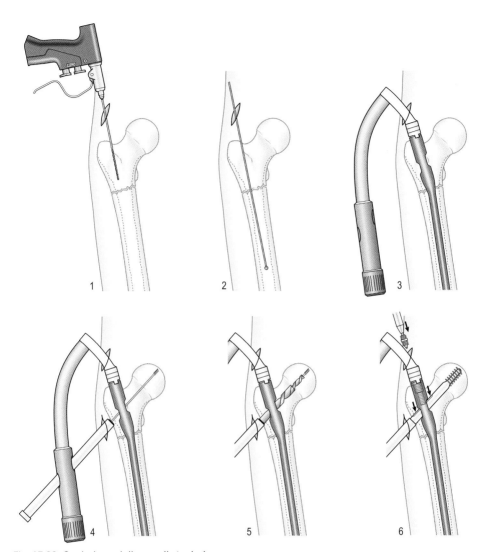

Fig. 17.32 Cephalomedullary nail: technique.

## Outpatient management

### Elderly patients

Management of elderly patients will vary considerably, depending on local preference. There are few advantages to the routine review of elderly patients after hip fracture surgery. The patient is advised that failure of a surgical construct or avascular necrosis will result in symptoms of pain, and that should their level of comfort deteriorate, they should seek help.

Salvage is generally with an arthroplasty. Conversely, in the absence of painful symptoms, it is rare to consider any further intervention.

### Young patients

In contrast, young patients may develop complications for which salvage may be offered before symptoms become marked (see box), and follow-up is therefore generally recommended.

**Outpatient management summary**

| Week | Examination | Radiographs | Additional notes |
|------|-------------|-------------|------------------|
| 2 | Wound check<br>Neurovascular status | AP and lateral hip | Consider revision fixation where there is loss of fixation |
| 8 | Assessment of range of movement<br>Lifting of restrictions where progressing to union | AP and lateral femur | Consider revision where there is loss of fixation |
| 26 | Exclusion of early features of avascular necrosis (AVN) | AP and lateral hip | Consider restricted weight-bearing or salvage surgery in the presence of AVN |

6-monthly or annual review thereafter for a total of 3 years with check radiographs to exclude AVN

# COMPLICATIONS

## *Early*

Local     Infection: Incidence is very low for cannulated screws or intramedullary nailing, but up to 5% for arthroplasty

Fixation failure: This is usually related to technical errors in surgery, or to pathological bone (e.g. rheumatoid arthritis, osteomalacia)

General     Fat embolism: This is associated with arthroplasty and nailing. Patients may develop intraoperative hypoxia during cement pressurization, or when a hip arthroplasty is reduced, as the femoral veins are straightened. Embolization is minimized by adequate canal lavage and drying

## *Late*

Local     Metalwork irritation: This may occur as a result of controlled fracture collapse and screw back-out

Avascular necrosis: AVN of the femoral head occurs in up to 10% of undisplaced fractures and 30% of displaced fractures. It results in radiographic sclerosis and pain, and is usually salvaged with THR. Osteotomy, arthrodesis or core decompression may be considered in young patients

Non-union: This occurs in 5% of undisplaced fractures but 25% of displaced fractures

Osteoarthritis: This occurs in around 25% of patients within 8 years

Dislocation: This is associated with arthroplasty. It is more common in THR than hemiarthroplasty, and with the posterior approach to the hip

General     Death: Mortality in the elderly is around 30% in the first year after fracture, a reflection of the frailty of the population sustaining this injury

## HIP DISLOCATION

Dislocation of the native hip (see Fig. 17.36) is usually posterior and commonly occurs following high-energy trauma, such as a motor vehicle collision or a fall from a height. In a dashboard impact to the knee (**a** on **Fig. 17.33**), transmitted forces may produce associated fractures of the patella, femoral shaft (**b**), hip (**c**) and the posterior wall of the acetabulum (**d**), and injury to the sciatic nerve (**e**). Less commonly, the hip may dislocate anteriorly following an abduction force to the femur.

Dislocation of a hip prosthesis, in contrast, usually follows the adoption of a position of flexion and internal rotation, such as when pulling on shoes or rising from a low seat. The majority of these dislocations are also posterior (**Fig. 17.34**).

## Emergency Department management

Dislocation of a native hip results from violent trauma and the patient should be appropriately assessed with a full primary and secondary survey (see Ch. 2). Associated injuries are common. Dislocation of a prosthetic hip is a low energy injury.

### Clinical features

- The limb is usually shortened, flexed and internally rotated (**Fig. 17.35**), although this deformity may be less evident if there is an associated femoral fracture (**a** on the figure).
- Carry out a careful secondary survey and examine the ipsilateral limb, particularly for associated injuries.

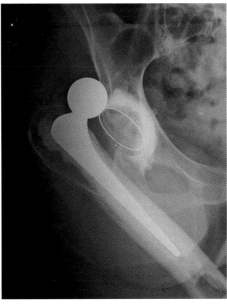

Fig. 17.34 Dislocation of a total hip replacement.

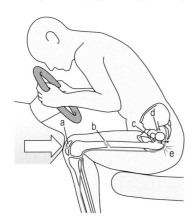

Fig. 17.33 Dashboard injuries. See text for details.

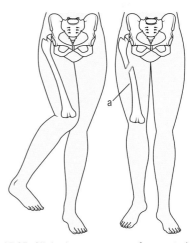

Fig. 17.35 Clinical appearance of a posterior hip dislocation. This may be less evident if the femur is fractured (a).

- The patient will be in severe pain and will not usually tolerate any passive movement of the hip.
- A sciatic nerve palsy is common after a posterior dislocation, as are femoral artery and nerve compromise in an anterior dislocation.

### Radiological features

- *AP pelvis* (**Fig. 17.36**): This is usually sufficient to make a diagnosis. In the more common posterior dislocation, the femoral head often appears small (as it is closer to the X-ray plate and is therefore less magnified) and overlaps the acetabular roof. Inspect carefully for associated fractures of the acetabulum, femoral head and femoral neck.

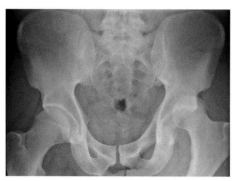

Fig. 17.36 Radiographic appearance of a posterior native hip dislocation.

- *CT*: This should be performed after reduction to assess the integrity of the acetabulum and femoral head, and to exclude incarcerated loose bodies. Small fragments within the condylar fossa usually have soft tissue attachments, are stable, and may be left, but loose fragments within the joint require surgical exploration and removal.

### Closed reduction

#### *Posterior dislocation of the hip joint (Fig. 17.37)*

The dislocated native hip should be reduced on recognition to minimize the risk of AVN. Reduction may be challenging and the key to success is complete muscle relaxation.

1. With the patient supine, an assistant should stabilize the pelvis while the hip is flexed to 90°. Place the patient's ankle under your arm, with your forearm under their calf, and your hands locked together. Keep your back straight and lift with your legs and hips. The femoral head is then lifted forwards into the acetabulum with gentle internal and external rotational movements. Reduction occurs with an obvious 'clunk' but this may be less striking if there is a large posterior wall fracture.

2. Alternatively, the reduction manœuvre may be easier with the patient placed on a stretcher on the floor: greater leverage can then be obtained by gripping the patient's leg between your knees, resting your forearms on your thighs, and flexing your knees.

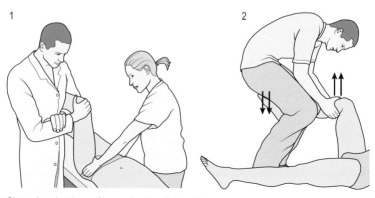

Fig. 17.37 Closed reduction of a posterior dislocation.

Following reduction, carefully assess stability by bringing the hip slowly back towards 90° and applying gentle downward pressure on the knee. Avoid dislocating the hip again, as this causes further articular scuffing. Instability is an indication for fixation of a posterior wall acetabular fracture.

### Anterior dislocation of the hip joint

With a well-anaesthetized patient and an assistant stabilizing the pelvis, flex the patient's hip and correct abduction and external rotation. This may result in reduction of the hip. Occasionally, the manoeuvre may convert an anterior dislocation into a posterior dislocation, which is then treated as above.

### Dislocated total hip replacement

The principles of management are the same as for a native hip (above). Reduction is performed in the Emergency Department under procedural sedation and analgesia, but complete muscle relaxation is not normally required. A light 'clunk' is often misinterpreted as a reduction but may merely indicate contact between the prosthetic head and the rim of the acetabular cup. Assess limb position and length if there is uncertainty. Perseverance will usually result in successful reduction. If the hip cannot be reduced, a general anaesthetic with muscle relaxation is required. On rare occasions, an open reduction of a dislocated THR is required, at which point the opportunity may be taken to revise any component malposition that has contributed to the dislocation.

### Immobilization and reassessment

Apply a knee extension split in order to prevent hip flexion (and therefore the risk of re-dislocation) while the patient is recovering from sedation. The splint can be removed once the patient is fully awake. A repeat assessment of the neurovascular status should be performed. Obtain repeat radiographs to ensure the reduction has been successful. After dislocation of a prosthetic hip, ensure the components remain well seated.

A CT scan is required after the reduction of a native hip dislocation to assess the femoral head and acetabulum, and to exclude intra-articular loose bodies.

### Inpatient referral

- Dislocated THR patients who are sedated or require physiotherapy assistance.
- Native hip dislocations – should be referred to the orthopaedic service.

### Outpatient follow-up

- Patients with a relocated prosthetic hip can be discharged from the Emergency Department if fully recovered from sedation and able to mobilize. They can be referred to an arthroplasty clinic.

## Orthopaedic management

### Open reduction of a dislocated native hip joint

Indications for open reduction are inability to achieve a congruent reduction by closed manipulation, concurrent fractures of the femoral head, neck or posterior acetabular wall, or retained loose bodies in the hip joint. A posterior (Kocher–Langenbeck) approach allows fixation of a posterior wall acetabular fracture, and the convenient exposure of the dislocated head and the sciatic nerve (p. 347). Femoral neck or shaft fractures can make reduction difficult and it may be easiest to fix these first prior to reducing the femoral head.

## Outpatient management

### Native hip joint dislocation

Mobilization depends on the assessment of stability at the time of reduction and any surgery performed. Where fixation of a posterior wall fracture has been required, protected weight-bearing may be instituted for 6 weeks. Otherwise, patients are allowed full weight-bearing but are restricted to active flexion to 90° in neutral rotation for 6 weeks to allow the posterior capsule to heal.

### Prosthetic hip dislocation

Patients should be schooled in the necessity of avoiding 'at risk' positions, particularly hip flexion and internal rotation, as well as high-risk manoeuvres, including pulling on shoes and socks, and rising from low seats. Those patients with recurrent instability should be considered for revision surgery.

## COMPLICATIONS

### Early

Local    Sciatic nerve palsy: This accompanies 10% of native hip dislocations and is managed expectantly unless it arises only after reduction or surgery in which case nerve entrapment is a possibility. Around one-third recover completely, one-third recover partially and one-third are permanent

### Late

Local    Avascular necrosis of the femoral head: This occurs in up to 10% of cases and arises from spasm and traction of the plexus of vessels around the hip. Reduction within 6 hours of injury reduces the incidence. AVN results in radiographic sclerosis, collapse and the development of osteoarthritis

Osteoarthritis: This occurs in around 25% of patients within 8 years

## FEMORAL HEAD (PIPKIN) FRACTURES

Fractures of the femoral head are generally, but not inevitably, associated with hip dislocation.

## Classification

### Pipkin classification

The Pipkin classification relates to the position of the fracture line and the presence of associated injuries (**Fig. 17.38**):

- Type 1: infrafoveal fracture.
- Type 2: suprafoveal fracture: within the weight-bearing portion of the head.
- Type 3: associated femoral neck fracture.
- Type 4: associated acetabular fracture.

## Orthopaedic management

Small or comminuted fragments should be excised; large fragments, particularly from the suprafoveal region, should generally be reduced and fixed. The surgical approach may be dictated by the requirement to fix an associated acetabular or femoral neck fracture. Otherwise, as the fragment is typically placed superoanteriorly, either a Smith-Peterson approach, a trochanteric osteotomy or a Ganz surgical dislocation are appropriate options. Fragments may be fixed with 2-mm titanium screws. This provides good compression between the low-profile screw head and the subchondral bone,

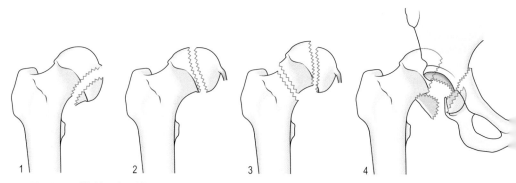

Fig. 17.38 Pipkin classification of femoral head fractures.

and will minimize interference with subsequent MRI images if there is a suspicion of AVN. Alternatively, headless screws may be suitable if the fragment has a sufficient depth of subchondral bone.

## PERIPROSTHETIC FRACTURES AROUND THE HIP

Implant-related fractures (termed periprosthetic when the device is a prosthetic joint rather than a trauma implant) are becoming increasingly common as the population ages and the prevalence of prosthetic joints and other implants increases. The management of these injuries is challenging: the patient population is usually elderly and frail, the fractures are often complex and multifragmentary, and the bone quality is often poor. The aim, as for hip fractures, is to perform a single operation that will allow the patient to be fully weight-bearing and rehabilitate without delay.

## Classification

### Vancouver classification

The Vancouver classification describes the position of the periprosthetic fracture and the stability of the femoral stem in the canal (**Fig. 17.39**):

- Vancouver A: Fractures of the trochanters that do not affect implant stability:
    - $A_G$: These occur at the greater trochanter.
    - $A_L$: These occur at the lesser trochanter.
- Vancouver B: Fractures around the femoral stem that may affect implant stability:
    - $B_1$: The implant remains stable, being well fixed to the bone of the proximal segment.
    - $B_2$: The implant is unstable.
    - $B_3$: The implant is unstable and the remaining bone stock is deficient.
- Vancouver C: Fractures below the level of the prosthesis, which remains stable and unaffected by the fracture.

## Emergency Department management

Patients should be assessed for comorbid conditions and treated carefully to optimize their preoperative medical condition.

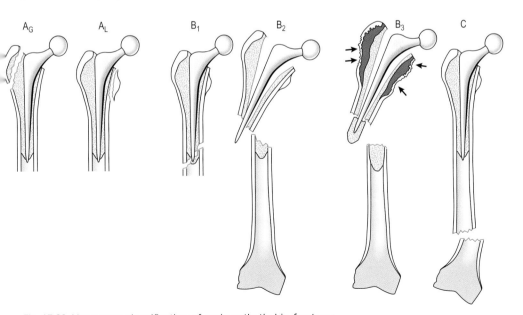

Fig. 17.39 Vancouver classification of periprosthetic hip fractures.

## Clinical features

The clinical presentation is the same as for a hip fracture (see Fig. 17.8). There is a history of previous THR surgery. A history of prodromal hip pain is suggestive of prior stem loosening.

## Radiological features

- *AP and lateral hip radiographs.*
- *AP and lateral femur radiographs.*

## Immobilization and reassessment

Most periprosthetic fractures are relatively stable while the patient is supine and do not require immobilization. However, an unstable and displaced fracture may require realignment after procedural sedation and analgesia, or a nerve block (p. 34). Realign the limb using gentle manual traction from the end of the table. Skin traction will maintain limb realignment and distal vascular supply (Fig. 18.6). After applying traction, reassess the *neurovascular supply* to the limb and obtain *repeat radiographs*.

## Inpatient referral

Refer all periprosthetic fractures to the orthopaedic service.

# Orthopaedic management

The Vancouver classification is helpful in directing treatment (**Table 17.1**).

**Table 17.1   Orthopaedic management of periprosthetic fractures around the hip**

| Vancouver type | Stability/bone quality | Management |
|---|---|---|
| A | Stable implant | Conservative management |
| B$_1$ | Stable implant | The implant remains well fixed to the proximal segment. The fracture is usually treated with open reduction and internal fixation. Be cautious about transverse fractures at the tip of the stem, which heal less reliably than fractures around the stem. Revision arthroplasty should be considered. |
| B$_2$ | Loose implant, normal bone | Where the implant is uncemented, or where there is cement fragmentation or loosening, a revision arthroplasty is inevitably required. This often comprises a long-stemmed revision implant or an endoprosthesis with an interference fit in the intact distal canal. However, where the implant is cemented, and is of a polished, tapered design, reconstruction can be successful even if the implant itself is loose. In this scenario, the cement mantle is often fractured approximately in line with the fractured bone, but the bone–cement interface of each main fragment remains intact. The fractured bone fragments and their attached cement can usually be reconstructed. The implant is then reinserted, with or without a fresh skim of cement, and is stable within its Morse taper |

**Table 17.1   Orthopaedic management of periprosthetic fractures around the hip—cont'd**

| Vancouver type | Stability/bone quality | Management |
|---|---|---|
| B$_3$ | Loose implant, deficient bone | There is typically an area of endosteolysis at the tip of the implant. These are challenging injuries and may require a long-stemmed revision implant, with reconstruction of the fracture and augmentation of the bone stock with structural bone graft. Alternatively, a proximal femoral endoprosthetic replacement with an interference fit in the intact distal canal can be used where the bone stock cannot be augmented |
| C | Femoral shaft fracture below a stable implant | An intramedullary nail cannot be used because of the presence of the femoral stem in the canal of the proximal femur. Two implants in close proximity are termed 'kissing implants' and result in a stress-riser in the intervening bone segment and a high risk of fracture; thus they are to be avoided. Plating techniques are therefore preferred, and the plate must extend proximally to overlap the stem of the femoral component |

### SURGICAL TECHNIQUE: Periprosthetic fracture fixation – Vancouver B (Fig. 17.40)

#### Patient set-up
Theatre set-up and positioning are as for hip arthroplasty (see Fig. 17.11). The equipment and expertise for both fracture fixation and prosthetic revision should be available.

#### Incision
The incision is placed laterally over the thigh and should extend from the greater trochanter to a point 20 cm distal to the tip of the fracture. The existing arthroplasty scar can often be incorporated; avoid 'tramline' incisions in close proximity to avoid the risk of intervening skin necrosis.

#### Approach: sub-vastus approach to the lateral femur
Internervous plane: This falls between vastus lateralis (femoral nerve) and biceps femoris (sciatic nerve).

The fracture is exposed through a sub-vastus approach by carefully lifting the vastus lateralis muscle forwards from the deep fascia of the thigh, the intermuscular septum and the femur. Perforating branches of the profunda femoris artery penetrate the septum in close proximity to the bone and should be identified and ligated.

#### Open reduction
The fracture is exposed and cleared of soft tissue and small fragments of bone or cement. A cemented implant may have become impacted in the fracture and is disengaged proximally by leg traction or tapping the tip of the implant if necessary. The cement mantle

*Continued*

and bone stock should be assessed carefully. If either is found to be deficient, a revision arthroplasty is likely to be more appropriate than fixation. If fixation is undertaken, the fracture fragments must be reduced anatomically. If this cannot be achieved, the problem is usually bone or cement fragments, or soft tissue interposition. These must be removed and the reduction perfected. Particular attention is paid to the medial cortex and the calcar of the femur. This acts as the main load-bearing structure during mobilization, and a defect here greatly increases the likelihood of construct failure. Large bone clamps are often used to aid reduction.

### Internal fixation – absolute stability

The fracture is usually oblique or spiral, and often multifragmentary. Several strips of fractured cortex together resemble the staves of a barrel and thus this configuration is often termed 'barrel-staved'. Initial fixation is usually with cerclage wires (Fig. 17.40). Simple 1.8-mm flexible wire is adequate, although braided cables may be preferred. The construct is then completed with the application of a lateral plate. A standard 4.5-mm broad AO plate with offset holes is ideal, although several more complex alternatives are available, including locking plates and systems that incorporate devices for gripping cerclage wires. Screw grip in the cortex of the shaft distally is usually satisfactory, but more proximally the bone is weaker and screws placed through the cement mantle, both in front of and behind the prosthetic stem, achieve better purchase. Where there is a large canal-filling uncemented implant, it may be impossible to use screws proximally, and then cerclage cables are required. These have a tendency to loosen by slipping distally, and should therefore be linked to the plate via holes or notches. The stability of the stem should then be assessed. If there is doubt, recementing the same stem, or a stem one size smaller, should be considered.

### Postoperative restrictions

Movement: Standard THR precautions should be taken.

Weight-bearing: Full weight-bearing is encouraged whenever possible. In specific cases – for example, a deficient medial cortex – protected weight-bearing may be preferred until union.

## Outpatient management

| Outpatient management summary | | | |
|---|---|---|---|
| **Week** | **Examination** | **Radiographs** | **Additional notes** |
| 2 | Wound check <br> Assessment of hip and knee movement <br> Neurovascular status | AP and lateral femur to ensure no early loss of reduction | Continue with physiotherapy |
| 6 | Assessment of hip and knee movement | AP and lateral femur to check early healing | Review weight-bearing status if necessary |
| 12 | | AP and lateral femur | If there is clinical and radiographic union, then discharge to routine arthroplasty follow-up |

Further assessments at 8-week intervals if required for delayed union

Average time to union=40 weeks

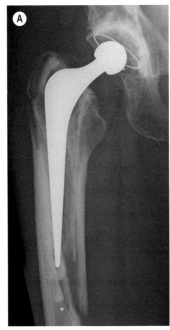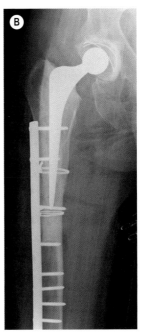

Fig. 17.40 Vancouver B2 periprosthetic fracture. **A**, Fracture around the stem. **B**, The bone–cement interface is intact and the fracture has been fixed with cerclage wires, plate and screws (see Table 17.1).

## ATYPICAL HIP FRACTURES

A small proportion of subtrochanteric fractures (around 5%) are classified as 'atypical' (**Fig. 17.41**) and share a number of characteristic features. These are:

- a history of long-term bisphosphonate therapy in 80% of cases
- a history of prodromal thigh pain (30%)
- an expanded, thickened cortex in the subtrochanteric region producing 'beaking' at the fracture
- a low-energy fracture
- transverse or short oblique orientation
- linear, non-comminuted morphology
- fracture healing that is typically delayed or incomplete.

The condition usually presents after a completed subtrochanteric fracture, but can present subacutely with prodromal hip or thigh pain, which may be unilateral or bilateral, with characteristic radiographic cortical thickening. An association with bisphosphonate treatment is thought to arise from impaired healing of microfractures from reduced osteoclast activity. However, amongst patients who are prescribed bisphosphonates, the risk of sustaining an atypical femoral fracture is considered to be very small compared with the likely benefits of drug therapy in terms of an overall reduced fracture risk.

## Orthopaedic management

- A complete fracture is stabilized with a cephalomedullary nail.
- An incomplete fracture, or an area of painful radiographic abnormality, is usually also nailed prophylactically.

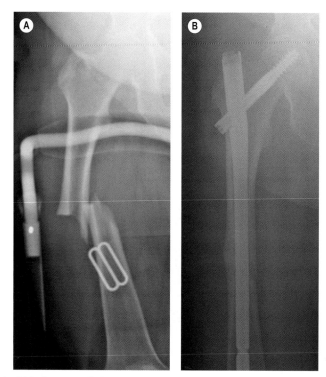

Fig. 17.41 Atypical hip fracture. **A**, Fracture in the subtrochanteric region with thickening of the lateral cortex. **B**, Fixation with a cephalomedulllary nail.

- Rheumatological advice is obtained, usually comprising:

  stopping the bisphosphonate

  continuing with calcium and vitamin D supplementation

  consideration of treatment with recombinant parathyroid hormone (teriparatide) to stimulate bone healing.

- Patients require an extended period of follow-up surveillance to ensure the fracture goes on to heal, and to monitor the contra-lateral femur.

## GENERAL PRINCIPLES

### Anatomy

The femur has three distinct regions: the hip, the shaft and the distal metaphysis. Proximally, the femoral head articulates with the acetabulum to form the hip joint, while distally, the femur broadens out to form the medial and lateral condyles, which articulate with the tibial plateau at the knee joint.

In the coronal plane, a line drawn between the centre of the femoral head and the centre of the knee joint forms the mechanical axis. A line drawn through the centre of the shaft is termed the anatomical axis of the bone; this lies lateral to the mechanical axis (**Fig. 18.1**). The angle between the anatomical axis and the mechanical axis at the knee is around 7°, and this relationship is important when considering the reduction of supracondylar fractures (see Fig.

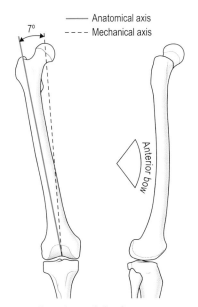

Fig. 18.1   Osteology of the femur.

18.36). In the sagittal plane, the shaft of the femur has a marked anterior bow, with a cortical thickening posteriorly called the linea aspera. This thickening carries insertions for several important muscles: gluteus maximus, vastus lateralis and medialis, the adductors (magnus, medius and minimus) and pectineus. Distally, the gastrocnemii arise from the posterior aspect of both femoral condyles before crossing the knee joint; in supracondylar fractures, this arrangement produces the characteristic extension of the distal fragment (see Fig. 18.30).

There are three large muscle compartments in the thigh (**Fig. 18.2**, **Box 18.1**).

The femoral artery divides in the anterior triangle of the thigh into the superficial femoral artery (SFA) and the profunda femoris (**Fig. 18.3**). The SFA courses through the medial compartment, passing through Hunter's canal and the adductor hiatus to enter the popliteal fossa. Here it becomes the popliteal artery and supplies the leg. The profunda femoris artery gives rise to perforating branches, which wrap around the femur posteriorly and supply the thigh musculature. These pierce the intermuscular septum at the linea aspera to enter the lateral compartment, where they can be torn by femoral fractures, or injured during lateral exposure of the femur. Nutrient vessels arise from these perforators and run along the posterior aspect of femur in the region of the linea aspera, arborizing to provide the endosteal and periosteal blood supply.

### Clinical assessment of the injured thigh (femur)

#### High-energy fractures

These fractures may be accompanied by other life-threatening injuries, which must be excluded by an initial *primary and secondary survey* (see Ch. 2). The femoral fracture itself can be associated with blood loss of over a litre in a

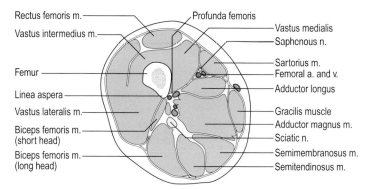

Fig. 18.2    Cross-sectional anatomy of the thigh. a, artery; m, muscle; n, nerve; v, vein.

---

### Box 18.1   Thigh muscle compartments

| | |
|---|---|
| **Anterior** | Quadriceps femoris |
| | Vastus lateralis |
| | Vastus medialis |
| | Vastus intermedius |
| | Rectus femoris |
| | Iliopsoas |
| | Sartorius |
| | Pectineus |
| **Medial** | Adductors |
| | Adductor magnus |
| | Adductor longus |
| | Adductor brevis |
| | Gracilis |
| | Obturator externus |
| **Posterior** | Hamstring muscles |
| | Biceps femoris |
| | Semitendinosus |
| | Semimembranosus |

closed fracture, and considerably more in an open fracture. This must be addressed as part of 'C – circulation and haemorrhage control' with realignment and traction.

### Low-energy osteoporotic fractures

These injuries have a very similar demographic to hip fractures, and the patient should initially be assessed and investigated in the same way

(p. 35). The fracture should then be immobilized with skin traction, as described below.

### Examination

*Look*

Assess for shortening and deformity of the limb, swelling of the thigh, open wounds and skin compromise. Inspect carefully for other injuries, particularly to the ipsilateral knee, hip and acetabulum (see Fig. 17.33).

*Feel*

Palpate for prominence of the bone ends. As you realign the limb and apply traction, you may feel crepitus.

*Move*

It will be apparent as you realign the limb that the femur does not move as one segment.

*Neurovascular assessment*

Assess sensation in the femoral and sciatic nerve distributions, and palpate for both the dorsalis pedis and posterior tibial pulses. Mark these with an indelible ink cross to allow later reassessment.

## Radiological assessment of the injured thigh (femur)

### Radiographs

- *AP and lateral views of the femur*: These should include the hip and knee joints. Repeat these after the application of traction or splintage (**Fig. 18.4**).

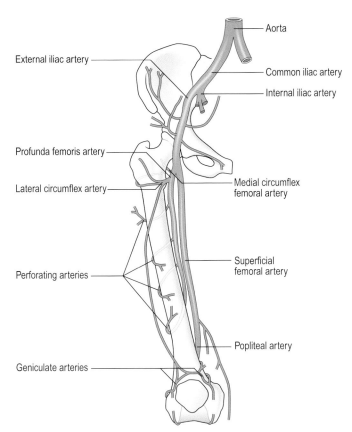

External iliac artery

Aorta

Common iliac artery

Internal iliac artery

Profunda femoris artery

Lateral circumflex artery

Medial circumflex femoral artery

Perforating arteries

Superficial femoral artery

Popliteal artery

Geniculate arteries

Fig. 18.3   Femoral blood supply.

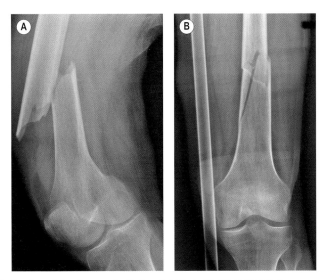

Fig. 18.4   Radiographs of the femur. **A**, Before traction. **B**, After traction.

## FEMORAL SHAFT FRACTURES

There is a bimodal distribution of injury: young, usually male, patients suffering high-energy trauma; and elderly, often female and osteoporotic patients, suffering low-energy falls. Within this latter demographic group, there is an increasing incidence of periprosthetic fractures related to hip and knee replacements, or previous fracture surgery.

## Classification
### AO classification
The femoral shaft is defined as the AO 32 region between the proximal segment (hip, AO 31) and the distal segment (condylar, AO 33) (see Fig. 1.21). Fractures of the shaft are often described in relation to proximal, middle and distal thirds. The proximal third is sometimes referred to as the subtrochanteric region (see Fig. 17.5). Shaft fractures of all long bones are classified similarly according to their pattern and degree of comminution (see Fig. 1.22).

## Emergency Department management
### Clinical features
- A careful history of the mechanism of injury is required. Where there is a history of high-energy trauma, an initial primary and secondary survey is mandatory to detect and treat other, potentially more urgent, injuries (see Ch. 2).
- Consider the other skeletal injuries that might have arisen, given the mechanism of injury (see Figs 17.33, 22.26) and exclude these.
- In the elderly, a thorough medical assessment is crucial in order to ascertain the cause of the fall and to identify potentially remediable medical problems (p. 35).
- There may be clear deformity, which should be reduced on recognition. Carefully assess the integrity of the skin, looking for lacerations and abrasions that would indicate an open fracture.

- Avoid unnecessary movement except to realign a deformed limb.
- Consider whether there is an acute vascular injury (p. 58). Palpate the dorsalis pedis and posterior tibial pulsations, and mark their locations with ink to allow later reassessment. Assess capillary refill to the toes.
- Examine the distal neurological status of the limb.

### Radiological features
- *AP and lateral views of the femur*: Ensure that both the hip and knee joints are included in the film or with additional views. Assess the femoral neck carefully: an occult hip fracture occurs in up to 5% of femoral shaft fractures. If there is uncertainty, a CT scan of the femoral neck should be obtained.

### Closed reduction and immobilization
Reduce the femur under procedural sedation and analgesia, or a femoral nerve block (see Fig. 2.12). Realign the limb using gentle manual traction from the end of the table. For pre-hospital retrieval, an emergency traction splint with a simple Velcro ankle strap and ratchet allows for the rapid application of traction (**Fig. 18.5**). However, initial definitive skin or skeletal traction is preferable in the resuscitation room, as it avoids skin complications and the requirement to change splints later. Skeletal stability is required for haemodynamic stability, and repeated movement of the bone ends can:

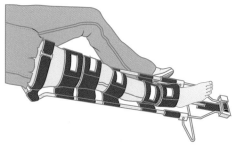

Fig. 18.5   Emergency traction splint.

- prevent clot formation or dislodge a clot, exacerbating haemorrhage
- cause the patient pain, exacerbating the physiological stress response
- release medullary fat, exacerbating fat embolism to the lungs
- compromise the skin, resulting in an open fracture.

Limb realignment will improve the *distal vascular supply* as kinks in the shortened femoral artery are straightened out.

### Reassessment
After applying traction, reassess the neurovascular supply to the limb and obtain repeat radiographs (see Fig. 18.4).

### Inpatient referral
Femoral shaft fractures require admission for surgical management.

## Orthopaedic management

### Non-operative
The management of femoral shaft fractures is almost invariably operative, with the use of an intramedullary nail in most instances. Where a delay of more than a few hours is expected, those traction devices that incorporate a simple webbing strap around the ankle must be converted to skin or skeletal traction to avoid local skin necrosis.

### Traction
Traction is used to alleviate pain, reduce bleeding and prevent further complications. By counteracting the strong pull of the quadriceps and hamstrings with a longitudinal force, the fractured ends of the femur are brought into alignment. Anatomical reduction of the bone ends is not usually achievable. The two main considerations are:

1. *How the limb is held*:
   a. *Skin traction*: This can be applied in the Emergency Department or on the ward, using simple equipment and without requiring anaesthesia.
   b. *Skeletal traction*: This method is employed if the traction is to be maintained for more than a few days or if the skin is compromised.

2. *How the longitudinal force is achieved*:
   a. *Splints*: Self-contained traction devices, such as the Thomas splint, are designed to exert counter-pressure against the ischium or groin. When used in this manner in the pre-hospital or emergency setting, they do not require weights.
   b. *Fixed traction*: This involves a simple pulley system with weight to pull the leg in a single direction. It can be applied to a Thomas splint to alleviate groin pressure.
   c. *Balanced traction*: This realigns the femoral fracture by the resultant vector of more than one traction force.

### Skin traction (Fig. 18.6)
1. Begin by providing adequate analgesia, and shaving the skin if required.

2. Position the spreader bar 10 cm from the heel, with the traction cords orientated towards the end of the bed.

3. Apply the tapes to the medial and lateral aspects of the lower limb, extending as far proximally as possible to minimize shear stresses on the skin. Some tapes are supplied with an adhesive backing; gradually peel off the protective backing and apply the adhesive face of the tape to each side of the limb in turn.

4. Secure with a crepe bandage.

Weights may be attached directly to the skin traction cords but usually additional support is provided by applying a Thomas splint (see Fig. 18.9).

### Skeletal traction (Fig. 18.7)
This is most commonly applied through a pin placed transversely in the proximal

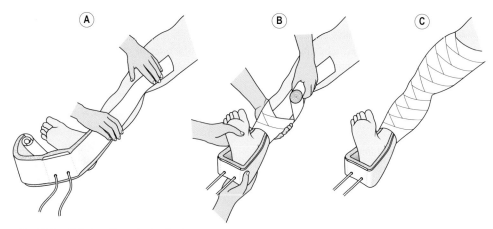

Fig. 18.6    Skin traction. **A,** Apply the tapes to the medial and lateral aspects of the limb. **B,** Secure with a crepe bandage. **C,** Completed skin traction.

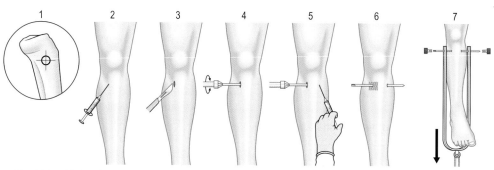

Fig. 18.7    Skeletal traction.

tibia, although the distal femur and the calcaneus are alternative sites. A Schanz pin is smooth, whereas a Denholm pin has threads on its middle section that achieve a more stable grip on the bone. This minor surgical procedure is performed under aseptic conditions following skin preparation and local draping.

1. Palpate the proximal tibia and find a point 2 cm posterior to the tibial tuberosity.

2. If the patient is not already under general anaesthesia, local anaesthetic is infiltrated at the lateral aspect of the proximal tibia, from the skin down to periosteum.

3. A small stab incision is made.

4. The pin is driven on a chuck handle through the lateral cortex and medullary canal of the bone with gentle rotational movements until it encounters the medial cortex.

5. The anticipated line of the pin is now assessed and further anaesthetic is infiltrated medially.

6. The pin is then advanced through the medial cortex. Be careful not to place your hand near the expected exit point of the pin when applying counter-pressure; the pin is extremely sharp and may move suddenly as it leaves the bone to penetrate your hand. Make a small stab incision over the tenting skin to allow the pin to come through, and apply a local dressing.

7. A stirrup or Tulloch Brown loop is used to apply traction to the pin, the sharp ends of which are protected with caps.

## Thomas splint

The Thomas splint is the most commonly used device for applying longitudinal traction in the

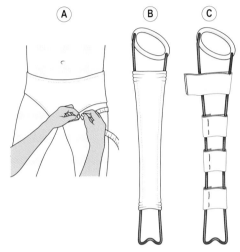

Fig. 18.8    Thomas splint: preparation.

case of a femoral fracture. It came to prominence during the First World War in the Battle of Arras, where its use was associated with a reduction in deaths related to open femoral fracture from 80% to 15%.

Older devices may have fixed rings; in this situation, select a size by measuring the circumference of the uninjured thigh and adding 5 cm to allow for swelling (**Fig. 18.8A**). The Thomas splint is first furnished with a sling to support the limb. Tube stockingette is most convenient (**Fig. 18.8B**) but multiple separate bandage slings secured to the bars with safety pins may be preferred (**Fig. 18.8C**).

Longitudinal traction is applied, and the splint is pushed up the leg until the ring reaches the ischial tuberosity (**Fig. 18.9A**). The cords are tied to the end of the splint. Conventionally, the medial cord (shown in grey) runs under the bar whilst the lateral cord (orange) runs over the bar to help control the tendency to lateral rotation of the limb (**Fig. 18.9B**). A windlass (of tongue spatulas or a metal rod) may be used to increase the amount of traction. The end of the Thomas splint is elevated on a pillow

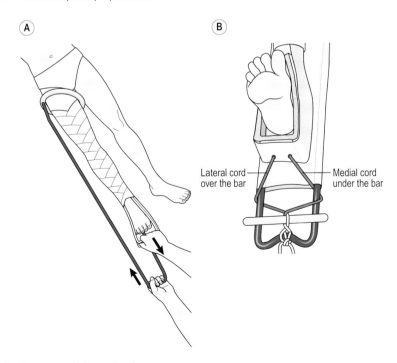

Lateral cord over the bar                Medial cord under the bar

Fig. 18.9    Thomas splint: application.

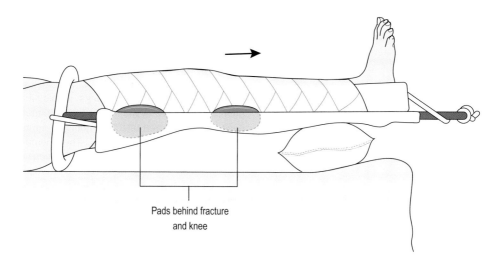

Pads behind fracture
and knee

Fig. 18.10   Thomas splint: padding.

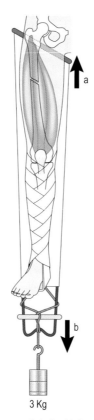

3 Kg

Fig. 18.11   Fixed traction with a Thomas splint. Ischial and perineal pressure (a) is alleviated by applying a traction weight (b).

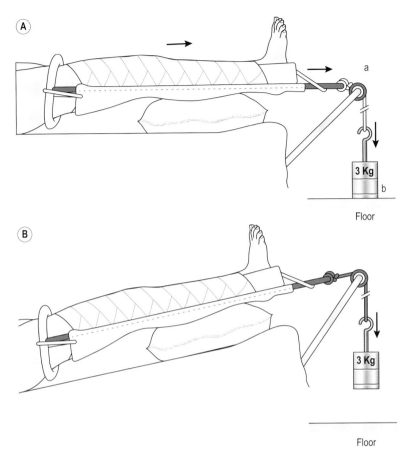

Fig. 18.12 Fixed traction. **A**, The traction weight tends to pull the patient towards the end of the bed; when the weight reaches the floor, traction is lost. **B**, Counteract this tendency by elevating the foot of the bed.

to reduce heel pressure. Pads are placed behind the fracture to act as a fulcrum to prevent posterior sag, and behind the knee to allow slight flexion (**Fig. 18.10**). The limb may be bandaged to the splint for further support.

### Fixed traction

The Thomas splint will maintain traction by counter-pressure of the ring against the ischial tuberosity, which may be useful if the patient is being transported (**a** on **Fig. 18.11**). However, perineal pressure sores will rapidly develop and must be avoided by applying 3 kg of traction weight to the end of the splint (**b**).

This may have the effect of gradually pulling the patient to the foot of the bed, at which point either the splint will rest on the pulley (**a** on **Fig. 18.12A**) or the weights will rest on the floor (**b**) and the traction effect will cease. Prevent this by raising the foot of the bed slightly (**Fig. 18.12B**). The traction apparatus should be inspected daily to ensure that the traction force is maintained and to check the skin, especially in the perineum, behind the upper thigh where

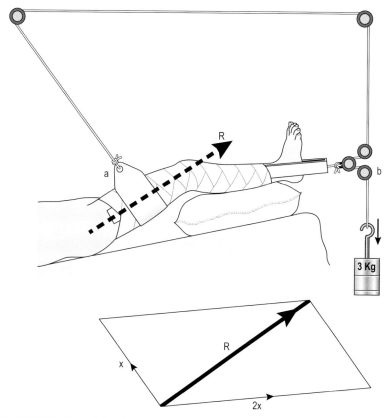

Fig. 18.13    Hamilton Russell traction.

it rests on the ring, around the traction tapes, at the bony prominences (particularly the fibular neck) and at the heel.

### *Balanced traction*

Balanced traction was originally developed to be used for definitive femoral fracture treatment and may still be preferred for temporary traction. The proximal segment of the femur has a tendency to flex at the hip as a result of the action of iliopsoas, and balanced traction aims to bring the distal fragment into alignment with it. In classic Hamilton Russell traction, a canvas sling (*a* on **Fig. 18.13**) is placed around the thigh, lifting it anteriorly (upwards).

Longitudinal traction is then applied to the leg and the force of this is effectively doubled by an arrangement of pulleys attached to the skin traction tape and the bed frame (**b**). The resultant vector (**R**) of these two traction forces is in the line of the femur.

### **Operative**

The majority of femoral fractures undergo operative fixation. Most shaft fractures are nailed, either antegrade or retrograde. Occasionally, plating may be preferred. The combination of a femoral shaft and neck fracture requires special consideration and is described separately below.

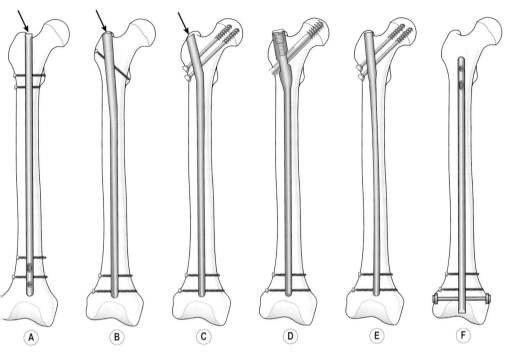

Fig. 18.14   Femoral nails. See text for details.

## Surgical techniques

### Intramedullary nailing

This is the preferred treatment for almost all femoral shaft fractures. It allows a closed reduction and percutaneous stabilization of the fracture with minimal morbidity, and the rapid mobilization of the patient avoiding the complications of recumbency (p. 39).

A wide variety of nails are available and each has its own idiosyncrasies. When viewed in an AP projection, the entry point may be at the piriformis fossa for a straight nail (**Fig. 18.14A**), at the tip of the greater trochanter (**Fig. 18.14B**), or lateral to the tip of the trochanter (**Fig. 18.14C**). Viewed in a lateral projection, most femoral nails have an anterior bow that corresponds to the curve of the femur (see Fig. 18.1), although the radius of this curvature differs from nail to nail; some are straighter than others. A cephalomedullary nail is one in which there is fixation in both the femoral head (Greek: *cephalus*, 'head') and the shaft; it is used where the fracture is very proximal, or in the elderly when there is a high risk of a subsequent hip fracture. It is also one of the options where a femoral shaft fracture and a hip fracture occur together (see below). Fixation in the head may comprise a single large lag screw (**Fig. 18.14D**), a helical blade or, in the case of a reconstruction (or 'recon') nail (**Fig. 18.14E**), two smaller screws. Although most femoral nails are implanted from the hip (anterograde), in certain circumstances insertion from the knee (retrograde) offers advantages (**Fig. 18.14F**). The surgeon must be thoroughly familiar with the device that has been chosen and the surgical steps required for its use before embarking on surgery.

## SURGICAL TECHNIQUE: Antegrade femoral nailing

### Surgical set-up (see Fig. 17.25)

Patient positioning is most commonly supine on the traction table, in a 'banana' position to allow ease of access to the start point. Alternatively, a lateral position may be preferred: this offers easier access to the start point but requires a horizontal perineal post, and it may not be prudent to turn severely injured patients on to their side. In either position, traction can be applied either via a boot or with skeletal traction via a Steinmann pin placed in the distal femur or proximal tibia.

### Closed reduction

Traction restores length and alignment, while turning the foot plate provides rotational correction.

Fluoroscopic images: Ensure clear identification of the entry point on optimized AP and true lateral image intensifier images (see Fig. 17.26). Assess the femoral neck carefully: an occult hip fracture occurs in up to 5% of femoral shaft fractures and will require a change of surgical plan (see Fig. 18.29). Assess fracture reduction – it should be possible to confirm that the femur is out to length by inspecting the fracture fragments on the image intensifier. Very occasionally, extensive comminution makes this impossible, and then the contralateral femur should be screened and measured as a template. When setting up the traction, rotation is initially addressed by ensuring the intercondylar axis of the knee (a line between the medial and lateral epicondyles) is horizontal, and the patella is pointing straight up. Fine corrections can then be made by inspecting the fluoroscopic images and assessing:

- Fracture fragment alignment (**Fig. 18.15A**): Inspect the position of any fracture spike and ensure it keys into the corresponding apex of the other fragment.
- Cortical appearance (**Fig. 18.15B**): The femur is not perfectly circular but has a teardrop cross-sectional shape because of the linea aspera posteriorly. Malrotation in transverse fractures will be evident as a mismatch in both femoral diameter and cortical thickness.

### Incision

A 3-cm incision is placed 10 cm proximal to the tip of the greater trochanter in line with the axis of the femur (**Fig. 18.16A**). No further dissection is required.

### Starting point

Grasp the greater trochanter and aim to bisect the position between your finger and thumb with the guide wire as it passes percutaneously through fascia and muscle to bone (**Fig. 18.16B**). Now assess the position of the guide wire tip fluoroscopically (**Fig. 18.17**).

- AP image: For a straight (piriformis entry) nail, the start point is at the piriformis fossa. The site of insertion of the piriformis tendon is directly in line with the centre of the medullary canal on the AP view of the femur, and slightly behind the highest point of the neck, so that, when resting on the correct start point, the guide wire tip overlaps the upper border of the neck by a few millimetres.
- For a trochanteric entry point nail, the start point is at the tip of the greater trochanter. A common error is selecting a start point that is too lateral when implanting a trochanteric entry nail, resulting in varus malalignment and incorrect lag screw position (see Fig. 17.30).
- Lateral view: The entry point is again in line with the femoral canal. Selecting an entry point that is too anterior risks a 'blowout' fracture of the proximal femur as the nail is impacted into an offset hole in the femur.

**Procedure (Fig. 18.18)**

1. Threaded guide wire insertion: A threaded guide wire is driven into the proximal femur and the position checked with fluoroscopy. Alternatively, an awl can be used to make an entry hole before introducing the guide wire.
2. Cannulated drill insertion: A drill is then passed over the wire.
3. Realignment with a reduction device: A reduction device can be advanced into the proximal fragment and used to manœuvre it in order to realign the fracture, usually by pushing the handle towards the patient's side and pulling up. The tip can occasionally be advanced right across the fracture.
4. Ball-tipped guide wire insertion: The guide wire can then be passed across the fracture and into the distal fragment. The ball tip should lie behind the patella and this position should be checked in both AP and lateral projections.
5. Measurement: The length of nail required is measured from the ball-tipped wire. Ensure that the measuring device is seated on bone at the entry point with fluoroscopy.
6. Reaming: A series of reamers is used sequentially to enlarge the medullary canal (see Fig. 5.25).
7. Nail insertion: Ensure that the nail is correctly and securely mounted on the jig before insertion. Repeated blows with a hammer allow controlled nail progression down the femur. If significant resistance is encountered, image the nail carefully; it may have caught on a fracture edge. Once the nail has reached its final depth, reassess the fracture site carefully to ensure correct rotational alignment and fracture reduction, and to check that the fracture site has not been distracted. If there is a gap of more than a couple of millimetres, release the traction to allow the gap to close. Carefully inspect the AP view of the hip again to ensure that a femoral neck fracture has not been revealed.
8. Locking screw insertion: If a fracture gap remains after releasing traction, insert the distal locking screw(s) and 'back-slap' the nail to close the gap. The proximal locking screw is then inserted using a drill guide placed through the jig.

**Post procedure**

Before the patient is removed from the table after either antegrade or retrograde nailing, check:

- Vascular supply: Both dorsalis pedis and posterior tibial pulses should have been marked at admission, and should now be reassessed (**Fig. 18.19A**).
- Rotational alignment: Flex each hip and knee to 90° in turn and compare the range of internal and external rotation (**Fig. 18.19B**). If there is a discrepancy of more than 10°, consider repreparing and revising the reduction and distal cross-screws.
- Limb length: Ensure that the pelvis is square on the table and compare limb length at the medial malleoli.
- Knee ligament stability: See page 423.

**Postoperative restrictions**

Movement: Full active movement at hip and knee is allowed.

Weight-bearing: Stable fracture patterns (A and B types with transverse configuration) allow load-sharing between the nail and the bone, and full weight-bearing will commence immediately. Comminuted patterns result in a load-bearing nail and some surgeons will prefer touch weight-bearing until callus is visible at 6 weeks.

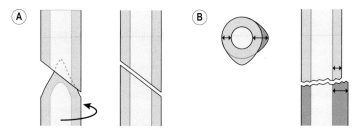

Fig. 18.15   Fluoroscopic fracture reduction.  This requires careful assessment of: **A**, fracture pattern and **B**, cortical width and thickness.

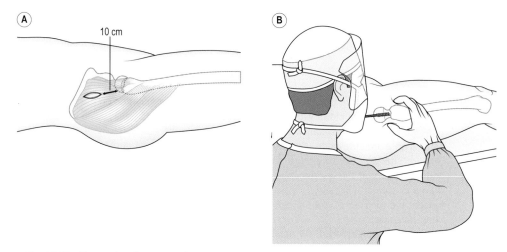

Fig. 18.16   Femoral nail: approach.

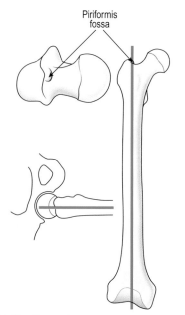

Fig. 18.17   Femoral nail: start point.

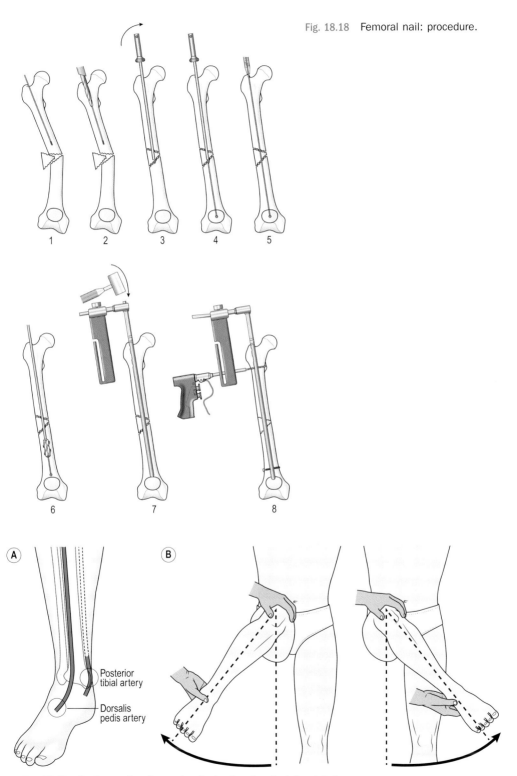

Fig. 18.18    Femoral nail: procedure.

Fig. 18.19    Postoperative femoral nail checks. See text for details.

---

### ✓ Technical tip

For distal freehand locking with 'perfect circles', the c-arm must be positioned such that the image shows the two holes in the sides of the nail as perfectly round and perfectly superimposed, to give the appearance of a single round hole. An elliptical hole indicates that the trajectory of the X-ray beam is oblique in relation to the nail. This can produce two types of ellipse, each of which requires correction of the X-ray beam in a certain plane.

- *Thin holes* (coronal plane; **Fig. 18.20A**): A vertical ellipse indicates that the c-arm is oblique to the nail. The c-arm must be repositioned so that the beam is perpendicular to the nail.
- *Flat holes* (axial plane; **Fig. 18.20B**): A flattened ellipse indicates that the c-arm is incorrectly rotated in the axial plane. Most commonly, the radiographer will have positioned the c-arm horizontally, whereas the nail will lie in slight external rotation.

The screw insertion technique is as follows:

1. *Stab incision*: Under fluoroscopic guidance, the scalpel is lined up with the centre of the perfect circle. A stab incision is made down to bone.

2. *Drilling*: The drill tip is positioned at the centre of the circle. The drill hand is then carefully raised so that the drill trajectory aligns with that of the X-ray beam and will therefore pass through the circles. If the tip of the drill slips at all, start again. The drill bit can be advanced smoothly through the outer cortex of the femur, through both holes in the nail, and on to the distal cortex. At this point, the depth should be measured against the guide; some tissue sleeves allow measurement from markings on the drill bit. Select a screw that is 5 mm longer than this measurement. Now drill through the far cortex, checking the depth markings on the drill bit against the guide to confirm screw length.

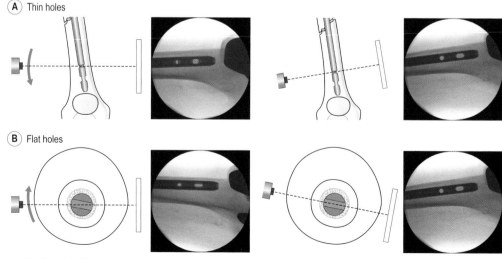

(A) Thin holes

(B) Flat holes

Fig. 18.20    Distal locking with 'perfect circles'.

3. *Screw insertion*: Wait until the screw is ready on the screwdriver. Without removing your gaze from the entry point, withdraw the drill, accept the screwdriver and smoothly insert the screw along the same trajectory. In good bone, one or two screws are usually sufficient, but in osteoporotic bone a locking bolt (see Fig. 18.14F) is more stable.

### Adjuncts to reduction

In addition to the reduction spoon (see Fig. 18.18), other reduction manœuvres include using an angled guide wire (**Fig. 18.21A**), applying external pressure with the aid of an assistant (**Fig. 18.21B**), pushing with a percutaneous wire (**Fig. 18.21C**) or, if necessary, opening the fracture and directly holding the fractured bone ends in apposition with clamps (**Fig. 18.21D**). In rare circumstances, such as when fluoroscopy is not available, the fracture can be opened and the nail inserted through the fracture, being passed through the proximal femur in a retrograde manner until it presents at the buttock, where it is delivered through a small incision (**Fig. 18.22A**). The fracture is then reduced and the nail driven back down across the fracture and into the distal segment (**Fig. 18.22B**).

### Retrograde nailing technique

The *indications* for retrograde femoral nailing include:

- *Ipsilateral femoral neck fracture* (see Fig. 18.29).
- *Ipsilateral acetabular fracture*: There may be concern over conflicting incisions, or difficulty in gaining access to the entry point (if the acetabular fracture is displaced) or in disrupting the acetabular fixation (if, unusually, this has been performed first).
- *Ipsilateral tibial fracture*: Both injuries can be addressed with intramedullary nails with one surgical set-up, through the same incision at the knee.
- *Ipsilateral patellar fracture*: Both injuries can be addressed through the same incision at the knee.
- *Bilateral femoral fractures*: Both fractures can be nailed in the same set-up, whereas antegrade nailing on traction requires two separate procedures.
- *Obesity*: This can often make anterograde nailing difficult.
- *Pregnancy*: Anterograde nailing requires more ionizing radiation close to the pelvis than does retrograde nailing.

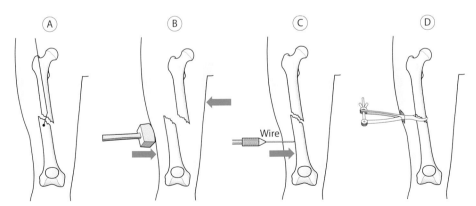

Fig. 18.21   Adjuncts to fracture reduction.

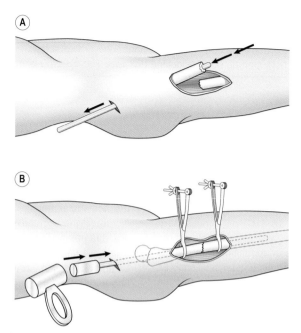

Fig. 18.22    Femoral nailing without live radiographs.

## SURGICAL TECHNIQUE: Retrograde intramedullary nailing

### Surgical set-up (Fig. 18.23)
The patient is placed supine on the operating table with the thigh resting on a sterile bolster and the knee flexed to 45°. The entire limb and hip are prepared to allow access to the groin for proximal locking.

### Closed reduction
Fluoroscopic images: The femoral neck should be imaged to ensure there is no concurrent fracture. The distal femur should also be screened carefully, as an intercondylar fracture extension may need to be addressed with lag screws before nailing. The fracture is then assessed.

Manual longitudinal traction is used to regain length, alignment and rotation, and must be maintained throughout the procedure.

- Varus or valgus alignment is adjusted by moving the foot laterally or medially (**Fig. 18.24A**).
- Flexion and extension are controlled by moving the bolster distally or proximally (**Fig. 18.24B**).

### Incision (Fig. 18.25)
A 15-mm incision is made through skin and joint capsule in line with the medial aspect of the patella tendon. This is effectively a medial parapatellar tendon arthrotomy.

## Start point

The entry point is directly in line with the medullary canal of the femur in both the AP and lateral projections. On the AP view (**Fig. 18.26A**), this is towards the medial side of the intercondylar notch. On the lateral image (**Fig. 18.26B**), the correct entry point lies just anterior to Blumensaat's line.

## Procedure

1.  Threaded guide wire insertion: A guide wire is introduced and placed on the entry point (**Fig. 18.26A,B**). This is then driven into the centre of the distal fragment (**Fig. 18.26C**).
2.  Cannulated drill preparation: A cannulated drill is then used to prepare the distal metaphysis (**Fig. 18.26D**).
3.  Ball-tipped guide wire insertion: The reamer and threaded guide wire are then removed and a long ball-tipped guide wire is passed across the fracture (**Fig. 18.26E**). Minor adjustments to reduction aid wire passage (**Fig. 18.26F**). The wire tip is passed into the proximal segment, proximal to the level of the lesser trochanter.
4.  Measurement: The guide wire depth is measured to provide nail length. Ensure that the measuring device is seated on bone at the entry point with fluoroscopy.
5.  Reaming: A series of reamers is used sequentially to enlarge the medullary canal (see Fig. 5.25).
6.  Nail insertion: Ensure that the nail is correctly and securely mounted on the jig before insertion. Repeated blows with a hammer allow controlled nail progression up the femur. If significant resistance is encountered, image the nail carefully; it may have caught on a fracture edge. Once the nail has reached its final depth, assess the fracture site again carefully to ensure correct rotational alignment and fracture reduction.
7.  Locking screw insertion: Unlike antegrade nailing, retrograde nail insertion does not usually cause fracture distraction. Distal locking is performed using the jig attached to the nail. In osteoporotic bone or in the face of extensive comminution, a bolt is preferred to screw(s) (**Fig. 18.26G**). Proximal locking is more challenging. An anterior-to-posterior screw is placed under fluoroscopic control, with careful blunt dissection to avoid the neurovascular structures in the anterior triangle of the thigh (**Fig. 18.26H**). A suture tied around the neck of the screw will assist in its retrieval if the screw becomes misplaced during insertion.

## Post procedure

Before the patient is removed from the table after either antegrade or retrograde nailing, check:

- Vascular supply: Both dorsalis pedis and posterior tibial pulses should have been marked at admission, and should now be reassessed (see Fig. 18.19A).
- Rotational alignment: Flex each hip and knee to 90° in turn and compare the range of internal and external rotation. If there is a discrepancy of more than 10° consider repreparing and revising the reduction and distal cross-screws (see Fig. 18.19B).
- Limb length – ensure the pelvis is square on the table and compare limb length at the medial malleolus.
- Knee ligament stability – see Chapter 19, p. 421.
- Postoperative restrictions are as for antegrade nailing, p. 397.

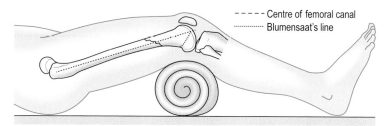

Fig. 18.23    Retrograde nail set-up.

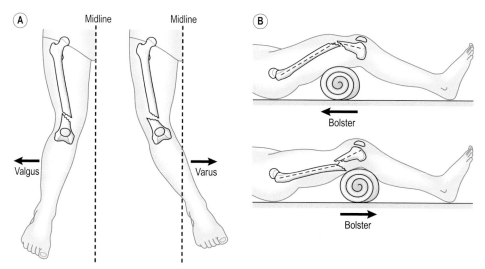

Fig. 18.24    Closed reduction for retrograde nailing. See technique box p. 402.

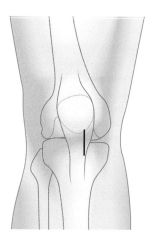

Fig. 18.25    Retrograde nail: incision.

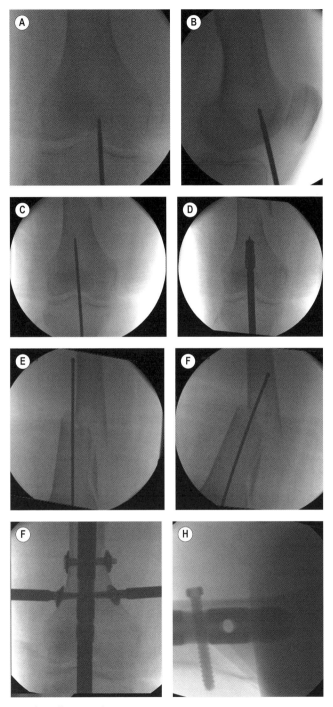

Fig. 18.26 Retrograde nail: procedure.

### External fixation (Fig. 18.27)

This is rarely appropriate for the definitive treatment of femoral fractures because of a high rate of pin site infection, loss of reduction, and muscular tethering that restricts knee movement. However, external fixation may be useful as temporary stabilization (so-called 'portable traction') in the context of gross contamination (such as military projectile or blast injuries) or as an alternative to traction where the patient is too physiologically unstable to undergo nailing (p. 28). The external fixation is then converted to a femoral nail as soon as practicable. If the fixator has been in place for more than a week, this may be done in stages to minimize the risk of infection. In the first procedure, the fixator pins are removed and the pin tracks are over-drilled, curetted and irrigated to remove colonizing organisms. The patient is then placed on traction for several days to allow the pin sites to heal over. Nailing is then performed as a second procedure.

### Plating (Fig. 18.28)

Femoral shaft fractures are rarely plated primarily, as a large incision and extensive soft tissue dissection are required, conferring an increased risk of infection. Additionally, plate fixation is biomechanically weaker than nailing with a higher risk of construct failure. However, it may be preferred in certain circumstances, such as in an open fracture where the exposure has already been performed by the injury. Anatomical reduction, absolutely rigid fixation and compression with lag screws should be carried out where possible.

### Treatment of combined femoral neck and shaft fractures

This combination of injuries occurs in approximately 5% of shaft fractures and merits separate consideration in view of the importance of the femoral head blood supply and viability. Three scenarios may pertain:

1. *The fracture is recognized preoperatively and is undisplaced.* A cephalomedullary nail can be used to fix both fractures with one implant. However, there is a risk of hip fracture displacement during nailing, and it is prudent to place heavy guide wires across the fracture (in front of and behind the intended path of the nail) to minimize this risk. The risk can be avoided altogether by first addressing the hip fracture with the implant best suited to that fracture (often a dynamic hip screw, DHS) and then addressing the shaft fracture with the implant best

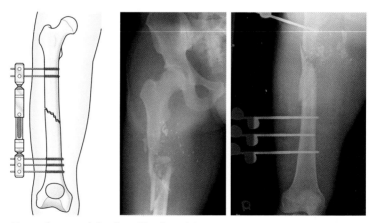

Fig. 18.27    Femoral external fixation. Simple uniplanar temporary external fixation of a military patient with a high-energy ballistic injury and soft tissue contamination.

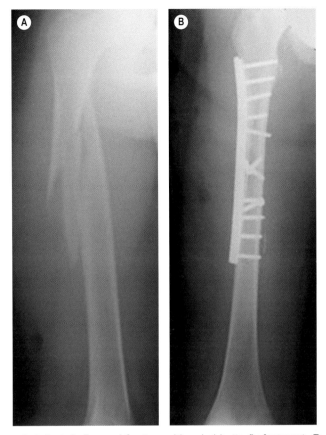

Fig. 18.28   Femoral plating. **A**, Femoral fracture with spiral butterfly fragment. **B**, Open anatomical reduction, lag-screw compression and neutralization femoral plating.

suited to that injury (a retrograde nail) (**Fig. 18.29**). Note that, in the case shown, the side-plate screws for the DHS have also been used to lock the nail proximally, linking the devices and increasing the strength of the construct. Alternatively, if plate fixation of the shaft is preferred, a long-plate DHS may address both injuries.

2. *The fracture is recognized after nailing and remains undisplaced.* Access to the hip fracture is impeded by the proximal end of the nail, but it is often possible to stabilize the hip with cannulated screws placed

immediately in front of and behind the femoral nail. Alternatively, the nail can be removed and replaced with one of the options above.

3. *The fracture is displaced.* Whether this is recognized preoperatively or postoperatively, there is a requirement to reduce and stabilize the fracture as soon as possible to protect the viability of the femoral head. An open reduction (via a Smith-Petersen approach (p. 345)) and DHS fixation (p. 365) is often preferred, with either a retrograde nail or a plate for the shaft fracture.

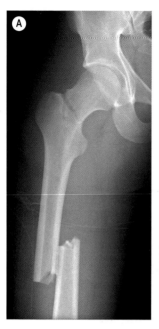 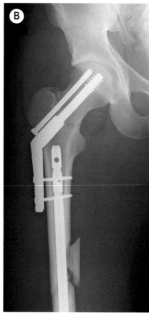

Fig. 18.29 Ipsilateral femoral neck and shaft fractures. **A**, Before treatment. **B**, Fracture has been treated with a dynamic hip screw and anti-rotation screw, the shaft fracture with a retrograde nail. Note that the implants overlap to prevent the creation of a stress riser.

## Outpatient management

### Femoral shaft fracture treated with intramedullary nail

| Outpatient management summary | | | |
|---|---|---|---|
| **Week** | **Examination** | **Radiographs** | **Additional notes** |
| 2 | Wound check<br><br>Hip and knee movement check<br><br>Neurovascular status | AP and lateral femur to ensure no early loss of reduction | Begin physiotherapy |
| 6 | Hip and knee movement check | AP and lateral femur to check early callus | If restrictions were applied, commence weight-bearing |
| 16 | Hip and knee movement check | AP and lateral femur | Ensure physiotherapy is continuing and that healing is progressing |
| 40 | | AP and lateral femur to assess union | If there is clinical and radiographic union, discharge |

Further assessments at 8-week intervals if required for delayed union

Average time to union = 40 weeks

# COMPLICATIONS

## Early

Local      Vascular injury: The femoral artery may be kinked and transiently obstructed following femoral fracture, particularly where there is shortening. Realignment and limb traction will often restore circulation but an arterial laceration or an intimal tear should be suspected if there is any subsequent circulatory abnormality (p. 59). The popliteal artery is at particular risk with injuries around the knee

Neurological injury: The sciatic nerve is at particular risk when femoral fractures are associated with a hip dislocation, and the common peroneal nerve is at particular risk with injuries around the knee

Associated injury: A femoral fracture is a distracting injury and a careful secondary survey in the Emergency Department, and then a tertiary survey on the ward, are required to exclude other injuries

Infection: This is extremely rare after closed femoral nailing (<1%) but is more common with open fractures and open surgery

General    Haemorrhage: This is addressed during resuscitation but the response to fluids, blood and blood products must be reassessed throughout the acute period (p. 25)

Fat embolism and acute respiratory distress syndrome (ARDS): While 30% of patients with a long bone fracture may suffer a period of perioperative hypoxaemia, the incidence of ARDS is <1%. The risk is greater in young patients with multiple injuries. Careful monitoring throughout the acute perioperative period is required (p. 28)

## Late

Local      Delayed-union or non-union: This is rare after closed nailing (<1%) but again is more common after open fractures and open surgery. Exchange nailing is successful in 80%, but exchange of the nail for a compression plate, with or without additional autogenous bone graft, may be required

Malunion: This is very uncommon following femoral nailing when meticulous attention is paid to the surgical procedure, as described above. However, external fixation or non-operative treatments are both associated with high rates of shortening and angulation

Knee joint stiffness: Significant stiffness is uncommon following surgical fixation where active mobilization has been instituted postoperatively. Where it does occur, intra-articular adhesions or tethering of the quadriceps muscle (which prevents it from sliding over the distal femoral shaft) is usually responsible. Where prolonged and vigorous physiotherapy is unsuccessful in gaining adequate knee flexion, a stepwise approach, including manipulation under anaesthetic (MUA), arthroscopic arthrolysis and open quadriceps release, with postoperative physiotherapy (and consideration of supervised

## COMPLICATIONS... cont'd

inpatient treatment using continuous passive motion equipment), is generally successful. Loss of extension may require passive splintage or even serial casting

General     Critical illness sequelae: Long-term systemic complications are very unusual after femoral fractures, unless the injury is accompanied by other severe injuries

## DISTAL FEMORAL (SUPRACONDYLAR) FRACTURES

Fractures of the distal femur are not as common as hip fractures but have a very similar bimodal distribution. There is a relatively small population of young adults suffering high-energy trauma, and a much larger population of older individuals with insufficiency fractures, an increasing proportion of whom have a fracture in relation to a knee replacement. These older individuals are as vulnerable as patients with hip fractures and should be managed according to the same principles of expeditious surgery, aiming for early full weight-bearing mobilization. The distal metaphyseal segment of these fractures usually rotates apex-posterior as a result of the action of gastrocnemius, and this often results in the proximal spike being pushed anteriorly, where it can erode through the quadriceps mechanism and skin if not reduced and fixed (**Fig. 18.30**). This makes non-operative treatment difficult, and most of these fractures are therefore treated operatively.

## Classification

### AO classification (Fig. 18.31)

The AO classification is most commonly used, describing extra-articular (type A), partial articular (type B) and complete articular (type C) patterns.

A-type fractures are 'metadiaphyseal' fractures that separate the metaphysis from the diaphysis. They are treated by securing these two elements together:

- A1: simple
- A2: metaphyseal wedge
- A3: complex metaphyseal fracture.

B-type fractures are partial articular fractures, involving a shear fracture of one or other of the condyles. They are treated with lag screws or antiglide plates:

- B1: lateral condyle
- B2: medial condyle
- B3: shear fracture of the posterior aspect of the femoral condyles, commonly termed a *Hoffa fracture*.

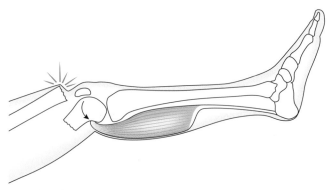

Fig. 18.30   Supracondylar fracture: displacement.

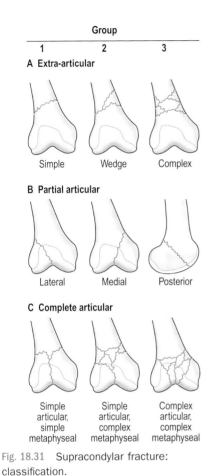

**Group**

| 1 | 2 | 3 |
|---|---|---|

**A Extra-articular**

Simple | Wedge | Complex

**B Partial articular**

Lateral | Medial | Posterior

**C Complete articular**

Simple articular, simple metaphyseal | Simple articular, complex metaphyseal | Complex articular, complex metaphyseal

Fig. 18.31 Supracondylar fracture: classification.

C-type fractures have both a metadiaphyseal separation and an intra-articular component. Both elements of the fracture must be addressed:

- C1: simple articular and simple metaphyseal
- C2: simple articular but complex metaphyseal
- C3: complex articular and complex metaphyseal (**Fig. 18.32**).

Subclassifications have also been added but are of little clinical relevance and have poor inter-observer reliability.

## Emergency Department management

### Clinical features

- High-energy fractures should be assessed and managed in the same way as described for femoral shaft fractures, with initial exclusion of life-threatening and other associated injuries, and concurrent resuscitation (see Ch. 2).
- Low-energy osteoporotic fractures have a similar demographic to hip fractures and the patient should initially be assessed and investigated in the same way (p. 35). The fracture should then be immobilized with a backslab, splint or skin traction.

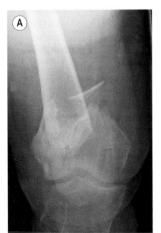
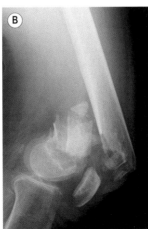

Fig. 18.32 Distal femoral fracture. This low supracondylar fracture is complex metaphyseal, with a simple intra-articular extension: AO 33C2.

## Radiological features

- *AP and lateral views of the knee.*
- *AP and lateral views of the femur:* Exclude a more proximal or femoral neck fracture.
- *CT:* If an intra-articular extension is suspected, a CT scan is often helpful.

## Closed reduction and immobilization

The limb should be realigned under procedural sedation and analgesia, if required. Where shortening and displacement are minimal, a knee extension splint may suffice. In more comminuted fractures, traction is more effective (p. 389).

## Inpatient referral

Supracondylar femoral fractures require admission for surgical management.

# Orthopaedic management

## Operative

Supracondylar fractures of the femur are almost always managed operatively. These fractures are often more complex than femoral shaft fractures as:

- angulatory deformities, particularly in the coronal plane, are less well tolerated the closer they are to the knee
- the cancellous bone of the distal metaphysis is weaker than the cortical bone of the shaft and fixation is more tenuous, particularly in the elderly

- fractures may extend distally into the knee joint
- an increasing proportion of these injuries occur in relation to a knee joint prosthesis.

These fractures can be fixed with a retrograde femoral nail, single or double plating or, in severely comminuted intra-articular fractures, joint replacement.

## Retrograde femoral nailing

Retrograde nailing (p. 402) has the advantages that the procedure can be performed percutaneously, and the intramedullary implant is mechanically stronger than a plate (Fig. 5.2). Where there is an intra-articular extension, it is often possible to lag the major components together (effectively converting a C-type fracture into an A-type fracture) and then stabilize the reconstructed metaphyseal segment to the diaphysis with a nail. Periprosthetic fractures are more challenging. A posterior cruciate ligament (PCL)-sparing knee joint prosthesis may have an adequate channel between the condylar elements to allow nailing, but it is important to check the shape and dimensions of the implant, as several types, particularly PCL-sacrificing designs, block access to the femoral shaft. Mechanical failure following retrograde nailing of distal femoral fractures often occurs as a result of the 'broomstick in a bucket' phenomenon (**Fig. 18.33**). The nail (broomstick) is held firmly in the proximal canal and remains well fixed, but the metaphysis (bucket)

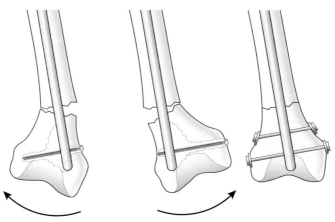

Fig. 18.33   'Broomstick in a bucket' phenomenon.

is trumpet-shaped, capacious and filled with weak cancellous bone. This metaphyseal block can progressively move, loosen and then fail around the nail. The likelihood of a 'broomstick in a bucket' failure can be reduced by using distal locking bolts instead of screws, and by using more than one bolt.

### Lateral plating

An angle-stable device (Fig. 18.38) is preferred where the distal fragment is small, or split by an intra-articular extension, or where access to the femoral canal is blocked by an implant. Options include a blade plate, a dynamic condylar screw (DCS) or a locked plate system. The first two devices are highly stable and published results are as good as, or superior to, those for locked plating. However, they require a larger exposure and surgical dissection, and are now infrequently used. Type A and C1 fractures have simple metadiaphyseal fracture lines, and these are best treated by (open) anatomical reduction and fixation with absolute stability and compression (Fig. 5.15). Type C2 and C3 fractures require a bridging technique and are often best fixed percutaneously.

### Combined medial and lateral plating

The addition of a medial plate adds considerable mechanical stability against medial collapse. Both plates can be applied together through an anterior approach, although percutaneous plating requires less dissection.

### Endoprosthetic replacement

Joint replacement (**Fig. 18.34**) is required when fixation is technically not feasible as a result of comminution or bone quality. It allows immediate weight-bearing mobilization.

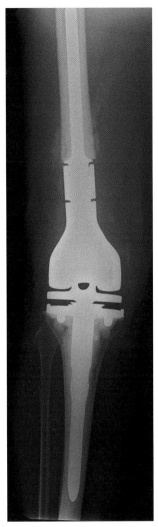

Fig. 18.34  Distal femoral replacement. This is the same fracture as is shown in Figure 18.32. The distal metaphyseal fragment was too small and comminuted to allow stable fixation. A distal femoral replacement allowed early ambulation.

## SURGICAL TECHNIQUE: Distal femoral locked plating

### Surgical set-up

Theatre set-up is as for retrograde nailing with a bolster under the knee, which is flexed to 45° (see Fig. 18.23).

### Closed reduction (see Fig. 18.24)

Longitudinal traction provides length, as well as correction of varus/valgus and flexion/extension.

Fluoroscopic image: Check the fracture reduction. The correct length of plate required can be confirmed fluoroscopically before draping the patient by holding the wrapped plate next to the limb.

### Incision

For percutaneous plating, the incision is short, curvilinear and lateral parapatellar, to expose the lateral aspect of the lateral femoral condyle (**Fig. 18.35A**). If there is an intercondylar split or a Hoffa fracture, a more extensive lateral parapatellar exposure will be required and a midline incision may be preferred. A simple A-type fracture that is to be stabilized rigidly will require a larger exposure to allow the fracture to be cleared and reduced anatomically.

### Approach

For percutaneous plating, there are no underlying structures at risk deep to the small wound illustrated; therefore sharp dissection can proceed down to the periosteum. A more extensive exposure will require a sub-vastus approach (p. 381).

### Open reduction (if required)

The articular fracture should be assessed, cleared of clot and bone fragments, and temporarily reduced and held with k-wires and clamps. Once the articular surface is anatomical, lag screws are used to provide definitive fixation and compression of the metaphyseal block (turning a C-type fracture into an A-type). A periosteal elevator is used to clear a path for the plate proximally.

### Internal fixation – absolute or relative stability (Fig. 18.35B,C)

The plate is passed up the lateral aspect of the femur in contact with the bone.

Distally, the plate should be drawn anteriorly and inferiorly until it lies against the 'vermilion border' of the lateral condyle where the (white) articular cartilage abuts the (red) periosteum. The distal metaphysis is trapezoidal in cross-section, and the lateral face of the femoral metaphysis slopes up and back at an angle of 10-20°. The plate must sit square against this face, and instruments passed through the jig are therefore passed at an angle towards the floor. Proximally, the plate should lie squarely on the lateral surface of the shaft. The subsequent sequence is pin–pin, lag–lag, lock–lock.

1. Pin–pin (**Fig. 18.36**): The fracture is reduced, and the plate is temporarily secured to the femur with a wire proximally and a second wire distally. The fracture reduction and the correct placement of the plate are confirmed on AP and lateral screening. Most plates have distal locking screws that project at an angle of around 95° from

the plate, corresponding to the mechanical axis of the knee. Thus, when the fracture has been reduced correctly, the distal guide wire will lie parallel to the articular surface of the femoral condyles in the AP projection. If there is a converging angle, the fracture is likely to be malaligned in varus, and similarly a diverging angle suggests valgus. Malrotation in the lateral projection is also common, with the fracture apex pulled posteriorly by the action of gastrocnemius. Again, this must be corrected at this stage. It may not be easy to establish a satisfactory reduction and correct plate position percutaneously, but it is an error to move on to the next stage unless this has been achieved; it is better to enlarge the exposure than accept malreduction.

2. Lag–lag: A lag technique may be helpful and should be considered at this point, but is not always required. Two scenarios should be considered:
   - Lagging (aligning) plate to bone (**Fig. 18.37A**): The first role is to assist in alignment of the main fragments. These can be 'pulled back' on to the plate using non-locked 'lag' screws proximally and distally.
   - Lagging (compressing) the fracture (**Fig. 18.37B**): Additionally, where there is a simple A-type fracture, the two fragments can be reduced anatomically and lagged together to achieve interfragmentary compression. This increases the rigidity of the construct; it will no longer be a 'bridging' technique and the fracture will heal by primary bone healing (Fig. 1.30). The remainder of the construct will need to provide absolute stability rather than relative stability. It is important to understand which technique is being employed and not to mix or confuse these (see Fig. 5.15).

3. Lock–lock: Once the fracture has been reduced and the plate applied correctly, further screws are placed to provide definitive fixation. Locking screws are used distally to grip the weak metaphyseal bone, whereas standard, non-locked screws are preferred proximally. Locked screws both above and below the implant result in an overly stiff construct and the risk of a non-union. The location of the screws determines the rigidity of the construct:
   - Where a bridging technique is employed for a comminuted fracture, screws placed well away from the fracture will allow some movement and callus healing (**Fig. 18.38A**).
   - Where a fracture has been anatomically reduced and compressed, movement is not desirable and screws should be positioned close to the fracture site (**Fig. 18.38B**).

### Postoperative restrictions

Movement: Unrestricted hip and knee movement is allowed.

Weight-bearing: Full weight-bearing is permitted whenever possible, particularly in the elderly, as they are at higher risk of the complications of recumbency. In specific cases – for example, a comminuted intra-articular fracture – protected weight-bearing may be preferred until union. In younger patients who are likely to load their construct more, protected partial weight-bearing is usually employed until callus is visible at the fracture site at between 6 and 10 weeks.

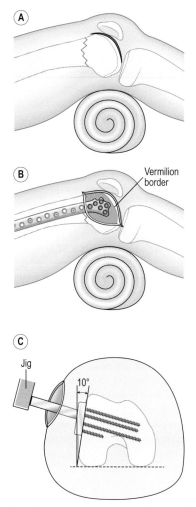

Fig. 18.35   Distal femoral locked plating: approach and plate positioning.

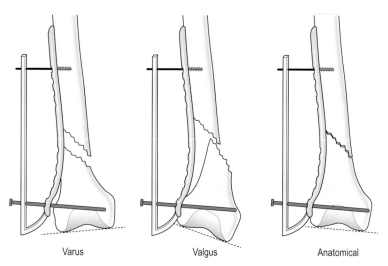

Fig. 18.36   Distal femoral locked plating: pin–pin.

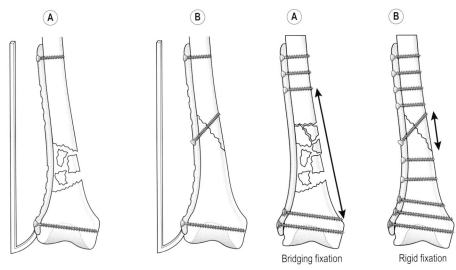

Fig. 18.37   Distal femoral locked plating: lag–lag.

Fig. 18.38   Distal femoral locked plating: lock–lock.

## Outpatient management

### Supracondylar fractures treated with plating

| Outpatient management summary | | | |
|---|---|---|---|
| **Week** | **Examination** | **Radiographs** | **Additional notes** |
| 2 | Wound check<br><br>Hip and knee movement check<br><br>Neurovascular status | AP and lateral femur to ensure no early loss of reduction | Begin physiotherapy |
| 6 | Hip and knee movement check | AP and lateral femur to check early callus | Review weight-bearing status if necessary |
| 12 | | AP and lateral femur | If there is clinical and radiographic union, discharge |

Further assessments at 8-week intervals if required for delayed union

Average time to union = 12 weeks

## GENERAL PRINCIPLES

### Anatomy

The knee is a complex hinge joint involving the femur, tibia and patella (**Fig. 19.1**). It is commonly conceptualized as having three compartments: medial, lateral and patellofemoral. Within the medial and lateral compartments, the curved *articular surfaces* of the femoral condyles slide over the flat surfaces of the tibial plateau. Filling the peripheries of each compartment are the crescentic medial and lateral *menisci* (**Fig. 19.2**). The menisci act principally to reduce articular cartilage point-loading by increasing the contact area between femur and tibia; they also contribute to joint stability. They are composed of parallel bundles of fibrocartilage arranged in circumferential bands. This cartilage is avascular except in the 'red zone' peripherally, where the menisci are secured to the capsule of the knee joint by the coronary ligaments. The *extensor mechanism* consists of the quadriceps muscle and tendon, the patella and the patellar tendon. The patella itself is a large sesamoid bone that articulates with the trochlea of the femur; it provides a lever arm that improves the biomechanical advantage of the quadriceps muscle.

### Cruciate ligaments

The two cruciate (Latin: 'crossing') ligaments lie deep within the intercondylar notch of the knee. These limit movement in the sagittal plane: the *anterior* cruciate ligament (ACL) stops the tibia sliding *anteriorly*, while the *posterior* cruciate ligament (PCL) stops the tibia sliding *posteriorly*. The ACL arises from the lateral wall of the notch and passes downwards and forwards to an insertion between the tibial spines. It has two bundles – the anteromedial and the posterolateral; the latter bundle is also important in restricting internal rotation. When rupturing, the ACL does so explosively, and the patient usually reports the sensation of a 'pop' from within the knee. In the ACL-deficient knee, the tibia displaces forwards (the basis of the Lachman test) and into internal rotation (the basis of the pivot shift test). The PCL arises from the medial wall of the notch and passes downwards and backwards to insert behind the tibial plateau. In the PCL-deficient knee, the tibia sags back and externally rotates.

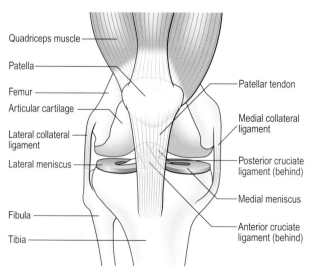
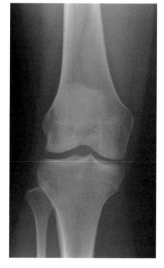

Quadriceps muscle
Patella
Femur
Articular cartilage
Lateral collateral ligament
Lateral meniscus
Fibula
Tibia

Patellar tendon
Medial collateral ligament
Posterior cruciate ligament (behind)
Medial meniscus
Anterior cruciate ligament (behind)

Fig. 19.1 Knee anatomy.

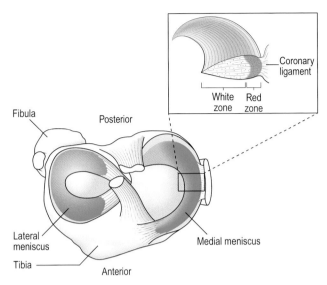

Fig. 19.2 Menisci.

## Collateral ligaments and posterolateral corner

The medial collateral ligament (MCL) and lateral collateral ligament (LCL) resist valgus and varus movements. The MCL arises from the medial femoral epicondyle. It has deep and superficial components, which insert into the medial aspect of the proximal tibia to resist valgus strain. The LCL runs from the lateral epicondyle and inserts into the head of the fibula to resist varus strain. The posterolateral corner (PLC) of the knee, consisting of popliteus, the popliteofibular ligament and biceps femoris, is considered functionally as an additional stabilizing structure.

---

### ✓ Key points

- The *anterior* cruciate ligament stops the tibia sliding *anteriorly*.

- The *posterior* cruciate ligament stops the tibia sliding *posteriorly*.

- The *medial collateral ligament* prevents *valgus* instability.

- The *lateral collateral ligament* prevents *varus* instability.

---

## Knee stability

The knee is supported by both static and dynamic stabilizers.

### Static stabilizers

- *Bone shape*: The femur, tibia and patella have somewhat conforming shapes.

- *Ligaments*: These are the ACL, PCL, MCL, LCL and PLC.

- *Joint capsule*: The capsule, particularly posteriorly, also contributes to knee stability.

- *Menisci*: These form hoops within the medial and lateral compartments, which act a little like the chocks placed on either side of a wheel to prevent it rolling, and help to resist sliding of the femur on the tibia.

### Dynamic stabilizers

- *Muscles crossing the knee joint*: The quadriceps anteriorly, and the hamstrings, biceps femoris and gastrocnemii posteriorly, are powerful stabilizers of the knee. Subjective knee instability is often related to poor muscular tone and control.

## Neurovascular anatomy (Fig. 19.3)

The superficial femoral artery traverses Hunter's canal and passes through the adductor hiatus to become the popliteal artery. It then runs vertically down the centre of the popliteal

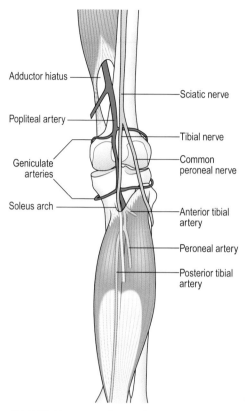

Adductor hiatus

Popliteal artery

Geniculate arteries

Soleus arch

Sciatic nerve

Tibial nerve

Common peroneal nerve

Anterior tibial artery

Peroneal artery

Posterior tibial artery

Fig. 19.3 Neurovascular anatomy.

nerve. The *tibial nerve* passes with the popliteal artery directly through the centre of the popliteal fossa to gain the deep posterior compartment of the leg, in which it supplies all of the muscles. It then passes behind the medial malleolus to supply the muscles and skin of the sole of the foot. The *common peroneal nerve* passes laterally under biceps femoris to pass around the neck of the fibula, where it can easily be injured. It then divides into the superficial and deep peroneal nerves. The superficial peroneal nerve passes through the lateral compartment (supplying the peroneal muscles in it) before passing through the deep fascia of the leg in the distal third of the leg to lie in the subcutaneous fat, where it can be injured in a lateral approach to the fibula. It supplies sensation to the dorsum of the foot, except the first web space. The deep peroneal nerve passes through the anterior compartment of the leg (supplying the muscles in it) before passing under the extensor retinaculum of the ankle (with the dorsalis pedis artery) to enter the foot and supply sensation to the first web space.

The *sural nerve* arises from branches of the tibial nerve and the common peroneal nerve in the popliteal fossa. It is a superficial structure and passes down the posterior aspect of the leg in the subcutaneous fat before passing around the lateral aspect of the ankle, where it supplies sensation to a small area of skin over the lateral aspect of the foot.

The *saphenous nerve* arises from the femoral nerve and passes, in the subcutaneous fat with the great saphenous vein, one hand's breadth posterior to the medial border of the patella. It can be damaged in a medial approach to the knee, resulting in a painful neuroma and reduced sensation over the medial malleolus of the ankle.

fossa to pass under the fibrous soleus arch before trifurcating into the posterior tibial artery (posterior compartment), the anterior tibial artery (anterior compartment) and peroneal artery (lateral compartment). The posterior tibial artery can be palpated further distally behind the medial malleolus, whilst the anterior tibial artery can be palpated after it has passed under the extensor retinaculum of the ankle and become the dorsalis pedis artery, over the dorsum of the foot. In the popliteal fossa, the popliteal artery gives off five geniculate branches medially and laterally, both above and below the joint, and the deep branch, which passes directly forwards into the joint. The popliteal artery is thereby 'crucified to the skeleton' behind the knee, and this lack of mobility makes it highly vulnerable to injury in knee dislocations.

The sciatic nerve divides just above the knee into the tibial nerve and the common peroneal

## Clinical assessment of the painful knee

### History

A detailed description of the mechanism of injury often points to the diagnosis. A common mechanism of injury is a blow to the lateral aspect of the knee, resulting in a valgus force.

This often leads to a rupture of the MCL (in younger patients) or a lateral tibial plateau fracture (more frequently in the elderly). A varus force is far less common but results in the opposite pattern of injuries. A twisting injury on a loaded knee suggests a tear of a meniscus or a rupture of the ACL. A description of a 'pop' and the rapid development of tight swelling are suggestive of an ACL rupture with a resultant haemarthrosis. The more gradual development of swelling over more than 4 hours is indicative of an effusion, often arising from a meniscal injury. Uncommonly, a forceful blow to the front of the tibia in sport or from a fall may result in a PCL rupture. A direct blow to the front of the knee or a twisting incident, particularly in a young woman, commonly results in a patellar subluxation or dislocation. In the elderly, a localized ligamentous or meniscal injury is unusual; joint line pain and an effusion generally represent an exacerbation of osteoarthritis.

Acute monoarthritis without a history of injury suggests a non-traumatic aetiology. The differential diagnoses are remembered as 'cat in bed = VIP' (p. 103). The most important pathology to exclude is a septic arthritis, suggested by progressively worsening and unremitting pain, generalized malaise, local heat and exquisite pain on attempted movement (p. 103).

## Examination

Knee examination follows the usual sequence of 'look, feel, move, special tests and neurovascular assessment', although modified slightly by first palpating the knee in extension, then assessing movements, and then palpating the knee at 90° of flexion. Knee examination is often limited in the emergency setting due to pain, and certain manœuvres may not be possible at the time of presentation.

### Look

Expose both lower limbs completely. Stand at the end of the examination trolley to compare the two sides and comment on:

- *Deformity*: There may be clear deformity or angulation after a dislocation or fracture.

- *Swelling*: This may be localized after an impact, or a generalized swelling suggesting fluid in the knee: either an effusion (usually developing over >4 hours after injury) or haemarthrosis (usually developing rapidly, within 4 hours).

- *Contusions or abrasions*: Contusions may not appear for several hours after acute injury. Extensive bruising usually indicates an uncontained haemarthrosis, which suggests a severe knee injury.

### Feel (knee extended)

- *Heat*: With the knee extended, palpate for generalized warmth and compare this to the other side.

- *Effusion*: A gross effusion will be obvious from inspection alone but there are also two specific tests:

  *Patellar tap*: In a large effusion, press down on the patella and note that it descends through the fluid within the knee before coming to an abrupt stop as it meets the trochlea of the femur.

  *Fluid sweep*: A more subtle effusion can be demonstrated as a fluid sweep. With the flat of your hand, sweep the fluid from the medial aspect of the knee and up through the suprapatellar pouch; watch the fluid fill the normal concavity to the lateral aspect of the patella, making this region convex. Now empty this pouch of fluid, sweeping it up and through the suprapatellar pouch to fill the medial concavity.

- *Patellar apprehension*: Palpate the medial retinaculum just to the inner aspect of the patella, which will be tender after a dislocation. Grasp the patella and gently move it laterally. Excessive movement, discomfort, or an expression of apprehension on the patient's face is suggestive of patellar instability.

### Move

Screen the hip and extensor mechanism, and then establish the *range of movement* present, comparing this with the uninjured knee (**Fig. 19.4**):

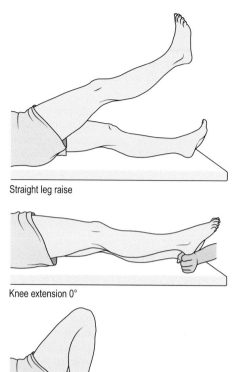

Straight leg raise

Knee extension 0°

Knee flexion 140°

Fig. 19.4 Screening movements.

- *Hip screening*: Roll the limb gently from side to side, keeping the knee straight, and observe for any indication of groin or hip pain, in order to exclude hip pathology presenting as referred pain at the knee.

- *Straight leg raise*: Ask the patient to lift the limb off the couch. Inability to do so may indicate an extensor mechanism disruption. If a straight leg raise cannot be performed, assist the patient by placing one hand under the thigh and the other under the heel, and lifting the straight leg 30 cm from the examination trolley. Ask the patient to maintain this position while you gradually remove support from the heel and maintain support to the thigh. After an extensor mechanism disruption the patient will not be able to

maintain this position. If the patient can hold a near-extension, albeit briefly, the extensor mechanism is grossly intact.

- *Knee extension*: Now allow the patient's heel to rest on your closed fist on the trolley and ask them to press the back of their knee down into the trolley. Inability to straighten the knee may result from a tight effusion or haemarthrosis, pain inhibition or a mechanical block arising from a meniscal tear. If the knee does not come straight, press gently over the front of the proximal tibia; the sensation of a rubbery mechanical block to extension is suggestive of a meniscal tear (usually a bucket-handle tear with an incarcerated fragment).

- *Knee flexion*: Finally, ask the patient to bend the knee fully. Inability to achieve full flexion is common, resulting from the presence of an effusion or simply the generalized irritability of an injured knee. Comparison with the uninjured limb is often described in terms of how close the patient can bring the heel towards the buttock. Leave the knee flexed to 90°.

### Feel (knee flexed)

- *Tenderness*: With the knee at 90°, palpate the anatomical structures of the knee in an orderly manner. Start at the tibial tuberosity and work proximally along the patellar tendon, patella and quadriceps tendon, looking for tenderness or a defect suggestive of an extensor mechanism disruption (tendon rupture or patellar fracture). Now palpate along both the medial and the lateral joint margins. Localized tenderness here is suggestive of a meniscal injury, while generalized joint line tenderness in a degenerative knee is more suggestive of an exacerbation of osteoarthritis. Tenderness medially is common; establish whether it is horizontally distributed (along the joint margin, suggesting a meniscal or joint injury) or vertically distributed (along the medial collateral ligament, suggesting an injury to this structure). Palpate below the joint line, along the proximal tibia both medially and laterally, to exclude the bony tenderness that might suggest a tibial plateau fracture. Palpate the fibular head, hamstrings and popliteal fossa.

## Special tests

Examine the knee for *ligamentous stability* and *meniscal pathology*, again starting with the uninjured knee for comparison. In a stepwise progression, the ligaments are examined:

1. the collaterals with varus and valgus stress tests
2. the ACL with Lachman's test and pivot shift test
3. the PCL with inspection for posterior sag and the posterior drawer test
4. the PLC with the dial test
5. the menisci with McMurray's test.

Examination proceeds as follows:

- *Collateral ligaments*: With the patient's ankle held firmly under your arm, place your hands around the proximal calf away from any areas of knee joint tenderness (**Fig. 19.5**). With the knee in full extension, push firmly medially and then laterally to stress first the MCL and then the LCL. Abnormal movement suggests an extensive (grade 3) ligamentous rupture. If the knee is stable in complete extension, now flex the knee to 30° (to relax the posterior joint capsule) and repeat the movement. Abnormal laxity in this position suggests a partial (grade 2) tear.
- *Anterior cruciate ligament*: Now perform Lachman's test (**Fig. 19.6**). Grasp the distal thigh with one hand to stabilize the limb with

30° of knee flexion. If the thigh is too big for your hand, place your knee under the thigh and press your hand down on top of the thigh. Grasp the proximal tibia with the other hand and pull firmly and sharply up and down in turn. On the normal side you will feel a few millimetres of movement but then a definite, firm end point as the ACL (pulling the tibia anteriorly) and the PCL (pushing back) engage. In an ACL disruption, the tibia moves forwards excessively and there is no clear end point. A confirmatory test for ACL deficiency is the *pivot shift test*. This is often difficult to perform in the acute setting and is most valuable in the knee clinic and on examination under anaesthesia. One hand grasps the patient's heel, allowing the knee to extend fully while applying an internal rotation force. The other hand is placed behind the upper calf, which pushes the tibia forwards and internally into a subluxed position in the ACL-deficient knee. The knee is now flexed slowly. At around 30° of flexion, the

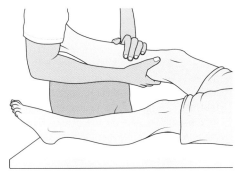

Fig. 19.5 Testing the collateral ligaments.

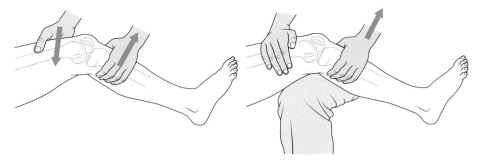

Fig. 19.6 Lachman's test.

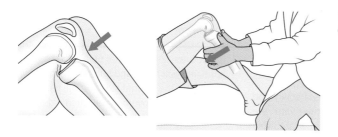

Fig. 19.7 Posterior sag and drawer test.

tibia is felt to shift backwards and externally into its anatomical position, a movement caused by the pull of the fascia lata, which engages during knee flexion.

- *Posterior cruciate ligament*: In a PCL disruption, with the knee flexed at 90°, the tibia is seen to *sag* back. This is confirmed with a *posterior drawer test*, in which the same posterior translation and lack of end point is demonstrated (**Fig. 19.7**). The *quads active test* is confirmatory; from a position of posterior sag, if the patient is asked to contract the quadriceps muscle, the tibia will be seen to be pulled forwards to its correct position.

- *Posterolateral corner*: Injury to the PLC is demonstrated by a positive *dial test* (**Fig. 19.8**). Place the patient prone with the knees flexed to 30° and apply passive external rotation to both feet. Repeat the same test at 90°. If there is increased external rotation of the foot on the injured side at 30°, the PLC is injured. If there is also increased external rotation of the foot on the injured side at 90°, there is a combined injury to the PLC and PCL.

- *Menisci*: Aim to provoke any meniscal instability using *McMurray's test* (**Fig. 19.9**). Grasp the knee with one hand, placing your fingers lightly over the 'soft spots' on the medial and lateral joint lines. Take the patient's foot in the other hand and gently flex the knee. Now exert a firm internal rotation force on the foot while extending the knee. Now flex the knee again and exert an external rotation force while extending. The sensation of a click or clunk at the joint margin, or a sharp pain, is suggestive of an unstable meniscal tear.

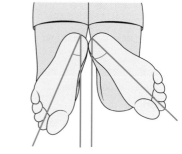

Fig. 19.8 Dial test.

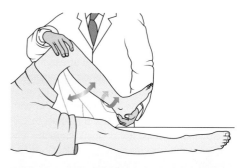

Fig. 19.9 McMurray's test.

### Neurovascular assessment

Palpate the dorsalis pedis and posterior tibial pulsations, and after a significant knee injury mark their locations with ink to allow later reassessment. Assess the capillary refill to the toes. A Doppler probe is used where there is an abnormal pulse. The ankle–brachial pressure index (ABPI) is a ratio of the systolic blood pressure when measured using the probe in the lower and upper limbs, and allows quantification of any subtle reduction in flow. An ABPI <0.9 is considered abnormal. Check for sensation in the distributions of the deep and superficial peroneal, and posterior tibial nerves (see Figs 3.20–3.22). Confirm active toe and foot dorsiflexion and plantar flexion.

## Radiological assessment of the painful knee

### Radiographs

- *AP and lateral views of the knee*: Orthogonal images (taken at 90°) are required after a significant knee injury to exclude a fracture. High-quality images are necessary for a full assessment. On the AP view (**Fig. 19.10A**), ensure that the knee is fully extended and there is no overlap of the femur and tibia. On the lateral view (**Fig. 19.10B**), the medial and lateral femoral condyles should be superimposed. Carefully inspect the outline of the femur, tibia, fibular head and neck, and patella, noting any *fractures*. Look for any defect in the articular surface that might indicate an *osteochondral fracture*. Small flakes of bone, indicating avulsion fractures, may be present at either pole of the patella, around the tibial plateau, or at the sites of origin of the MCL or LCL.

  The *Segond fracture* (**Fig. 19.11**) is a small avulsion fracture of the lateral aspect of the tibial plateau, which in itself is innocuous but is pathognomonic of an ACL disruption.

  The *Pellegrini–Stieda* lesion (**Fig. 19.12**) is calcification within the MCL at its femoral origin and is indicative of previous MCL injury.

  A *fabella* (**Fig. 19.13**; Latin: 'little bean') is a well-circumscribed ossicle in the gastrocnemius head behind the knee and is a normal structure, although it is often mistaken for a fracture.

  A *bipartite patella* is a normal variant that is commonly mistaken for a patellar fracture. Occurring in 1% of the population, it arises from two ossification centres that have failed to fuse. It occurs most often in the superolateral quadrant of the patella, and radiographically has smooth, rounded edges and no displacement. If the features are suspicious, it is important to correlate the site of this abnormality with any bony tenderness.

  Note the position of the patella on the lateral radiograph: a *high-riding patella* is suggestive of a patellar tendon injury.

  Examine the *soft tissue shadows* for an effusion or a haemarthrosis (see Fig. 20.6), or a fleck of bone in the joint space representing a probable osteochondral fragment.

- *Skyline view* (**Fig. 19.14**): This view of the patellofemoral joint is taken with the knee flexed and the beam orientated along the long axis of the patella. It can be helpful for assessing a vertical fracture of the patella, but is more commonly used for outpatient assessment of patellofemoral anatomy.

### CT

CT provides more detail for preoperative planning of intra-articular fractures.

### MRI

This is highly sensitive in identifying disruptions of ligaments and cartilage, and is useful for preoperative planning.

### Angiography

The selective use of angiography (or CT angiography) is helpful in identifying arterial disruption or an occult intimal tear (Fig. 3.23). However, it is not required when there is a critically ischaemic limb after a severe knee injury: this is an indication for surgical exploration, the lesion being predictably at the level of the knee dislocation. Its routine use in the clinically well-perfused limb is controversial, and careful clinical monitoring is usually considered optimal management. Selective angiography based on an ABPI of <0.9 is recommended.

## Aspiration

Whilst aspiration is not routinely performed after knee injury in the Emergency Department, it is indicated in two situations:

- Where there is a tight haemarthrosis: Aspiration can provide considerable pain relief. It also helps in diagnosis, frank blood

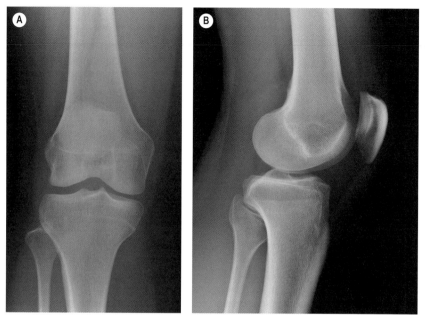

Fig. 19.10 Normal radiographs of the knee. **A**, AP view. **B**, Lateral view.

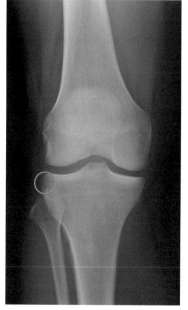

Fig. 19.11 Segond fracture.

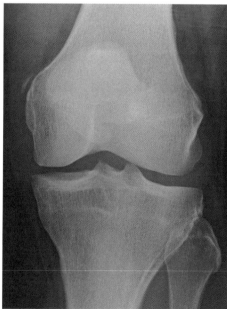

Fig. 19.12 Pellegrini–Stieda lesion.

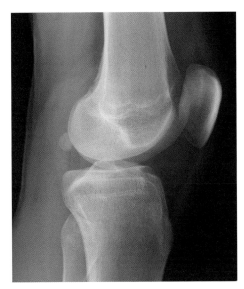

Fig. 19.13 Fabella.

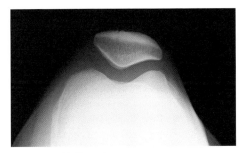

Fig. 19.14 Skyline view.

indicating the presence of an ACL disruption in 85% of cases. The other causes of a frank haemarthrosis are an intra-articular fracture, capsular tear or a very peripheral bucket-handle tear of a meniscus.

● Where there is suspicion of infection: A sample can be obtained for microbiology.

The technique of aspiration is described on page 112.

## KNEE DISLOCATION

Knee (tibiofemoral) dislocation usually results from a high-energy mechanism of injury, although low-energy stumbles can result in complete knee dislocation in the morbidly obese.

Associated neurovascular injury is common. Most cases of ligament disruption do not present with obvious deformity; indeed, up to two-thirds of all complete knee dislocations have reduced spontaneously before presentation to hospital. A careful clinical assessment after knee injury is mandatory to avoid missing a significant disruption. Subsequent management relies on clear identification of the injured structures, and is influenced by the age, health and sporting aspirations of the patient.

## Classification

### Schenck (or Knee Dislocation) classification

This describes which anatomical structures have been torn:

● *KD I*: One cruciate ligament plus one collateral ligament.

● *KD II*: Both cruciates but neither collateral (very rare).

● *KD III*: Both cruciates and either the MCL or LCL, recorded as:

*KD IIIM*: MCL injuries.

*KD IIIL*: LCL injuries.

● *KD IV*: Fracture dislocations of the knee.

## Emergency Department management

### Clinical features

● Obtain a detailed history of the injury. Did the knee feel or look dislocated at any point?

● Ask what happened to the patella. Often patients will say they have a knee dislocation when in fact they mean a patellofemoral dislocation.

● Carry out a thorough examination of the knee, paying particular attention to ligamentous stability and any distal neurovascular compromise.

### Radiological features

● *AP and lateral knee radiographs* (**Fig. 19.15**): These may demonstrate a dislocation but are often surprisingly normal.

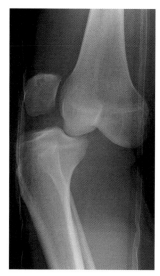

Fig. 19.15 Knee dislocation.

referred urgently for orthopaedic and vascular surgical assessment. A critically ischaemic limb will require emergency surgical exploration. Partial compromise, suggested by a diminished pulse volume, slow capillary return or an ABPI <0.9, may indicate an intimal tear, which could progress rapidly to a critically ischaemic limb. Serial careful examinations are required, and in selected patients angiography may be indicated.

Neurological compromise after closed dislocation does not in itself mandate urgent surgical exploration unless the abnormality was not present prior to manipulation; these injuries are usually a neurapraxia or axonotmesis (p. 50), and are managed expectantly.

## Closed reduction

If there is obvious deformity on presentation, it should be reduced immediately under procedural sedation. Apply gentle but firm longitudinal traction with pressure over the displaced proximal tibia until the knee is felt to reduce with a soft 'clunk'. An experienced examiner should take this opportunity to assess the ligamentous integrity of the knee, if this has not already been established. Rarely, an irreducible dislocation may be caused by the femoral condyle 'button-holing' through the capsule: this requires surgical exploration.

## Immobilization and reassessment

After closed reduction, the limb is immobilized in 30° of knee flexion in a full-leg plaster backslab (see p. 72). If there was no deformity at presentation, an extension knee splint may be preferred. A careful reassessment of knee congruity and neurovascular integrity is required after reduction.

## Inpatient referral

Patients with a knee dislocation are referred for inpatient assessment. Those who have any evidence of vascular compromise should be

## Orthopaedic management

Knee dislocations are generally stabilized surgically, with primary repair (with or without graft augmentation) of the collateral ligaments/PLC, and reconstruction of the cruciates. Timing of surgery depends on the individual circumstances and surgeon's preference.

- *Emergency surgery* is required where there are contaminated wounds or critical ischaemia. Temporary stabilization with a transarticular frame may be necessary before vascular shunt or repair, or where the soft tissues are compromised. However, there is a high rate of stiffness, and early repair of the collateral ligaments and early movement are preferred where feasible.

- *Early surgery* (within 1 or 2 weeks of injury) is often preferred, as this allows early, supervised mobilization with satisfactory outcomes. However, where there is capsular disruption, arthroscopic surgery carries a danger of fluid extravasation and compartment syndrome, and so early cruciate reconstruction has to be performed open. The presence of a bucket-handle meniscal tear is a relative indication for early surgery, in order to allow meniscal repair.

- *Staged surgery* is often optimal, with early collateral ligament (and meniscal) repair, a period of physiotherapy to regain range of movement, and then reassessment and cruciate repair at 8 to 12 weeks.

- *Delayed surgery* may be preferred. Once the capsule has healed (after 3 weeks), the knee can be reassesed, the collaterals repaired (or, often, reconstructed), with arthroscopic cruciate reconstruction. Delayed surgery carries a greater risk of knee stiffness (arthrofibrosis) and instability.

## Surgical techniques

The technique and procedure depend on the grade of dislocation. Preoperative MRI is used to confirm the nature of the injury and identify any associated meniscal or osteochondral injury.

- *KD I: ACL + MCL*: The MCL will usually heal spontaneously over 6–8 weeks, converting this into an isolated ACL injury, which can then be treated electively by arthroscopic reconstruction. The patient is provided with a hinged knee brace, and active range of movement exercises are commenced early.

- *KD I: ACL + LCL/PLC*: Early exploration and repair of the LCL/PLC is performed, usually with open reconstruction of the ACL. Augmentation of the LCL/PLC repair with graft may be added if the tissues are attenuated. Some surgeons prefer to stage this surgery.

- *KD II and III: bicruciate injuries*: Early open surgery within 2 weeks is preferred. Allograft is used for the PCL, most commonly tendo Achilles allograft. The ACL may be reconstructed from hamstring or patellar tendon autograft. In KD IIIM, a single midline incision is used, and the MCL is repaired, advanced or reattached with suture anchors. In KD IIIL injuries, a midline incision is used for the cruciate reconstruction, and a separate posteromedial incision is employed for exposure of the LCL/PLC. The anatomy can be markedly distorted, and careful identification and protection of the common peroneal nerve are required.

- *KD IV: fracture dislocations*: These are challenging injuries to treat. Plain radiographs, a CT scan of the bony injury and an MRI of the soft tissue injury can all assist in preoperative planning. Surgery aims to achieve reduction and fixation of the fracture, intraoperative assessment of the stability of the knee, and subsequent ligament reconstruction as required.

## Outpatient management

A carefully supervised and staged physiotherapy regime is important to minimize stiffness, while protecting the repaired and reconstructed ligaments from unprotected stressing and failure. Early active flexion, for example, can result in stretching of a PCL graft. While local protocols will vary, the sequence of drills is generally to regain range of movement first, then begin closed-chain muscle strengthening exercises, before moving on to open-chain and proprioceptive training, and finally sport-specific coaching.

---

### COMPLICATIONS

*Early*

| | |
|---|---|
| Local | Vascular injury: The popliteal artery is commonly injured and careful serial clinical assessment and selective use of angiography are required |
| | Neurological injury: Both the posterior tibial nerve and common peroneal nerve are at risk |

*Continued*

## COMPLICATIONS... cont'd

### Late

Local    Instability: Persistent functional instability can occur even after early surgery, and may require further ligamentous reconstruction or osteotomy

Stiffness: Arthrofibrosis is common and very difficult to overcome. Arthroscopic arthrolysis and manipulation under anaesthesia are offered for loss of flexion, while loss of extension is treated with nocturnal extension splintage

Muscle weakness: The common peroneal nerve is most commonly injured. With expectant management, one-third will return to normal spontaneously, one-third will recover partially, and one-third will remain severely abnormal. Persistent foot drop is treated with functional bracing or later tendon transfers

## ISOLATED KNEE LIGAMENT INJURIES

Injury to isolated knee ligaments is much more frequent than complete knee dislocation, and commonly follows a blow to the knee or a twisting fall in sport. Tears can be partial or complete.

## Classification

Knee ligament injuries are classified according to the amount of laxity and instability caused. There are a number of similar classifications; the preferred ones are listed here.

### Medial and lateral collateral ligaments

Classifications of injury are based on the stability of the knee to valgus stress (MCL) and varus stress (LCL), assessed both at 30° and in full extension:

- Grade 1: There is tenderness over the ligament on palpation but no laxity on stress testing, indicating only a partial injury.
- Grade 2: There is abnormal laxity to varus/valgus stress with the knee held in 30° of flexion, indicating ligament rupture. However, the knee is stable in extension, indicating that other knee stabilizers (including the

cruciates and posterior knee joint capsule) are intact.

- Grade 3: There is abnormal laxity to varus/valgus stress both in extension and 30° of flexion. This usually indicates a more extensive injury to other stabilizers.

### Anterior cruciate ligament

Classification is based on the distance by which the tibia can be translated forwards in relation to the femur on Lachman's testing, although the presence or absence of a definite end point, and a different examination from the uninjured side, are probably more important:

- Grade 1: <5 mm
- Grade 2: 5–10 mm
- Grade 3: >10 mm

### Posterior cruciate ligament

Classification is based on the amount of posterior translation that can be demonstrated on posterior drawer testing at 90° of knee flexion:

- Grade 1: The anterior tibial cortex remains clearly in front of the femoral condyle.
- Grade 2: The tibia can be pushed back to the level of the femoral condyle.
- Grade 3: The tibia can be made to sag behind the femoral condyle.

# Emergency Department management

## Clinical features

The two most common single ligament injuries are to the MCL and the ACL. Each has a typical history:

- The MCL is disrupted in a valgus injury to the knee, often from a blow from the lateral aspect, such as a rugby tackle. There is immediate pain medially. There is little or no initial swelling or bruising, although a modest local swelling or an effusion may develop gradually over several hours.

- An ACL rupture typically occurs in a twisting injury to a loaded knee, such as when skiing or pivoting on a planted leg. There is often a sensation of a 'pop' with severe pain, followed by the rapid development of marked swelling. This is maximal within 4 hours and is caused by a haemarthrosis.

The rarer isolated LCL injury is caused by a varus force to the knee, and is particularly associated with common peroneal nerve injury. An isolated PCL injury is very rare, but may be caused by a direct blow to the shin.

A full, careful knee examination is required (see p. 421).

## Radiological features

- *AP and lateral knee radiographs*: These are required to exclude a bony injury. A Segond fracture (see Fig. 19.11), a small avulsion flake fracture from the lateral tibial plateau, is virtually pathognomonic of an ACL rupture. An avulsion fracture from the tip of the fibula is highly suggestive of an LCL/PLC injury. Avulsion of the tibial spine (Fig. 19.16) may be seen as a variant of an isolated cruciate injury in younger patients.

## Immobilization and reassessment

Isolated ligamentous injuries rarely require formal immobilization but patients may find a canvas extension splint and crutches helpful.

## Outpatient follow-up

Isolated ligament injuries are referred for review at the orthopaedic outpatient clinic at around 7-14 days to allow swelling to subside.

# Orthopaedic management

## Medial collateral ligament

Grade 1 and 2 MCL disruptions will almost inevitably heal over 6–8 weeks without the need for further intervention. No form of bracing is required, and patients can usually be discharged directly to a supervised physiotherapy programme. Grade 3 MCL disruptions should arouse suspicion of other ligamentous injuries and warrant reassessment to exclude other instability as function returns.

## Lateral collateral ligament

LCL injuries and fibular head avulsions are usually treated operatively with repair, fixation or graft augmentation as appropriate.

## Anterior cruciate ligament

The ACL has virtually no ability to heal. ACL disruptions often occur in young, athletic individuals who are likely to be symptomatic if left untreated. The risks and benefits of an ACL reconstruction should be discussed. The timing of surgery is important: there is a higher incidence of secondary medial meniscal tears if surgery is delayed for more than 6 months. An initial programme of physiotherapy rehabilitation will allow a return of a normal range of movement prior to surgery, and 'prehabilitation' exercises may assist in postoperative recovery. If patients are sedentary, or over the age of 35, there is a greater chance that they will be asymptomatic, despite lack of the ACL, and surgery is less commonly required. In those patients for whom surgery is planned, and in whom clinical examination is inconclusive, a preoperative MRI scan may assist in confirming the diagnosis and excluding other injuries, such as a meniscal tear.

## Posterior cruciate ligament

Isolated PCL injuries are rare. The PCL has some capacity to heal and a non-operative rehabilitation protocol, including avoidance of early active flexion, may be recommended. Grade II and III injuries with symptomatic instability, particularly involving hyperextension, may benefit from PCL reconstruction after initial rehabilitation. The results of PCL reconstruction are generally less predictable than those of ACL surgery.

## TIBIAL SPINE FRACTURES

This is effectively an avulsion injury at the tibial insertion of the ACL and follows the same type of twisting injury. It is most common in children but also occurs in young adults. Avulsion of the PCL insertion at the posterior aspect of the tibial plateau is rare, and is seen as an incongruity of the posterior tibial cortex.

## Classification

### Meyers and McKeever classification (Fig. 19.16)

- Type I: Undisplaced.
- Type II: Partially displaced; anterior elevation of the eminence.
- Type III: Entire eminence involved:

  IIIA: Entire eminence lies above its bed, out of contact with the tibia.

  IIIB: Eminence is rotated, as well as elevated.

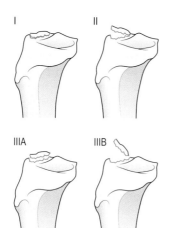

Fig. 19.16 Meyers and McKeever classification of tibial spine fractures.

## Emergency Department management

### Clinical features

- Obtain a detailed history of the injury. There is usually a history of a sporting twist or fall in a child or young adult.
- There will be a tense haemarthrosis.
- Carry out a thorough examination of the knee, paying particular attention to ligamentous stability and any distal neurovascular compromise.

### Radiological features

- Plain AP and lateral radiographs of the knee will demonstrate the injury.
- A CT scan will confirm the size of the fragment and the degree of comminution and displacement.

### Immobilization

The knee should be placed in a knee extension splint and the patient restricted to non-weight-bearing with crutches.

### Inpatient referral

All tibial spine fractures warrant orthopaedic review.

## Orthopaedic management

### Non-operative

Undisplaced fractures can be managed with extension casting or splintage for 6 weeks, with careful radiographic review to ensure that there is no displacement.

### Operative

Reduction and fixation are indicated where there is displacement, a block to extension or instability on Lachman's testing. Arthroscopic reduction and fixation with a cannulated, partially threaded screw (or transosseous suture) is preferred, although open reduction is occasionally required.

## MENISCAL INJURIES

Acute meniscal tears typically occur in young patients after a twisting injury to a flexed, loaded knee. Sporting injuries predominate but tears following falls and even standing up from a crouched or cross-legged position are relatively common. Tears resulting in an unstable, mobile segment can cause persistent mechanical pain and irritation to the knee, while a large bucket-handle tear can become incarcerated in the intercondylar notch and block extension: the locked knee. A chronic bucket handle tear may move into and out of this incarcerated position intermittently, producing symptoms of recurrent locking. There is usually a good history of a 'click' or 'clunk' with knee movement, followed by a sensation of release. Surgery is usually required to address these tears. In older patients, pre-existing degenerative meniscal tears are common, and twisting injuries usually result in an exacerbation of this degenerative process rather than causing a new discrete tear. Time, analgesics and physiotherapy are often sufficient to allow these to resolve.

## Classification

Meniscal tears are classified by their appearance (**Fig. 19.17**):

A. radial

B. parrot-beak

C. horizontal cleavage

D. longitudinal

E. bucket-handle.

Bucket-handle tears represent longitudinal tears that have become displaced centrally.

## Emergency Department management

### Clinical features

● Enquire about the mechanism of injury, and any subsequent mechanical block to *extension* (locking) that might indicate a displaced meniscal tear. Inability to achieve full *flexion* is due to pain inhibition and effusion and does not constitute locking.

● Enquire about pre-existing symptoms suggestive of osteoarthritis.

● Conduct a careful examination of the knee; establish in particular the range of movement, any rubbery block to full extension, and any joint margin tenderness.

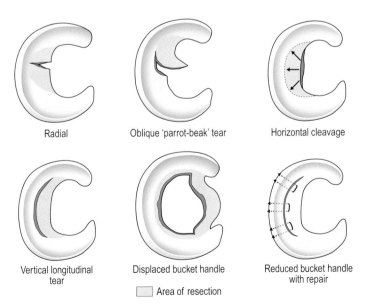

Radial

Oblique 'parrot-beak' tear

Horizontal cleavage

Vertical longitudinal tear

Displaced bucket handle

Reduced bucket handle with repair

☐ Area of resection

Fig. 19.17 Meniscal injuries.

- A modest effusion may develop over several hours or even days after injury.

- A tense haemarthrosis at presentation may result from a 'red' zone meniscal tear but is more likely to be due to an ACL disruption.

- The McMurray test is helpful in identifying meniscal irritability but is not always tolerated immediately after injury.

### Radiological features

- *AP and lateral knee radiographs*: Obtain AP and lateral radiographs after any significant knee injury. These may be entirely normal.

### Immobilization

Treatment in the Emergency Department aims to limit discomfort with analgesia, a temporary knee extension splint and crutches.

### Inpatient referral

- An acutely locked knee is suggestive of a bucket-handle tear. Not only is this highly disabling, but also meniscal repair is most successful acutely and prompt referral to the on-call orthopaedic service is appropriate. Do not attempt to unlock the knee by manipulation in the Emergency Department.

---

 **Key point**

The term 'locked knee' has a specific meaning in the context of knee injuries. It implies a physical block to knee extension. Presenting acutely, this will be evident as a rubbery block to passive knee extension. A long-standing unstable tear may present with intermittent locking, and the patient will complain of a recurrent 'click' or sense of something moving in the knee to cause the locking, and then another 'click' later as the fragment reduces back into position and the knee unlocks. Locking is not a sense of transient catching or instability; nor is it a failure to achieve full flexion.

---

### Outpatient follow-up

- Patients with a likelihood of an acute meniscal tear but who can achieve knee extension are referred to the orthopaedic clinic.

- Older patients with clear clinical and radiographic features of degenerative knee arthritis can be referred directly for physiotherapy rehabilitation.

## Orthopaedic management

### Non-operative

Most young patients who complain of joint line tenderness but still have full extension after a twisting injury experience gradual spontaneous resolution of their symptoms over 2 or 3 weeks without further investigation or treatment, implying that the injury was a non-specific soft tissue injury (p. 442). An MRI scan may be required where there is ongoing uncertainty.

### Operative

Indications for arthroscopy include:

- *Locked knee*: This should be evaluated arthroscopically. Irreparable or extensively damaged meniscal tears are resected. Bucket-handle tears in the red (vascularized) zone of the meniscus are repaired, most commonly using an 'all inside' suture technique (**Fig. 19.17**). The success of this technique diminishes with time; aim to perform the repair within 3 or 4 weeks of injury. An MRI may be helpful preoperatively to exclude associated injuries, such as an ACL tear, which could be treated at the same operation.

- *Ongoing joint line tenderness*: Marked, localized and persistent discomfort at the joint margin associated with a sense of catching, and a positive McMurray's test suggests a meniscal tear. This can be addressed with arthroscopic resection or repair. If there is any uncertainty over the aetiology of the pain, an MRI is helpful.

## QUADRICEPS AND PATELLAR TENDON RUPTURES

The extensor mechanism of the knee consists of the quadriceps tendon, the patella, the

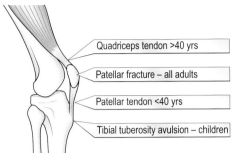

Fig. 19.18 Extensor mechanism injuries.

patellar tendon and the tibial tuberosity. Quadriceps tendon ruptures generally occur around 2 cm above the patella in degenerative tissue in the over-forties (**Fig. 19.18**). Other risk factors include chronic renal disease, diabetes, inflammatory joint disease, and steroid or quinolone antibiotic use. Patellar tendon ruptures generally occur in the under-forties and may follow a sporting injury or pre-existing degeneration. In children, the tibial tuberosity may be avulsed, or may be affected by traction apophysitis (Osgood–Schlatter's disease; p. 603). Fractures and dislocations of the patella are addressed in separate sections below.

## Emergency Department management
### Clinical features
- There is usually a history of a stumble in which the quadriceps muscles have contracted forcefully to prevent a fall, or indeed a history of a fall with sudden uncontrolled knee flexion.
- Recent treatment with ciprofloxacin, or previous injection of steroid into or around the tendon increases the risk of tendon rupture.
- The patient often reports a sudden pain or 'pop' from the front of the knee.
- On inspection of the knee, there may be a defect in the contour of the quadriceps tendon or patellar tendon, with some surrounding soft tissue swelling.

- Palpation will reveal a defect in the surface of the tendon (which is more obvious when the knee is flexed) and local tenderness.
- The patient will be unable to perform a straight leg raise.

### Radiological features
- *AP and lateral knee radiographs*: Careful inspection of plain radiographs may show a soft tissue defect, a flake of avulsed patella or, in the case of a patellar tendon rupture, a high-riding patella. Compare the length of the patella with the length of the tendon (the distance between the tibial tuberosity and the distal pole of the patella). This is termed the Insall–Salvati ratio (normal range 0.8–1.2). Where this is <0.8, it is referred to as 'patella alta', and in this context is suggestive of tendon rupture. A ratio of >1.2 is termed 'patella baja' and can be a late complication of patellar tendon injury and surgery.
- *Ultrasound scan*: This is far more sensitive than plain radiographs and will confirm the diagnosis if there is doubt.

### Immobilization
The knee is immobilized in a knee extension splint and the patient is provided with crutches.

### Inpatient referral
Patients with extensor mechanism disruption should be referred to the orthopaedic service. Patients are permitted to weight-bear with their splint, and may be able to return on a planned basis.

## Orthopaedic management
### Non-operative
Partial tears (diagnosed with ultrasound scanning) with an intact straight leg raise can be managed in a hinged knee brace, with movement restricted to 30° of flexion, for 8 weeks.

### Operative
Ruptures of the quadriceps tendon or the patellar tendon are treated operatively.

## SURGICAL TECHNIQUE: Quadriceps tendon or patellar tendon repair

### Surgical set-up
The patient is placed supine. A tourniquet is usually avoided as this impairs mobilization of the quadriceps tendon.

### Incision
A 20-cm midline anterior knee incision is made, centred so as to expose the ruptured tendon and the patella.

### Procedure
The tendon is identified and held with a Kocher's clamp. Two non-absorbable, strong sutures are placed in the avulsed tendon end with a Krackow-type whipstitch (see Fig. 21.52). The stitches are loaded cyclically to ensure they are tight. Three parallel 2.5-mm drill holes are placed longitudinally through the patella. The drill holes should be placed such that the tendon will be reattached in its anatomical position. If the holes are drilled too anteriorly, the patella will be tilted in towards the femoral trochlea, increasing patellar contact pressures and causing pain. A Hughson suture passer is used to draw the suture ends through the drill holes: two through the central hole and one to each side (**1** on **Fig. 19.19**). The sutures are drawn tight and tied firmly (**2**). The knee can now be flexed carefully to 45° and the repair inspected. If the repair holds well without gapping, the patient can be allowed 30° of knee flexion during healing.

A protection wire (**Fig. 19.20**) is sometimes used to supplement patellar tendon repair, although with modern sutures this is rarely necessary. The wire is passed through transverse drill holes placed just below the midpoint of the patella, and through the tibial tuberosity *before* placement of the sutures (to avoid damaging these). The position of the patella should be assessed carefully on lateral fluoroscopy and compared to the uninjured knee; it is very easy to over-tighten the protection wire, resulting in patella baja. The patient is warned that the wire will often be found to have broken on later radiographs, although routine removal is usually unnecessary.

### Postoperative restrictions
Movement: Patients are restricted to 0–30° of knee movement in a hinged knee brace for 8 weeks. They should begin isometric quads exercises immediately.

Weight-bearing: Patients may be allowed full weight-bearing during this time.

1

2

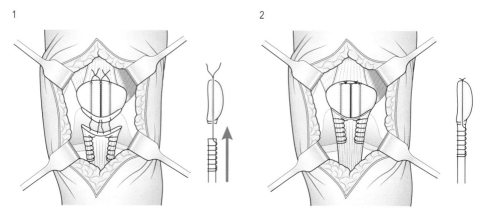

Fig. 19.19 Patellar tendon repair.

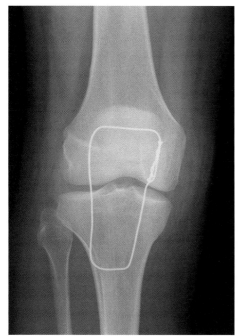

Fig. 19.20 Patellar tendon protection wire.

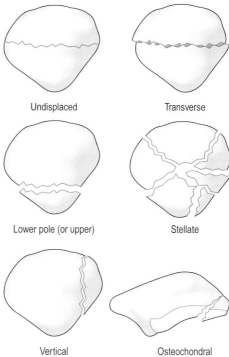

Undisplaced      Transverse

Lower pole (or upper)      Stellate

Vertical      Osteochondral

Fig. 19.21 Patellar fracture types.

## PATELLAR FRACTURES

Patellar fractures occur commonly after a stumble with quadriceps contraction, a fall on to the point of the knee, or a dashboard strike in a motor vehicle collision; occasionally, they are found in association with other injuries (Fig. 17.33).

## Classification

Patellar fractures are classified according to their morphology (**Fig. 19.21**).

## Emergency Department management

### Clinical features

- Look particularly for open wounds, tenderness and deformity of the patella.

- The patient will be unable to perform a straight leg raise.

- Exclude other injuries (see Fig. 17.33).

## Radiological features

- *AP and lateral knee radiographs* (**Fig. 19.22**): Assess fracture displacement. Exclude a bipartite patella.

- *Skyline knee radiograph*: This may show a vertical or osteochondral fracture (**Fig. 19.23**). Skyline radiographs are often uncomfortable and difficult to obtain after acute injury, and are only indicated where the patella remains undisplaced and the diagnosis is uncertain.

### Immobilization

The knee should be immobilized in an extension knee splint; weight-bearing is allowed with the aid of crutches.

### Outpatient follow-up

- Undisplaced fractures can be referred to the fracture clinic.

### Inpatient referral

- Displaced patellar fractures should be referred to Orthopaedics.

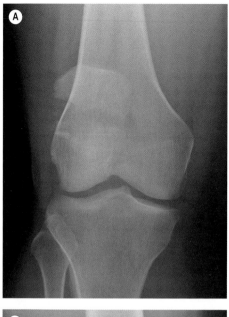

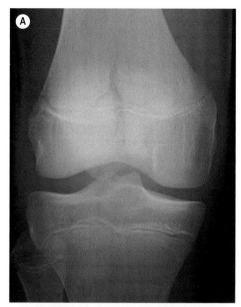

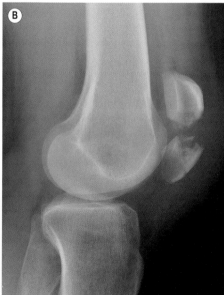

Fig. 19.22 Transverse patellar fracture with some comminution. **A**, AP view. **B**, Lateral view.

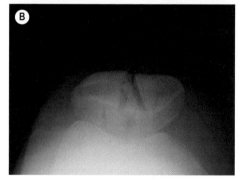

Fig. 19.23 Minimally displaced vertical fracture. **A**, AP view. **B**, The articular congruity is confirmed on the skyline view.

## Orthopaedic management

### Non-operative management

Undisplaced fractures, particularly vertical fractures, can be managed non-operatively in a hinged knee brace, fully weight-bearing, for 6 weeks.

### Operative

Most fractures of the patella are displaced and intra-articular, and are therefore treated operatively.

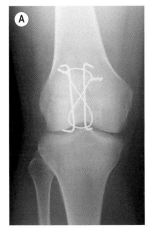 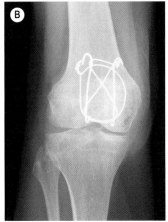 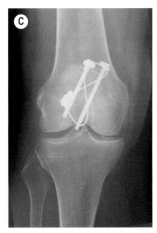

Fig. 19.24 Patellar fixation techniques. **A**, Conventional construct with two longitudinal k-wires with a figure-of-eight, commonly used for transverse fractures. **B**, Same construct with an additional cerclage wire for a more comminuted or stellate fracture. **C**, Use of two lag screws. The figure-of-eight wire has been placed behind the screws here, but is often passed through the cannulation of the screw.

## Surgical techniques

Several techniques are described. The most widely used is the tension band technique (p. 95). Modifications to this technique (**Fig. 19.24**) include the use of:

- interfragmentary screws
- a cerclage wire around the circumference of the patella, especially in stellate fractures
- cannulated screws instead of longitudinal wires, with the cerclage wire threaded through the central cannulation.

Other surgical strategies are occasionally required:

- *Fragment excision*: Where there is a small or comminuted fracture at either pole of the patella, repair may be more secure if the

## SURGICAL TECHNIQUE: Tension band wire fixation of a patellar fracture

### Surgical set-up
The patient is placed supine. A tourniquet is not usually required.

### Incision
The patella is exposed through a longitudinal incision.

### Open reduction
The fracture fragments are cleared and reduced. Reduction is aided by passing a finger through the rent in the retinaculum and feeling the articular surface alignment. The reduction is held with reduction forceps and checked with fluoroscopy.

### Internal fixation – absolute stability (Fig. 19.25)
1. Longitudinal K wires – retrograde: Longitudinal k-wires are used to prevent fracture translation. These can be driven across the fracture from one end of the patella.

*Continued*

Alternatively, a more accurate position in the bone can be achieved with the use of double-ended wires. Firstly, the wires are passed retrograde from the fractured bone surface through the proximal fragment until just the tips of the wires are protruding beyond the fractured surface.

2. Longitudinal k wires – antegrade: The fracture is then held reduced with a clamp and the wires are driven antegrade through the distal fragment.

3. Figure-of-eight tension band: Compression at the joint surface is achieved with a figure-of-eight wire, looped behind the k-wires. This is passed through the quadriceps and patellar tendons, and as close to the bone and the wires as possible; this placement is aided by use of a 14G intravenous cannula.

4. Cutting the wires: The wire is tightened and twisted (see Fig. 5.21). The longitudinal wires are then bent at one end, rotated so that the curved end points back into the tendon, and hammered into place. The other end of the wires is also bent, or (to ease future removal) cut flush with the surface of the tendon.

The rents in the patella retinaculum are repaired last. If a solid repair has been achieved, the knee is brought into 60° of flexion to check the integrity of the fixation. If this is satisfactory, the patient can be allowed 45° of knee flexion during healing. If there is doubt about the integrity of the repair, a period of knee extension may be necessary.

### Postoperative restrictions

Movement: A 0–45° range of movement is permitted.

Weight-bearing: Full weight-bearing in a hinged knee brace is allowed.

fragment is excised and the injury treated as for a quadriceps or patellar tendon avulsion.

- *Patellectomy*: Occasionally, multifragmentary, stellate fractures are unreconstructable and excision of the entire patella and direct suture of the quadriceps tendon to the patellar tendon is unavoidable.

## Outpatient management

### Operative and non-operative patellar fractures

| Outpatient management summary | | | |
|---|---|---|---|
| **Week** | **Examination** | **Radiographs** | **Additional notes** |
| 1 | Wound check<br><br>Neurovascular status | AP and lateral knee | Allow a restricted range of movement in a knee brace; range is dependent on fracture configuration and fixation, and is often 0–45°. Allow full weight-bearing |
| 6 | Range of movement check<br><br>Check for tenderness at fracture site | AP and lateral knee | If the fracture is united and pain-free, then discharge the patient to physiotherapy. If there are issues, review at 8 weeks |

Further assessments at 2–4-week intervals if required for delayed union

Average time to union = 6 weeks

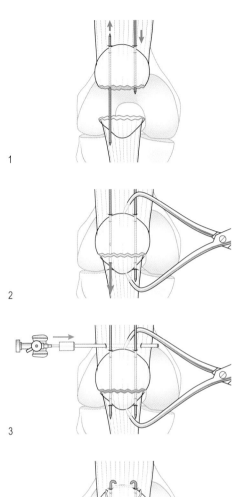

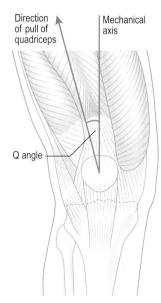

Fig. 19.26 The 'Q' angle.

Fig. 19.25 Patella tension band wire.

## PATELLAR DISLOCATION

Patellar dislocation is a common knee injury. Some patients will present with the clear deformity of a lateral patellar dislocation, but many patellae will have reduced spontaneously before presentation. Many individuals, particularly young, hypermobile women with a large 'Q' angle (see below), will have a history of previ-ous patellar dislocation or subluxation, and will recognize the injury themselves. Often, however, it may be unclear to patients what happened and they will describe the whole knee 'giving way'.

## Pathoanatomy of patellofemoral stability

The patella is vulnerable to instability, particularly lateral dislocation. This is partially because the direction of pull of the quadriceps muscle is slightly lateral to the mechanical axis of the limb; this is termed the quadriceps (or Q) angle (**Fig. 19.26**). The patella is held in place by a combination of static and dynamic stabilizers:

### Static stabilizers
- The sides of the trochlea of the femur are formed from the femoral condyles. The size and shape of the lateral femoral condyle in particular is important.
- The medial retinaculum of the knee joint capsule is reinforced by a thickening, the medial patellofemoral ligament (MPFL), which limits lateral movement of the patella.

*Dynamic stabilizers*

● The most distal component of the quadriceps muscle, vastus medialis obliquus (VMO), exerts a medially directed pull to maintain patellar position.

# Emergency Department management

## Clinical features

● There is tenderness of the medial patellar retinaculum and a positive patellar apprehension test.

● Exclude knee joint (tibiofemoral) instability.

## Radiological features

● *AP and lateral knee radiographs*: The patellar dislocation may be evident on plain radiographs. However, radiographs are often entirely normal if the patella has been reduced, although, on close inspection of the soft tissues, a loose body may be seen within the knee. This may represent an osteochondral fragment that has been detached from the articular surface of the patella or trochlea.

● *Skyline knee radiograph*: Skyline views may be helpful for later evaluation of instability but rarely offer useful additional information in the acute setting.

## Closed reduction

A dislocated patella is reduced under procedural sedation. The manœuvre is rarely difficult and simply consists of placing the thumbs over the lateral aspect of the patella and pushing it medially and anteriorly into the femoral trochlea.

## Immobilization and reassessment

The knee is immobilized for comfort in an extension knee splint. If a reduction has been performed, reassess the neurovascular status.

## Outpatient follow-up

● The patient is referred for review in an outpatient clinic.

# Orthopaedic management

## Non-operative

Almost all patellar dislocations are managed non-operatively, with rapid weaning from bracing within the first week or two as comfort allows, and early active physiotherapy rehabilitation.

## Operative

Surgical intervention is indicated in the presence of:

● *Open injuries*, to debride and close the wound.

● *Loose intra-articular bodies*, usually osteochondral fragments from either the patellar or trochlear articular surface. These are usually small and are retrieved arthroscopically. Rarely, a fragment of lateral femoral condyle will be large enough to warrant reduction and fixation.

● *Recurrent patellar instability*. This can be addressed on an elective basis with a number of stabilization procedures.

## Surgical techniques

Recurrent instability can be addressed with a variety of procedures:

● *MPFL reconstruction*: This aims to reconstruct a check-rein to lateral subluxation, usually using a hamstring graft placed between the medial femoral condyle and the patella.

● *Proximal realignment*: There are a number of modifications of the Insall procedure, which involve a lateral retinacular release and a medial retinacular or VMO advancement.

● *Distal realignment*: Where the tibial tuberosity is excessively lateral compared to the trochlea groove (high TT–TG measurement), resulting in a high Q angle, an osteotomy can be performed to medialize and advance the tuberosity.

## NON-SPECIFIC SOFT TISSUE KNEE INJURY

Numerically, most patients with knee pain presenting to the Emergency Department have either:

● Non-specific soft tissue injury (a sprain) with no definable structural abnormality.

● Exacerbation of pre-existing osteoarthritis of the knee: These patients often have joint-line tenderness from degeneration of both the articular and the meniscal cartilages, but very rarely have a surgically treatable meniscal tear or ligamentous injury.

# Emergency Department management

## Clinical features

These typically stem from a low-energy fall or a sporting collision. Be particularly suspicious of any high-energy mechanism of injury, such as a motorcycle collision or a fall from a height. A history of pre-existing arthritis is important.

A full, careful clinical examination is required to exclude:

- a knee dislocation or fracture
- an isolated knee ligament rupture
- an extensor mechanism disruption
- dislocation of the patella (with or without spontaneous reduction)

- a locked knee following a bucket-handle meniscal tear.

## Outpatient follow-up

A non-specific soft tissue knee injury is a diagnosis of exclusion. Where the history is benign and the examination has excluded structural injury, patients should be discharged with advice to rest, apply ice and elevate ('RICE advice'), and begin early active mobilization. Referral to physiotherapy may be appropriate.

A full examination may not be possible in the Emergency Department owing to pain or swelling. Where suspicion of a structural injury remains, re-examination after 7–14 days, once the swelling and pain have abated, is often far more rewarding. Such patients should be referred to an orthopaedic clinic for review, with the provision of analgesia, crutches and a knee extension splint for comfort.

## GENERAL PRINCIPLES

### Anatomy

The proximal tibial metaphysis consists of two condyles – medial and lateral – separated by the tibial spines (**Fig. 20.1**). The articular surface of the medial plateau is concave, whereas that of the lateral plateau is convex. These articular surfaces of the tibia are covered, and to some extent protected, by the medial and lateral menisci (see Fig. 19.2). The proximal and distal articular surfaces of the tibia (at the knee and ankle) are parallel, and are orthogonal to the long axis of the tibia in the coronal plane. Angular deformity is not tolerated as well as in the femur or humerus, where the ball-and-socket joints can compensate. The plateau has a posterior slope of 10°.

The tibial shaft is triangular in cross-section. The anteromedial surface is subcutaneous and the soft tissue envelope around a tibial fracture is therefore highly vulnerable. Open fractures are relatively common, as is the requirement for complex soft tissue reconstruction after injury (p. 41). The lateral and posterior faces of the tibia are covered in the four fascial compartments of the leg (see Fig. 3.8), and tibial fractures may result in swelling of the muscle within these, resulting in acute compartment syndrome (p. 45).

Posterior to the knee joint is the popliteal fossa and its traversing neurovascular structures (see Fig. 19.3). These are immobile and thus highly vulnerable after a proximal tibial fracture and during surgery. Below the level of the trifurcation, the three vessels (the anterior and posterior tibial arteries and peroneal artery) pass through the anterior, posterior and lateral compartments, respectively, and remain vulnerable to injury in tibial fracture. The common peroneal nerve is closely applied to the fibular neck as it traverses from the popliteal fossa to the anterior compartment, and is vulnerable to direct and indirect injury here.

## Clinical assessment of the injured leg

Anatomically, the leg is that part of the lower limb below the knee; the proximal segment of the lower limb is termed the thigh. Because the anteromedial surface of the tibia is subcutaneous, tibial fractures are usually apparent at admission as a clinical deformity or as an open injury.

### History

Tibial fractures often follow sporting injuries and falls. Where a tibial fracture has occurred after high-energy injury, initial primary and secondary surveys and appropriate investigations should be carried out to exclude life-threatening injury.

### Examination

*Look*

Assess for deformity and shortening of the limb, swelling of the leg, open wounds and skin compromise. Inspect carefully for other injuries, particularly to the ipsilateral knee and ankle.

*Feel*

Palpate for prominence of the bone ends. As you apply traction and realign a deformed limb, you may feel crepitus.

*Move*

It will be apparent as you realign the limb that the tibia does not move as one segment. Assess active movements at the ankle and toes.

*Neurovascular assessment*

● Palpate for both the dorsalis pedis and posterior tibial pulses. Mark these with an indelible ink cross to allow later reassessment.

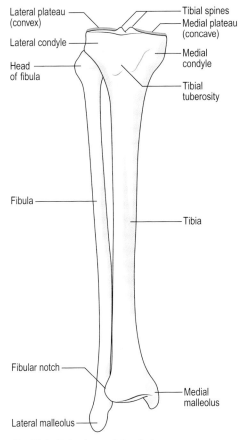

Lateral plateau (convex)
Lateral condyle
Head of fibula
Fibula
Fibular notch
Lateral malleolus
Tibial spines
Medial plateau (concave)
Medial condyle
Tibial tuberosity
Tibia
Medial malleolus

Fig. 20.1 Osteology of the leg.

- Assess very carefully for the signs and symptoms of *compartment syndrome* and consider the insertion of a compartment monitor (Fig. 3.7). Note that these features are not the same as the signs and symptoms of an acutely dysvascular limb.

## Radiological assessment of the injured leg

### Radiographs

- *AP and lateral views of the tibia and fibula*: These should include both the knee and the ankle. Films are taken with the patient supine and the knee straight.

- *Additional views*: Additional AP and lateral views of the knee or ankle joints, centred

on the joint line, may be required to assess intra-articular fractures or fracture extensions.

### CT
The fracture configuration of complex and bicondylar plateau fractures is better appreciated on axial imaging, which assists in preoperative planning. CT is not required for tibial shaft fractures.

### MRI
Complex plateau fractures, particularly in young patients, may be associated with substantial meniscal tears or ligamentous injury, and on occasion both a CT and an MRI are required.

### Angiography (or CT angiography)
This may be required in selected patients with impaired circulation (p. 58).

## TIBIAL PLATEAU FRACTURES
Tibial plateau fractures are severe intra-articular injuries of the knee. There is a bimodal distribution, with complex fractures occurring after high-energy injuries in the young, and low-energy insufficiency fractures occurring in the elderly. Plateau fractures occur within a vulnerable 'soft tissue envelope', which must be monitored and protected. Complications, such as infection, wound dehiscence, neurovascular injury and compartment syndrome, are more common after high-energy injury. Good outcomes are dependent on avoiding these surgical complications and restoring the mechanical axis of the limb.

## Classification
### Schatzker classification
The Schatzker classification defines the fracture in relation to the involvement of the medial and lateral condyles (**Fig. 20.2**).

I. *Split fracture of the lateral plateau*: These fractures are seen principally in young patients after a valgus injury.

II. *Split-depression fracture of the lateral plateau*: This is the most common type, and

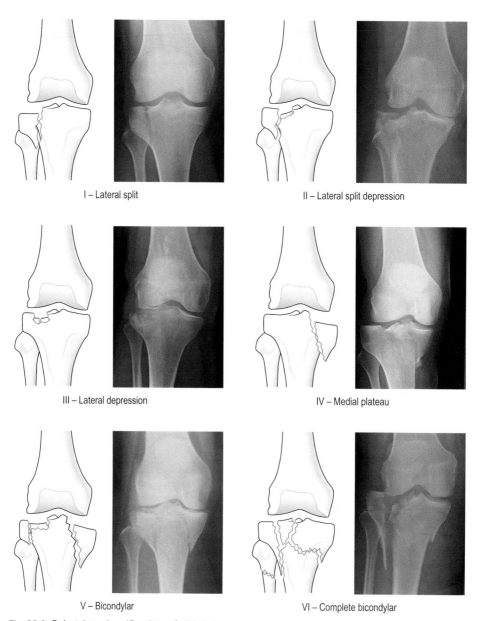

I – Lateral split

II – Lateral split depression

III – Lateral depression

IV – Medial plateau

V – Bicondylar

VI – Complete bicondylar

Fig. 20.2 Schatzker classification of tibial plateau fractures.

is most commonly seen in middle-aged and elderly patients after low-energy injuries.

III. *Depression fracture of the lateral plateau*: These are uncommon fragility fractures; with regular use of axial imaging, it is clear

that most fractures that appear to be type III on plain radiographs are actually type II.

IV. *Medial plateau fracture*: These are often high-energy injuries, which occur following a varus load to the knee. They may be

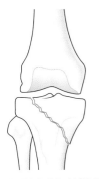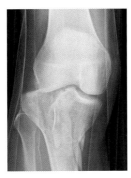

Fig. 20.3 AO 41B3.3 fracture.

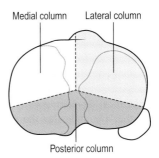

Fig. 20.4 Three-column concept.

fracture-dislocations in which the medial condyle remains correctly located under the medial femoral condyle, while the lateral condyle and tibial shaft are subluxed laterally and proximally.

V. *Bicondylar fracture*: This injury is extremely rare, involving both condyles but preserving the tibial spines.

VI. *Complete bicondylar fracture with metadiaphyseal separation*: This fracture typically follows a high-energy injury and, in addition to being a technically complex fracture to reduce and fix, has the highest rate of soft tissue complications.

### AO classification

The AO classification follows the universal pattern of describing extra-articular injuries as type A, partial articular injuries as type B, and complete articular injuries as type C (see Fig. 1.23). There are a number of groups and subgroups, which are principally useful for research. There is, however, one subtype that is of particular interest but is not represented in the Schatzker system, and that is the B3.3 fracture/dislocation of the knee. This is a medial condylar fracture that exits into the lateral compartment of the knee (**Fig. 20.3**). It is highly unstable and requires careful assessment and surgery (see Table 20.1).

### Three-column concept

The tibial plateau is classically considered to have two columns: medial and lateral. However,

the three-column concept draws attention to a posterior column, which, in Schatzker type V and VI fractures, may need to be reduced and fixed separately (**Fig. 20.4**).

## Emergency Department management

Tibial plateau fractures often present as knee injuries (p. 420).

### Clinical features

- Establish the mechanism of injury causing the fracture. A fall, or a blow to the outer side of the knee, in sport or even following a collision with a large dog, is common.

- High-energy injuries are often associated with severe injury to the soft tissue envelope around the knee; carefully assess the integrity of the skin and the distal neurovascular status.

- Tenderness will be found on palpation of the proximal tibia, often accompanied by swelling. Bruising will evolve gradually.

- Consider the possibility of an acute *compartment syndrome* (p. 45).

### Radiological features

- *AP and lateral knee radiographs*: The majority of tibial plateau fractures are clearly shown on plain films. However, more subtle fractures can be difficult to appreciate. Helpful radiographic features in uncertain cases include:

    The clarity of the joint surface: The joint line should be clear and smooth, with an uninterrupted white cortical line. Particularly in the elderly, minor impaction fractures are appreciated as the loss of this appearance (compare the lateral and medial joint lines in **Fig. 20.5**).

A lipohaemarthrosis (**Fig. 20.6**): The presence of a 'fat–fluid level' on a lateral view of the knee indicates the presence of both fat and blood within the capsule of the knee, which is pathognomonic of an intra-articular fracture. In contrast, homogenous fluid may represent a haemarthrosis (most commonly, a rupture of the anterior cruciate ligament), an effusion or pus.

- *CT*: Most complex tibial plateau fractures require a CT scan for preoperative planning.

- *MRI*: An MRI is useful where a combination of a tibial plateau fracture and a significant ligamentous or meniscal injury is anticipated.

### Closed reduction, immobilization and reassessment

Deformed limbs should be gently brought back into anatomical alignment before plain films are taken. An above-knee backslab is required if the limb has been realigned (see p. 72). In

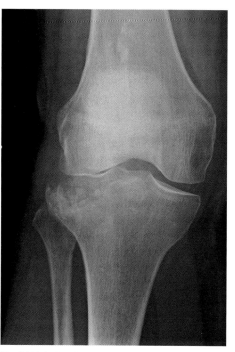

Fig. 20.5 Schatzker II fracture of the tibial plateau.

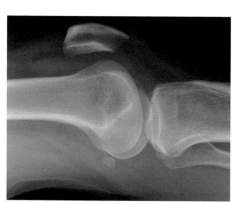
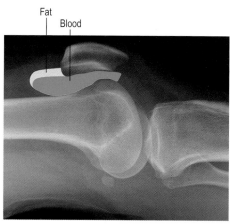

Fig. 20.6 Lipohaemarthrosis. Note the sharp delineation at the blood/fat interface level, most clearly seen when the radiograph is viewed in the same orientation as it was taken in. In this case the patient was supine.

minimally displaced fractures, a removable extension knee splint is often sufficient. Reassess the neurovascular supply to the limb.

## Inpatient referral

- All tibial plateau fractures should be referred to the orthopaedic service.

# Orthopaedic management

## Non-operative

Undisplaced or minimally displaced plateau fractures, which are usually Schatzker types I–III, can sometimes be managed non-operatively in a knee brace, and should be non-weight-bearing.

## Operative

Most plateau fractures are displaced and unstable, and require surgery. The aims of surgery are:

- To restore coronal alignment and axial stability: This has the most significant effect on outcome.
- To reduce and compress the articular surface: A step or gap >2 mm is widely considered to be the limit of acceptable displacement.

Plateau fractures are demanding fractures to manage, and surgery should only be undertaken by surgeons with the appropriate expertise. Although most plateau fractures are stabilized by primary internal fixation with plates, staged management with the initial application of a spanning external fixator may be indicated in the context of heavily contaminated open wounds, vascular injury, or tenuous viability of the soft tissue envelope (see Fig. 20.32). High-energy fractures are associated with compartment syndrome of the leg, and pressure monitoring (see Fig. 3.7) or repeated clinical assessment is required both before and after surgery.

## Surgical approaches to the tibial plateau

There are four principal surgical approaches to the tibial plateau; the choice of approach is dictated by the type of fracture. The antero-

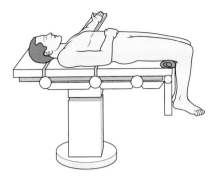

Fig. 20.7 Tibial plateau surgery: patient set-up.

lateral and posteromedial approaches can be performed with the patient supine and the knees flexed over the end of the operating table (**Fig. 20.7**). The extended posteromedial approach can also be performed in this position, but is also commonly performed with the patient in a lateral or prone position. The direct posterior approach is rarely used, and requires the patient to be placed prone.

### Anterolateral approach (Fig. 20.8)

The patient is positioned supine with the knee flexed to 90°. A tourniquet is used. A longitudinal midline incision is made, and may be curved posteriorly at its proximal end. A lateral parapatellar approach is made through the extensor mechanism, elevating a full-thickness flap that leaves only bone, fat pad and meniscus behind. A submeniscal arthrotomy is made through the coronary ligament to expose the lateral plateau fracture.

### Posteromedial approach (Fig. 20.9)

The incision is based over the palpable posterior edge of the tibia. Blunt dissection through fat is performed to avoid injury to the great saphenous nerve and vein. The pes anserinus (Latin: 'goose's foot'; the insertion of the hamstring tendons) crosses the proximal tibia. The pes may be retracted to allow the plate to be slid underneath it or divided. If it is divided, marking sutures can be placed in the tendons and used for repair during closure. The gastrocnemius is elevated posteriorly to expose the posteromedial corner of the tibia and the fracture.

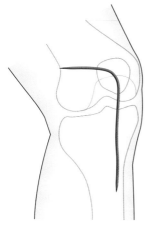
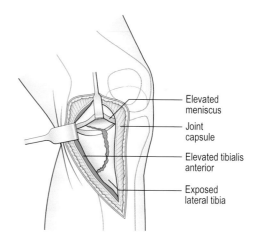

Elevated
meniscus

Joint
capsule

Elevated tibialis
anterior

Exposed
lateral tibia

Fig. 20.8 Anterolateral approach.

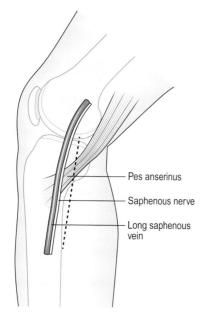
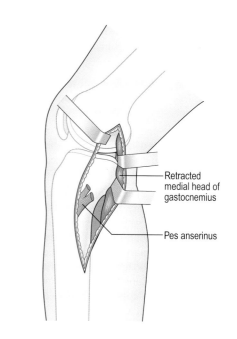

Pes anserinus

Saphenous nerve

Long saphenous
vein

Retracted
medial head of
gastocnemius

Pes anserinus

Fig. 20.9 Posteromedial approach.

### Extended posteromedial approach (Fig. 20.10)

This allows exposure of the entire posterior aspect of the tibia. The posteromedial incision is made as above, and extended transversely across the popliteal fossa. The medial head of gastrocnemius is retracted or, if necessary, released to allow an extensive submuscular plane to be developed.

### Direct posterior approach

This approach is used occasionally for avulsion fractures at the posterior cruciate ligament insertion or for access to the popliteal vessels, but is not commonly chosen for tibial plateau fractures. It involves a 'boat race' or 'lazy S' incision over the popliteal fossa. A formal dissection of the short saphenous vein (in the superficial plane) and of the popliteal artery,

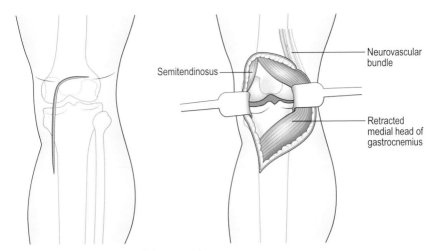

Fig. 20.10 Extended posteromedial approach.

vein and tibial nerve (in the deep plane) is then required. Ligation of the medial geniculate branches allows the neurovascular bundle to be retracted laterally. This exposes the posterior joint capsule, which is then divided to expose the knee joint.

## Surgical techniques

### Plate fixation

- *Unicondylar fractures* (AO B-type, Schatzker I–IV) are fixed by compression screws or buttress plating. The fracture and joint surface are exposed, cleared of clot and bone fragments, reduced, and then provisionally fixed and compressed with k-wires and bone clamps. Three or four lag screws with washers, or a contoured, low-profile buttress plate, are then applied to provide compression. Screws placed under the articular surface are described as a raft, but in fact are rather more like rafters holding up a roof. These 'rafters' are supported at one end by the plate and at the other end by the intact condyle of the tibia, and so do not need to be locked.

- *Bicondylar fractures* (AO C-type, Schatzker V and VI) are approached through separate incisions and the two condyles are buttressed individually (**Fig. 20.11**). The medial fragment is usually the larger, and is approached first via a posteromedial inci-

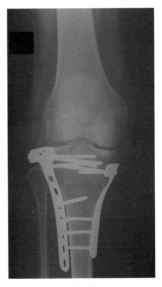

Fig. 20.11 Bicondylar plating.

sion. There is usually a clear posteromedial spike and this cortical fracture line can be 'keyed in' with confidence. The fragment is buttressed with a posteromedial plate (either a precontoured plate or a 3.5-mm dynamic compression plate is suitable) and becomes the 'keystone' on to which the remainder of the plateau fracture is reduced. The lateral condyle is then exposed and fixed through the anterolateral approach.

● *Posterior column fractures* are usually approached through an extended postero-medial incision. Only very rarely is a formal posterior (popliteal fossa) approach required. The patient can be placed prone, lateral, or supine with the knees flexed over the table edge.

These techniques are summarized in **Table 20.1**.

### Percutaneous screws

Simple split (type I) fractures can often be reduced closed by ligamentotaxis. Similarly, depressed (type II) fractures can often be

**Table 20.1    Plate fixation of tibial plateau fractures**

| Fracture type | Approach | Internal fixation |
| --- | --- | --- |
| Schatzker I | Percutaneous | Minimally displaced split fractures that can be elevated percutaneously, often with the assistance of a varus force to the knee, can be fixed with percutaneous cannulated screws (**Fig. 20.12**) |
| | Anterolateral | If open reduction has been required, an anterolateral buttress plate is usually applied |
| Schatzker II–III | Percutaneous | Depressed fractures can be reduced percutaneously with punches under fluoroscopic or arthroscopic control. The fracture is then fixed with percutaneous screws. A contained void is often left just under the joint, and calcium phosphate cement can be used to support the articular surface (**Fig. 20.13**) |
| | Anterolateral | Where an open reduction is required, a lateral buttress plate, with a 'raft' of screws placed under the reconstructed plateau, is used |
| Schatzker IV | Posteromedial | The fracture line is usually in the sagittal plane and a direct medial approach is used to apply a low-profile medial buttress plate |
| AO B3.3 | Posteromedial ± anterolateral | A careful assessment of the preoperative CT may reveal incarcerated fracture or meniscal fragments within the fracture. An initial lateral arthrotomy or arthroscopy may be required to remove these. A medial approach is then made and the fracture is reduced and compressed with a buttress plate. The fracture line in the lateral plateau is appraised critically. Any persistent gapping of the fracture or widening of the plateau suggests ongoing interposition of bone fragments or incarceration of the lateral meniscus |

| Table 20.1 | Plate fixation of tibial plateau fractures—cont'd | |
|---|---|---|
| Fracture type | Approach | Internal fixation |
| Schatzker V–VI | Posteromedial then anterolateral | Type V and VI fractures typically consist of a large medial or posteromedial plateau fragment, variable involvement of the tibial spines, and a comminuted and displaced lateral plateau. Entirely undisplaced medial condyle fragments can be fixed from the lateral side using intraoperative clamp compression and then fixation with a locked plate but, more commonly, double plating through two incisions is required. A posteromedial incision allows access to the large 'keystone' fragment, which can usually be reduced to an anatomical position with the posterolateral cortex. A buttress plate is applied (**Fig. 20.14A**). A separate anterolateral exposure is then performed, and the rest of the plateau is reduced on to this keystone. The articular surface is stabilized and compressed with lag screws (**Fig. 20.14B**) and then a lateral plate (often locking) is inserted (**Fig. 20.14C, D**). In the example shown in **Figure 20.14**, a third dynamic compression plate has been used anteriorly to secure an avulsed tibial tuberosity |

elevated percutaneously under fluoroscopic or arthroscopic control. A punch is inserted through the fracture line or a 'trap door' created under the tibial flare (**Fig. 20.13A**). These fractures can then be stabilized by large (7-mm) percutaneous cannulated screws (**Fig. 20.13B, C**). Calcium phosphate cement is often injected percutaneously as a bone graft substitute to fill the resulting defect (**Fig. 20.13D**).

### External fixation

Fine wire frames can be used for complex fractures with severe soft tissue damage. Small arthrotomy incisions are used to reduce the fracture and allow interfragmentary compression screw placement. The major fragments are then compressed using olive wires. Finally, the area of metadiaphyseal comminution is bridged with the frame. Frame treatment is principally indicated for management of complications, including infection, malunion and non-union.

### Arthroscopic surgery

Minimally displaced type I–IV fractures can be seen clearly with an arthroscope. This allows percutaneous reduction of the fracture under arthroscopic view prior to percutaneous fixation (**Table 20.1**).

## Outpatient management

Management will vary depending on the fracture 'personality', stability of the fixation, and age and state of health of the patient. A hinged knee brace is usually worn to restrict range of movement to 0–90°. Complex intra-articular fractures of the lower limb may require 12 weeks of non-weight-bearing. This period is reduced where the fracture is simple, bone quality good and fixation secure, and the patient is a reliable non-smoker.

Elderly patients may not be able to mobilize at all with weight-bearing restrictions and pragmatically are usually allowed full weight-bearing after percutaneous reduction and fixation of type II fractures.

### ✓ Key point

Bicondylar plating through a *single* midline anterior incision, with the elevation of both medial and lateral flaps, requires significant stripping and may compromise the blood supply to the wound edges and the fracture fragments. This is colloquially referred to as a 'dead bone sandwich' and has an increased rate of wound dehiscence and infection.

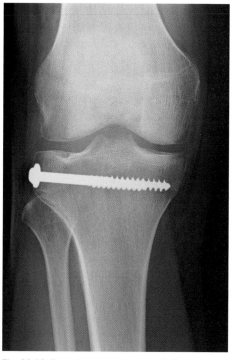

Fig. 20.12 Percutaneous screws: Schatzker I (split).

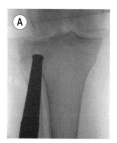 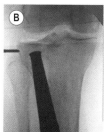 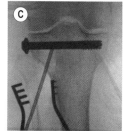 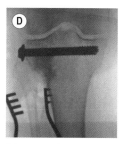

Fig. 20.13 Percutaneous fixation of a Schatzker II fracture. **A**, Elevation with a punch through a cortical window. **B**, Secured with a 3.2-mm guide-wire. **C**, Fixed with cannulated screws. **D**, CaPO4 cement. See **Table 20.1** for details.

## COMPLICATIONS

### *Early*

Local    Vascular injury: The popliteal artery is 'crucified to the skeleton' behind the knee and may be injured (Fig. 19.3)

Neurological injury: Both the common peroneal and tibial nerves are at risk of injury. This is usually a neurapraxia or axonotmesis and usually resolves spontaneously, at least in part

*Continued*

## COMPLICATIONS... cont'd

Wound dehiscence and infection: These are more common after a single midline incision followed by both medial and lateral exposure, or an incision placed directly over plates. It may also occur after extensive incisions through a devitalized soft tissue envelope

Compartment syndrome: This is most common after high-energy type VI fractures (p. 45)

### Late

Local     Delayed union or non-union: This occurs most commonly at the metadiaphyseal junction where there is comminution or inadequate stability. Management is with revised compression plating, with or without additional autogenous bone graft

Post-traumatic osteoarthritis: Although radiographic joint space narrowing is relatively common after plateau fractures, the rate of conversion to a total knee replacement is <5%, and is usually related to failure to regain coronal stability

Stiffness: Post-traumatic arthrofibrosis is common and may require surgical release

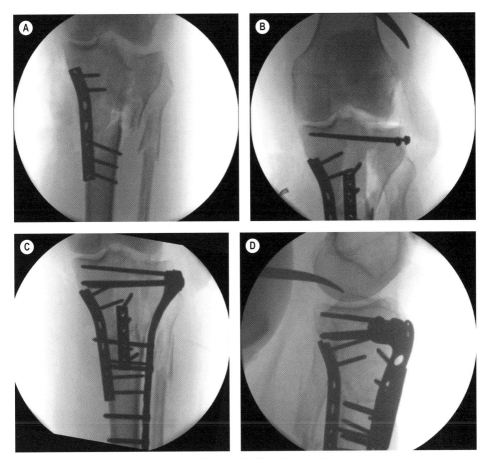

Fig. 20.14 Plate fixation. Schatzker VI. See **Table 20.1** for details.

## TIBIAL SHAFT FRACTURES

The tibial shaft is vulnerable to direct injury (in falls, collisions and direct blows) and indirect injury (twisting and bending forces). It can also be affected by stress fractures in military recruits, runners and dancers. Fractures of the proximal and distal thirds have a different mechanical behaviour from mid-shaft fractures and caution is required when fixing these. The vulnerability of the soft tissue envelope, particularly anteromedially, and the threat of compartment syndrome both require careful consideration.

## Classification

### AO classification

The AO universal classification of fractures is applied (see Fig. 1.21). Some configurations have particular implications:

- A fracture of the *proximal third* will have a tendency to collapse into valgus and flexion before, during or even after fixation and should be managed cautiously.

- Very *distal fractures* are also relatively unstable.

- A tibial fracture with an *intact fibula* will have a tendency to collapse into varus. There is a higher rate of non-union. Consideration should be given to fixing these fractures, even if they are initially undisplaced.

## Emergency Department management

### Clinical features

- A careful history of the mechanism of injury is required. A description of a direct or indirect force will allow an appreciation of the amount of soft tissue damage present and the likelihood of other injuries.

- There may be clear deformity, which should be reduced on recognition. Carefully assess the integrity of the skin, looking for lacerations and abrasions that would indicate an open fracture.

- Avoid unnecessary movement except to realign a deformed limb.

- Consider whether there is an acute vascular injury (p. 58). Palpate the dorsalis pedis and posterior tibial pulsations, and mark their locations with ink to allow later reassessment. Assess the capillary refill to the toes.

- Consider whether there is an acute *compartment syndrome* and think about inserting a compartment monitor (see Fig. 3.7). The clinical features of compartment syndrome are different from those of an acutely dysvascular limb and are:

  i  Pain out of proportion to the injury sustained.

  ii  Pain on passive stretching of the muscles within the affected compartment. The anterior compartment is most commonly affected, so passive plantar flexion of the ankle and toes is unexpectedly painful.

  iii  Paraesthesia and hypoaesthesia in the distribution of the nerves travelling through the affected compartment. Check the distributions of the superficial peroneal, deep peroneal and tibial nerves. Do not be falsely reassured by normal sensation in the saphenous distribution (femoral nerve) (see Figs 3.20–3.22).

  iv  Reduced power in the muscles within the affected compartment. There is most commonly weakness of foot and hallux dorsiflexion (anterior compartment) and foot eversion (lateral compartment).

  v  Tight and tense feel on palpation of the affected compartment.

### Radiological features

- *AP and lateral tibia and fibula radiographs* (**Fig. 20.15**): The knee and ankle should be included. The fracture is normally easy to identify but careful attention should be given to the possibility of an intra-articular extension.

### Closed reduction

The tibia should be realigned without delay under procedural sedation. An anatomical reduction is not required, but the tibia should be out to length and straight, in neutral rotation, and with no areas of bony prominence under the skin. Reduction is achieved with gentle traction first (**Fig. 20.16**). The thumbs are then used to palpate the subcutaneous tibial crest at the level of the fracture to assess adequacy of the reduction, and to correct any residual translation.

## Immobilization and reassessment

An above-knee backslab is applied with 20° of knee flexion in order to control rotation (see p. 72). The first web space of the foot should be in line with the patella. Note that a below-knee backslab is insufficient, as it will not control rotation at the fracture (see p. 73). Reassess the neurovascular status and obtain repeat radiographs in cast (**Fig. 20.17**).

## Inpatient referral

- Refer all tibial shaft fractures to the orthopaedic service.
- The presence of an acute vascular injury or a compartment syndrome is a surgical emergency.

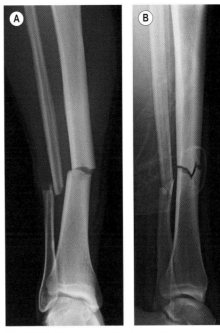

Fig. 20.15 Tibial shaft fracture. Simple, transverse mid-diaphyseal fractures of both tibia and fibula. **A**, AP view. **B**, Lateral view.

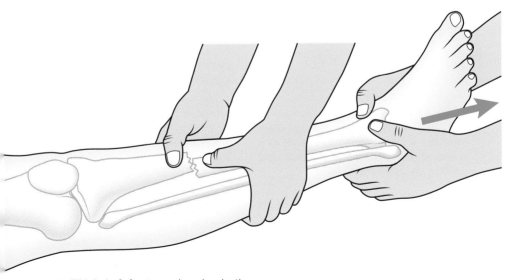

Fig. 20.16 Tibial shaft fracture: closed reduction.

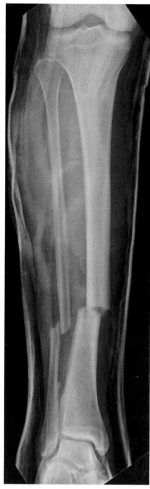

Fig. 20.17 Tibial shaft fracture: plaster backslab.

- Open fractures require specialist management and should be referred urgently to a centre with appropriate orthopaedic and plastic surgical facilities.

## Orthopaedic management

### Non-operative

- Closed, undisplaced, neurovascularly intact fractures of the tibia and fibula may be suitable for non-operative management in cast (**Fig. 20.18**).

- Minimally displaced fractures with <10° of coronal, sagittal or rotational deformity and <10 mm of shortening may also be considered.

An above-knee cast is worn for 4–6 weeks until some callus becomes visible at the fracture site. This is then exchanged for a patellar tendon-bearing (PTB) cast for a further 6 weeks, and then a below-knee cast for 4 weeks. Weight-bearing is allowed from 4 weeks. Time to union is around 16 weeks. Careful clinical and radiographic monitoring is required to ensure that the fracture does not displace during this period. Small corrections in angulation can be made with cast wedging.

### Plaster wedging

Small angulatory deformities during plaster management can be addressed with plaster wedging, although conversion to surgical fixation usually provides a more predictable outcome (**Fig. 20.19**).

1. Mark the cast at the level of the deformity, using the radiographs as a guide.

2. The plaster should be left intact at the apex of the fracture. This acts as a hinge to correct the deformity. For example, where there is apex-medial angulation only (normal lateral film), the plaster should remain intact medially. Where there is lateral angulation along with posterior angulation, the apex will be posterolateral, and this is where the plaster should remain intact.

3. Saw the cast circumferentially seven-eighths of the way round, leaving only the small section at the apex. Spring the cast open on this hinge by 2 cm, wedging it open with a small piece of cork. Check radiographs are now taken, with further correction as required. Once alignment is adequate, the cast is completed.

### Operative

Most tibial shaft fractures are managed operatively. Emergency surgery is required in the presence of an acute compartment syndrome or a critically ischaemic limb and definitive

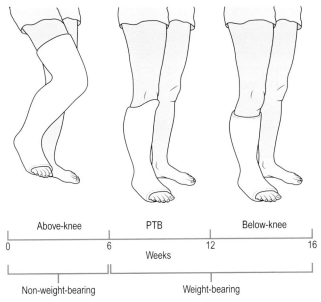

Fig. 20.18 Tibial shaft: non-operative management plan. PTB, patellar tendon-bearing.

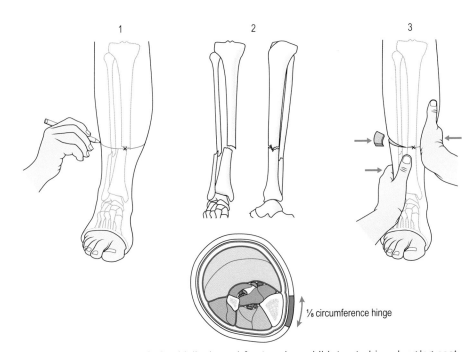

Fig. 20.19 Plaster wedging. **A**, A mid-diaphyseal fracture in a child, treated in a long-leg cast, has displaced into varus. **B**, The cast has been wedged to restore alignment.

fixation of the fracture can usually be performed at the same procedure. Open fractures are managed as an emergency or urgently, depending on the degree and nature of contamination present. Patients with severe multiple injuries may not be stable enough to undergo definitive treatment immediately, and consideration should be given to temporary external fixation (**Fig. 20.31**).

Concurrent fibular fractures should generally be ignored; they heal well once the tibia has been stabilized. In very distal injuries where both tibia and fibula are fractured at the same level, it is tempting to plate the fibula to aid reduc-

tion. However, the ankle joint is usually stable and fibula plating increases the stiffness of the construct and the chance of a non-union of the tibia.

## Surgical techniques

Most tibial fractures are managed by intramedullary nailing, although plates and external fixators are also used.

### Intramedullary nailing (Fig. 20.20)

Nailing is used almost universally for tibial fractures because it allows minimally invasive

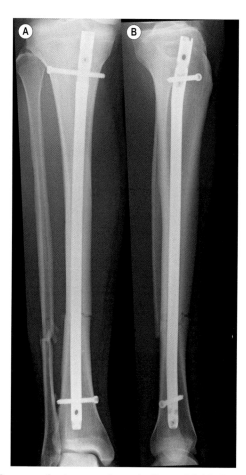

Fig. 20.20 Tibial nail. The same fracture as shown in Figure 20.15, fixed with a locked, intramedullary nail. **A**, AP view. **B**, Lateral view.

surgery, without exposure or stripping of the fracture or the periosteum, with a construct that is biomechanically intrinsically very stable (p. 98). Reaming is almost always employed, as it allows the implantation of larger, stronger nails with stronger screws, and is associated with greater union rates than unreamed nails (p. 100). Primary nailing of open fractures after adequate assessment and debridement is usually appropriate.

## SURGICAL TECHNIQUE: Tibial nailing for mid-shaft or distal fractures

### Surgical set-up
Tibial nailing is performed on traction or freehand over a bolster:

- Traction table (**Fig. 20.21A**): The patient is positioned supine on the table; the uninjured leg is placed in a gutter support with the hip and knee both flexed to 90°. The injured limb rests over a bolster placed behind the distal femur so as not to compress the popliteal fossa. The foot is secured to a traction plate and held with adhesive tape. Alternatively, a Denholm pin or wire can be placed through the calcaneus to control the foot.
- Freehand with a radiolucent triangle (**Fig. 20.21B**): The patient is supine, with the uninjured leg resting on the table. The injured leg rests over a radiolucent triangle, with the foot secured and controlled by an assistant.
- Semi-extended position: the patient is supine with the knee extended or slightly flexed, resting on a low radiolucent block to allow a retropatellar or parapatellar approach. This is particularly helpful with proximal tibial fractures. Specific instrumentation can make surgery easier.

Rehearse taking AP and lateral fluoroscopic images to ensure an adequate reduction has been achieved, and that no equipment or table attachments obscure the c-arm.

### Reduction
It is essential to achieve an accurate reduction during reaming and nailing. If reaming is performed in a malreduced tibia, the nail will follow the same path and leave the tibia malaligned. The application of traction, then rotational correction, is often sufficient to reduce the fracture. A fracture that remains displaced after set-up on traction can be realigned by:

- The application of varus/valgus stress or flexion/extension to the fracture by an assistant. Pushing with a blunt object such as a mallet is used to allow fluoroscopic evaluation (**Fig. 20.22A**).
- The use of a percutaneously applied reduction clamp, placed through stab incisions, for oblique or spiral fractures (**Fig. 20.22B**).

It is essential for any technique, even simple external pressure with a mallet, to be maintained until the nail is fully inserted.

### Incision (Fig. 20.23)
For mid-shaft or distal fractures, a small transverse or longitudinal incision is made over the medial aspect of the proximal patellar tendon and the capsule opened longitudinally to expose the proximal tibia.

*Continued*

Proximal tibial fractures behave differently and the incision may be made over the lateral aspect of the patellar tendon (see below).

### Start point

The correct start point is crucial and is judged on AP and lateral images. If the guide-wire position is changed to improve its position on one fluoroscopic view, the orthogonal view must also be checked before proceeding.

For mid-shaft and distal fractures (**Fig. 20.24**):

- AP image: The start point is at the medial edge of the patella tendon, and is approximately at the mid-point of the proximal metaphysis.
- Lateral image: The start point is at the corner between the plateau and anterior cortex.

For proximal fractures:

- These behave differently and require separate consideration (see below).

### Procedure (Fig. 20.25)

1. Threaded guide-wire insertion: After the starting point is checked fluoroscopically, a threaded guide wire is passed into the proximal tibia. The trajectory of this wire in the coronal plane is judged by placing the thumb and index finger on the tibial crest in the mid-shaft and aiming between them (**Fig. 20.24**). In the sagittal plane, pulling back on the wire driver will deliver the wire tip anteriorly.
2. Cannulated drill insertion: A drill is then passed over the wire into the centre of the metaphysis to prepare the entry point.
3. Ball-tipped guide-wire insertion: The flexible guide wire is then passed across the fracture and into the distal metaphysis. During guide-wire insertion, there is a tendency for the wire to become snagged on the posterior cortex; the wire tip can be steered anteriorly using the reduction spoon. The correct finish point for the wire tip is at the physeal scar, in line with the centre of the talus, not the centre of the tibial metaphysis.
4. Measurement: A measuring device is used to select the correct length of nail; the accuracy of this measurement is improved by taking a *lateral* fluoroscopic image of the measuring device in place at the level of the knee.
5. Reaming: Sequential reamers are used to enlarge the endosteal space. To avoid burning the bone or the reamer becoming stuck, these should be sharp, used at full speed and advanced gradually and continuously, while not being allowed to stop at one level. If pressure or a reduction clamp was required to achieve perfect reduction, this continues to be applied during reaming and nailing. As the reamer is withdrawn, the guide wire is grasped with a clamp to prevent displacement. Cortical 'chatter' at the isthmus indicates that the correct width of reamer has been achieved. A nail is selected that is 1 mm smaller in diameter.
6. Nail insertion: The nail is implanted with hammer blows until fully seated. If there has been more than 1 mm of fracture distraction during nailing, and the fracture is transverse, consideration is given to releasing traction, locking distally and then back-slapping to reduce the fracture. Be cautious: in a comminuted, oblique or spiral fracture, this may cause shortening and displacement.

7. Locking: The nail should be cross-locked to control length and rotation. Proximally, this is done through the jig. Distally, this is done freehand using a 'perfect circles' technique (see Fig. 18.20). Two or more screws are used in very proximal or distal fragments to maintain alignment.

**Post procedure**
The wounds are closed and the insertion of a compartment pressure monitor should be considered.

**Postoperative restrictions**
Movement: A full range of knee and ankle movement is encouraged.

Weight-bearing: Full weight-bearing is permitted unless there is a specific concern regarding the stability of the fracture.

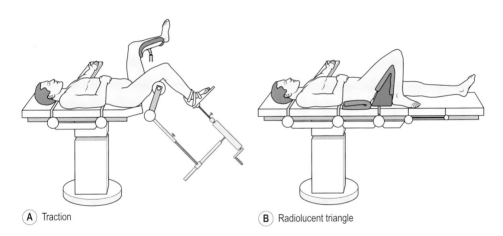

(A) Traction

(B) Radiolucent triangle

Fig. 20.21 Tibial nail: set-up.

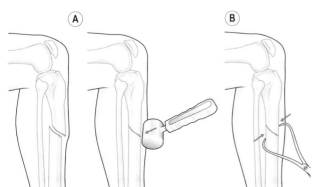

Fig. 20.22 Tibial nail: reduction.

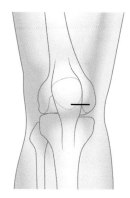

Fig. 20.23 Tibial nail: a horizontal incision in Langer's lines is shown. A vertical incision may be preferred.

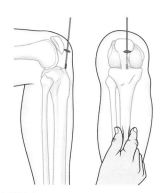

Fig. 20.24 Tibial nail: identifying the correct start point and trajectory.

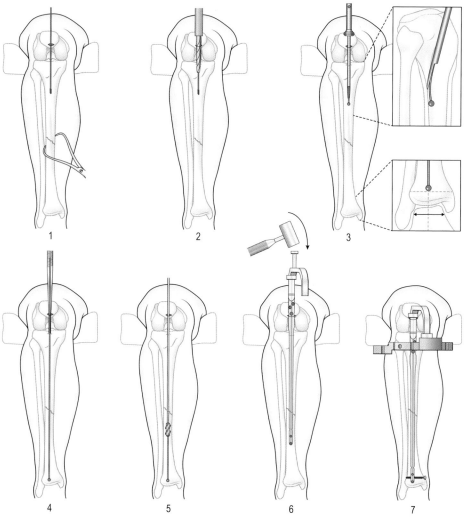

Fig. 20.25 Tibial nail: procedure. See surgical technique box (p. 461).

## Considerations in proximal tibial fractures (Fig. 20.26)

Very proximal tibial fractures have a tendency to displace into flexion and valgus. The nail grips the metaphysis at its entry point but does not lie against the cortex at the level of the fracture. This allows the fragment to rotate until the lateral and posterior cortices meet the nail. A number of surgical techniques are used to ensure adequate alignment when nailing:

1. *Lateral starting point*: A lateral parapatellar start point will allow the nail to rest against the lateral cortex of the proximal fragment, resisting the valgus rotational moment, and is often all that is required to prevent valgus collapse.

2. *Blocking screws*: These are bicortical screws, inserted before reaming and nailing. A blocking screw blocks the incorrect path of the nail and forces it in a different direction, resulting in correct alignment. An alternative way to conceptualize this is to think of the screw acting as an artificial 'cortex' in an optimal position. In the proximal tibia, blocking screws are placed laterally to prevent valgus, and posteriorly to prevent flexion.

3. *'Stitch' plate*: Open reduction of the fracture through a small incision, and the application of a two- or four-hole unicortical plate before nailing, will maintain alignment in both coronal and sagittal planes.

4. *Semi-extended nailing*: Setting up the patient in 90° of knee flexion can in itself cause fracture flexion. Longer instruments are available that allow nailing with the knee in extension via a parapatellar or suprapatellar incision.

## Considerations in distal tibial fractures

The same situation of a narrow nail in a broad metaphysis (a 'broomstick in a bucket'; see Fig. 18.33) exists at the distal tibia. This is not usually as much of a problem as it is proximally; the distal fracture can normally be held in correct alignment manually, with a percutaneous reduction clamp, or with external pressure with a mallet or other blunt pusher, during nailing, and held with multiple multiplanar locking screws (**Fig. 20.27**). However, the use of blocking screws or a stitch plate can, on occasion, be helpful.

## Distal intra-articular extensions

Fractures that extend into the ankle joint require separate consideration (**Fig. 20.28**). Where the fracture is completely undisplaced, a standard nailing technique with careful fluoroscopic monitoring of the fracture is usually successful. Where the fracture is displaced, or becomes displaced intraoperatively, reduction and the placement of lag screws (**Fig. 20.28B**) in the metaphysis will often recreate a stable metaphyseal block, which then allows successful nailing (**Fig. 20.28C, D**).

## Segmental fractures

A tibial shaft fracture at two levels is well suited to nailing. There is often a theoretical concern that the intercalated fragment will spin within the leg as it is reamed. This does not occur unless the fragment has been completely stripped of soft tissue in a devastating open injury. One of the fractures will usually heal promptly, while the second fracture may go on to delayed or even non-union and require revision surgery – usually exchange nailing. This occurs as a result of the change in the biomechanical environment that occurs during healing. Initially, small amounts of movement occur at both fracture sites, and this diminishes with fracture healing. When one fracture unites, all the movement is redirected to the second fracture and this can disrupt the process of healing.

## Plating of tibial fractures (Fig. 20.29)

Very proximal or distal fractures, particularly those with intra-articular extensions, can be difficult to reduce and hold with nailing, and a locked plate may be preferred. The disadvantages are the requirement for a relatively large incision, soft tissue dissection at the level of the fracture, and insufficient strength of the implant to allow weight-bearing. In the shaft of the tibia, the disadvantages are such that plating is very rare compared with nailing.

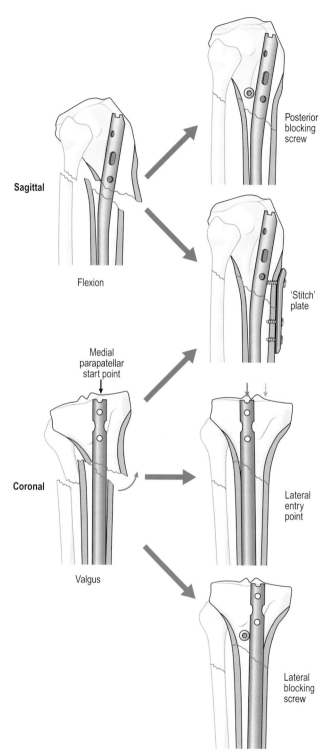

Fig. 20.26 Considerations in proximal tibial fractures.

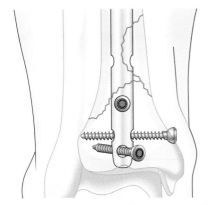

Fig. 20.27 Multiplanar cross-locking screws in distal tibial fractures.

## Monoaxial external fixators

These are used temporarily for evacuation from remote settings, or in the context of highly contaminated, blast or aquatic wounds, or in the multiply injured patient for damage-limitation surgery. It should be noted that the majority of open fractures are most appropriately treated with expert debridement and wound management, followed by primary definitive fixation. Where a monoaxial fixator is used, early conversion to a nail or circular frame is required, as the monoaxial fixator will not provide sufficient stability for definitive tibial fracture treatment, and is associated with a high rate of pin-track infection.

Four parallel pins are placed through stab incisions in the 'safe corridor' (**Fig. 20.30**) over the subcutaneous anteromedial tibial surface, in a near–near–far–far configuration (p. 97). Pins are placed close to the sagittal plane (**Fig. 20.31**).

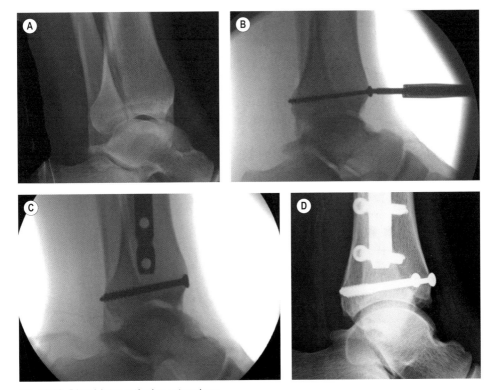

Fig. 20.28 Distal intra-articular extensions.

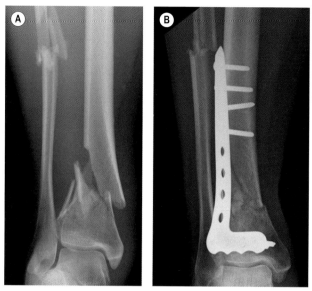

Fig. 20.29 Plating of distal tibial fractures. **A,** Comminuted fracture in the metadiaphyseal region. **B,** The fracture was stabilized with an anterolateral locking plate. An intramedullary nail would have been an appropriate alternative technique.

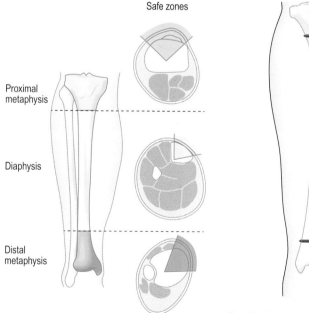

Safe zones

Proximal metaphysis

Diaphysis

Distal metaphysis

Fig. 20.30 Safe corridors for pin insertion in the tibia.

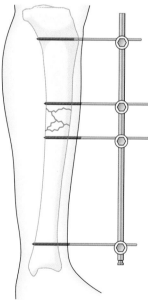

Fig. 20.31 Monoaxial external fixator.

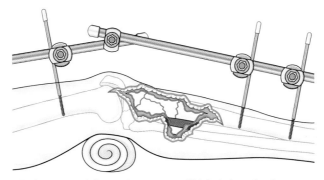

Fig. 20.32 Transarticular external fixator for an open tibial plateau fracture.

Where the fracture extends towards or into the tibial plateau, the knee joint is bridged by placing further pins in the sagittal plane in the distal femur (**Fig. 20.32**).

Where the fracture extends towards or into the tibial plafond, the ankle joint is bridged with a spanning fixator (**Fig. 20.33**). A Denholm pin is placed transversely through the tuberosity of the calcaneus, following the same procedure as for placement of a tibial traction pin (see Fig. 18.7). An A-frame will control length and coronal plane movement and is suitable for short-term use. However, if longer-term use is anticipated, a cross-bar is added to control sagittal plane movement, and consideration should be given to controlling forefoot equinus with a foot plate or pins in the first and fifth metatarsals.

### Fine wire circular frames
Circular frames are indicated principally for fractures with extensive bone or soft tissue loss where acute shortening can be used to allow simplification and often closure of the soft tissue defect, with subsequent lengthening or bone transport through distraction osteogenesis. Some surgeons will

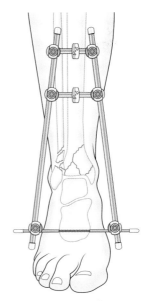

Fig. 20.33 A-frame external fixator.

prefer a frame for the management of very proximal or distal fractures. Mid-shaft fractures are rarely treated acutely with a fine wire frame.

## Outpatient management

| Outpatient management summary | | | |
|---|---|---|---|
| **Week** | **Examination notes** | **Radiographs** | **Additional notes** |
| 2 – post surgery | Wound check <br><br> Neurovascular status | AP and lateral tibia | Permit early weight-bearing mobilization if the construct is stable |
| 6 | Range of movement check at knee and ankle | AP and lateral tibia | Note that this attendance may not be required in a simple fracture |
| 16 | Range of movement check | AP and lateral ankle | If the fracture is united and the patient is walking without pain, then discharge |
| Further assessments at 4-week intervals if required for delayed union | | | |
| Average time to union of closed tibial shaft fracture = 16 weeks | | | |

## COMPLICATIONS

### *Early*

Local

Compartment syndrome: This complication should be anticipated, and either continuous monitoring or close clinical observation instituted both before and after surgery. Once a diagnosis of compartment syndrome is made, there should be no delay in performing emergency four-compartment fasciotomy (Fig. 3.8)

Neurovascular injury: This is associated with high-energy fractures. Damage to all of the three vessels in the leg requires emergency revascularization surgery (Fig. 3.24). Damage to two vessels (the 'one-vessel leg') is a relative indication for exploration and grafting; the improved vascularity may assist fracture healing and soft tissue recovery

General

Fat embolus (p. 28): This is extremely unusual after tibial nailing

# COMPLICATIONS... cont'd

## *Late*

Local

Delayed-union or non-union: This is rare after closed nailing (<1%) but is more common after open fractures and open surgery. Exchange nailing is successful in 95% of cases but exchange of the nail for a compression plate, with or without additional autogenous bone graft, may be required

Malunion: This is very unusual after nailing but routine after non-operative or monoaxial frame treatment

Joint stiffness: This is rare after nailing with early active movement but extremely common after plaster cast treatment, particularly that affecting the hindfoot

Knee pain: This occurs in around 40% of patients after tibial fracture regardless of the method of treatment, but is particularly associated with nailing. Predisposing factors include a prominent nail and a trans-patellar tendon dissection. Half of these resolve after removal of the nail

## GENERAL PRINCIPLES

### Anatomy

#### Osseoligamentous anatomy (Figs 21.1–21.2)

The ankle joint is comprised of the tibia, fibula and talus. The distal tibial metaphysis flares out to form the *plafond* (French: 'ceiling') of the ankle joint, the medial malleolus and the posterior malleolus. The distal fibula is called the *lateral malleolus* and rests within the *incisura* – a groove on the posterolateral aspect of the tibia. The medial and lateral malleoli and the plafond together form a *mortise* – a carpentry term used to describe a stable slot – into which fits the talar dome. The intrinsic stability of these congruent articular surfaces is reinforced by a number of ligaments (**Box 21.1**):

- The *distal tibia and fibula* are bound by a collection of ligaments referred to as the syndesmosis. This constitutes the anterior and posterior inferior tibiofibular ligaments (AITFL and PITFL), the interosseous ligament (IOL) and the interosseous membrane. The AITFL inserts on to the tubercle of Chaput on the tibia, and the tubercle of Wagstaffe on the fibula. Rotational ankle injuries often result in rupture of this ligament, or avulsion

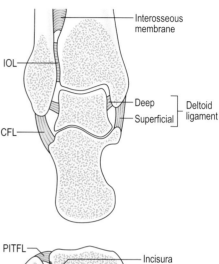
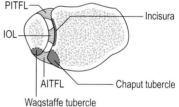

Fig. 21.2 Cross-sectional anatomy. AITFL, anterior inferior tibiofibular ligament; CFL, calcaneofibular ligament; IOL, interosseous ligament; PITFL, posterior inferior tibiofibular ligament.

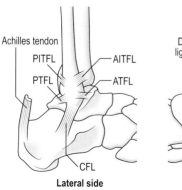
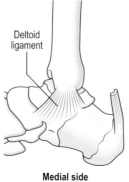

Fig. 21.1 Osseoligamentous anatomy. AITFL, anterior inferior tibiofibular ligament; ATFL, anterior talofibular ligament; CFL, calcaneofibular ligament; PITFL, posterior inferior tibiofibular ligament; PTFL, posterior talofibular ligament.

## Box 21.1   Ankle ligaments

| | |
|---|---|
| **Lateral ligaments** | Anterior talofibular ligament (ATFL) |
| | Calcaneofibular ligament (CFL) |
| | Posterior talofibular ligament (PTFL) |
| **Syndesmosis** | Anterior inferior tibiofibular ligament (AITFL) |
| | Interosseous ligament |
| | Interosseous membrane |
| | Posterior inferior tibiofibular ligament (PITFL) |
| **Medial ligaments** | Deltoid ligament |
| | Deep component inserts into the talus |
| | Superficial component inserts into the talus and calcaneus |

fractures of one or other of its insertions. In children, especially, the Tillaux fracture is important (see Fig. 21.17). The PITFL inserts on to the posterior malleolus, and rotational fractures also commonly result in ruptures of this ligament or 'Volkmann's fractures' of the posterior malleolus (see Fig. 21.15).

- On the *medial side*, the deltoid (Greek: 'triangular') ligament arises from the tip of the medial malleolus. A deep component passes distally within the joint to insert into the talus, and is the principal restraint to lateral movement, while a superficial component inserts into a broad area of the talus and calcaneus.

- On the *lateral side*, the lateral collateral ligament (or ligament complex) also has a number of separate components arranged in a broad inverted triangle. The anterior talofibular ligament (ATFL) passes anteriorly to the talar neck and is very commonly ruptured in ankle sprains. The calcaneofibular ligament (CFL) passes vertically down to insert into the calcaneus, while the posterior talofibular ligament (PTFL) passes obliquely backwards.

The body of the talus (described on p. 518) is semicircular when viewed in the sagittal plane. When viewed in the coronal plane, it has a rectangular cross-section that is broader anteriorly than it is posteriorly. As a result, the talus fills the mortise fully in dorsiflexion but is looser in plantar flexion, allowing some inversion and eversion to occur. This may result in an abnormal-looking joint space on an ankle radiograph taken in plantarflexion.

## Traversing structures

Tendons, vessels and nerves cross the ankle joint in three groups:

- *Anterior to the ankle joint*: The muscles of the anterior compartment of the leg and their neurovascular bundle run under the extensor retinaculum. Most medially is the large tendon of tibialis anterior, then extensor hallucis longus (EHL). Lateral to EHL is the anterior tibial artery, which, on entering the dorsum of the foot, becomes the dorsalis pedis artery. It is accompanied by the deep peroneal nerve. Lateral to this bundle are the tendons of extensor digitorum longus and peroneus tertius. The superficial peroneal nerve, having penetrated the deep fascia in the distal third of the leg (where it is vulnerable to injury during ankle fracture surgery) passes superficial to the retinaculum in the subcutaneous plane.

- *Behind the lateral malleolus*: The tendons of peroneus longus and brevis (the muscles of the lateral compartment of the leg) pass behind the lateral malleolus within a retaining sheath. In the superficial subcutaneous plane passes the sural nerve. Its course is variable, and lies close to the midpoint between the tip of the fibula and the point of the heel (see Fig. 22.30).

- *Behind the medial malleolus*: The muscles of the deep posterior compartment of the leg and their neurovascular bundle pass behind the medial malleolus in a constant arrangement best recalled using the mnemonic *Tom, Dick and very nervous Harry*: the tibialis posterior tendon, flexor *d*igitorum longus tendon, posterior tibial *a*rtery (palpable here) and *v*ein, tibial *n*erve, and flexor *h*allucis longus tendon. The most posterior structure is the Achilles tendon (tendo Achilles, or TA), which arises from the three muscles of the posterior compartment (the two heads of gastrocnemius, and soleus, together termed the triceps surae). The Achilles tendon inserts into a broad area of the calcaneal tuberosity.

## Clinical assessment of the painful ankle

### History

Ankle injuries most commonly arise from a simple twisting fall, with the foot inverting or everting under the loaded tibia, resulting in an ankle sprain (p. 514), ankle fracture (p. 479), Achilles tendon rupture (p. 514) or tendon dislocation (p. 515). A high-energy mechanism with axial loading (such as a fall from a height) may result in a pilon fracture: a much more severe injury (see p. 506). The atraumatic presentation of ankle monoarthritis raises the possibility of a septic arthritis or gout (p. 103).

### Examination

#### Look

Inspect for swelling, deformity and the presence of abrasions or lacerations that might indicate an open fracture. Bruising may not be evident until a few hours after the injury.

#### Feel

Carefully palpate around the ankle in a sequential manner to identify any localized bony or ligamentous tenderness. This begins by descending the lateral, then medial aspects of the leg and

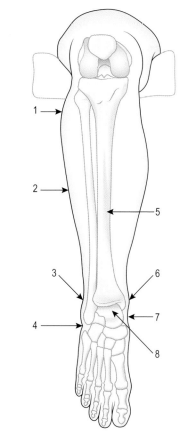

Fig. 21.3 Examination: feel.

ankle, before assessing the foot, and finally palpating for specific tenderness in the syndesmosis and Achilles tendon (**Fig. 21.3**):

- *Lateral side*:
  1. Start just below the knee by palpating the fibular head and neck.
  2. Work down the full length of the fibular shaft. Tenderness in the fibular neck or shaft should prompt full-length radiographs of the leg in order not to miss a Maisonneuve fracture (Fig. 21.14).
  3. Palpate the lateral malleolus.
  4. Palpate the AITFL, ATFL, CFL and PTFL in turn by working sequentially anterior, distal and posterior to the lateral malleolus.

- *Medial side*:

  5. Again, begin proximally on the medial side and palpate the tibial shaft, working distally to:
  6. The medial malleolus
  7. The deltoid ligament.

- *Anterior aspect*:

  8. Palpate across the front of the ankle joint between the medial and lateral malleoli assessing for the presence of local heat or swelling.

- *Posterior aspect*:

  Palpate the heel and Achilles tendon (p. 514).

- *Foot*:

  Palpate the foot (p. 521) especially the base of the fifth metatarsal, fractures of which frequently present as an ankle injury.

- *Syndesmosis*:

  Injuries to the syndesmosis can be identified with the 'squeeze test': grasp the tibia and fibula together in the middle third of the leg and squeeze firmly but gently (**Fig. 21.4**). Pain at the syndesmosis is indicative of a ligamentous injury there.

### Move (Fig. 21.5)

Begin with active movements by asking the patient to dorsiflex and plantar-flex the foot. Then measure the range of passive movement. Ensure the knee is flexed to prevent any restriction in ankle movement caused by gastrocnemius (which crosses both the knee and ankle joints).

- *Dorsiflexion/plantar flexion (ankle joint)*: Cradle the forefoot with one hand and place your index finger along the sole of the foot to gauge the angle of movement. Place the index finger and thumb of the other hand on the talar neck, and as you dorsiflex and plantar-flex the ankle, confirm that this movement is occurring at the ankle joint, rather than in the midfoot. A stiff (or even fused) ankle can be associated with considerable upward and downward movement of the forefoot, but it will be clear that this is

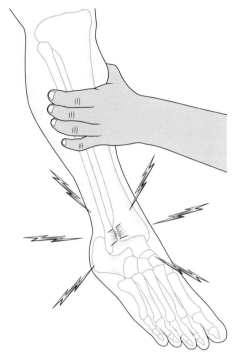

Fig. 21.4 Examination: squeeze test.

happening at the mid-tarsal level, distal to the talar neck.

- *Inversion/eversion (subtalar joint)*: Move your hand to cradle the heel whilst leaving the other resting on the talar neck. Firmly move the heel into inversion and eversion. Most movement occurs distal to the talus (at the subtalar joint), but when there is stiffness here, some inversion and eversion movement will be appreciated at the ankle joint.

- *Pronation and supination (midfoot joints)*: Leaving one hand to support the heel, take hold of the forefoot with the other and assess the range of pronation and supination at the combined midfoot joints.

### Neurovascular assessment

Palpate the dorsalis pedis and posterior tibial artery pulsations, and after a significant ankle injury mark their locations with ink to allow later reassessment. Assess the capillary refill to the toes. Check for sensation in the distributions

| Ankle joint | Subtalar joint | Midfoot |
|---|---|---|

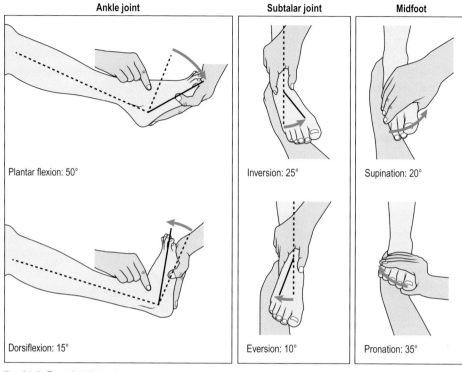

Plantar flexion: 50° — Inversion: 25° — Supination: 20°

Dorsiflexion: 15° — Eversion: 10° — Pronation: 35°

Fig. 21.5 Examination: move.

of the deep and superficial peroneal, and tibial nerves (see Fig. 3.20–3.22). Confirm active toe and foot dorsiflexion and plantar flexion.

## Radiological assessment of the painful ankle

### Radiographs

A standard ankle series comprises three radiographs:

- AP ankle (**Fig. 21.6**): This is taken with the foot in neutral (see Fig. 21.10). It allows assessment of the plafond, the medial malleolus, lateral malleolus, posterior malleolus and talus, and also the congruity of the ankle joint. Several measurements are noted (see below).

- Mortise view: An AP radiograph taken in 20° of internal rotation, allowing a better view of the lateral joint space and the lateral process of the talus.

- Lateral ankle view: The talar dome should appear in perfect profile. Two separate

arcs representing the medial and lateral aspects of the dome, seen on the same lateral view, denote an oblique view (**Fig. 21.7**). Note the talus and its dome, and its congruity with the plafond, as well as the posterior malleolus. Many fibular fractures are in the coronal plane and are most easily discerned on the lateral view.

A number of radiographic measurements are described for ankle radiographs (**Fig. 21.8**). These are not wholly reliable and vary considerably with rotation, but you should assess the following features.

On the AP view:

- Superior and medial clear space: These spaces should be equal. A larger medial clear space indicates talar shift and an incongruent ankle joint. The limit of normal is usually taken as a medial clear space of 5 mm, or a difference between the superior and medial spaces of >2 mm. The medial clear space can only be assessed with the

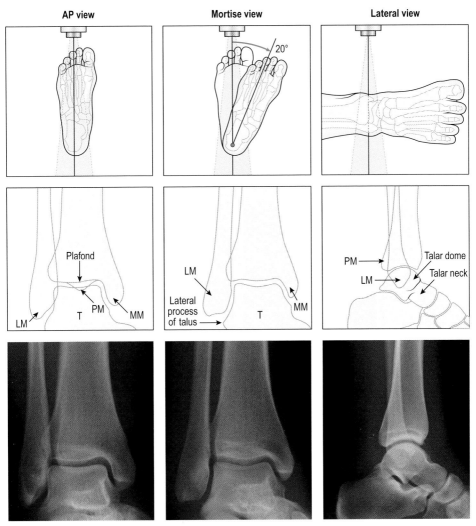

Fig. 21.6 Ankle series of radiographs: AP, mortise and lateral views. LM, lateral malleolus; MM, medial malleolus; PM, posterior malleolus T, talus.

foot in neutral, as plantar flexion will result in some apparent increase in the width of this space (see 'Key point' on p. 479 and Fig. 21.10).

- *Lateral (tibiofibular) clear space*: This indicates the engagement of the fibula in the incisura and should also be <5 mm. A larger gap indicates diastasis of the syndesmosis.

- *Tibiofibular overlap*: This is often cited but is highly variable with rotation; it is usually >5 mm on an AP view.

On the mortise view:

- *'Fibular nipple sign'*: This is similar to Shenton's arc in the hip, indicating that the curves of the fibular and tibial articular surfaces are congruent at the mortise.

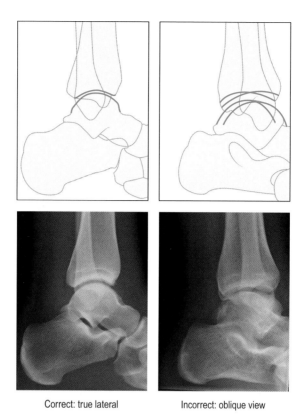

Correct: true lateral      Incorrect: oblique view

Fig. 21.7 Correct and incorrect ankle lateral views.

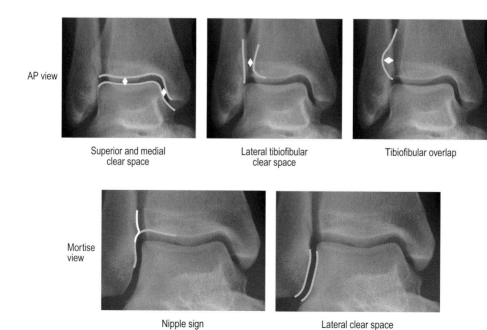

AP view

Superior and medial
clear space

Lateral tibiofibular
clear space

Tibiofibular overlap

Mortise
view

Nipple sign

Lateral clear space

Fig. 21.8 Radiographic landmarks of the ankle.

- *Lateral clear space*: This should consist of the two parallel lines of the articular surfaces of the fibula and the lateral process of the talus. Fibular shortening is best appreciated as an increase in the lateral clear space distally, just above the lateral process of the talus, when compared to that space immediately lateral to the talar dome.

Other abnormalities on the ankle series that should be excluded include:

- fractures of the base of the fifth metatarsal
- fractures of the lateral process of the talus
- osteochondral fractures of the talar dome
- navicular fracture.

---

###  Key point

The surface of the talus that articulates with the tibia is frustral in shape, and is narrower posteriorly than anteriorly (**Fig. 21.9**). Radiographs of the ankle must be taken with the ankle plantigrade (in neutral flexion/ extension), so that the broader anterior part of the talus is grasped within the mortise (between the malleoli). With the ankle plantar-flexed (in equinus), the narrower posterior aspect of the talus is within the mortise and the medial clear space can appear to be abnormally wide. **Figure 21.10** shows a fracture of the fibula with an apparently increased medial clear space, suggestive of talar shift (**Fig. 21.10A**). Closer inspection of the lateral view shows that this radiograph was taken with the ankle in plantar flexion. When this is corrected to a neutral, plantigrade position (**Fig. 21.10B**), the mortise is shown to be congruent. This is a stable ankle fracture (see below).

---

#### *Additional views*
- *AP and lateral views of the tibia and fibula*: Full-length radiographs of the leg are required where there is suspicion of a proximal fracture, particularly of the fibular neck or shaft (see Fig. 21.14).

- *Stress view*: Where there is uncertainty regarding ankle stability, a radiograph can be taken either while an external rotation force is applied to the dorsiflexed foot, or with the patient lying in the lateral position so that gravity exerts the same force. This may demonstrate an increased medial clear space. However, stress views are known to have a high false-positive rate and considerable caution is required in their interpretation.

### CT
This is rarely required for an ankle fracture but is invaluable for the assessment of, and preoperative planning for, pilon and triplane fractures (see Fig. 21.47).

### MRI
This may be helpful in identifying osteochondral injuries to the talar dome, and in assessing chronic ligamentous instability. MRI does not have a major part to play in the assessment of acute ankle injuries.

## ANKLE FRACTURES

Ankle fractures are extremely common injuries presenting to the Emergency Department, usually resulting from a simple twisting fall, jump or sporting collision. A higher-energy mechanism of injury (a motor vehicle collision or high fall) should raise the suspicion of a pilon fracture.

## Classification

Three classification systems are popular and are commonly used. The Pott's classification provides a simple shorthand, while the AO/ Weber system is widely adopted for description of the injury to the fibula. The Lauge-Hansen classification is more complex, yet helpful in planning surgery.

### Pott's classification
Pott's classification (**Fig. 21.11**) is simple and remains in common use despite its significant shortcomings. It describes the number of

Anterior

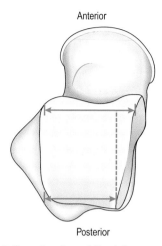

Posterior

Fig. 21.9 Superior view of the talus.

malleoli involved in the fracture: thus a uni-malleolar fracture is generally understood as describing an isolated fracture of the lateral malleolus, a bimalleolar fracture is one involving both medial and lateral malleoli, while a trimalleolar fracture additionally involves the posterior malleolus.

## Weber classification

The Weber classification (**Fig. 21.12**) is simple and easily applied. It also forms part of the *AO universal classification system*, which addresses ankle fractures as a separate region: 44. The fracture types are classified according to the level of the fibular fracture in relation to the syndesmosis:

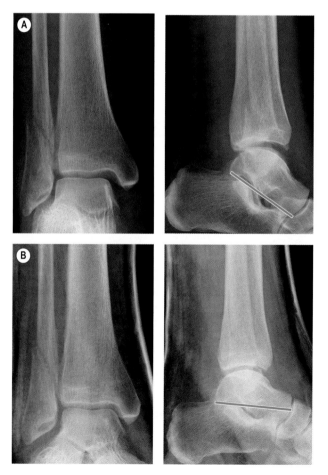

Fig. 21.10 Ankle radiographs.
**A**, Plantar-flexed.
**B**, Plantigrade. See Key Point box on p. 479 for details.

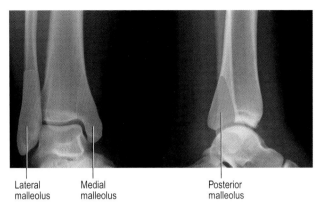

Lateral          Medial          Posterior
malleolus        malleolus       malleolus

Fig. 21.11 Pott's classification of ankle fractures.

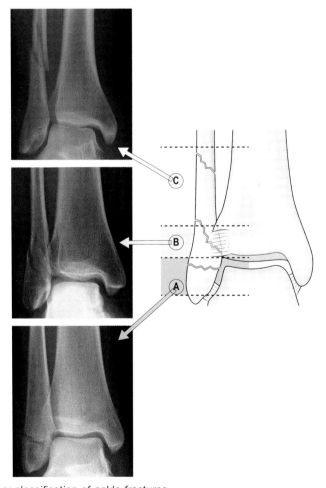

Fig. 21.12 Weber classification of ankle fractures.

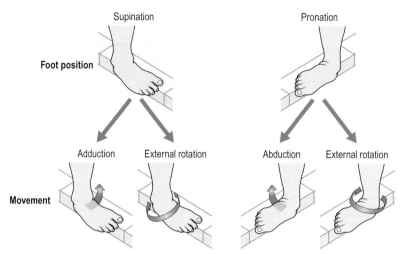

Fig. 21.13 Lauge-Hansen classification of ankle fractures.

- *Type A* fractures are infrasyndesmotic, and are usually avulsion fractures occurring after an inversion injury.
- *Type B* fractures are trans-syndesmotic and are the most common type, occurring after torsional injuries.
- *Type C* fractures are suprasyndesmotic and are less common; they may represent more of a challenge in terms of reduction and fixation.

Groups and subgroups of the AO classification are described and are principally useful for research.

## Lauge-Hansen classification

The Lauge-Hansen classification (**Fig. 21.13**) was developed through producing experimental fractures in cadavers and is mechanistic, aiming to describe the force vectors that produced the injury, and the severity of the injury in terms of a progression through a characteristic series of fractures or ligament ruptures. The first word in the classification describes the position of the foot at the time of injury – either pronation or supination. The second word describes the movement of the hindfoot – either adduction, abduction or external rotation. This results in four groups of fractures:

- supination–adduction (SAD), a pure inversion injury
- supination–external rotation (SER), inversion injury with external rotation
- pronation–abduction (PAB), a pure eversion injury
- pronation–external rotation (PER), eversion injury with external rotation.

For each group, there is a sequence of stages of injury, which are numbered. Although not all fractures pass through each stage as described, the classification system is helpful in planning management (see Figs 21.23–26).

## Eponymous fractures

A number of eponymous terms remain in common use:

- *Maisonneuve fracture* (**Fig. 21.14**): This is a medial ankle injury (either a medial malleolar fracture or a deltoid ligament rupture) associated with a high fibular fracture, and is highly unstable. It is a trap for the unwary: failure to examine or X-ray the proximal fibula will lead to this type of injury being missed.
- *Volkmann's fracture* (**Fig. 21.15**): This is a posterior malleolar fracture.

- *Dupuytren's fracture-dislocation* (**Fig. 21.16**): This is a highly unstable fracture (Lauge-Hansen PER IV; Fig. 21.25).

- *Tillaux fracture* (**Fig. 21.17**): This is a fracture of the tubercle of Chaput, typically in an individual approaching skeletal maturity.

## Emergency Department management

### Clinical features

- Establish the history of the injury, in particular the mechanism and energy transfer involved.

- If the ankle is clearly deformed, it should be realigned immediately to preserve the soft tissue envelope and neurovascular structures.

- Examine the ankle carefully and systematically (p. 474), noting any breach in the skin, swelling, and areas of bony or ligamentous tenderness.

- Bruising may not be apparent immediately after injury

- Examine the foot and Achilles tendon (p. 514 and p. 521).

### Radiological features

- *AP, lateral and mortise ankle radiographs.*

- *AP and lateral views of the tibia and fibula*: These views are needed if proximal injury is suspected.

#### *Ottawa ankle rules*

The Ottawa ankle rules provide a framework for radiographic assessment. Radiographs

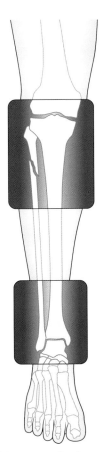

Fig. 21.14 Maisonneuve fracture.

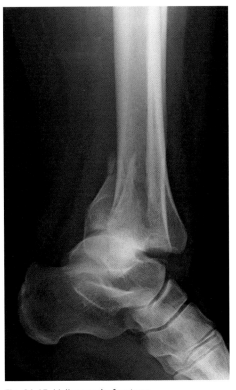

Fig. 21.15 Volkmann's fracture.

are indicated if there is pain in the ankle region and:

- bony tenderness of the malleoli – defined as the posterior edge or tip of either the medial or the lateral malleolus, *or*
- inability to bear weight through the injured foot at any point following injury.

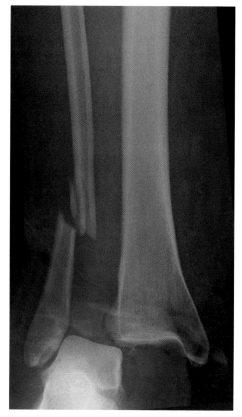

Fig. 21.16 Dupuytren's fracture-dislocation.

In addition, where there is any tenderness of the proximal two-thirds of the fibula, obtain full-length views of the leg.

### Radiograph assessment

When assessing an ankle radiograph decide:

1. Are the radiographs of adequate quality (see Figs 21.6–21.10)?
2. Is there a fracture? If so, which structures are affected?
3. Is the talus displaced in the mortise?
4. Is the syndesmosis widened?
5. Is the plafond involved? A pilon fracture is more serious than a simple ankle fracture.
6. Is the posterior malleolus fractured? If so, what percentage of the joint surface is on the displaced fragment?

---

### ✓ Key point

The term *syndesmosis* represents the ligamentous connection between the distal tibia and fibula (see Figs 21.1–21.2). The term *diastasis* represents disruption of the ligaments that causes the fibula to separate from the tibia, and results in widening or a visible gap on radiographs (see Fig. 21.16).

---

### Decision-making in ankle fractures: stable or unstable?

In the Emergency Department, decide whether an ankle fracture is:

- congruent
- stable.

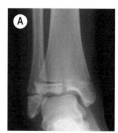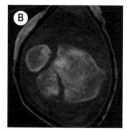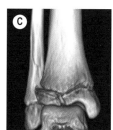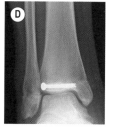

Fig. 21.17 Tillaux fracture. **A**, AP view. **B**, CT. **C**, Three-dimensional view. **D**, Screw fixation.

**Key point**

The complex anatomy, variety in fracture morphology, and multitude of treatment options can make the management of ankle fractures intimidating. Remember a single, key, principle: *The talus must sit in a congruent position in the mortise beneath the tibia, and remain there until fracture union.*

If a treatment achieves this aim, the patient is likely to have a favourable outcome. In contrast, subluxation of the talus within the mortise, termed *talar shift*, denotes instability and a poor outcome (**Fig. 21.18**).

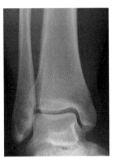
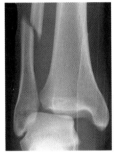
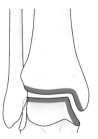
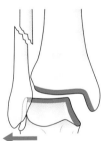

Fig. 21.18 Talar shift.

## Stable ankle fractures

Stable fractures have a *congruent mortise* that will remain so during fracture healing. These are treated non-operatively, even when there is some displacement of the fracture fragment itself. Stable ankle fractures include:

- isolated lateral malleolus fractures, with no medial fracture or deltoid ligament rupture

- isolated avulsion fractures of the tip of the fibula (Weber A)
- isolated fractures of the medial malleolus.

## Unstable ankle fractures

An unstable fracture implies that the mortise is not congruent, or that it could become incongruent before fracture healing. Management is usually with surgery. Unstable ankle fractures include those with:

- *Clinical deformity*: These are clearly clinically deformed or dislocated at presentation.
- *Radiographic deformity*: There is displacement of the mortise (talar shift) on the AP and/or mortise radiographs.
- *Unstable fracture pattern*: Certain fracture patterns are known to be unstable, although they can occasionally present with a congruent mortise on the initial radiographs. These include:
  — Bimalleolar fractures.
  — Trimalleolar fractures.
  — High fibular fractures (Weber C – suprasyndesmotic and Maisonneuve fractures): These have a high chance of being unstable. Even where the medial malleolus is intact, be suspicious of a deltoid ligament rupture.

### Immobilization of stable fractures

Patients with stable ankle fractures do not require specific immobilization, but are usually provided with a removable orthosis (moonboot), analgesia and crutches for comfort and to aid mobilization. They are instructed to keep the foot elevated for as much of the time as possible, preferably above the level of the heart. Where an orthosis is not available, a plaster backslab may be applied for comfort, although the patient will have to remain non-weight-bearing (the plaster slab will crumble under weight). This is converted to an orthosis or weight-bearing cast at the earliest opportunity.

### Closed reduction and immobilization of unstable fractures

A displaced ankle fracture should be reduced without delay in the Emergency Department in

##  Key point

It can be difficult to determine whether the ankle is stable or not. The most common source of uncertainty is where there is a lateral malleolar fracture with a congruent mortise but no fracture of the medial malleolus. Stability in this situation relies on the integrity of the *deep deltoid ligament*, which cannot be seen on the radiographs. This is the distinction between a *stable* (SER II, Fig. 21.23) and an *unstable* (SER IV, Fig. 21.18) fracture. Unfortunately, the clinical examination does not provide a conclusive distinction between the two. Deltoid ligament swelling, tenderness or bruising implies a deltoid ligament injury but may arise from a tear of the superficial deltoid only, with stability still being maintained by the deep deltoid. Stress views are used in some centres but these have a high false-positive rate. MRI scans of the deltoid are often not readily available and are difficult to interpret. Pragmatically, provided there is no talar shift on the plain radiographs, patients should be provided with an orthosis (moon boot) and allowed to mobilize fully weight-bearing. The radiographs are repeated at 1 week. If there is no talar shift, the ankle is considered stable.

order to minimize the soft tissue injury (**Fig. 21.19**). Remember that where the bone has fractured, the collateral ligaments will remain intact. During the reduction manoeuvre, the malleoli will faithfully follow the talus, and so *in essence, reduction is a case of realigning the foot and talus with the tibia.*

1. *Patient position*: Procedural sedation and/or analgesia are usually required. The patient lies supine, with the thigh resting on a plaster tray bolster (see Fig. 4.13) or supported by an assistant.

2. *Radiographs*: Begin by assessing the initial radiographs to define the main direction of displacement; this will guide hand placement (Fig. 21.19). The most common direction is lateral displacement with or without posterior subluxation.

3. *Reduction manoeuvre*:

   Posterior displacement and rotation: apply traction and lift the heel anteriorly. Still grasping the hindfoot, correct any rotation, aligning the first web space of the foot with the patella. Note that little force is required (**Fig. 21.19A**).

   Lateral displacement: apply the palm of one hand over the lateral malleolus and push medially. The other hand rests proximally on the ankle, providing gentle counter-pressure (**Fig. 21.19B**).

   Medial displacement: apply the palm over the medial malleolus and push laterally. The other hand rests proximally over the lateral ankle as counter-pressure (**Fig. 21.19C**).

Over-correction is difficult or impossible in the majority of ankle fractures, as there is usually an intact periosteal hinge on the fractured fragments that provides an end-point to the reduction manoeuvre.

4. *Clinical assessment*: The gross appearance of the ankle should be restored to normal, with the first web space of the foot aligned with the patella.

5. *Backslab application*: The reduction is maintained during plaster application by holding the big toe while the thigh rests on the bolster (see Fig. 4.13). Once the slab is in place, mould it by reapplying the forces used to achieve the reduction. Ensure that the ankle is held in a plantigrade (neutral flexion/extension) position by resting the foot against the abdomen of the plasterer (**Fig. 21.20**). Knee flexion at this point relaxes the gastrocnemius and makes it easier to attain the correct position.

6. *Reassessment*:

   Repeat radiographs are taken (**Fig. 21.21**). If the manoeuvre has not resulted in reduction of the mortise, the procedure should be repeated.

   Check the cast proximally and distally for appropriate padding.

   Reassess the neurological status.

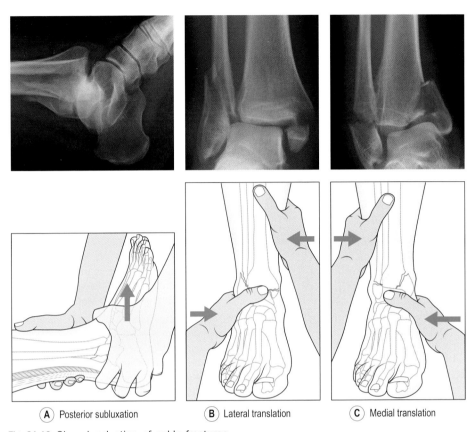

(A) Posterior subluxation    (B) Lateral translation    (C) Medial translation

Fig. 21.19 Closed reduction of ankle fractures.

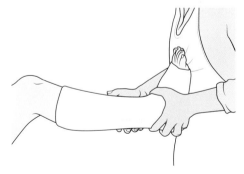

Fig. 21.20 Ankle fracture cast moulding.

### Inpatient referral

- Unstable ankle fractures.
- Open fractures.
- Neurovascular compromise.

### Outpatient follow-up

- Patients with stable fractures are allowed to bear weight as tolerated in an orthosis, are provided with crutches, and are referred for orthopaedic fracture clinic assessment.

## Orthopaedic management

A good outcome can be expected when the talus is held congruently in the mortise until fracture union. This can be achieved in a number of ways.

### Non-operative

- All closed, stable ankle fractures are managed non-operatively.

- Unstable fractures in the elderly may be considered for non-operative treatment, provided that adequate reduction can be achieved closed, and there is a willingness to accept the requirement for close supervision and the possibility of late displacement needing surgery. A full cast is applied and frequent radiographic review is performed.

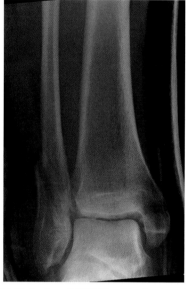

Fig. 21.21 Reduced SER IV ankle fracture in cast. (Same fracture as in Fig. 21.19B.)

### Application of a full below-knee plaster

Reduction is performed under *general anaesthesia* using the technique detailed on page 485. However, for a full cast, the patient's position is altered to aid application (**Fig. 21.22**):

1. *Position*: The patient is placed supine on the operating table with the knee flexed over the edge of the table and a sandbag behind the thigh. Adjust the table height so that you can steady the foot with your knee. Before plaster application, carry out a reduction rehearsal.

2. *Wool application*: Apply wool roll to the limb, making sure that the malleolar prominences are well covered.

3. *Plaster application to calf*: Without hurrying, follow wool application with 2–3 15-cm plaster bandages from the level of the tibial tubercle to just above the ankle.

4. *Plaster application to ankle*: Smooth the plaster well down and then quickly apply two 15-cm plaster bandages to the foot and ankle. The toes may be steadied with your knee. On completion, you should be left with a plaster that is setting at the calf, but is quite soft and mouldable at the foot and ankle.

5. *Reduction and moulding*: Now repeat the reduction manœuvre and hold the limb in the reduced position until the plaster has

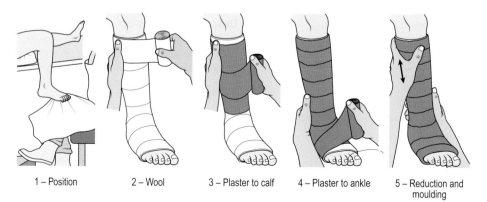

| 1 – Position | 2 – Wool | 3 – Plaster to calf | 4 – Plaster to ankle | 5 – Reduction and moulding |

Fig. 21.22 Full below-knee cast application. See text for details.

set. Steady the forefoot with your knee (to keep the ankle in a neutral (plantigrade) position) and ease your hands slightly upwards and downwards to prevent local indentation of the plaster.

Check the position of the fracture fluoroscopically and, if necessary, repeat the procedure. Take precautions to avoid swelling and its effects by elevating the limb and, if necessary, splitting the plaster (see p. 79). The plaster should be examined for slackness as swelling subsides over the course of the next few days and weeks. If it becomes slack, it must be changed with care to prevent displacement of the fracture, and a further general anaesthetic may be necessary. Radiographs should be taken weekly; remanipulation under anaesthesia or internal fixation may have to be considered if there is any displacement. The patient may be mobilized non-weight-bearing with crutches. Plaster fixation is maintained until radiographic union.

## Operative

Ankle fractures can be stabilized with a variety of screws, plates, wires and nails; the optimal configuration will depend on the age and health of the patient and on fracture morphology. While most fractures can be treated early, extensive soft tissue swelling, bruising or blistering at the site of planned incisions is an indication for delayed surgery (after 5–10 days) or the use of a percutaneous technique.

Four components of ankle anatomy should be considered for surgical fixation:

- *Lateral malleolus*: The lateral malleolus is the crucial lateral buttress against talar displacement. It will need to be brought back out to length and stabilized. If the syndesmotic ligaments are intact, this will complete the stabilization of the lateral buttress.
- *Medial malleolus*: If displaced, the medial malleolus is reduced and fixed.
- *Posterior malleolus*: Fixation is required if there is posterior subluxation of the talus. This is more likely when the fragment comprises >25% of the joint surface on the lateral radiographs.

- *Syndesmosis*: Incompetence of the syndesmotic ligaments may be clear from preoperative radiographs or may be detected after fibular fixation. Diastasis is addressed by stabilizing the fibula anatomically within the incisura to allow ligament healing.

The Lauge-Hansen classification is helpful for guiding fracture management. Careful assessment of the mechanism of injury and the fracture morphology will allow, firstly, an appreciation of which structures have been injured, and secondly, determination of the steps that have to be taken to address these injuries.

### Supination–external rotation (SER) fracture (Fig. 21.23)

This is the most common variant, accounting for 75% of all ankle fractures, and resulting from a typical twisting inversion injury (see Fig. 21.13).

- *Stage I*: There is a rupture of the AITFL (ankle sprain), or avulsion fracture from either the tubercle of Chaput (Tillaux fracture) or (rarely) the tubercle of Wagstaffe. A sprain is treated conservatively (see above), as is an avulsion fracture, unless there is a substantial intra-articular fragment, in which case reduction and fixation may be justified (Fig. 21.17).
- *Stage II*: There is an oblique fracture of the fibula with a classical long posterior spike. This is often best seen on the lateral radiograph. This fracture is the very common, stable 'Weber B' ankle fracture and is treated conservatively.
- *Stage III*: Either the posterior malleolus fractures or the PITFL and capsule tear.
- *Stage IV*: The medial malleolus fractures obliquely or the deltoid ligament tears as the talus continues to rotate in the mortise. This is the most common unstable ankle fracture. Surgical treatment begins with lateral malleolar reduction and fixation. The fibular fracture is usually oblique and simple, and appropriately treated by lag screw compression, with 1/3 tubular plate neutralization (see 'Surgical technique', p. 498). A fibular nail is an alternative that may reduce

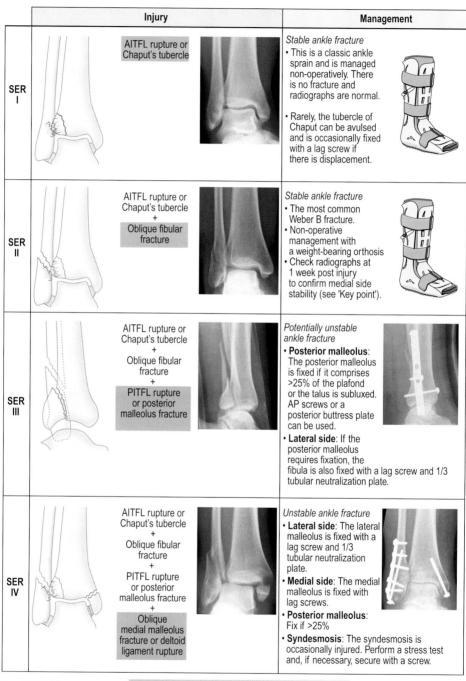

|  | Injury | Management |
|---|---|---|
| SER I | AITFL rupture or Chaput's tubercle | *Stable ankle fracture*<br>• This is a classic ankle sprain and is managed non-operatively. There is no fracture and radiographs are normal.<br>• Rarely, the tubercle of Chaput can be avulsed and is occasionally fixed with a lag screw if there is displacement. |
| SER II | AITFL rupture or Chaput's tubercle + Oblique fibular fracture | *Stable ankle fracture*<br>• The most common Weber B fracture.<br>• Non-operative management with a weight-bearing orthosis<br>• Check radiographs at 1 week post injury to confirm medial side stability (see 'Key point'). |
| SER III | AITFL rupture or Chaput's tubercle + Oblique fibular fracture + PITFL rupture or posterior malleolus fracture | *Potentially unstable ankle fracture*<br>• **Posterior malleolus**: The posterior malleolus is fixed if it comprises >25% of the plafond or the talus is subluxed. AP screws or a posterior buttress plate can be used.<br>• **Lateral side**: If the posterior malleolus requires fixation, the fibula is also fixed with a lag screw and 1/3 tubular neutralization plate. |
| SER IV | AITFL rupture or Chaput's tubercle + Oblique fibular fracture + PITFL rupture or posterior malleolus fracture + Oblique medial malleolus fracture or deltoid ligament rupture | *Unstable ankle fracture*<br>• **Lateral side**: The lateral malleolus is fixed with a lag screw and 1/3 tubular neutralization plate.<br>• **Medial side**: The medial malleolus is fixed with lag screws.<br>• **Posterior malleolus**: Fix if >25%<br>• **Syndesmosis**: The syndesmosis is occasionally injured. Perform a stress test and, if necessary, secure with a screw. |

Fig. 21.23 Management of **supination–external rotation (SER) fractures**. AITFL, anterior inferior tibiofibular ligament; PITFL, posterior inferior tibiofibular ligament.

soft tissue dissection and complications. Medial fracture fixation is conventionally carried out with two parallel partially threaded screws. A deltoid ligament rupture does not require repair, provided the mortise is reduced.

## Pronation–abduction (PAB) fracture (Fig. 21.24)

This is a pure eversion injury, comprising 10% of ankle fractures.

- *Stage I*: Either the deltoid ligament tears or there is an avulsion fracture of the medial malleolus with a transverse orientation. An isolated medial malleolar fracture is usually managed conservatively.

- *Stage II*: Both the anterior and posterior inferior tibiofibular ligaments (or their attachments) fail.

- *Stage III*: The fibula fractures in compression, resulting in a comminuted fracture above the syndesmosis. This fracture is often not amenable to interfragmentary lag screw compression and neutralization because of comminution, and either a bridging technique with a stronger plate (e.g. a

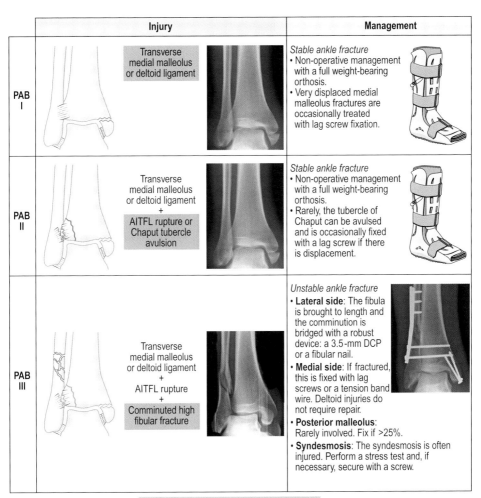

| | Injury | Management |
|---|---|---|
| PAB I | Transverse medial malleolus or deltoid ligament | *Stable ankle fracture* • Non-operative management with a full weight-bearing orthosis. • Very displaced medial malleolus fractures are occasionally treated with lag screw fixation. |
| PAB II | Transverse medial malleolus or deltoid ligament + AITFL rupture or Chaput tubercle avulsion | *Stable ankle fracture* • Non-operative management with a full weight-bearing orthosis. • Rarely, the tubercle of Chaput can be avulsed and is occasionally fixed with a lag screw if there is displacement. |
| PAB III | Transverse medial malleolus or deltoid ligament + AITFL rupture + Comminuted high fibular fracture | *Unstable ankle fracture* • **Lateral side**: The fibula is brought to length and the comminution is bridged with a robust device: a 3.5-mm DCP or a fibular nail. • **Medial side**: If fractured, this is fixed with lag screws or a tension band wire. Deltoid injuries do not require repair. • **Posterior malleolus**: Rarely involved. Fix if >25%. • **Syndesmosis**: The syndesmosis is often injured. Perform a stress test and, if necessary, secure with a screw. |

Fig. 21.24 Management of **pronation–abduction (PAB) fractures**. AITFL, anterior inferior tibiofibular ligament; DCP, dynamic compression plate.

dynamic compression plate, DCP), or a fibular nail may be required. Judging fibular length is more difficult and requires careful (fluoroscopic or open) assessment. Syndesmosis instability is relatively common and should be addressed with a screw.

## Pronation–external rotation (PER) fracture (Fig. 21.25)

This is a relatively unusual injury, accounting for 5% of ankle fractures, but both the Maisonneuve (PER III) and Dupuytren's (PER IV) fractures are highly unstable.

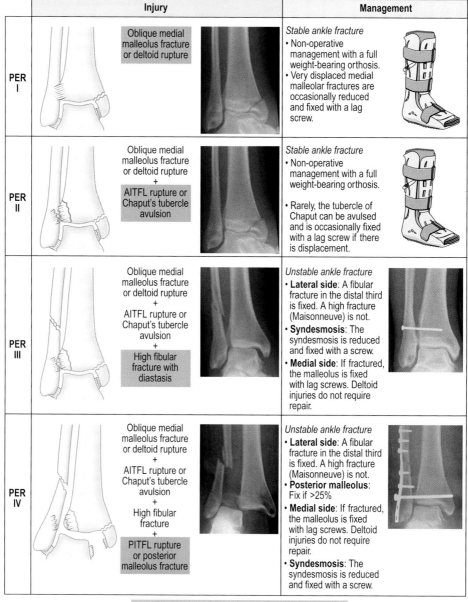

| | Injury | Management |
|---|---|---|
| **PER I** | Oblique medial malleolus fracture or deltoid rupture | *Stable ankle fracture* <br> • Non-operative management with a full weight-bearing orthosis. <br> • Very displaced medial malleolar fractures are occasionally reduced and fixed with a lag screw. |
| **PER II** | Oblique medial malleolus fracture or deltoid rupture <br> + <br> AITFL rupture or Chaput's tubercle avulsion | *Stable ankle fracture* <br> • Non-operative management with a full weight-bearing orthosis. <br> • Rarely, the tubercle of Chaput can be avulsed and is occasionally fixed with a lag screw if there is displacement. |
| **PER III** | Oblique medial malleolus fracture or deltoid rupture <br> + <br> AITFL rupture or Chaput's tubercle avulsion <br> + <br> High fibular fracture with diastasis | *Unstable ankle fracture* <br> • **Lateral side**: A fibular fracture in the distal third is fixed. A high fracture (Maisonneuve) is not. <br> • **Syndesmosis**: The syndesmosis is reduced and fixed with a screw. <br> • **Medial side**: If fractured, the malleolus is fixed with lag screws. Deltoid injuries do not require repair. |
| **PER IV** | Oblique medial malleolus fracture or deltoid rupture <br> + <br> AITFL rupture or Chaput's tubercle avulsion <br> + <br> High fibular fracture <br> + <br> PITFL rupture or posterior malleolus fracture | *Unstable ankle fracture* <br> • **Lateral side**: A fibular fracture in the distal third is fixed. A high fracture (Maisonneuve) is not. <br> • **Posterior malleolus**: Fix if >25% <br> • **Medial side**: If fractured, the malleolus is fixed with lag screws. Deltoid injuries do not require repair. <br> • **Syndesmosis**: The syndesmosis is reduced and fixed with a screw. |

Fig. 21.25 Management of **pronation–external rotation (PER) fractures**. AITFL, anterior inferior tibiofibular ligament; PITFL, posterior inferior tibiofibular ligament.

- *Stage I*: The rotating talus produces an oblique fracture of the medial malleolus or ruptures the deltoid ligament.
- *Stage II*: The AITFL ruptures.
- *Stage III*: There is a spiral or oblique high (Weber C) fracture of the fibula, which may be as proximal as the fibular neck (Maisonneuve fracture). The orientation of the fracture is opposite to that of the SER fracture, running from low posteriorly to high anteriorly.
- *Stage IV*: Infrequently, the PITFL fails (or the posterior malleolus fractures), the interosseous membrane tears and gross diastasis occurs (the Dupuytren fracture-dislocation of the ankle).

In stages III or IV, the fibular fracture itself is usually fixed if it is within the lower third of the fibula. This aids accurate reduction of length and prevents a syndesmosis screw from compressing the fibula shaft towards the tibia, which causes the lateral malleolus to move laterally, displacing the talus. Fractures in the proximal two-thirds of the fibula do not require fixation (indeed, this is to be avoided because of the extent of muscular dissection required

and the risk to the peroneal nerves), but the diastasis and ankle joint instability do. The difficulty of reducing the syndesmosis surgically is often under-appreciated; it involves careful reversal of the shortening, posterior translation (and occasionally external rotation) of the fibula in the tibial incisura. Direct visualization may allow a more accurate reduction (see 'Surgical technique', p. 502). The medial malleolus is fixed as for an SER fracture, with two parallel partially threaded screws.

### Supination–adduction (SAD) fracture (Fig. 21.26)

This injury accounts for 10% ankle fractures and results from an inversion injury, with the lateral structures failing in tension and the medial malleolus failing by vertical shear.

- *Stage I*: There is a tear of the lateral ligament complex (simple ankle sprain), or an avulsion fracture of the tip of the lateral malleolus (Weber A fracture). The fibular fracture is often a small avulsed fragment that can be ignored; if larger, it can be stabilized using a lag screw, a tension band technique or occasionally standard plating.

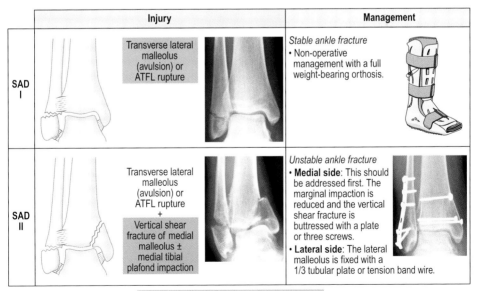

| | Injury | | Management |
|---|---|---|---|
| SAD I | Transverse lateral malleolus (avulsion) or ATFL rupture | | *Stable ankle fracture*<br>• Non-operative management with a full weight-bearing orthosis. |
| SAD II | Transverse lateral malleolus (avulsion) or ATFL rupture<br>+<br>Vertical shear fracture of medial malleolus ± medial tibial plafond impaction | | *Unstable ankle fracture*<br>• **Medial side**: This should be addressed first. The marginal impaction is reduced and the vertical shear fracture is buttressed with a plate or three screws.<br>• **Lateral side**: The lateral malleolus is fixed with a 1/3 tubular plate or tension band wire. |

Fig. 21.26 Management of **supination–adduction (SAD) fractures**. ATFL, anterior talofibular ligament.

- *Stage II*: The adducting talus strikes the medial malleolus, causing a classical vertical shear fracture, often with an area of impaction of the medial plafond. Unlike the other types of ankle fracture, operative treatment begins with the medial malleolus. The impacted plafond is assessed and reduced through the fracture, and supported if necessary with graft. The vertical shear injury is then compressed and stabilized with a buttress plate or multiple screws (see 'Surgical technique', p. 504).

## Surgical techniques

### Fibular plate

The plate may be placed laterally or posteriorly. A lateral position is a little easier technically but does result in the plate sitting in a subcutaneous location, where it may cause later wound discomfort. The distal metaphyseal screws pass medially and must not penetrate the far cortex into the ankle joint. They achieve the highest pull-out strength if orientated to form a triangle (**Fig. 21.27A**) or if the distal screw is placed longitudinally (**Fig. 21.27B**).

A posterior position allows the plate to function as a buttress plate in SER IV fractures. This location also allows screws to be directed in a posteroanterior direction; the screws can be bicortical and therefore longer, and this orientation can be useful in particularly poor bone. This position is often used when there has been a posterolateral incision for posterior malleolus plating (**Fig. 21.28**). The posterior location does, however, result in a small incidence of peroneal tendon irritation.

Whereas 1/3 tubular plates are ideal for neutralization and buttress modes, a bridging technique (e.g. for more comminuted PAB fractures) requires greater strength and a 3.5-mm DCP plate is usually selected (**Fig. 21.29**).

Locked fibular plates have been developed for osteoporotic bone. There is reportedly a higher incidence of soft tissue complications and their role has not yet been clarified.

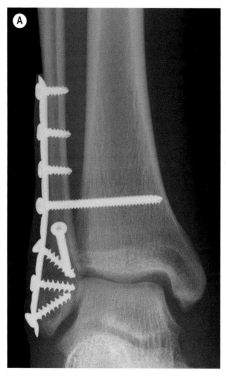
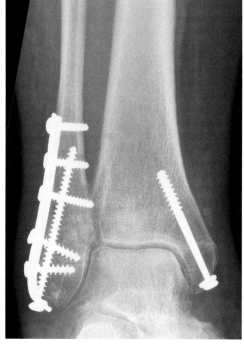

Fig. 21.27 Fibular plate: lateral position.

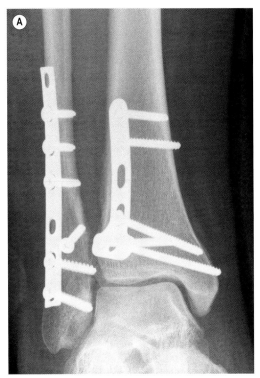 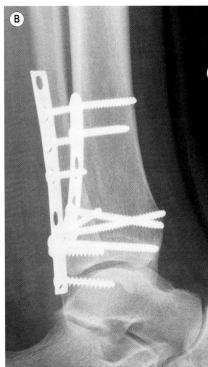

Fig. 21.28 Fibular plate: posterior position. The posterolateral approach has been used to fix both the posterior malleolus with a buttress plate, and the fibular fracture with a lag screw and neutralization plate.

### Fibular nail (Fig. 21.30)

A fibular nail allows percutaneous reduction and stabilization of lateral malleolar fractures and has particular advantages where there is osteoporotic bone, diabetes, neuropathy and swollen or contused skin, which are associated with an increased rate of complications after open reduction and fixation (ORIF). Whereas fibular ORIF requires anatomical reduction and fixation of the fibular cortex to achieve a congruent mortise, a nail entails accurate fluoroscopic mortise reduction but some cortical displacement can be accepted. The fracture unites by secondary bone healing with callus.

### Medial malleolar fracture fixation

Isolated medial malleolar fractures, even with modest displacement, are treated non-operatively, provided that there is no talar shift. It is customary to fix the medial malleolus after

lateral malleolar fixation in bimalleolar injuries. Parallel lag screws are usually adequate, but small, comminuted or osteoporotic fragments are more reliably fixed with a tension band technique (p. 95). The proximal end of the tension band wire is looped over a small fragment screw with washer inserted into the supramalleolar region; the distal section is passed through the deltoid ligament with the aid of an intravenous cannula (**Fig. 21.31**).

### Posterior malleolar fracture fixation

These are considered significant where there is posterior talar subluxation, which is more likely where the fragment comprises >25–35% of the articular surface. Posterior malleolar fixation will often address any syndesmotic instability, as the PITFL usually remains intact and attached to the fragment. Reduction can be achieved with:

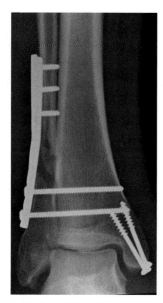

Fig. 21.29 Fibular bridge plate.

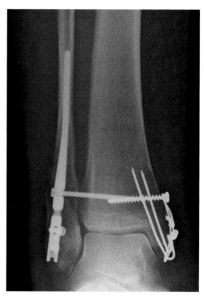

Fig. 21.31 Medial malleolus tension band wire.

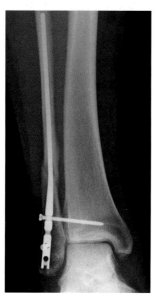

Fig. 21.30 Fibular nail with callus.

- *Closed ligamentotaxis*: Dorsiflexion of the ankle joint alone may be sufficient to achieve reduction. Fixation is percutaneous with partially threaded lag screws from the front.

- *Percutaneous manipulation* (**Fig. 21.32**): A fragment that is irreducible with ligamentotaxis alone can often be reduced percutaneously with a periosteal elevator or large reduction forceps (inserted with cautious respect for the neurovascular anatomy of the region posterior to the tibia), before placement of AP percutaneous screws.

- *Open reduction with posterior buttress plate* (**Fig. 21.33**): A direct visual reduction of the cortex can be achieved with the patient placed prone, via the posterolateral approach (p. 509). This can be helpful where bone quality is poor or the fragment is expected to be difficult to reduce. The fragment is provisionally held with a k-wire before buttress plate fixation. The fibula can be plated through the same incision.

## Syndesmosis fixation

- *Indication*: Syndesmosis fixation is indicated in three scenarios:
  1. *Fibula fracture in its proximal two-thirds* (a PER or Maisonneuve fracture; see Fig. 21.14). There is usually clear diastasis on the presentation (or

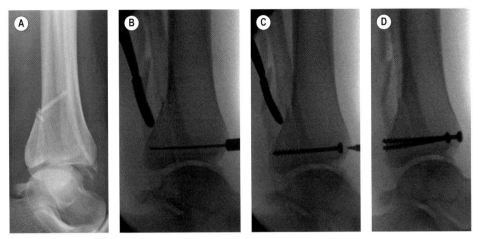

Fig. 21.32 **A**, Posterior malleolar fracture with posterior talar subluxation. **B**, The malleolus has been reduced percutaneously with a periosteal elevator. Through an anterior stab incision, a drill hole has been placed just above the joint and a depth gauge inserted. **C**, The fracture is fixed and compressed with a partially threaded 3.5-mm cancellous lag screw. **D**, Completed fixation with two screws. Note that the talus is now congruent.

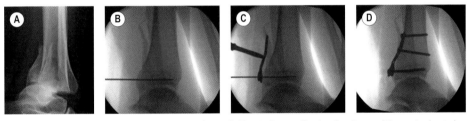

Fig. 21.33 Posterior malleolus: buttress plate. **A**, Posterior malleolar fracture with posterior talar subluxation. **B**, The malleolus has been reduced open through the posterolateral approach, and stabilized temporarily with a k-wire. **C**, A buttress plate is applied. **D**, Completed fixation with lag screws distally through the plate. Note that the talus is now congruent. The fibula was subsequently fixed through the same incision (see Fig. 21.28).

subsequent) radiographs. The fibular fracture does not need to be explored or fixed; doing so is unnecessary and puts the peroneal nerve at risk. Instead, the mortise is reduced and stabilized directly. The technique of mortise reduction is controversial. Closed screw placement is associated with a high rate of malreduction, as it is often difficult on plain fluoroscopy to show clearly whether or not the fibula has been returned to the incisura. Open reduction is often preferred.

2. *Fibular fracture in the distal third with clear diastasis* (see Fig. 21.16): The fibular fracture is reduced and fixed, and a syndesmosis screw is placed. The fibular fixation will usually ensure adequate syndesmotic reduction, and a separate open reduction of the syndesmosis is not usually required.

3. *Fibular fracture in the distal third with diastasis revealed only on intraoperative stress testing* (see Fig. 21.41): If clear opening of the syndesmosis is shown after fibular fixation, a syndesmosis screw is placed through the plate.

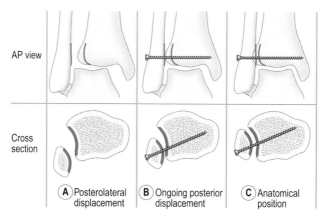

Fig. 21.34 Diastasis reduction. See text for details.

Again, the syndesmosis itself does not require open exploration.

- Reduction: Anatomical reduction is essential but is not easy either to achieve or to judge. The fibula tends to shorten and sublux laterally and posteriorly from the incisura (**Fig. 21.34A**); when performing a closed fixation, it is easy to clamp and fix the fibula in a subluxed position, as the AP fluoroscopic image may look deceptively normal (**Fig. 21.34B**). Direct visualization of the 'Mercedes–Benz' sign provides confirmation of an anatomical reduction (**Fig. 21.34C**) (see 'Surgical technique', p. 502).

- *Fixation method* (see Fig. 21.27): The number of screws (one or two), their size (3.5 or 4.5 mm), and number of cortices (three or four) is controversial but unimportant. A 'tightrope' suture construct is preferred by some. The results of these techniques are comparable. There is no indication that routine screw removal results in any clinical benefit. Screws left in situ may undergo late fatigue failure. This is asymptomatic and patients should be advised that future radiographs may demonstrate a broken screw. Pragmatically, if removal of the screw is planned, a 4.5-mm screw head is larger and easier to locate.

## SURGICAL TECHNIQUE: Open reduction and internal fixation of SER IV (Weber B) ankle fracture

The fibula is addressed first, followed by the medial and posterior malleoli if required.

### Surgical set-up (Fig. 21.35)

The patient is placed supine, with a bolster under the ipsilateral buttock. A tourniquet may be preferred. Place the injured ankle on a radiolucent box to allow easy AP and lateral fluoroscopic images to be taken without moving the limb. Rehearse the fluoroscopic images to ensure adequate space for the c-arm.

### Orthopaedic equipment

- Small fragment set.
- Pointed and serrated reduction clamps.
- 1/3 tubular plate.
- 1.6-mm k-wires.

### Lateral incision and approach

Make a longitudinal incision over the lateral malleolus, centred on the fracture (**Fig. 21.36A**). Perform blunt dissection through subcutaneous fat, to avoid injury to the superficial peroneal nerve, which is variably encountered at this level. The periosteum is dissected back from the fracture edge by a millimetre or two to allow inspection and clearance of the fracture margin (**Fig. 21.36B**). Gently exaggerating the external rotation deformity may allow easier clearance of clot and bone fragments from the fracture site.

### Open reduction of the fibula

Reduction requires that the distal fragment is pulled out to length and is internally rotated. The majority of the reduction is gained when the assistant applies traction, inversion and internal rotation on the foot. Anatomical reduction can then be perfected in one of three ways (**Fig. 21.37**):

1. Application of a pointed reduction clamp to the distal metaphysis allows direct manipulation.
2. A serrated reduction clamp is applied directly to the fracture. If rotation and compression are applied with the clamp, the two fractured surfaces can be made to slide past each other into reduction.
3. Occasionally, a transverse fracture will be encountered and will be difficult to reduce with these techniques. Greater power can be achieved by placing a reduction clamp directly on to each fracture fragment, to allow these to be separated and reduced.

A pointed reduction clamp is then applied obliquely across the fracture to maintain reduction. Reduction is assessed fluoroscopically with careful inspection of the normal radiographic features, particularly the fibular length, nipple and lateral joint space (Fig. 21.8).

### Internal fixation of the fibula – absolute stability (Fig. 21.38)

A lag screw is placed orthogonally across the fracture (see Fig. 5.7). A 1/3 tubular plate is precontoured to the shape of the fibula and applied as a neutralization plate, with at least three cortical screws above and three cancellous screws below the fracture. The metaphyseal screws should be placed in a triangular configuration or with a longitudinal screw (see Fig. 21.27). Ensure that the distal cancellous screws do not enter the joint.

### Medial incision and approach (Fig. 21.39)

The medial malleolus is exposed through a longitudinal incision centred over the fracture, taking care to avoid injury to the saphenous vein and nerve. The fracture is cleared of debris and clot. A flap of periosteum is usually folded into the superior edge of the fracture and this is removed with forceps or dental pick.

### Medial malleolus reduction and fixation – absolute stability (Fig. 21.40)

The fragment is reduced anatomically. Holding this reduction can be achieved with a small pointed reduction clamp, one tine of which is placed in a drill hole positioned 2 cm above the fracture. A 1.6-mm k-wire may also be placed to stabilize the fragment. The fracture is then held with two partially threaded cancellous screws. The screws should pass perpendicular to the fracture and must avoid entering the joint. Carefully assess their position on the fluoroscopic images. A small or comminuted fragment may be held more securely by a tension band wire looped around a screw (see Fig. 21.31).

### Syndesmosis assessment

Syndesmosis instability is uncommon in SER fractures, but should be excluded fluoroscopically by a direct lateral pull on the fibula with a reduction clamp (**Fig. 21.41**); if there is a clear opening of the syndesmosis, a syndesmosis screw is placed.

### Postoperative restrictions

Movement: The patient is provided with an orthosis (moon boot) to allow early active range of movement exercises.

Weight-bearing: The patient is usually allowed full weight-bearing.

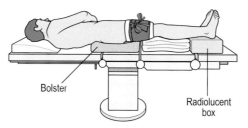

Bolster

Radiolucent box

Fig. 21.35 Ankle fractures: set-up.

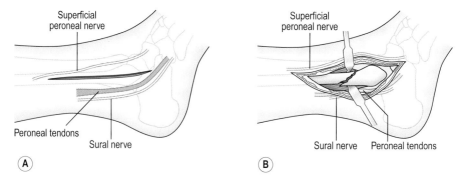

Superficial peroneal nerve

Peroneal tendons

Sural nerve

(A)

Superficial peroneal nerve

Sural nerve    Peroneal tendons

(B)

Fig. 21.36 Lateral malleolar fractures: incision and approach.

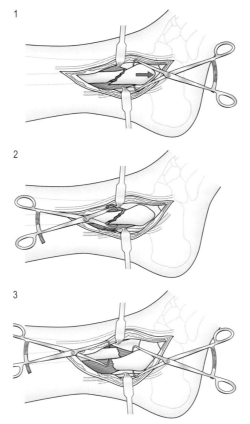

1

2

3

Fig. 21.37 Lateral malleolar fractures: reduction. See technique box (p. 498) for details.

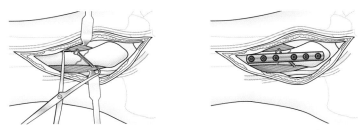

Fig. 21.38 Lateral malleolar fractures: fibular leg screw and neutralization plate.

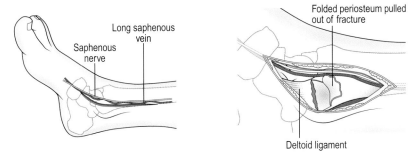

Fig. 21.39 Medial malleolar fractures: incision and approach.

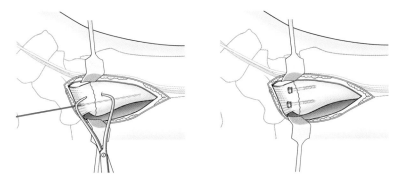

Fig. 21.40 Medial malleolar fractures: reduction and fixation.

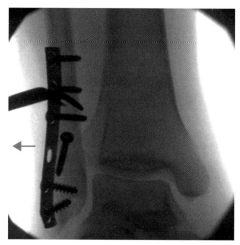

Fig. 21.41 Intraoperative stress testing of the syndesmosis.

## SURGICAL TECHNIQUE: Open reduction of the syndesmosis (PER III/Maisonneuve)

### Surgical set-up

The patient is placed supine, with a bolster under the ipsilateral buttock. A thigh tourniquet is used. Place the injured ankle on a radiolucent box to allow easy AP and lateral fluoroscopic images without moving the limb.

### Orthopaedic equipment

- Small fragment set.
- Large ball-spike clamp
- 2-mm k-wire.

### Incisions and approach

- *Syndesmosis*: A 4-cm longitudinal incision is made directly anteriorly over the inferior tibiofibular joint. The fat is dissected bluntly to avoid injury to the superficial peroneal nerve. The extensor retinaculum is incised. As the syndesmosis has been torn open, the ankle joint and syndesmosis are now exposed. The ATFL is seen to be torn or avulsed, and there is a clear space between the fibula and tibia (**Fig. 21.42A**).
- *Lateral ankle*: A separate longitudinal incision is made over the lateral aspect of the fibula just above the level of the syndesmosis for placement of the reduction clamp and fixation screw.
- *Medial ankle*: A small stab incision is required for the application of the reduction clamp.

### Open reduction and internal fixation

The syndesmosis and incisura are cleared of clot and the articular surfaces of the talus, tibia and fibula are identified. A percutaneous 2-mm k-wire is placed in the lateral malleolus as a joystick, to allow the fibula to the moved distally, anteriorly and with some internal rotation (to correct an externally rotated position) (**Fig. 21.42B**). The ankle is held plantigrade throughout the reduction and fixation, without dorsiflexion or plantar flexion. In this position, the talus fills the mortise fully, whereas if the foot is allowed to plantar-flex, the narrower posterior part of the talus is engaged and the reduction is more difficult to judge. Anatomical reduction is confirmed by a 'Mercedes–Benz' sign of the congruent articular surfaces formed by the fibula, tibia and talus (**Fig. 21.42C**).

The tines of a large ball spike clamp are applied to maintain this reduction, and the reduction is confirmed fluoroscopically. Assess the mortise view carefully to confirm fibular length, using the lateral joint space and the fibula nipple as references. Note that the position of the fibula in the incisura is posterior to the midline of the tibia, and that the orientation of the clamp, as well as the trajectory of the fixation screw, must be in 20° of external rotation (see Fig. 21.34). The drill is passed in this trajectory, 3cm above the tibial plafond, passing through three cortices (lateral fibula, medial fibula and lateral tibia, but not the medial tibial cortex). The depth is measured and the screw inserted (**Fig. 21.42C, D**). The syndesmosis cannot be over-tightened. The final construct should be evaluated on lateral fluoroscopy to confirm that the screw has successfully passed through the centre of the fibula into the tibia. In the figure shown, the view has been taken in the plane of the screw (20° of internal rotation) rather than as a true lateral; note that the talar dome is not seen in true profile.

### Postoperative restrictions

Movement: The patient is provided with an orthosis (moon boot) to allow early active range of movement exercises.

Weight-bearing: There is a lack of consensus. Some surgeons may prefer to keep the patient non-weight-bearing for 8weeks.

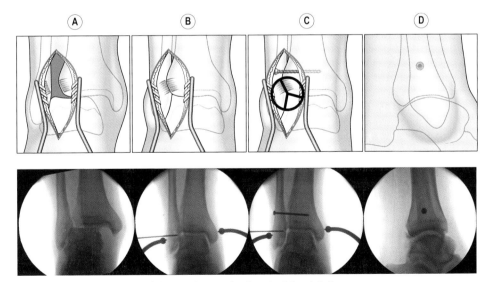

Fig. 21.42 Open reduction of the syndesmosis. See text for details.

**SURGICAL TECHNIQUE: Open reduction and internal fixation of an SAD II ankle fracture**

The medial malleolus is addressed first, followed by the lateral side if required.

### Surgical set-up (see Fig. 21.35)

The patient is placed supine, with a bolster under the ipsilateral buttock. A thigh tourniquet is used. Place the injured ankle on a radiolucent box to allow easy AP and lateral fluoroscopic images without moving the limb. Rehearse the fluoroscopic images to ensure adequate space for the c-arm.

### Orthopaedic equipment

- Small fragment set.
- Osteotomes.
- Bone graft or bone graft substitute may be required.

### Medial incision and approach (see Fig. 21.39)

The medial malleolus is exposed through a longitudinal incision centred over the fracture, taking care to avoid injury to the saphenous vein and nerve. The length of this incision should take into account the planned fixation technique; a longer incision will be required for a plate.

### Open reduction and internal fixation of the medial side – absolute stability (Fig. 21.43)

1. Reduction requires that the large medial malleolar shear fragment (**Fig. 21.43A**) is levered out from above so that the impacted region can be assessed (**Fig. 21.43B**). Clear the fracture of clot and bone fragments.
2. Impaction is corrected by passing an osteotome over the impacted region 1 cm above the articular surface.
3. Levering this down brings the plafond into an anatomical reduction against the talar dome (**Fig. 21.43C**). If the reduced subarticular segment is particularly frail, the void may be filled with graft (conveniently taken from the proximal tibial metaphysis) or graft substitute. However, the reduced region is usually large enough to be supported by screws, in which case no graft filling is required. The medial malleolar fragment is now reduced and temporarily held with k-wires.
4. The shear fracture can be compressed and buttressed with a plate (**Fig. 21.43D**), or alternatively with three screws (Fig. 21.26). The most proximal screw sits at the apex of the fracture and holds this in a reduced position, preventing failure through shear. The use of a washer at the apex is often helpful, and is colloquially termed a 'one-hole plate'.

### Internal fixation of the fibula

A large fibular fragment can be fixed with a plate or nail. A small or undisplaced fragment may be managed non-operatively, or secured with a tension band technique.

### Postoperative restrictions

Movement: The patient is provided with an orthosis (moon boot) to allow early active range of movement exercises.

Weight-bearing: If there has been significant marginal impaction, weight-bearing is restricted for 6 weeks.

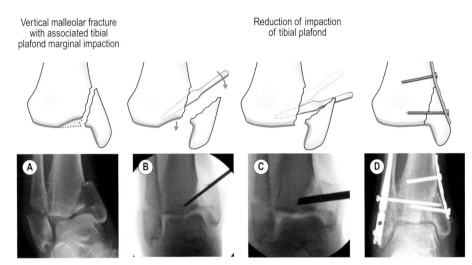

Fig. 21.43 Supination–adduction II fracture fixation.

## Outpatient management

### Weight-bearing

Patients with stable ankle fractures treated non-operatively can begin full weight-bearing as soon as comfortable. Most operatively treated fractures should also be allowed full weight-bearing postoperatively unless there is a specific concern. However, patients with altered neuromuscular perception and control are at risk of fixation failure and should be kept non-weight-bearing until fracture union. This includes patients with:

- diabetic (or other) peripheral neuropathy (union is often delayed)
- psychiatric disorders
- nerve or spinal cord lesions.

In addition, many surgeons protect certain constructs, including:

- syndesmosis fixation, with non-weight-bearing for 8 weeks
- fractures with substantial intra-articular components, such as a large posterior malleolus (>25%) that has been fixed, with non-weight-bearing for 6 weeks.

| Outpatient management summary | | | |
|---|---|---|---|
| **Week** | **Examination** | **Radiographs** | **Additional notes** |
| 1 – post surgery | Wound check<br>Neurovascular status | AP and lateral ankle | Permit early mobilization if the construct is stable |
| 1 – non-operative treatment | Examination after 1 week of weight-bearing to ensure no instability or displacement | AP and lateral ankle | If there is no displacement, continue to allow full weight-bearing in an orthosis (moonboot) until the fracture is united |
| 6 | Range of movement check<br>Check for tenderness at fracture site | AP and lateral ankle | If the patient is pain-free, then discharge |
| Further assessments at 2–4-week intervals if required for delayed union | | | |
| Average time to union = 6 weeks | | | |

## COMPLICATIONS

### *Early*

Local    Wound dehiscence or necrosis: This may occur where the soft tissue envelope has been compromised preoperatively. The use of percutaneous techniques, judiciously timed surgery and avoidance of tourniquets all reduce the risk. Infection is initially treated with wound debridement, suppressive antibiotic treatment and late removal of metalwork as required

### *Late*

Local    Delayed union or non-union: This is rare after surgically treated ankle fractures. Revision compression plating, with or without additional autogenous bone graft, may be required

Malunion: This usually results if the fibula has been left shortened and malrotated, and revision fixation is required. Occasionally, an osteotomy is needed if the fracture has already united

Post-traumatic arthritis: Arthritis may occur after both soft tissue injuries and fractures, and may take several years to become apparent. The incidence is related to grade and severity of the fracture, and is almost inevitable if the ankle mortise has not been reduced. Ankle arthroplasty or fusion may be required

## PILON FRACTURES

Pilon fractures are severe injuries to the ankle region that are quite different from ankle fractures. They are *intra-articular* fractures of the plafond caused by an axial load. Pilon fractures (French: 'pestle') are so named because the plafond is injured by the talus punching up into it, much as a pestle is used to crush and grind ingredients in a mortar. The history is usually one of a high-energy motor vehicle collision or fall from a height. Pilon fractures are associated with a considerable insult to the *soft tissue envelope*, and it is the soft tissues that usually define the type and timing of surgery, and the risk of acute complications.

## Classification

### Ruedi and Allgower classification

The Ruedi and Allgower classification is a simple description of three stages of severity (**Fig. 21.44**):

- Type I – undisplaced intra-articular fracture
- Type II – displaced intra-articular fracture
- Type III – comminuted or impacted fracture.

### AO classification

The AO universal classification of fractures describes distal tibial fractures as region 43 with three types (**Fig. 21.45**): type A are extra-articular fractures (which are distal tibial fractures rather than pilon fractures), B are partial articular fractures and C are complete articular fractures. Type C fractures are divided into three groups, reflecting the nature of the fracture line(s) in the metaphyseal and articular regions:

- C1 – simple metaphyseal, simple articular
- C2 – complex metaphyseal, simple articular
- C3 – complex metaphyseal, complex articular.

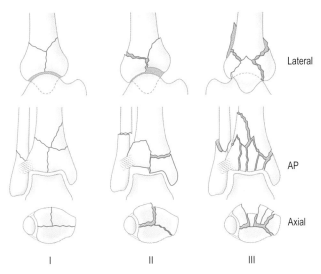

Lateral

AP

Axial

I          II          III

Fig. 21.44 Ruedi and Allgower classification of pilon fractures.

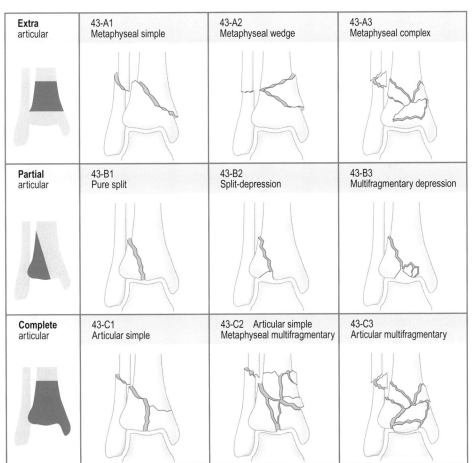

| **Extra** articular | 43-A1 Metaphyseal simple | 43-A2 Metaphyseal wedge | 43-A3 Metaphyseal complex |
| --- | --- | --- | --- |
| **Partial** articular | 43-B1 Pure split | 43-B2 Split-depression | 43-B3 Multifragmentary depression |
| **Complete** articular | 43-C1 Articular simple | 43-C2  Articular simple Metaphyseal multifragmentary | 43-C3 Articular multifragmentary |

Fig. 21.45 AO classification of distal tibia fractures.

# Emergency Department management

## Clinical features

- The mechanism of injury is usually high-energy. Exclude other associated injuries that may require urgent treatment.
- Obvious deformity of the ankle should be reduced on recognition.
- A careful examination of the leg, ankle and foot is required, including an assessment of the integrity of the skin and the neurovascular state of the limb.
- The soft tissue envelope in particular requires careful assessment. Swelling and contusion are common. Skin blistering, both clear and haemoserous (p. 40), will often develop over several hours.

## Radiological features

- *AP and lateral ankle radiographs*: The extent of the injury is usually indicated clearly on the plain films. However, accurate mapping of the various fragments is challenging.
- *CT scan*: This is invaluable for preoperative planning (see Fig. 21.47).

## Closed reduction

Emergency Department reduction of a pilon fracture requires realignment of the limb. The hindfoot should be brought in line with the tibia, and any rotation should be corrected. Articular congruity will rarely be re-established and can usually only be achieved with operative fixation.

## Immobilization and reassessment

A below-knee backslab should be applied (p. 70), followed by a careful clinical reassessment and check radiographs. The leg must be elevated to lie above the heart.

## Inpatient referral

- All pilon fractures should be referred to the orthopaedic service.

# Orthopaedic management

## Non-operative

Simple, undisplaced pilon fractures are rare but may be treated non-operatively, particularly in elderly patients. They do, however, require careful and regular review, as they are intrinsically unstable and may displace.

## Operative

Most pilon fractures are treated operatively. *Timing* of surgery will depend on the expertise available and the condition of the soft tissues. Early surgery may be appropriate in the initial phase if swelling and bruising are minimal, and where the necessary expertise and facilities are available. However, injudicious surgery through a compromised soft tissue envelope may lead to disastrous wound complications. If there is any concern, or when a delay is anticipated, a *staged protocol* with initial application of a bridging external fixator (see Fig. 20.34) will allow temporization for transfer, imaging and surgical planning ('span, scan and plan'). The frame should re-establish length and alignment of the limb, and the pin sites must be positioned well away from the planned surgical incisions and plate positions. Additional fixation of the fibula before transfer to another surgeon is to be avoided, as the wound will limit the subsequent options. Definitive surgical reconstruction is then performed at 5–14 days.

Regardless of timing, the aims of surgery are to:

- reconstruct the articular surface of the plafond
- restore the alignment of the mortise
- protect the soft tissue envelope.

## Surgical techniques

*A-type fractures*

From a surgical fixation perspective, these are distal tibial fractures rather than pilon fractures. Depending on the size of the fragment, they are treated with intramedullary nailing or distal tibial plates (see Fig. 20.29).

*B-type fractures*

Definitive surgery for B-type fractures is with percutaneous screws or buttress plating, with or without grafting of the defect (**Fig. 21.46**).

*C-type fractures*

In C-type fractures, the plafond usually separates into a number of common fragments,

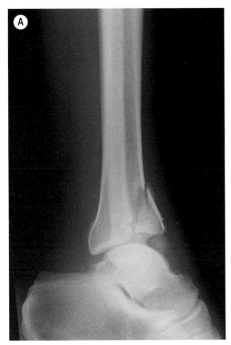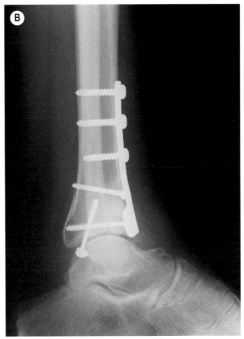

Fig. 21.46 B-type pilon fracture: buttress plate. **A**, Anterior impaction and incongruity. **B**, The articular surface was reduced, the resulting defect was grafted with a bone block (held with a screw), and a buttress plate applied with lag screws distally.

which can only be completely assessed with CT (**Fig. 21.47**):

- An *anterolateral fragment* bearing the tubercle of Chaput.
- A *medial fragment* bearing the medial malleolus.
- The *posterior malleolus*.
- A *die-punch fragment*, which has typically been driven proximally into the centre of the metaphysis. It has no soft tissue attachments and cannot therefore be reduced by traction or ligamentotaxis. Its impacted central position blocks the reduction of the remaining fragments.
- A variable number of *small, comminuted fragments* of bone that are too small to be incorporated into the reconstruction, but that must be identified and removed before the main fragments can be reduced.

Surgery is conveniently performed under traction using a femoral distractor or an external fixator. The location of the fracture lines and the fracture configuration govern the incision, or combination of incisions, used for the approach. Three main approaches allow the fixation of most pilon fractures (see below). For displaced C3 fractures, sequential exposures may be required. Where there is a displaced posterior malleolar fragment, it is often easiest to use the posterolateral approach first and then buttress it. This then becomes the keystone, on to which the remainder of the plafond is reconstructed through one of the anterior approaches (**Fig. 21.48**), in a manner analogous to the sequence of steps for fixing a bicondylar tibial plateau fracture. Fibula fixation or nailing, either before or after completing the tibial fixation, adds additional stability to the construct.

- *Posterolateral approach to the ankle* (**Fig. 21.49**): This approach allows access to the posterior malleolar fragment and fibula through the same incision. The patient is

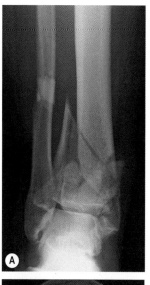
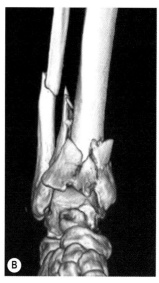
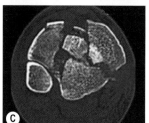
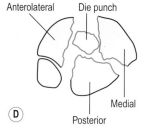

Fig. 21.47 C-type pilon: fracture assessment. **A**, Plain AP radiograph of a C3-type pilon fracture, showing the complexity of the injury. **B**, Three-dimensional CT reconstruction of the same ankle. **C**, Axial sections allow the fragments to be identified for preoperative planning. **D**, These usually follow a predictable pattern.

Anterolateral    Die punch

Medial

Posterior

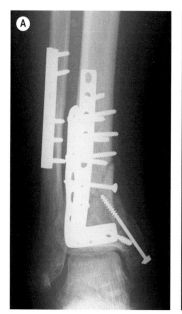
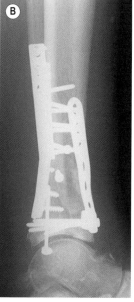

Fig. 21.48 C-type pilon: the same fracture as is shown in Figure 21.47. Postoperative radiographs after fracture union with posterior and anterolateral plates on the tibia. **A**, AP view. **B**, Lateral view.

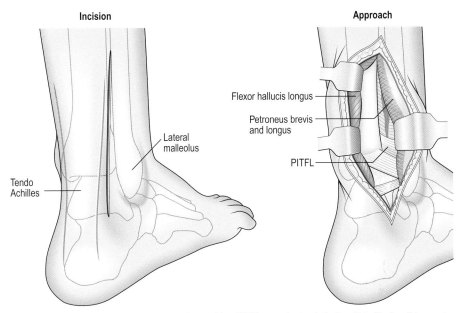

**Incision**

Tendo
Achilles

Lateral
malleolus

**Approach**

Flexor hallucis longus

Petroneus brevis
and longus

PITFL

Fig. 21.49 Posterolateral approach to the ankle. PITFL, posterior inferior tibiofibular ligament.

placed prone or lateral. The 10-cm incision lies midway between the lateral border of the Achilles tendon and the posterior border of the lateral malleolus, starting in line with the tip of the lateral malleolus. Blunt dissection prevents injury to the short saphenous vein and sural nerve. A plane is developed between the peroneal tendons laterally (superficial peroneal nerve) and the Achilles tendon medially (tibial nerve) to reveal the belly of flexor hallucis longus (tibial nerve). The flexor hallucis is elevated, starting at its lateral border and progressing medially, to reveal the posterior malleolus, which is reduced and buttressed. The posteromedial neurovascular bundle is retracted safely with the flexor hallucis muscle belly medially. If the fibula requires fixation, the peroneal sheath is incised and the tendons are retracted medially to allow a posterior plate to be inserted. If the patient is prone, they will now need to be repositioned supine for the anterior approach.

- *Anterolateral approach to the ankle* (**Fig. 21.50**): The 'workhorse' approach for most

pilon fractures, this incision allows access to the anterolateral fragment and also good visualization of the joint surface. The patient is placed supine. The incision is positioned immediately lateral to the extensor digitorum longus tendon to the little toe, and extends beyond the ankle joint distally to allow visualization of the joint surface. Blunt dissection avoids injury to the superficial peroneal nerve and exposes the deep fascia and extensor retinaculum, which are then divided. The major cortical fragments are progressively reduced and temporarily secured with k-wires or clamps, to restore tibial length. The fracture is opened to expose the die-punch fragment, which is cleared and reduced on to the posterior malleolus. It may be held with a threaded k-wire, which can be left within the bone permanently (incarcerated k-wire). The remaining fragments are then reduced and compressed. A contoured, low-profile locking plate can then be passed proximally in the submuscular plane to secure the definitive fixation (Fig. 21.48). Alternatively, an

**Incision**          **Approach**

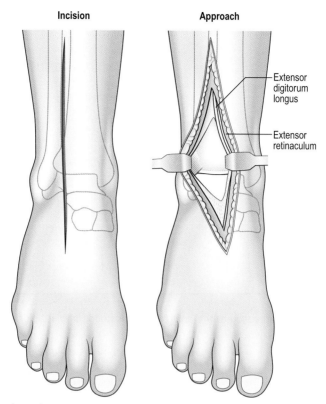

Extensor
digitorum
longus

Extensor
retinaculum

Fig. 21.50 Anterolateral approach to the ankle.

external fixator or ring frame may be used for definitive treatment, with or without prior articular lag screw placement.

- *Anteromedial approach to the ankle*: The incision is placed over the tibialis anterior tendon; it may be extended linearly towards that tendon's insertion in the navicular, or curved posteriorly distal to the medial malleolus. The extensor retinaculum is divided as above and the fracture is exposed by passing either medial to the tibialis anterior tendon, or lateral to the extensor hallucis tendon. Caution is required between these two tendons, as this approach risks injury to the deep peroneal nerve and anterior tibial artery.

- *Direct medial approach*: It is prudent to avoid extensive incisions directly over the medial subcutaneous border of the tibia, but small incisions can be made to allow the

percutaneous insertion of screws or small medial buttress plates, typically 1/3 tubular or 2.7-mm plates.

- *Lateral malleolar fixation*: This provides additional stability to the construct. Use of a posterolateral incision or a percutaneous fibular nail minimizes the degree of soft tissue disruption.

### Unreconstructible C-type fractures

Occasionally, the condition of the soft tissue envelope or the degree of comminution at the articular surface precludes safe fixation. In this situation, the ankle can initially be stabilized with an 'A-frame' external fixator until the soft tissues recover. This may take several weeks. Subsequent primary fusion of the ankle joint provides alignment and stability. The use of a blade plate through the posterolateral approach minimizes the risk to the soft tissues.

# Outpatient management

| Outpatient management summary | | | |
| --- | --- | --- | --- |
| **Week** | **Examination** | **Radiographs** | **Additional notes** |
| 1 – post surgery | Wound check<br>Neurovascular status | AP and lateral ankle | Immobilize in a cast or boot orthosis until the wounds are stable |
| 6 | Clinical and radiographic review | AP and lateral ankle | Begin gentle active ankle joint mobilization |
| 8–12 | Clinical and radiographic review | AP and lateral ankle | If the fracture has united, begin weight-bearing and passive and resisted ankle mobilization |
| 26 | Clinical and radiographic review | AP and lateral ankle | Ensure that the fracture is consolidating and stable |

Further assessments at 4-week intervals if required for delayed union

Average time to union = 12 weeks, depending on comminution and soft tissue damage

## COMPLICATIONS

### Early

Local    Wound dehiscence or necrosis: This may occur where the soft tissue envelope has been compromised preoperatively. The use of percutaneous techniques, judiciously timed surgery and avoidance of tourniquets all reduce the risk. Infection is initially treated with wound debridement, suppressive antibiotic treatment and late removal of metalwork as required. Wound dehiscence may require coverage with a flap

### Late

Local    Delayed-union or non-union: This occurs most commonly in the metadiaphyseal region when there has been comminution. Revised compression plating, with or without additional autogenous bone graft, may be required

Malunion: This occurs most commonly with non-operative or external fixator treatment

Post-traumatic arthritis: Some degree of arthritis is almost inevitable after high-grade pilon fractures, with high rates of stiffness and swelling. Analgesia, bracing or surgery (ankle fusion) may be required

## ANKLE SPRAINS

The majority of ankle injury presentations to the Emergency Department are ankle sprains. The aim of clinical assessment is to rule out any significant bony injury and to ensure that the ankle joint remains stable and congruent.

## Classification

Common ankle sprains include:

- *Lateral ankle sprains (SAD I injuries)*: These result in pain over the lateral ligamentous complex, particularly the ATFL and CFL, following an inversion injury. Local swelling and bruising are common, with tenderness anterior and inferior to the lateral malleolus. Radiographs may reveal a small fleck of bone at the tip of the fibula, demonstrating an avulsion fracture.

- *Syndesmosis sprains ('high ankle sprain' or SER I injuries)*: These are rarer but more severe; they result in tenderness over the AITFL and a positive squeeze test (see Fig. 21.4).

- *Deltoid ligament sprains (PER I injuries)*: These are uncommon but are the result of a forced eversion injury. Always be suspicious of a Maisonneuve type injury (see Fig. 21.14).

## Emergency Department management

Use the Ottawa ankle rules (p. 483) to help guide the requirement for radiographs. Once a fracture has been excluded clinically or radiographically, treatment is with rest, ice, compression bandaging and elevation (RICE). Immobilization in an orthosis (moon boot) or cast, and the use of crutches are occasionally required for short-term symptom control. Active range of movement exercises should begin early.

Recurrent ankle sprains give rise to the typical radiographic appearance of a 'footballer's ankle', with multiple old avulsion fractures and flakes of calcification that can occur medially, laterally or anteriorly.

## ACHILLES TENDON RUPTURE

Achilles tendon ruptures commonly occur after a sudden push-off in sport or following a simple trip with forced dorsiflexion of the foot against a contracting calf muscle.

## Emergency Department management

### Clinical features

- Patients are usually over the age of 30 and there is often a history of previous Achilles tendonitis.

- There is usually a clear history of pain in the back of the heel during activity or a fall, although occasionally, very sedentary individuals will complain simply of reduced power in the foot.

- Patients often report the feeling of a sudden explosive pain in the back of the ankle, as if they had been kicked.

- Ask about predisposing factors for tendinopathy, including local or systemic steroid treatment, inflammatory joint disease or the recent use of quinolone antibiotics.

- The Achilles tendon is most easily examined with the patient prone or kneeling, with the feet over the edge of the table (Fig. 21.51).

- Examine the uninjured side first for comparison and then carefully palpate along the length of the injured tendon. A clear tender defect in the contour of the tendon is diagnostic of a complete tendon rupture. This will be more evident if the tendon is gently stretched by passively dorsiflexing the foot.

- An area of swelling and tenderness is more difficult to assess and may represent a partial rupture.

- The Simmonds' (or Thompson's) test is performed by gently squeezing the belly of the calf muscle; in a positive test, the foot does not plantar-flex (**Fig. 21.51**).

- Pain and tenderness in the belly of the triceps surae (calf) muscle, with no tendon abnormality or defect, is suggestive of a muscular tear. This is treated symptomatically with analgesia and early mobilization.

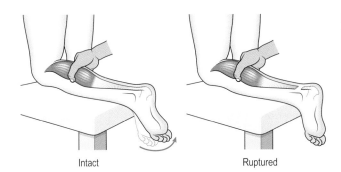

**Fig. 21.51** Simmonds' (Thompson's) test.

Intact        Ruptured

## Radiological features

- *Ultrasound scan*: An ultrasound scan is helpful where the diagnosis is in doubt or a partial rupture is suspected.

## Immobilization and outpatient follow-up

The patient is provided with a backslab in equinus (plantar flexion) or an equinus brace, with crutches, and referred to the orthopaedic clinic.

## Orthopaedic management

### Non-operative

Most Achilles tendon ruptures are managed non-operatively. The principle is to immobilize the foot in a position of equinus initially, in order to bring the two ruptured tendon ends together, and then to allow the gradual adoption of a neutral foot position as the tendon heals and regains strength. This can be achieved with serial casts (e.g. 4 weeks equinus, 4 weeks semi-equinus and 2 weeks neutral) or with an orthosis (boot) with heel wedges (e.g. 4 weeks with a 3-cm wedge, 2 weeks with a 1.5-cm wedge and 2 weeks in neutral). The advantage of an orthosis is that the patient is able to weight-bear immediately and is not reliant on crutches. There is probably some biological advantage to loading the Achilles tendon during healing. A partial tear is managed in similar fashion.

### Operative

There is little advantage in acute Achilles tendon repair in the majority of patients, although there are advocates for intervention in high-level athletes in order to allow an earlier return to training. Set against this is a small incidence of wound dehiscence and infection, and sural nerve injury. Surgery is usually reserved for patients who suffer a re-rupture, and those presenting late (more than 2 weeks) after rupture.

### Surgical techniques

Surgery is performed with the patient prone. A para-midline incision is placed slightly medially to avoid the sural nerve and to prevent a scar over the back of the heel. The paratenon is incised and the two ends of the Achilles tendon dissected free of scar tissue. If the two ends can be approximated without tension, a Krackow suture is placed in each end (see 'Technical tip') and the two sutures are tied together. If there is a defect, a turndown flap of triceps tendon, or a length of flexor hallucis longus tendon, is used to bridge this gap, weaving the graft through the distal stump. The paratenon is carefully closed as a separate layer. Alternatively, a number of percutaneous suture techniques have been described. A small incidence of suture failure and sural nerve entrapment is reported.

## PERONEAL TENDON DISLOCATION

Acute dislocation of the peroneal tendons is uncommon but may present following an eversion injury to the ankle. The tendons dislocate from their normal position in a shallow groove behind the lateral malleolus, either with a retinacular tear, or with avulsion of the entire sheath from the bone. The tendons will usually snap back into position with return of the foot to a neutral position.

## ⊘ Technical tip

A Krackow suture (**Fig. 21.52**) is an invaluable grasping suture for large tendons, and is used for repair of the Achilles tendon, patella tendon, quads tendon and biceps tendon as well as in the preparation of grafts.

1. Begin by passing the suture up through one torn end of the tendon.

2. Each bite of tendon passes through the loop of the previous bite, in order to lock the suture and reduce the risk of it tearing out.

3, 4. Further bites are taken progressively further from the tendon end, each locking with the last.

5. After four bites, a transverse bite takes the needle to the other side of the tendon.

6. A second line of locked sutures is now placed running distally, and finished by emerging from the torn tendon end. Pull firmly on the suture ends and load these cyclically to ensure the bites are snugged down and tight.

7, 8. The other tendon end is secured with another Krackow suture. The two ends are then tied firmly together to complete the repair. In a transosseous repair (for patellar tendon avulsion, for example), two separate pieces of suture material are used to produce two sets of Krackow sutures, with four suture ends. These are then fed through bone tunnels and tied together (see Fig. 19.19).

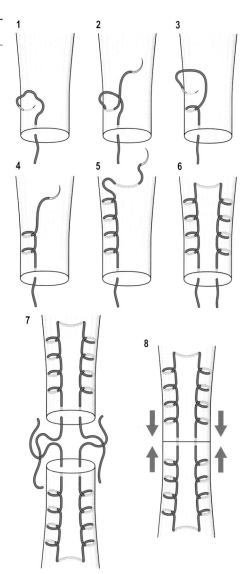

Fig. 21.52 Krackow suture.

## Emergency Department management

### Clinical features

- The patient will give a history of injury and a clear description of something snapping around the back of the lateral malleolus.

- Examination will identify local tenderness over the tendons, and pain and apprehension on resisted active eversion.

- It may be possible to demonstrate snapping of the tendons around the lateral malleolus with ankle movement.

- Exclude a fracture of the fibula and a rupture of the Achilles tendon.

### Outpatient follow-up

The patient should be provided with an orthosis (boot) or a backslab and crutches, and referred for orthopaedic assessment.

## Orthopaedic management

### Non-operative

Most cases of peroneal tendon dislocation can be treated non-operatively with 6 weeks in a cast or orthosis with the foot in slight plantar flexion and inversion to detension the peroneal tendons and steer them into the peroneal groove.

### Operative

Patients with ongoing peroneal tendon instability are offered surgical stabilization. This consists of an exposure of the posterior edge of the fibula and inspection of the retinaculum and groove. A shallow groove can be addressed by elevating the periosteum clear, deepening the groove with a burr and then replacing the periosteum. The avulsed sheath and retinaculum are then repaired back down to the bed with suture anchors. The patient is advised to remain non-weight-bearing with the foot in an equinus position in an orthosis for 6 weeks, before beginning a phased rehabilitation programme.

## GENERAL PRINCIPLES

### Anatomy

The foot is a highly complex structure, comprising 26 bones, 33 joints and more than 100 muscles, tendons and ligaments. These are conveniently considered in three regions separated by two major articulations (**Figs 22.1–22.2**):

1. *The hindfoot*: This comprises the talus and calcaneus.

2. *The midfoot*: This comprises the navicular and cuboid, and the three cuneiforms: medial, intermediate and lateral.

3. *The forefoot*: This comprises the metatarsals and phalanges.

The hindfoot articulates with the midfoot via *Chopart's joint*, and the midfoot articulates with the forefoot via the midtarsal or *Lisfranc joint*.

### Talus

The talus (Latin: 'ankle'), also known as the astragalus (Greek: 'ankle'), is remarkable for three reasons: 60% of its surface is covered in cartilage (**Fig. 22.3**), it has no tendon attachments, and it has a tenuous retrograde vascular supply (**Fig. 22.4**). Like the scaphoid and the femoral head, the talus is at particular risk of avascular necrosis after fracture. It is comprised of a body (with the lateral and posterior processes), a neck and a head.

The talar body is frustral in shape: a cone cut obliquely. It is almost semicircular when viewed in the sagittal plane. Viewed in the coronal plane, it has a rectangular cross-section that is broader anteriorly than posteriorly. As a result, the talus fills the mortise fully in dorsiflexion, providing ankle stability in heel-strike and stance, but is looser in plantar flexion, allowing some inversion and eversion to occur. The talar body carries the posterior and lateral processes. The *posterior process* has two tubercles, between which runs the tendon of flexor hallucis longus. In 50% of people, the lateral tubercle of the posterior process forms a separate *os trigonum*, which arises from a separate ossification centre and can be mistaken for a fractured fragment. Compare the lateral radiographs in **Figures 22.7** and **22.37**. The *lateral process* (seen most clearly on the mortise view of the ankle) can commonly be fractured in eversion injuries of the ankle (see Fig. 22.12).

The talar neck anteriorly terminates in the head, which articulates with the navicular.

### Articulations and blood supply

The talus contributes to three important articulations: with the tibia (ankle joint), navicular (talonavicular joint) and calcaneus (subtalar joint). The subtalar joint comprises three articular facets. The middle and anterior facets are separated from the posterior facet by the tarsal canal, which ends laterally in the trumpet-shaped tarsal sinus. The vascular supply to the talus arises from the three arteries of the leg (**Fig. 22.4**):

1. Branches of the dorsalis pedis (anterior tibial) artery supply the dorsum of the neck and head.

2. The posterior tibial and peroneal arteries anastomose as the artery of the tarsal canal, which supplies the body of the talus in a retrograde manner.

3. The posterior tibial artery also contributes a minor additional supply to the body via the deltoid ligament and capsular attachments.

This largely retrograde vascular supply is vulnerable to disruption in talar neck and body fractures.

### Calcaneus

The calcaneus has a complex shape, consisting of a tuberosity, an anterior process, and a medial process known as the sustentaculum tali (Latin: 'support for the talus') (**Fig. 22.5**).

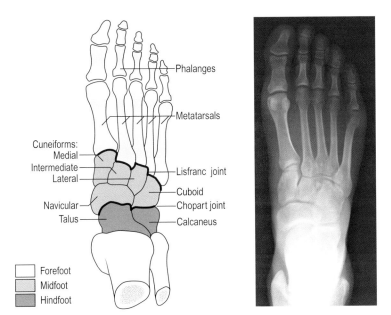

Fig. 22.1 Foot osteology AP view.

Phalanges

Metatarsals

Cuneiforms:
Medial
Intermediate
Lateral

Lisfranc joint

Cuboid
Chopart joint
Calcaneus

Navicular
Talus

Forefoot
Midfoot
Hindfoot

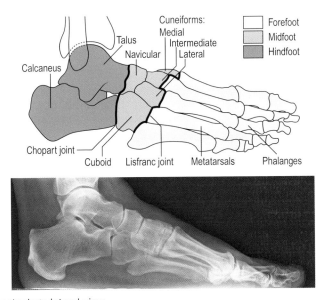

Cuneiforms:
Medial
Intermediate
Lateral

Forefoot
Midfoot
Hindfoot

Talus
Navicular

Calcaneus

Chopart joint
Cuboid    Lisfranc joint    Metatarsals    Phalanges

Fig. 22.2 Foot osteology lateral view.

The calcaneus articulates with the talus via the subtalar joint, which comprises a large posterior facet, a medial facet on the sustentaculum, and a smaller anterior facet. The subtalar joint is traversed by the tarsal canal, which broadens into the tarsal sinus laterally; the canal and sinus form a hollow between the calcaneus and talus that has no articular cartilage but contains the artery of the tarsal canal, and the talocalcaneal ligament. The calcaneus articulates with the cuboid via the calcaneocuboid joint (CCJ).

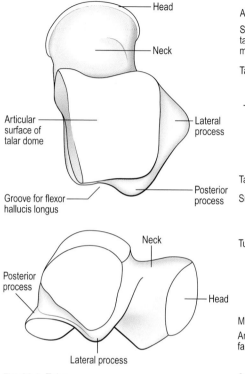

Head

Neck

Articular surface of talar dome

Lateral process

Groove for flexor hallucis longus

Posterior process

Neck

Posterior process

Head

Lateral process

Fig. 22.3 Talus.

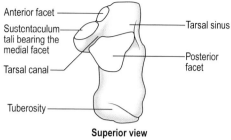

Anterior facet

Sustentaculum tali bearing the medial facet

Tarsal canal

Tuberosity

Tarsal sinus

Posterior facet

**Superior view**

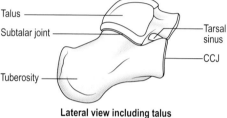

Talus

Subtalar joint

Tuberosity

Tarsal sinus

CCJ

**Lateral view including talus**

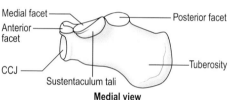

Medial facet

Anterior facet

CCJ

Sustentaculum tali

Posterior facet

Tuberosity

**Medial view**

Fig. 22.5 Calcaneus. CCJ, calcaneocuboid joint.

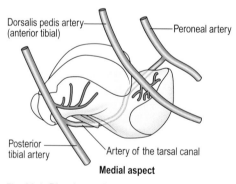

Dorsalis pedis artery (anterior tibial)

Peroneal artery

Posterior tibial artery

Artery of the tarsal canal

**Medial aspect**

Fig. 22.4 Blood supply to the talus.

## Navicular

The navicular (Latin: 'boat-like') is the keystone of the medial longitudinal arch of the foot. Its name derives from the proximal articular surface, which is concave and articulates with the talar head. In some respects, this joint, which is reinforced by articulations with the calcaneus and with the calcaneonavicular (spring) ligament, resembles a ball-and-socket joint, allowing limited movement in all three planes. The navicular has a prominent medial tuberosity that is the point of insertion of the tibialis posterior muscle. Fractures of the tuberosity must be distinguished from the *os naviculare*, which is an un-united secondary ossification centre, and radiographically is rounded and well corticated.

## Cuboid

The cuboid is the centre point of the lateral column of the foot. It links the Chopart and Lisfranc joints, and spans the naviculocuneiform joints.

## Cuneiforms

The cuneiform (Latin: 'wedge-shaped') bones articulate with the three distal articular

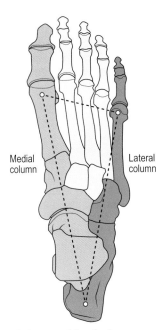

Medial column

Lateral column

Fig. 22.6 Columns of the foot.

surfaces of the navicular, and are important in creating the intrinsically stable shape of the Lisfranc joint.

## Columns of the foot

Biomechanically, the foot is considered to comprise a medial column, a lateral column and a middle column (**Fig. 22.6**). The relative lengths of these columns is important; a change in one will disrupt the architecture of the others. The foot is considered to have a weight-bearing triangle with principal contributions from the calcaneus and the heads of the first and fifth metatarsals.

## Toes

The great toe is termed the hallux. Both the hallux and the little toe are at increased risk of injury because of their vulnerable positions at the borders of the foot.

## Clinical assessment of the painful foot

### History

Foot injuries are a common presentation to the Emergency Department. Injury occurs via three broad mechanisms:

1. *Twisting injury*: The ankle and foot are vulnerable to rotational injury. The common simple inversion injury can result in malleolar fracture, a lateral foot sprain, or a fracture of the base of the fifth metatarsal. Be suspicious of more severe torsional injuries, which can result in the 'nutcracker' injury (see Fig. 22.33) or a Lisfranc dislocation (see Fig. 22.36).

2. *Axial compression injury*: The hindfoot is vulnerable to compression fracture following a fall from a height. Calcaneal or talar injury should raise suspicion of concurrent injuries in the axial skeleton as a result of proximal force transfer (see Fig. 22.26).

3. *Crush injury*: Toes injuries often present after being crushed by a heavy object or when a patient inadvertently kicks a hard object. These are relatively minor injuries but may involve the nail or joint. In contrast, high-energy crush injuries to the midfoot, particularly those involving the Lisfranc articulation, can be devastating, and may result in compartment syndrome of the foot (p. 549).

## Examination

### Look

Inspect the foot for deformity, swelling, abrasions or lacerations. Bruising may appear some hours after injury. Look particularly at the sole of the foot: bruising tracking through to the sole is indicative of a structural injury, such as a calcaneal fracture or Lisfranc injury.

### Feel

Begin by palpating the ankle to exclude any injury to the malleoli or collateral ligaments (p. 474). Then progress to palpating the bones of the foot from proximal to distal.

- *Hind foot*: Palpate the dorsum of the foot over the talar head and neck. Palpate the heel over the calcaneus. Pain on palpation of the heel pad may indicate either a bone or soft tissue injury; squeezing the calcaneus by grasping its sides suggests a bony injury (see Fig. 1.24).

- *Midfoot*: Continue by palpating over the dorsum of the midfoot, noting the congruity and any tenderness of Chopart's joint, the navicular, cuboid and cuneiforms, and the Lisfranc joint.

- *Forefoot*: Complete the palpation of the metatarsals, metatarsophalangeal joints and toes in turn.

### Move

Assess the range of movement of the ankle, subtalar and midtarsal joints. This is described in detail on page 475.

### Neurovascular assessment

Palpate the dorsalis pedis and posterior tibial artery pulsations, and after a significant foot injury mark their locations with ink to allow later reassessment. Ascertain the capillary refill to the toes. Check for sensation in the distributions of the deep and superficial peroneal, and tibial nerves (see Figs 3.20–3.22). Confirm active toe and foot dorsiflexion and plantar flexion.

## Radiological assessment of the painful foot

### Radiographs of the foot (Fig. 22.7)

A standard foot series of three radiographs is required:

- *AP*: The sole of the foot rests flat on the plate. This view shows the medial column of the foot clearly.

- *Oblique*: The lateral aspect of the foot is lifted off the plate by 45°. This view shows the lateral column of the foot more clearly.

- *Lateral*: The patient is turned laterally with the lateral side of the foot resting on the plate. The talar dome and ankle joint are seen in clear profile. Ensure rotation is correct (see Fig. 21.7). The hindfoot, and dorsal or plantar displacement of the midfoot and forefoot, are best appreciated on this view.

### Radiographic markers in the foot series

Injuries to the midfoot are often subtle, but a number of radiographic lines allow assessment of the relationship between the mid- and forefoot.

On the *AP* view:

- The *lateral* aspect of the *first metatarsal* should be aligned with the *lateral* border of the *medial cuneiform* (**Fig. 22.8A**).

- The *medial* aspect of the *second metatarsal* should be aligned with the *medial* border of the *middle cuneiform* (**Fig. 22.8B**).

On the *oblique* view:

- The *medial* borders of the *third and fourth metatarsals* should be aligned with the *medial* borders of the *lateral cuneiform and cuboid*, respectively (**Fig. 22.8C**).

### Radiographs of the calcaneus

Suspected calcaneal fractures require assessment with two views.

- *Lateral foot or ankle radiograph*: Inspect the outline of the calcaneus, including the anterior process, where fractures are most commonly missed. Calcaneal fractures can be subtle and a clear fracture line is not always present. The overall morphology of the calcaneus is altered by a compression fracture and can be assessed by measuring two radiographic angles:

  *Bohler's angle* (**Fig. 22.9**): This is measured from the highest points of each of the anterior process, posterior facet and tuberosity. Normal is >20°.

  *Gissane's crucial angle* (**Fig. 22.10**): This is the intersection between the posterior facet and the anterior process. Normal is <105°.

- *Harris's axial view* (**Fig. 22.11**): This allows assessment of the medial column, lateral displacement and posterior facet displacement. The patient lies supine with the foot dorsiflexed. The X-ray beam is directed cephalad.

## TALAR FRACTURES

The talus transmits all of the body weight to the foot and fractures are most commonly caused by a fall from a height or a rapid deceleration injury with foot dorsiflexion. It has a tenuous vascular supply, and avascular necrosis is a well-recognized complication of talar neck fractures.

AP foot

Oblique foot

Lateral foot

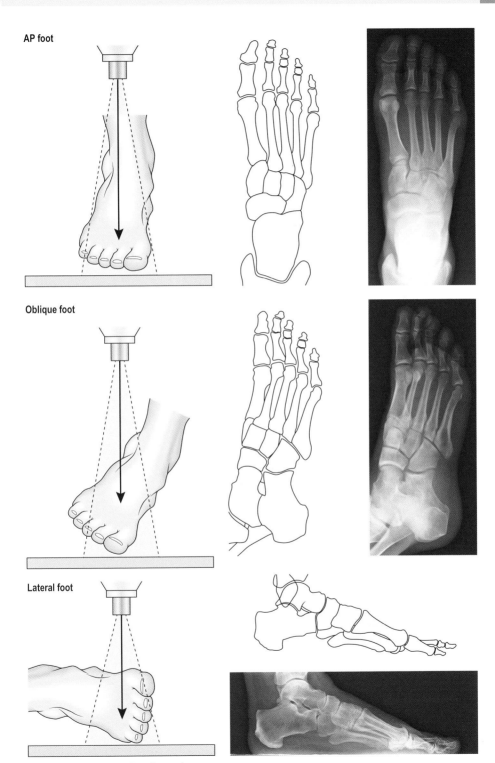

Fig. 22.7 Foot series of radiographs.

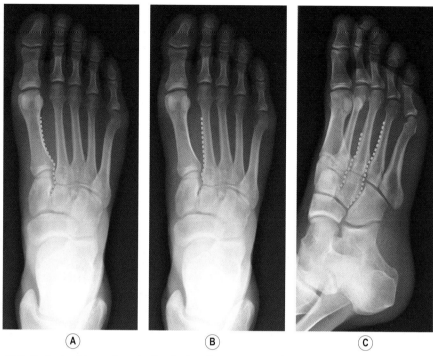

Fig. 22.8 Radiographic markers in the foot series.

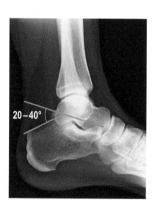

Fig. 22.9 Bohler's angle.

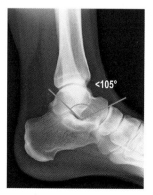

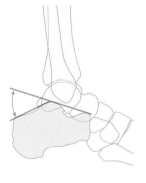

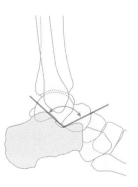

Fig. 22.10 Crucial angle of Gissane.

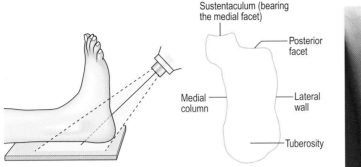
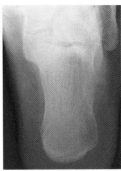

Fig. 22.11 Harris's view.

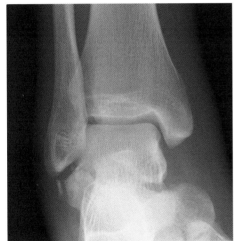

Fig. 22.12 Lateral process fracture.

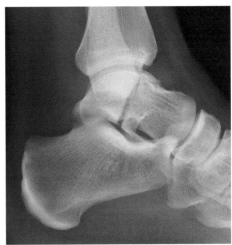

Fig. 22.13 Talar body fracture.

## Classification

### Anatomical location

Fractures are described according to the anatomy of the talus:

- *Lateral process* fractures (**Fig. 22.12**): These are ankle eversion injuries caused by a fall, and are commonly associated with snowboarding.

- *Posterior process* fractures: These are relatively unusual but should not be confused with an *os trigonum* which has a smooth, rounded cortical outline.

- *Talar body* fractures (**Fig. 22.13**): These split fractures result in an incongruent ankle joint and are usually treated operatively.

- *Talar dome* fractures: These are osteochondral impaction fractures, from the medial or lateral superior surface of the talar dome, often resulting from ankle inversion or eversion injuries.

- *Talar neck* fractures: These are especially important because injury to the retrograde blood supply of the talus can render the body avascular.

### Hawkins classification

Talar neck fractures are further described according to the Hawkins classification (**Fig. 22.14**). The mechanism is classically an axial load through a dorsiflexed foot, and commonly

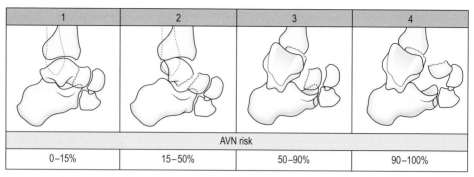

| 1 | 2 | 3 | 4 |
|---|---|---|---|
| AVN risk | | | |
| 0–15% | 15–50% | 50–90% | 90–100% |

Fig. 22.14 Hawkins classification of talar neck fractures. AVN, avascular necrosis.

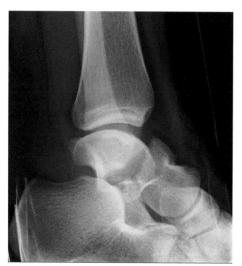

Fig. 22.15 Hawkins type 2 fracture.

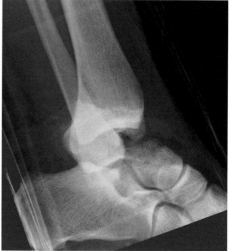

Fig. 22.16 Hawkins type 3 fracture.

occurs in motor vehicle collisions, when the impact transmitted through a foot pedal forces the talar neck against the anterior tibial margin. It is classically exemplified by the famous but now rare 'aviator's astragalus': a talar fracture caused by a pilot bracing his forefeet against the rudder bar of his crashing aeroplane at the moment of impact.

- *Type 1*: Undisplaced fracture.
- *Type 2*: Displaced fracture with subluxation of the subtalar joint. The talar body is flexed. The head maintains its relationship with the navicular (**Fig. 22.15**).

- *Type 3*: Displaced fracture with dislocation of both the subtalar and ankle joints. The talar body is completely extruded posteriorly, and is steered medially around the back of the medial malleolus so that the fractured neck surface points laterally. The talar body lies subcutaneously behind the medial malleolus and results in rapid skin compromise. Open injuries are common. This is a surgical emergency (**Fig. 22.16**).
- *Type 4*: Additional dislocation of the talonavicular joint (added by Canale and Kelly). This is rare but, as with type 3, it results in a dislocated and subcutaneous talar body.

## Emergency Department management

### Clinical features

- There is usually a history of significant limb injury.
- High-energy mechanisms of injury may suggest other important associated injuries and the patient should undergo full primary and secondary surveys (see Ch. 2).
- Assess the skin carefully, as a displaced talar body will cause blanching and later skin necrosis. This is a surgical emergency.
- Talar body dislocation is often an open injury, and indeed the talus may be extruded through the wound.

### Radiological features

- *AP and lateral ankle radiographs* (see Fig. 21.6): Inspect the talar outline carefully on all views, looking for subtle discontinuity of the lateral or posterior processes, or the more important fractures of the talar body or neck. Assess the congruity of the ankle, subtalar and talonavicular joints. Note an os trigonum, which may initially be misinterpreted as a fracture.
- *Foot series of radiographs*: Talar fractures are not infrequently associated with other foot injuries. Acquire additional views if there is clinical suspicion.
- *CT*: Fractures are more comprehensively assessed with CT because of the complex shape of the talus and the difficulty in assessing even apparently minor lateral or posterior process fractures. In displaced injuries, the CT is obtained after closed reduction.

### Closed reduction

#### Hawkins 1 fractures
These do not require any reduction.

#### Hawkins 2 fractures
The talar body is usually in a flexed position and often subluxed posteriorly in relation to the calcaneus. The ankle joint remains congruent and the overall alignment of the foot is usually good, with little skin compromise. The talar body can rarely be manipulated back into posi-

tion closed and this should not be attempted in the Emergency Department. Operative open reduction and fixation is usually required.

#### Hawkins 3 and 4 fractures
In fracture types 3 and 4, the talar body dislocates backwards and rotates around the medial malleolus to become extruded posteromedially. It can be hard to reduce it from this position, but *urgent closed reduction* is required, as the medial skin will be under considerable tension and will necrose rapidly. Reduction is performed in the Emergency Department under procedural sedation and analgesia, or in theatre under general anaesthesia (**Fig. 22.17**).

1. *Foot position*: The knee is flexed to 90° to relax the gastrocnemius. The assistant's hands behind the patient's thigh provide counter-traction. Grasp the heel to dorsiflex, evert and distract the ankle. This opens a space for the talar body to be relocated. More powerful traction can be applied via a Denholm pin through the calcaneus. A second assistant can hold the heel position while the reduction manœuvre is performed.
2. *Reduction manœuvre*: The dislocation is then reduced by placing the heel of the hand over the prominent talus and pushing anteriorly and laterally.

### Immobilization and reassessment
A below-knee *backslab* is applied (p. 70). Undisplaced fractures can be treated with an orthosis. A *CT scan* allows assessment of the reduction, the fracture and any incarcerated loose bodies.

### Outpatient follow-up
- Entirely undisplaced fractures of the lateral or posterior processes can be referred to the fracture clinic.

### Inpatient referral
- Talar body or neck fractures.
- Displaced lateral or posterior process fractures.
- Open fractures or injuries with neurovascular impairment.

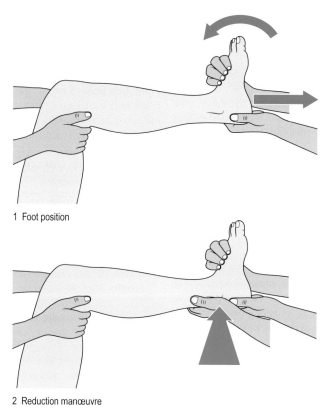

1 Foot position

2 Reduction manœuvre

Fig. 22.17 Hawkins type 3/4 reduction.

## Orthopaedic management

### Non-operative

- Undisplaced or minimally displaced fractures of the lateral or posterior processes can be managed symptomatically in a cast or removable orthosis (moon boot), *fully weight-bearing*, until union at around 6 weeks.

- *Undisplaced* talar *body* or *dome* fractures, and *Hawkins type 1* fractures of the talar neck, are also treated non-operatively in an orthosis, *non-weight-bearing* for 6 weeks.

### Operative

#### *Lateral and posterior process fractures*

Large fragments may be amenable to open reduction and internal fixation. Fractures of the posterior process may, uncommonly, snag the flexor hallucis longus tendon and inability to extend the hallux is an indication for exploration. Small or comminuted fragments may benefit from excision, which can be performed late if the patient complains of ongoing symptoms after an initial period of rehabilitation.

#### *Talar body fractures*

These are usually intra-articular, involving the ankle joint, and are reduced and fixed, either percutaneously or open. A medial malleolar osteotomy may be required for adequate visualization of the fracture. Mini-fragment and headless screws are commonly used.

#### *Talar dome fractures*

These are treated with open reduction and fixation with mini-fragment screws if the fragment is large and displaced. If the fragment is small and comminuted, excision is required.

## Talar neck fractures

The talar neck can be treated by closed or open means:

- *Percutaneous*: This is applicable only to undisplaced type 1 fractures. These are usually treated non-operatively but there may be a preference for surgical fixation to prevent displacement.
- *Open reduction*: This may be performed via an anteromedial incision, or combined anteromedial and anterolateral incisions:
  i   Anteromedial: The incision is placed just medial to tibialis anterior and exposes the medial aspect of the neck and body.
  ii  Anterolateral: The incision is placed just lateral to the extensor tendons (extensor digitorum longus and peroneus tertius) and exposes the lateral aspect of the neck and the tarsal sinus.

Combined incisions risk additional damage to the vascular supply from the arteries of the tarsal sinus and tarsal canal, but do allow complete assessment and correction of the displacement, which is often rotational.

Fixation is with screws or plates:

- *Anterior to posterior screw fixation* (**Fig. 22.18A**): This is often preferred if an anatomical reduction has been achieved via a single anteromedial incision and can be performed with cannulated screws. The screw heads are recessed into the talar head, as otherwise they risk impinging on the talo-navicular joint.
- *Posterior to anterior screw fixation* (**Fig. 22.18B**): This orientation of the screws is biomechanically stronger and can be inserted without injury to the talonavicular joint. Surgery is percutaneous via a small incision placed just lateral to the Achilles tendon. Both AP and PA orientation of screws risks some shortening of a comminuted talar neck with subsequent alteration of foot biomechanics.
- *Mini-fragment plate fixation* (**Fig. 22.18C**): Mini-fragment plates (placed medially, laterally or both), often with additional lag screws, ensure an anatomical reduction without shortening of the neck.

# Outpatient management

The patient is managed non-weight-bearing in an orthosis until fracture union. Close subsequent follow-up is important to exclude avascular necrosis of the talar body

The *Hawkins sign* is a zone of subchondral osteopaenia of the talar dome that is evident 6–8 weeks after injury. It is caused by bone resorption in a region with preserved or re-established vascularity, and is associated with a good outcome. Conversely, osteosclerosis of the talar body, which can be confirmed on MRI, suggests avascular necrosis and is associated with collapse and pan-talar arthritis. A prolonged period of non-weight-bearing is controversial but may minimize this collapse.

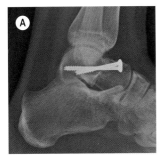 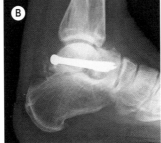 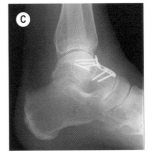

Fig. 22.18 Talar neck fracture fixation. **A**, Anterior to posterior screw fixation. **B**, Posterior to anterior screw fixation. **C**, Mini-fragment plate fixation.

## COMPLICATIONS

### *Early*

Local | *Wound dehiscence and infection*: These are inevitably more common after open fractures, particularly if the talus has been extruded. The risk is reduced by appropriate surgical timing, meticulous soft tissue handling, and minimizing the degree of dissection around the talar neck

*Compartment syndrome of the foot*: See page 549

### *Late*

Local | *Avascular necrosis*: The risk is related to the degree of initial fracture displacement and Hawkins grade:

- 1: 0–15%
- 2: 15–50%
- 3: 50–100%
- 4: up to 100%.

The degree of collapse may be minimized by a prolonged period of non-weight-bearing. Salvage is with fusion

*Post-traumatic osteoarthritis*: Ankle and/or subtalar stiffness and discomfort are common

*Delayed union*: This is frequently encountered, particularly after higher grades of talar fracture

*Malunion*: This may follow compression screw treatment with loss of length of the medial column of the foot. A varus deformity of the hindfoot is common

## SUBTALAR DISLOCATION

Subtalar dislocation is often misconstrued as an ankle fracture dislocation, presenting as pain and deformity following an inversion injury during sport. The calcaneus dislocates medially in relation to the talus, with rupture of the talo-calcaneal ligament. Occasionally, the calcaneus dislocates laterally.

## Emergency Department management

### Clinical features

- There is pain and deformity of the hindfoot, which is usually displaced medially.

- Careful clinical examination reveals that the ankle is enlocated, and the deformity is distal to this joint.

### Radiological features

- *AP and lateral ankle radiographs*: These are usually sufficient to confirm the diagnosis (**Fig. 22.19**).

### Closed reduction, immobilization and reassessment

Urgent closed reduction is performed in the Emergency Department under procedural sedation and analgesia. The knee is flexed to 90° to relax the gastrocnemius, and the ankle is plantar-flexed. Traction is applied to the heel

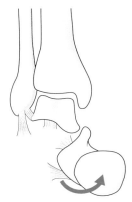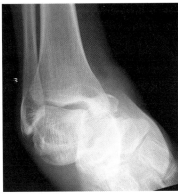

Fig. 22.19 Subtalar dislocation.

and the deformity is exaggerated to unlock the calcaneus. The deformity is then reduced with gentle pressure over the calcaneus and counter-pressure over the lateral malleolus. Reduction occurs with a satisfying clunk. A below-knee backslab is applied (p. 70). The neurovascular status of the limb is reassessed and repeat radiographs are required.

### Inpatient referral
- Patients with subtalar dislocation require orthopaedic review.

## Orthopaedic management

A CT scan will confirm reduction and exclude any associated fracture or incarcerated loose bodies. Failure to achieve an anatomical reduction is an indication for operative exploration. The reduced subtalar joint is usually highly stable and management is normally non-operative with careful radiographic monitoring.

## TALAR DISLOCATION

Rarely, the entire talus can be completely extruded from the ankle mortise, and comes to lie subcutaneously in an anterolateral position in front of the ankle. If the injury is closed, it results in severe tenting and compromise of the skin, and this is a surgical emergency. Manipulative closed reduction is required. However, the skin is often torn at the time of injury, and the dislocation is often open, occasionally with extrusion of the talus.

### Closed reduction (Fig. 22.20)
1. *Foot position*: Forceful plantar flexion and inversion to the foot are applied.
2. *Reduction manoeuvre*. The talus lies with its posterior pole facing laterally, and is therefore reduced by firm pressure directed medially and posteriorly.

## CALCANEAL FRACTURES

Most calcaneal fractures are high-energy injuries caused by a fall from a height, occurring in men of working age. These are impaction-type fractures exacerbated by a substantial overlying soft tissue injury. They result in considerable disability and are challenging injuries to treat, with a relatively high complication rate.

## Classification
### Essex-Lopresti classification
The Essex-Lopresti classification was developed on the basis of plain radiographs to describe intra-articular and extra-articular fractures of the calcaneus. The classification focuses on whether there is extension into, and displacement of, the posterior facet joint. Fractures that do not involve the posterior facet are considered to be extra-articular fractures.

#### Extra-articular fractures
- *Anterior process*: These fractures occur after a twisting fall and are often misdiagnosed

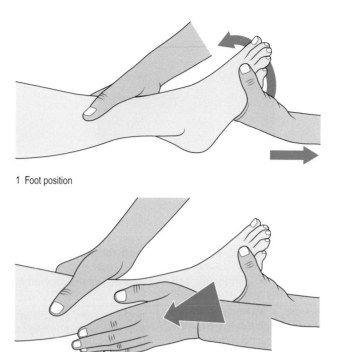

1  Foot position

2  Reduction manœuvre

Fig. 22.20  Reduction of a dislocated talus.

as ankle sprains. They may involve the calcaneocuboid joint.

- *Tuberosity fractures*: These are most commonly impaction fractures sustained after a
  fall. They are usually stable.

- *Achilles tendon avulsion fractures* (see Fig.
  22.29): These occur in osteoporotic bone
  and are similar to a tongue-type fracture.
  They can result in considerable pressure on
  the heel skin and should be reduced as an
  emergency.

- *Sustentacular fractures*: These may be mistaken for a medial ankle sprain.

### Intra-articular fractures

The two terms used by Essex-Lopresti to
describe intra-articular fractures are still in
common usage:

- *tongue type*
- *joint depression*.

Understanding the difference between these
requires an appreciation of the way in which the
calcaneus fractures along predictable *primary*
and *secondary* fracture lines:

- The *primary fracture line* (of Palmer) (**Fig.
  22.21**): The inferior surface of the talus
  strikes the posterior facet like an axe, splitting it obliquely into two fragments. The
  fracture starts in the tarsal sinus at the
  crucial angle of Gissane on the lateral wall.
  The fracture propagates posteromedially
  across the posterior facet until it reaches
  the medial wall behind the sustentaculum
  tali. This results in two fragments:

  The *anteromedial* fragment, bearing the
  sustentaculum, anterior and medial facets,
  and the remaining medial part of the
  posterior facet. This is often termed the
  *constant fragment*, as it holds its
  anatomical relationship with the talus.

  The *posterolateral* fragment, bearing the
  tuberosity and lateral portion of the
  posterior facet, which displaces to become
  shortened and lateralized (see Fig. 22.25).

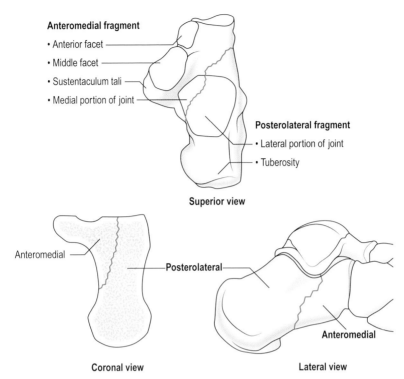

Superior view

**Anteromedial fragment**
- Anterior facet
- Middle facet
- Sustentaculum tali
- Medial portion of joint

**Posterolateral fragment**
- Lateral portion of joint
- Tuberosity

Anteromedial — Posterolateral —

**Coronal view**

Anteromedial

**Lateral view**

Fig. 22.21 Primary fracture line of Palmer.

- The *secondary fracture line* (**Fig. 22.22**): A secondary line emanates from the first, splitting the *posterolateral* fragment into two pieces. There are two types:

*Tongue type*: The secondary fracture line passes backwards and splits the tuberosity into two pieces: a superior fragment consisting of both the posterior facet articular surface and the superior part of the tuberosity; and an inferior fragment consisting of the remainder of the tuberosity. The superior fragment has the appearance of a tongue (see Fig. 22.29).

*Joint depression*: The secondary line travels superiorly and detaches the posterior facet from the tuberosity. The posterior facet, which is now free of any attachment, can be driven downwards into the substance of the calcaneus (see Fig. 22.27). The thin lateral wall of the calcaneus may also fracture away from the tuberosity (lateral wall blowout fracture).

## Sanders classification

The Sanders classification has largely superseded the Essex-Lopresti system for planning operative treatment (**Fig. 22.23**). It is more detailed, reflecting the fact that the primary fracture line can often consist of two or more separate fracture lines breaching the articular surface. The classification describes the number and disposition of these fracture line(s) through the posterior facet, as seen on CT scan. The *number* of fragments is first indicated by a numeral:

I. all undisplaced fractures

II. two fragments

III. three fragments

IV. any comminuted fracture.

The *location* of the primary fracture line(s) through the posterior facet is then indicated by a letter:

A. a fracture through the lateral portion of the posterior facet

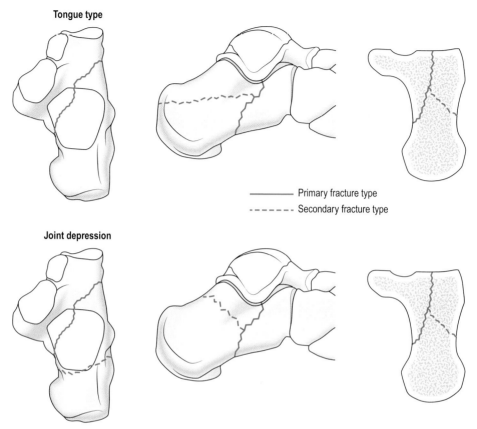

**Tongue type**

Primary fracture type
Secondary fracture type

**Joint depression**

Fig. 22.22 Secondary fracture lines. Note that, in the coronal view, both types of secondary fracture appear the same.

B. **a fracture through the middle of the posterior facet**

C. **a fracture passing medially, at the neck of the sustentaculum.**

In type II fractures there is only one fracture line and a single letter is allocated (e.g. IIB). Type III fractures have two fracture lines and are therefore given two letters (e.g. IIIAB; **Fig. 22.24**). Types I and IV do not have letter allocations.

## Displacement of calcaneus fractures

The primary and secondary fracture lines tend to result in predictable displacement of the calcaneus, leading to:

- *incongruity* of the *posterior facet* articular surface (*a* on **Fig. 22.25**)
- loss of *length and height* of the calcaneus (*b*)

- increase in *heel width* (*c*)
- *varus malalignment* of the tuberosity (*d*)
- *subfibular impingement* from the lateral wall fragment, which entraps the peroneal tendons (*e*).

## Emergency Department management

### Clinical features

- There is usually a history of a high-energy mechanism, such as a fall from a height, and other associated injuries must be excluded by primary and secondary surveys (see Ch. 2).

- Commonly associated injuries include ipsilateral fractures of the tibia, femur and hip, and fracture of the spine (**Fig. 22.26**); 10% of calcaneal fractures are bilateral.

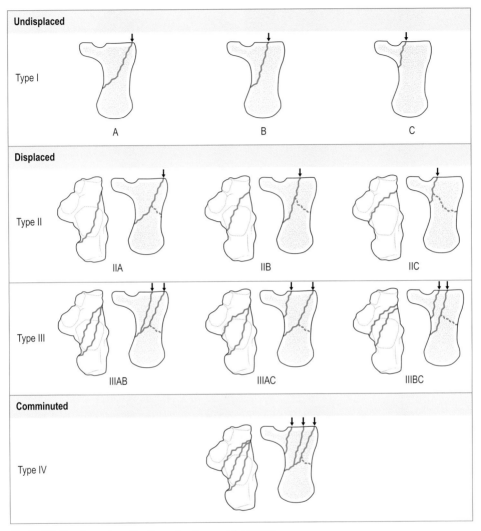

| | | | | |
|---|---|---|---|---|
| **Undisplaced** | | | | |
| Type I | A | B | C | |

| | | |
|---|---|---|
| **Displaced** | | |
| Type II | IIA | IIB | IIC |

| | | |
|---|---|---|
| **Type III** | IIIAB | IIIAC | IIIBC |

| | |
|---|---|
| **Comminuted** | |
| Type IV | |

Fig. 22.23 Sanders classification of calcaneal fractures.

- Important medical history includes diabetes, peripheral neuropathy and smoking.
- Examine the skin to look for deformity, swelling and open wounds (open fractures are usually medial burst injuries).
- Bruising in the sole of the foot is virtually pathognomonic.
- Excessive pain and swelling in the foot may indicate a foot compartment syndrome (p. 549).

### Radiological features

- *Lateral calcaneus radiograph*: Inspect the outline of the calcaneus, including the anterior process, where fractures are most commonly missed. Assess the degree of flattening of the calcaneus by measuring the angles of Bohler and Gissane (see Figs 22.9–22.10). The 'double density' sign (**Fig. 22.27**) is an increased density within the calcaneal body due to depression of a portion of the posterior facet.

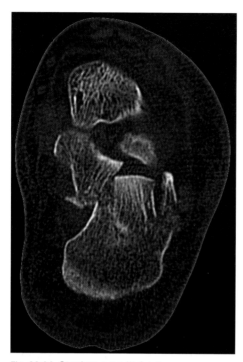

Fig. 22.24 Sanders type III fracture.

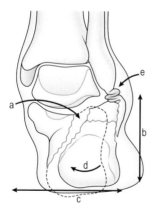

Fig. 22.25 Intra-articular calcaneal fracture displacement.

- *Harris view*: This will often display greater displacement than the lateral view (**Fig. 22.28**).
- *CT*: A CT scan is invaluable for displaced calcaneal fractures and allows assessment according to the Sanders classification.

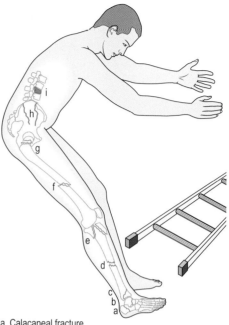

a Calacaneal fracture
b Talar neck fracture          f Midshaft femur
c Pilon fracture               g Femoral neck
d Midshaft tibia               h Acetabulum/pelvis
e Tibial plateau fracture      i Spine compression fractures

Fig. 22.26 Axial load injuries.

### Closed reduction and immobilization

There is no closed reduction manœuvre for calcaneal fractures but they should be immobilized in a below-knee backslab.

### Inpatient referral

- All displaced calcaneal fracture are referred to Orthopaedics.

### Outpatient follow-up

- Undisplaced fractures are treated with a *non-weight-bearing* orthosis and referred to the fracture clinic.

## Orthopaedic management

The indications for surgery remain somewhat controversial. Young, healthy, non-smoking patients with displaced fractures are likely to have a better outcome with surgery. The risks of complications are higher in patients who smoke and who have systemic disease, particularly diabetes and vasculopathy.

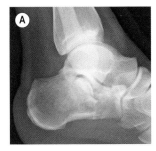
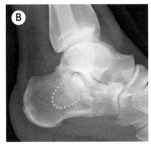

Fig. 22.27 Double density sign. **A**, Lateral radiograph of the hindfoot showing a displaced 'joint depression' calcaneal fracture. **B**, The depressed fragment is highlighted to show the region of the calcaneus that is 'doubly dense'.

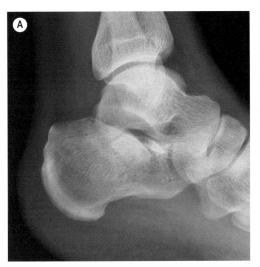
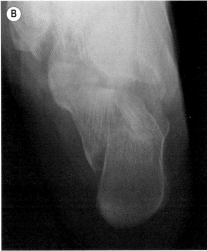

Fig. 22.28 Importance of the Harris view. **A**, The lateral radiograph can look relatively normal, however the posterior facet is incongruent and both the Bohler's and Gissaine's angles are abnormal. **B**, The Harris view clearly shows a displaced intra-articular fracture.

## Non-operative

Non-operative management is indicated for most extra-articular fractures and for undisplaced intra-articular fractures. Patients are provided with an orthosis (moon boot) and crutches, with *non-weight-bearing* restrictions until fracture union at between 6 and 10 weeks.

## Operative

### Urgent operative management

This is indicated for tuberosity avulsion fractures and tongue-type fractures where there is internal pressure on the heel skin (**Fig. 22.29**); blanching or discoloration is a warning sign of dysvascular skin, which may ulcerate and is very difficult to reconstruct once lost.

### Intra-articular fractures

Operative management aims to:

- restore the *congruity* of the *posterior facet* articular surface
- restore the *length, width and height* of the calcaneus
- restore the *coronal alignment* of the tuberosity (particularly avoiding varus)
- relieve *impingement* between the lateral wall fragment and the tip of the fibula.

Surgery risks further insult to the vulnerable soft tissues over the lateral aspect of the heel. The approach must avoid causing ischaemic necrosis of the lateral heel skin (which

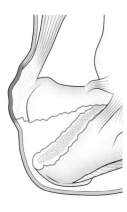

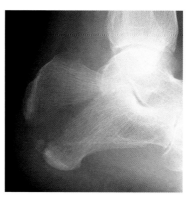

Fig. 22.29 Tongue-type fracture causing skin compromise.

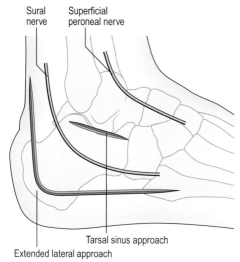

Sural nerve    Superficial peroneal nerve

Tarsal sinus approach

Extended lateral approach

Fig. 22.30 Approaches to the calcaneus.

is supplied by a branch of the peroneal artery) and injury to the sural nerve. The classical extended lateral approach offers an excellent exposure of the calcaneus, although there is a small risk of flap edge necrosis and infection (**Fig. 22.30**). Minimal access techniques, including the tarsal sinus approach and various percutaneous and arthroscopically assisted techniques, are also used to minimize the soft tissue dissection. In the face of extensive swelling and bruising, surgery is often delayed for 5–14 days to allow elevation and icing, until wrinkles appear in the skin over the lateral heel.

## Surgical techniques

### Open reduction and internal fixation – extended lateral approach

This approach is based on the concept of the angiosome – a three-dimensional volume of skin and tissue that is supplied by a source artery. Placing an incision between angiosomes, rather than through one, prevents necrosis of the skin distal to the incision. The extended lateral incision is safe if the lower portion is made along the junction between the thick plantar heel skin (calcaneal branch of the posterior tibial artery) and the softer lateral heel skin (calcaneal branch of the peroneal artery). Sharp dissection continues down to bone and all soft tissue is raised as a single flap. The lateral aspect of the calcaneus is exposed (**Fig. 22.31**):

1.  The lateral wall (which is often loose) is removed or elevated to expose the depressed lateral joint fragment. This is elevated or removed in turn, to expose the constant fragment (the anteromedial fragment bearing the sustentaculum tali). The fracture is cleaned and debrided of clot and bone fragments.

2.  The tuberosity is reduced with the aid of a lever and heavy threaded guide wire to restore the medial column of the calcaneus by levering down, medially and into neutral alignment. This also restores the height and length of the tuberosity, and narrows the heel. The threaded guide pin is advanced into the constant fragment to secure the reduction.

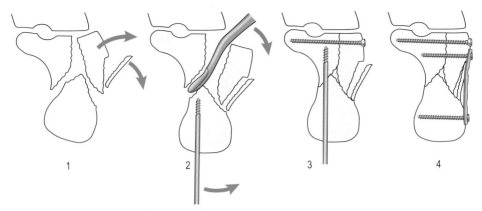

Fig. 22.31 Joint depression fracture fixation.

3. The lateral joint fragment is then replaced to reconstruct the posterior facet joint anatomically. This reduction is held and compressed with a lag screw passed under the posterior facet and into the constant fragment.

4. Finally, the lateral wall of the calcaneus is replaced and a low-profile plate is implanted. Screws are inserted into the tuberosity, anterior process and subarticular region. The void in the centre of the calcaneus does not usually need to be filled, as metaphyseal bone will spontaneously fill the defect.

### Tarsal sinus approach

This is a less invasive approach (see Fig. 22.30), which affords an excellent view of the subtalar joint, but with a smaller incision and more limited access to the calcaneal tuberosity. An oblique incision is made over the tarsal sinus, starting just distal to the tip of the fibula. The incision lies between the peroneal tendons and sural nerve inferiorly, and the peroneus tertius and extensor digitorum longus superiorly. The fascia is divided in line with the skin, leaving the peroneal tendons within their sheath distally. The posterior facet joint is exposed. If a plate is to be used, a periosteal elevator is used to lift the peroneal sheath, periosteum and skin away from the lateral wall of the calcaneus. The fracture is reduced and fixed as above.

### Fusion

Where there is extensive posterior facet comminution, articular reconstruction may not be feasible. Reconstruction of the height and width of the calcaneus and a primary fusion may provide the best results.

## COMPLICATIONS

### *Early*

Local | Wound dehiscence and infection: These are the principal complications of operative treatment. Deep infection can result in calcaneal osteomyelitis, which can be difficult or impossible to salvage. The risk is minimized by appropriate surgical timing, meticulous soft tissue handling and, potentially, the use of minimal access techniques

*Continued*

## COMPLICATIONS... cont'd

### Late

| | |
|---|---|
| Local | Post-traumatic osteoarthritis: Subtalar stiffness and lateral hindfoot discomfort is common. Subtalar fusion is effective in this situation |
| | Lateral subfibular impingement: Persistent displacement of the lateral wall can result in impingement of the peroneal tendons under the tip of the fibula |
| | Altered foot size: Widening of the heel is common, particularly after non-operative management |

## MIDFOOT FRACTURES

Torsional or rotational forces applied to the foot stress the stability of the medial and lateral columns, and may cause (tensile) avulsion fractures or compression fractures.

## Classification

Midfoot fractures are described mechanistically according to whether the force has been principally tensile or compressive.

### Avulsion fractures

Torsional or tensile forces applied to the midfoot can result in capsular tears of the many joints in this region (a foot sprain), or small avulsion fractures of the surfaces of one or other of the bones. These are visible radiographically as small flakes of bone.

### Compression fractures

Torsional or compressive forces applied to the midfoot can result in compression fractures, particularly of the navicular (**Fig. 22.32**) or cuboid. These are important, as they may disrupt the length of the medial or lateral column of the foot (see Fig. 22.6). The classic 'nutcracker' injury occurs with a forceful lateral stress to the foot, and comprises a compression fracture of the cuboid (compression injury to the lateral column) with an associated avulsion fracture (or dislocation) of the navicular (tension injury to the medial column) (**Fig. 22.33**). Simple fractures of the navicular body often occur in line with the intercuneiform joint, indicating the line of passage of the causative force. These are often undisplaced.

## Emergency Department management

### Clinical features

- There will usually be a history of a twisting injury to the foot, a fall from a height or a motor vehicle collision.

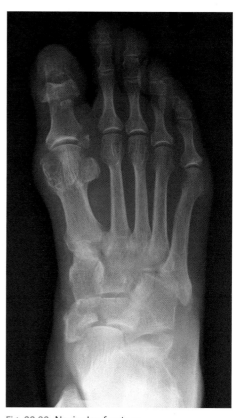

Fig. 22.32 Navicular fracture.

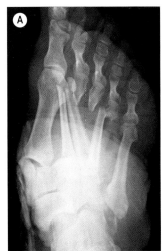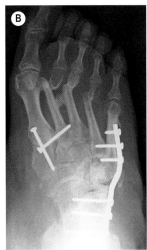

Fig. 22.33 'Nutcracker' fracture. **A**, Severe open fracture-dislocation of the foot following a motorcycle collision. A nutcracker compression fracture of the cuboid in the lateral column is accompanied by a dislocation of the Lisfranc articulation in the medial column. There are associated metatarsal fractures. **B**, The lateral column was brought out to length, bridged and bone-grafted. The medial column was stabilized with lag screws.

- Repetitive or unaccustomed activity may indicate a stress fracture, usually of the navicular or cuboid.
- There will be pain and swelling, with later bruising, around the foot.
- Palpate the ankle and foot carefully to identify any localized bone or joint tenderness, or any deformity.
- It is essential to exclude a *Lisfranc injury* (p. 542).

### Radiological features
- *Foot series*: These are essential in any significant foot injury.
- *AP and lateral ankle radiographs*: These may offer additional information where there is hindfoot or ankle tenderness or swelling.
- *CT*: CT is often invaluable for preoperative planning.

### Reduction, immobilization and reassessment
Where there is a simple avulsion fracture or foot sprain, and the architecture of the foot remains undisrupted and stable, treatment is symptomatic with rest, ice, compression and elevation (RICE). If the patient has difficulty mobilizing, an orthosis (moon boot) may be helpful.

Deformity is not common, but any gross deformity should be reduced under procedural sedation and analgesia. A below-knee backslab is then applied (p. 70), and the foot reassessed clinically and with repeat radiographs.

### Inpatient referral
- Fracture dislocations and tarsal body fractures are referred to Orthopaedics.

### Outpatient follow-up
- Minor avulsion fractures can be referred to the fracture clinic.

## Orthopaedic management
### Non-operative
- Assess foot stability; if there is any doubt whether the foot is mechanically stable, investigate further with stress views, CT or MRI.

- Simple foot sprains, with or without avulsion flake fractures, are treated non-operatively with reassurance and a removable orthosis, if required.

### Operative

- Large avulsion fragments, particularly those of the navicular tuberosity and those representing the tibialis posterior insertion, are often reduced and fixed where technically feasible.
- Navicular body fractures are usually undisplaced and can be fixed with a percutaneous lag screw.
- Fractures and dislocations, particularly 'nutcracker' injuries, are intrinsically unstable. Surgery aims to restore the length of the affected column, using structural bone graft where required. Stability often requires the injured segment to be bridged with a plate on the column, and severely damaged joints often need a primary fusion.

## TARSOMETATARSAL (LISFRANC) INJURIES

These are severe midfoot injuries. They are famously easy to miss because the radiographic features may be subtle, but early diagnosis is crucial, as a neglected injury often results in severe and incapacitating midfoot instability and deformity. The injury arises from a severe torsional or translational force applied across the tarsometatarsal (Lisfranc) joint, classically described as occurring when a rider falls from a horse, leaving the forefoot entrapped in the stirrup. This results in disruption of the normal stabilizers of the joint (**Fig. 22.34**):

- *Osseous stability*: The second metatarsal base keys into the cuneiforms when viewed in the AP plane.
- *Ligamentous stability*: There are a number of strong ligamentous stabilizers, including (a) the *Lisfranc ligament*, which runs from the medial cuneiform to the base of the second metatarsal; (b) the tarsometatarsal ligaments; and (c) the intermetatarsal ligaments between second and fifth metatarsal bases. Note that there is no direct ligamentous attachment between first and second metatarsals.

## Classification

### Quenu and Kuss classification

The most commonly used classification is a simple description of the direction of instability, described by Quenu and Kuss (**Fig. 22.35**):

- *Homolateral*: All five rays are displaced in the same direction (usually laterally).
- *Isolated*: One or two rays are displaced while the others remain stable.
- *Divergent*: The rays are displaced in different directions.

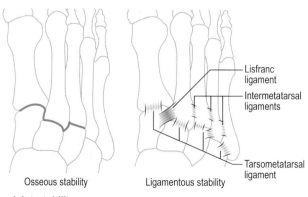

Osseous stability    Ligamentous stability

Fig. 22.34 Lisfranc joint stability.

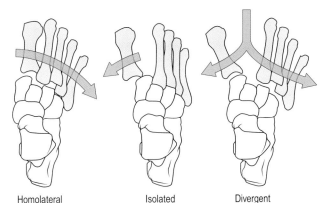

Fig. 22.35 Quenu and Kuss classification of tarsometatarsal (Lisfranc) injuries.

Homolateral            Isolated            Divergent

## Emergency Department management

### Clinical features

- There will be a history of a torsional or plantar flexion injury to the midfoot. This can be as benign as an awkward stumble over a step, resulting in twisting and loading of the forefoot, but usually a more powerful force is involved, such as when the forefoot is run over, or is entrapped while remainder of the foot rotates.

- There will be tenderness and swelling of the midfoot.

- Bruising in the sole of the foot is highly suggestive of a significant structural injury.

- There may be prominence of the metatarsal bases, which will reduce back down with pressure: the 'piano key' sign.

- There is usually pain on stressing the forefoot and inability to weight-bear.

### Radiological features

- *Foot series*: There may be clear deformity (see **Fig. 22.38**), but often only subtle features betray this severe injury:

  *Displacement* of the tarsometatarsal joint. There is disruption to the normal alignment on the AP film (**Fig. 22.36**), or dorsal displacement of the metatarsal bases on the lateral view (**Fig. 22.37**).

  *Flake fractures* at the base of the second metatarsal, indicating an avulsion injury to the Lisfranc ligament.

- *Stress views*: Where the initial radiographs do not show displacement but there is suspicion that the injury is more than a 'midfoot sprain', stress views can be obtained in the Emergency Department or under anaesthesia (manipulation under anaesthesia, or MUA). The forefoot is stressed laterally while an AP film is taken.

- *CT*: This may demonstrate deformity, or flake fractures particularly at the plantar aspects of the metatarsal bases.

- *MRI*: This can be used to assess the integrity of the Lisfranc ligament.

### Closed reduction and immobilization

These are occasionally required for gross deformity in order to protect the soft tissue envelope. Under procedural sedation, gentle traction is applied to the forefoot (*a* on **Fig. 22.38**) and pressure is applied to the metatarsal bases to reverse the deformity (*b*). A backslab is applied (p. 70).

### Inpatient referral

- Confirmed instability of the tarsometatarsal joint should be referred to Orthopaedics.

### Outpatient follow-up

- Midfoot sprains with no suggestion of displacement or instability are managed symptomatically in an orthosis for comfort.

- The patient should be advised to return for review if discomfort persists.

## Orthopaedic management

### Non-operative

Patients without displacement, but who have suspicious features such as metatarsal base fractures or bruising in the sole of the foot, may be managed non-operatively in the first instance, with non-weight-bearing mobilization in an orthosis (moon boot) and regular radiographic review. Alternatively, they may be subjected to MUA.

### Operative

Patients with clear displacement on the initial radiographs or stress films are managed operatively (**Fig. 22.39A**). A longitudinal incision over

the first intermetatarsal space is used. Careful dissection allows identification and protection of the dorsalis pedis artery and deep peroneal nerve. The disrupted joints are easily identified and should be cleared of incarcerated bone or soft tissue fragments. The Lisfranc joint, and the first and second metatarsal bases, are all reduced anatomically and held with clamps and k-wires (**Fig. 22.39B–C**). These three articulations are then stabilized in turn with lag screws (**Fig. 22.39D–F**). Small, region-specific plate systems are also occasionally used. Reduction of the medial column usually results in reduction of the lateral column when the intermetatarsal ligaments remain intact, but where the fluoroscopic assessment suggests persisting subluxation, a second incision can be made over the fourth metatarsal to allow exploration and reduction. The lateral column is more mobile than the medial, and is therefore stabilized with percutaneous k-wires rather than screws.

If there is extensive articular damage to the metatarsal bases or cuneiforms, a primary fusion of the medial column may prevent later post-traumatic arthritic pain. Some surgeons advocate a primary fusion in all cases.

## Outpatient management

In order not to place stress across the reconstituted Lisfranc joint, the patient is kept non-weight-bearing, or allowed only to weight-bear through the heel in an off-loader orthosis, for 8 weeks. Progressive weight-bearing mobilization and physiotherapy are then permitted. Lateral column k-wires, if used, are removed at 4–6 weeks. The medial column fixation is left undisturbed unless there is pain or prominent

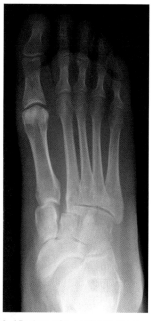

Fig. 22.36 AP view of a Lisfranc injury.

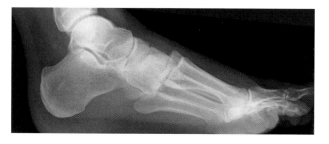

Fig. 22.37 Lateral view of a Lisfranc injury.

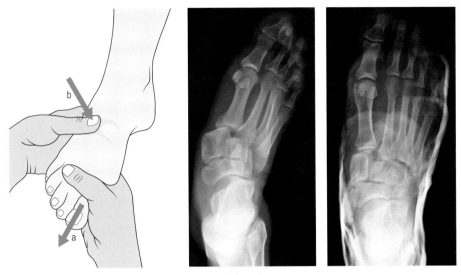

Fig. 22.38 Closed reduction of a homolateral dislocation.

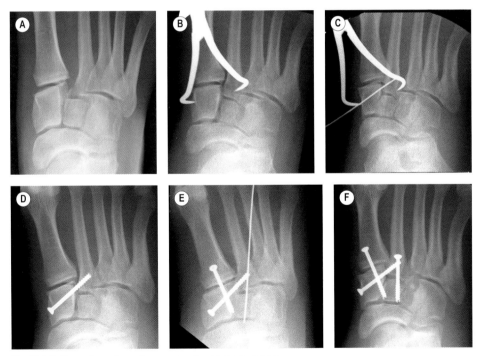

Fig. 22.39 Operative steps for repair of a Lisfranc injury.

metalwork. Late post-traumatic arthritis is salvaged with fusion.

## METATARSAL FRACTURES

These are very common injuries, resulting from twisting, crushing, or dropping a heavy object on the foot. Displacement is usually minimal because the metatarsals are splinted to each other at their bases, at their heads (by the transverse intermetatarsal ligament), and by the fascia of the intrinsic muscle compartments that lie between each ray. Stress fractures can follow repetitive or unaccustomed activity. The 'march fracture' of the second metatarsal is classically seen in military recruits who are suddenly exposed to regular long training marches, and is often most clearly appreciated several weeks after injury when callus becomes visible (**Fig. 22.40**).

## Classification

Metatarsal fractures are described according to the fracture position: the affected ray, and whether the fracture is of the base, shaft, neck or head. They are also described in terms of morphology, often being oblique. The first ray is larger and stronger than the remainder and is rarely fractured in isolation.

### Base of fifth metatarsal

The base of the fifth metatarsal is somewhat different, as it is only supported on one side and is subjected to traction and torsional forces. Fractures are considered in three zones (**Figs 22.41–22.42**):

- *Zone 1*: Avulsion fractures of the fifth metatarsal tuberosity, distal to the intermetatarsal joint. This is the site of insertion of the peroneus brevis tendon and plantar fascia, which exert traction in an ankle inversion injury.

- *Zone 2*: Jones fractures. These were first described by Sir Robert Jones after he sustained this fracture dancing. The fracture line enters the intermetatarsal joint between the fifth and fourth metatarsals.

- *Zone 3*: Proximal diaphysis fractures. These are less common than zone 1 and 2

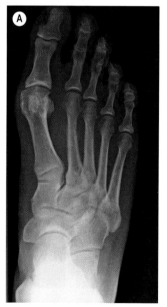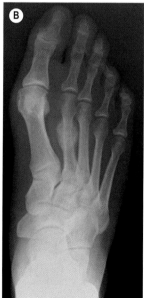

Fig. 22.40 Metatarsal stress fracture. **A**, The initial radiograph often shows little more than a barely discernible crack. **B**, The healed fracture 3 months later is obvious.

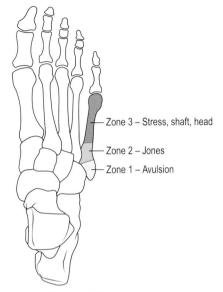

Zone 3 – Stress, shaft, head

Zone 2 – Jones

Zone 1 – Avulsion

Fig. 22.41 Base of fifth metatarsal fracture zones.

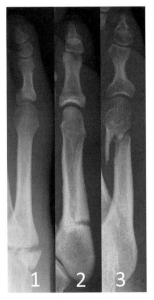

Fig. 22.42 Radiographs of fifth metatarsal fracture zones.

fractures, and may be stress fractures in athletes, who present with a history of prodromal pain. Many of these fractures do, however, arise from simple twisting injuries.

## Emergency Department management

### Clinical features
- The patient will complain of localized pain and difficulty mobilizing.
- Patients with no history of trauma, but a recent increase in their level of activity, should be suspected of having a stress fracture.
- There will be localized tenderness on palpation, and variable swelling and bruising.
- Where there are multiple metatarsal fractures with excessive swelling, there may be an acute compartment syndrome of the foot (p. 549).

### Radiological features
- *Foot series*: These will allow confirmation of the fracture(s) and an assessment of the level of displacement. When inspecting the base of the fifth metatarsal, do not misinterpret the well-corticated and rounded shadows of the accessory bones of the peroneal tendons (os peroneum of the peroneus longus, and os vesalianum of the peroneus brevis) as zone 1 fractures; in children, do not mistake the physis for a fracture (see Fig. 23.14).

### Immobilization
Patients with isolated, minimally displaced fractures can be provided with a removable orthosis (moon boot) for comfort, and may be allowed to mobilize weight-bearing as tolerated. Patients with multiple fractures may require a backslab and high elevation.

### Inpatient referral
- Patients with multiple or open fractures, or neurovascular abnormalities, should be referred to Orthopaedics.

### Outpatient follow-up
- Most metatarsal fractures are managed non-operatively and referred to the fracture clinic.

## Orthopaedic management

### Non-operative

Most traumatic and stress metatarsal fractures can be managed with reassurance and advice to mobilize progressively, dispensing with any orthosis as soon as pain allows. There is no evidence that non-weight-bearing is helpful.

### Operative

Operative management of metatarsal fractures is rare, but indications include open fractures where the approach has already been performed in the course of debridement. Although isolated, closed fractures are rarely fixed; multiple displaced metatarsal shaft fractures may progressively drift laterally, and may benefit from surgery. As the relationship between the metatarsals is usually preserved by the inter-metatarsal ligament, it is sometimes only necessary to fix the second ray. This can be achieved by plating via a longitudinal dorsal incision or with a longitudinal retrograde k-wire.

### *Fifth metatarsal base fractures*

In selected high-demand athletic patients, early primary fixation may be considered. However, in the majority of patients, surgery is required only in the uncommon event of a painful non-union. Jones fractures in zone 2, and fractures in zone 3, are more prone to non-union, as they occur in a relatively hypovascular area of bone. This region is also subject to movement between a well-supported, immobile, proximal segment and a mobile, distal segment. Intra-medullary screw compression is a simple and effective treatment.

### METATARSOPHALANGEAL JOINT AND TOE INJURIES

The metatarsophalangeal (MTP) joints and the toes can be injured by being hyperextended, crushed, or caught or stubbed. Patients may present with an avulsion or impaction fracture around a joint. The first and fifth toes are most commonly injured because of their more vulnerable position at the border of the foot. A dislocated joint is usually caused by a high-energy mechanism of injury. Acute fractures of the sesamoid bones under the first MTP joint can occasionally occur as the result of a jump or fall from a height.

## Emergency Department management

### Clinical features

- The patient will complain of pain, swelling and tenderness around the affected toe.
- Palpate carefully to assess for localized tenderness, joint congruence and stability.
- Crepitus suggests a fracture.
- Assess the sensation and capillary refill of the affected toe.
- A nailbed injury, in particular to the hallux, may require assessment in the same way as a nailbed injury to the finger (p. 285).

### Radiological features

- *Foot series*: Assess joint congruence and cortical outline.

### Reduction and immobilization

A fractured toe or a dislocated MTP joint can be reduced under a regional block (as for the hand; Fig. 2.8) or light procedural sedation, by gentle traction and reversal of the deformity. The use of a pen can be helpful in addressing deformities at the base of the phalanx (see Fig. 13.26). The injured toe is splinted to its neighbour with buddy strapping, as for finger injuries. A removable orthosis (moon boot) is often helpful for mobility.

### Inpatient referral

- Open or irreducible injuries, or fractures that are unstable, should be referred to Orthopaedics.

### Outpatient follow-up

- Patients with MTP joint sprains can be discharged with advice.
- Dislocated joints that have been reduced and are congruent should be reviewed in the fracture clinic.

## Orthopaedic management

### Non-operative

The majority of MTP joint and toe injuries are managed non-operatively with strapping, splintage and gradual mobilization.

## Operative

MTP joint fracture dislocations with incarcerated fragments or joint incongruity can be explored and washed out, and then stabilized. Unstable toe fractures that are not successfully immobilized with buddy strapping may require operative fixation. Where there is a large periarticular fragment causing joint incongruity or instability, this is fixed with mini-fragment screws. Comminuted fractures or persistently unstable joints are splinted straight with a longitudinal k-wire, as for the equivalent finger injury.

# COMPLICATIONS

## Late

Local    Post-traumatic osteoarthritis: Persistent fusiform swelling, stiffness and discomfort are common after toe dislocation or fracture. Salvage is with localized fusion

# COMPARTMENT SYNDROME OF THE FOOT

Compartment syndrome is the development of swelling within an indistensible anatomical space, resulting in increased pressure and tissue hypoperfusion. Swelling in the foot can be rapid and extensive, and most commonly follows crushing injuries and multiple tarsal or metatarsal fractures. Rarely, it can occur after isolated calcaneal fracture. Its management is controversial, as, unlike in the leg, only a small volume of muscle is affected. Moreover, the contained neurovascular structures are not traversing the compartment to a distal region, unlike injuries to the leg or arm, in which the foot and hand are at risk. Untreated, foot compartment syndrome may result in toe flexion contractures that can be addressed later simply by flexor tenotomy, and many trauma surgeons consider the treatment of foot compartment syndrome by fasciotomy to be worse than the condition itself.

## Anatomy

There are four indistensible osteofascial compartments in the foot. Although some texts refer to up to nine compartments, several of these are functionally confluent. These compartments contain the muscles of the foot:

1. medial (containing abductor hallucis and flexor hallucis brevis)

2. lateral (containing abductor digiti minimi and flexor digiti minimi brevis)

3. interosseous (four)

4. central: consists of three spaces:

   a. superficial (containing flexor digitorum brevis)

   b. central (containing flexor accessorius)

   c. deep (containing adductor hallucis).

Within these compartments are also the terminal branches of the tibial nerve: the *medial plantar nerve* (supplying the muscles of the medial compartment and flexor digitorum brevis) and *lateral plantar nerve* (supplying the remaining muscles), with their accompanying arteries. These nerves also supply sensation to the medial and lateral aspects of the plantar surface of the forefoot, respectively.

## Emergency Department management

### Clinical features

- The patient will have a grossly swollen and tight foot.

- There will be generalized pain on palpation and on toe movement, particularly toe extension (which stretches the muscles of the plantar aspect of the foot).

- There may be altered sensation over the plantar aspect of the forefoot.

### Radiological features

- *Foot series*: Radiographs will often show multiple tarsal or metatarsal fractures, and gross soft tissue swelling.

### Inpatient referral

- Patients with suspected foot compartment syndrome should be referred for orthopaedic assessment.

## Orthopaedic management

### Non-operative

- Constrictive dressings should be removed and the foot should be splinted and elevated to the level of the heart (but not higher).
- Ice or a cryotherapy device is applied.
- Fractures of the tarsus should be evaluated and treated on their merits.
- Intravenous opiate analgesia is often required for pain control.

### Operative

- This is controversial in the foot, as it is not clear that the outcome following fasciotomy is better than the outcome of non-operative management, and many feel the treatment is worse than the condition.
- Pressure monitoring may provide corroborative information if surgery is intended. A 'safe' pressure level for the foot has yet to be defined, and the level established for the diagnosis of leg compartment syndrome (a $\Delta P$ >30 mmHg; p. 45) is often used. Each of the four compartments should be measured.
- If surgery is thought to be appropriate, fasciotomies may be performed using two or three incisions (**Fig. 22.43**):

  Two longitudinal dorsal incisions are based over the second and fourth metatarsals. These allow decompression of the interosseous compartments, and, through them, access to the central, medial and lateral compartments.

  A medial incision, which is transverse and positioned just distal and anterior to the medial malleolus, may provide easier access to the medial and central compartments.

- The wounds are left open, and usually require split skin grafting at the time of second-look surgery at 48 hours.

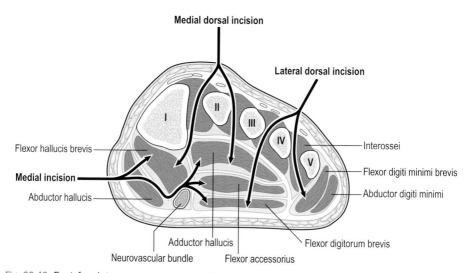

Fig. 22.43 Foot fasciotomy compartment release.

# COMPLICATIONS

### Early

Local    Wound dehiscence and infection: It is rarely possible to close the dorsal fasciotomy wounds, and skin grafting is usually required. This can be vulnerable to later abrasion

### Late

Local    Post-traumatic pain, stiffness and numbness: The foot is rarely normal after an injury of this severity, regardless of method of treatment

Toe stiffness: Surgical exposure of the extensor tendons commonly results in adhesions and restricted toe flexion

Toe flexion contractures: Fibrosis of the intrinsic muscles results in curled toes. These can be addressed later with flexor tenotomies and fusions

## FOOT SPRAINS

The majority of minor foot injuries presenting to the Emergency Department are simple foot or toe sprains. The aim of clinical assessment is to rule out any significant bony or ligamentous injury.

## Classification

Foot sprains are described according to anatomical location.

- *Midfoot sprains*: These result from a simple fall, twist or sporting collision, and cause pain over the midfoot.
- *Turf toe*: This is a sprain of the MTP joint, usually of the hallux, caused by a hyperextension injury. There is typically a history of a slip and fall, occasionally with an opponent then falling on the foot.

## Emergency Department management

### Clinical features

A foot sprain is a diagnosis of exclusion, and must be differentiated from more serious injuries such as a fracture, or an unstable injury of the Lisfranc joint. Certain features should *arouse suspicion*:

- A history of a high-energy fall, collision or sporting incident.
- Inability to bear weight through the foot.
- The presence of plantar bruising: Blood tracking through to the sole is indicative of a significant injury such as a Lisfranc injury or calcaneal fracture.
- Local bony tenderness or deformity on palpation.
- Forefoot pain on stressing: Gently stress the midfoot in pronation and supination (see Fig. 21.5), and in abduction/adduction while the hindfoot is stabilized. Look for pain or excessive movement of the injured tarsometatarsal joint when compared to the uninjured side.

Conversely, a foot which has no localized tenderness after a mild injury, and which permits midfoot stressing and a single-foot heel raise, is unlikely to have a significant structural injury.

### Radiological features

- *Foot series*: Where there is local tenderness, a series of foot radiographs should be obtained to exclude a fracture, particularly subtle flake fractures in the Lisfranc joint.

- *Weight-bearing foot radiographs*: If the patient can stand on the affected foot, radiographs taken with full weight-bearing may reveal dynamic instability at, for example, the Lisfranc joint.

- *Stress films*: Where there is pain, swelling and bruising, but no abnormality on plain radiography, an AP radiograph taken with the application of an abduction and plantar flexion stress may reveal dynamic instability.

- *CT*: Where there is continued suspicion of a fracture, a CT may reveal subtle flake fractures.

- *MRI*: Persistent pain or clinical suspicion occasionally warrants an MRI scan to exclude an occult fracture or ligamentous injury.

## Management

Once a fracture has been excluded clinically or radiographically, treatment is with rest, ice, compression bandaging and elevation (RICE). Immobilization in an orthosis (moon boot) or cast and the use of crutches are occasionally required for short-term symptom control and mobility. Active range of movement exercises should begin early.

## TRAUMA IN THE SKELETALLY IMMATURE

Many of the principles of adult fracture management are equally applicable to the paediatric setting. Initial *resuscitation* and pain management take priority (p. 21). Fracture management then follows the same principles of *reduce–hold–move* (p. 15). However, not only does the immature skeleton heal rapidly and remodel, but also children have a tolerance of limb immobilization not shared by the adult population. This skews most treatment towards a non-operative approach.

## THE UNIQUE PROPERTIES OF CHILDREN'S BONES

### Bone structure and growth

The anatomical regions of the *skeletally immature* bone are shown in **Fig. 23.1**:

- Epiphysis: The region on the articular side of the physis. Within the epiphysis is the *secondary ossification centre*.

- Physis (growth plate): A highly specialized cartilaginous (radiolucent) band between epiphysis and metaphysis. This structure provides longitudinal growth.

- Metaphysis: The widening region between the diaphysis and physis. The cortex is thinner than in diaphyseal bone.

- Diaphysis: The tubular mid-section of a long bone. The cortex is uniform and thick. The diaphyses have often begun ossifying prenatally at loci termed the *primary ossification centres*.

- Apophysis: Apophyses are peripheral areas in specific bones that form as secondary ossification centres and usually act as attachments for muscle and ligament.

## Physis (growth plate)

The normal physis (Fig. 23.1) is a complex structure in a state of continual cellular activity, and is responsible for generating longitudinal growth in the bone. Chondrocytes (cartilage cells) in the proliferative zone undergo division (mitosis) and become stacked into columns. The cells hypertrophy and then begin to degenerate, leaving behind a matrix that becomes calcified. The five histologically distinct zones are described in **Box 23.1**.

The physis is a site of potential structural weakness and is reinforced by an encircling fibrous layer: the *ring of Lacroix*. Underlying the ring of Lacroix is the *groove (or ring) of Ranvier*, a triangular region containing chondroblasts. This is responsible for the increase in width of the physis with growth.

## PHYSEAL INJURIES

Despite the ring of Lacroix, the physis is weaker than the surrounding bone and ligaments. This makes it vulnerable to injury, disruption usually occurring within the zones of hypertrophy and provisional calcification (Fig. 23.1). Healing is rapid, but permanent structural damage can result in *premature arrest* of the growth plate in around 2% of fractures. Fractures that stray into the proliferative and resting zones carry a higher chance of growth arrest due to disruption of the germinal cells.

- *Partial arrest* causes growth to cease in the damaged region, while the healthy portion of the physis continues to grow. This results in progressive deformity, particularly if the region of partial arrest is placed peripherally rather than centrally (**Fig. 23.2**).

- *Complete arrest* will result in a shortened bone. This may cause a length discrepancy in relation to an adjacent bone in the same limb (e.g. radius in relation to the ulna) or compared with the contralateral limb (resulting in leg length discrepancy).

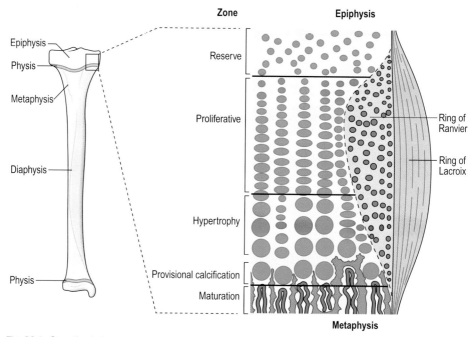

Fig. 23.1 Growth plate.

## Box 23.1 Histological zones of the physis

Epiphyseal side

Zone of reserve: A layer of randomly distributed, quiescent chondrocytes waiting for hormonal signals to commence mitosis

Zone of proliferation: Rapidly dividing chondrocytes stacked on one another, taking on a flattened appearance and forming columns

Zone of hypertrophy: Enlarged chondrocytes, absorbing lipids, glycogen and alkaline phosphatase

Zone of provisional calcification: Chondrocytes undergoing apoptosis (controlled cell death), leaving behind a matrix, which is then ossified

Zone of maturation: Ossified bone undergoing organization

Metaphyseal side

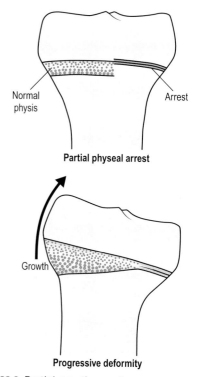

Fig. 23.2 Partial growth arrest.

## Salter–Harris classification of physeal fractures

This classification system of physeal fractures is useful in planning treatment and has prognostic value for predicting later growth disturbance (**Fig. 23.3**). The acronym SALTER may be helpful for remembering this system:

I  **S**traight across: The fracture line passes straight across the physis, and does not involve the bone of the epiphysis or metaphysis (**Fig. 23.4**).

II  **A**bove: The fracture line leaves a fragment of metaphyseal bone (the Thurston Holland fragment) above the physis. This is the most common type of fracture (**Fig. 23.5**).

III  **L**ower: The fracture line passes distally into the joint, resulting in an epiphyseal fragment that is lower than the physis (**Fig. 23.6**).

IV  **T**hrough: The fracture line passes through the metaphysis, physis and epiphysis (**Fig. 23.7**).

V  **E**radication: This is a compression injury, causing little displacement but considerable damage to the structure of the physis.

VI  **R**ing of Ranvier injury: This type was added to the classification system later and is sometimes referred to as the 'lawnmower injury'. It is an abrasion injury that results in the loss of peripheral bone and physis.

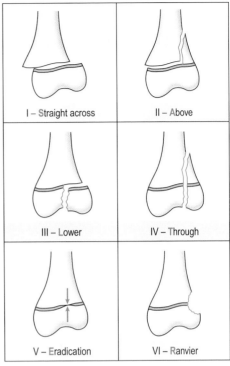

Fig. 23.3 Salter–Harris classification of physeal fractures.

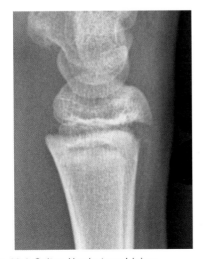

Fig. 23.4 Salter–Harris type I injury.

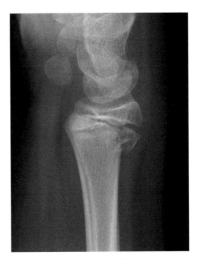

Fig. 23.5 Salter–Harris type II injury.

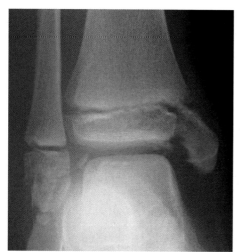

Fig. 23.6 Salter–Harris type III injury.

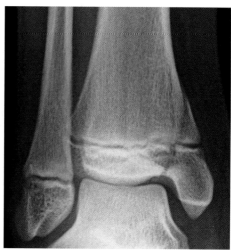

Fig. 23.7 Salter–Harris type IV injury.

## Early management of physeal injuries

### Type I and II injuries

Fractures that are undisplaced or minimally displaced are managed non-operatively with casting. Displaced type I or II fractures should be gently manipulated within the first 5 days, bearing in mind the great potential for remodelling (see below). To avoid late loss of position, it is often advisable to secure a manipulated type I or II fracture with a transphyseal smooth k-wire. These carry very little risk of physeal damage if placed with care (see Fig. 24.21).

Manipulation of type I or II physeal fractures *after 5 days* greatly increases the risk of physeal damage and growth arrest, as healing has already commenced. If a good initial position is lost or the injury presents late after 5 days, the poor position is usually best accepted in the expectation that remodelling will improve the position. Osteotomies can be performed later to correct residual deformity if remodelling is insufficient.

### Type III and IV injuries

These intra-articular injuries should be addressed with prompt, anatomical reduction and fixation to reduce the risk of physeal arrest and joint surface disruption. This often constitutes open reduction of the intra-articular component, with fixation that does not cross the physis (**Fig. 23.8**).

### Type V injuries

These injuries cannot be improved surgically and can only be monitored for the development of partial or complete physeal arrest. Salvage surgery in these situations is described below.

### Type VI (Peterson) injuries

These occur when the physis has been exposed to peripheral abrasion: for example, being dragged along a road surface. The principles of treating open fractures apply. The damage to the physis is often very significant.

## Follow-up of physeal injuries

Careful long-term follow-up (18–24 months) is required for those injuries at high risk of physeal arrest. High-risk fractures include:

- Salter–Harris types III, IV, V and VI
- high-energy physeal fractures of any type
- distal femoral physeal fractures
- proximal tibial physeal fractures.

The latter two are included, as disturbance of these rapidly growing physes can have very significant clinical consequences.

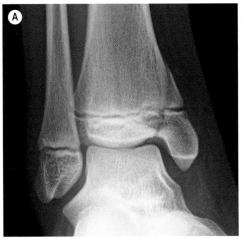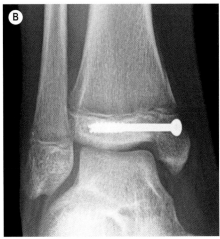

Fig. 23.8 Salter–Harris type IV injury with screw fixation. **A**, The fracture line passes through the physis. **B**, After fixation with a transverse screw in the epiphysis, avoiding the physis.

Growth should be monitored clinically and radiographically. An irregularity in the growth plate may be visible on plain films before the development of clinical deformity. MRI is an invaluable tool for more accurate assessment of the physis and should be considered if there is any suspicion of growth disturbance at follow-up. Intervention is best performed before noticeable deformity or joint incongruity occurs. It is determined by the age of the child and extent of the physeal closure, and consists of either:

- *Physeal preservation*: Occasionally, only a small area of partial arrest is seen in the form of a 'bony bar' – a bridge of bone that crosses the physis and causes tethering. This can be excised (the Langenskiöld procedure) to allow uniform growth of the affected physis. This technique works best for small (<30%), peripheral bars. Larger bars and those located centrally are less successfully treated with this technique.
- *Physeal ablation*: When the bony bar is not amenable to excision, then the physeal arrest is completed by ablating the remaining intact physis, in order to avoid the development of

further deformity. This technique is termed *epiphysiodesis*.

If a complete physeal arrest has occurred, epiphysiodesis of other (uninjured) bones may be necessary to avoid the development of deformity or length discrepancy.

## Late surgery for deformity secondary to growth arrest

The presentation of established, unacceptable degrees of deformity will require realignment surgery to correct mechanical axes and joint alignment. This can be done acutely with osteotomy and fixation, or gradually with an external fixator.

In **Figure 23.9**, a Salter–Harris type III injury of the medial malleolus (**Fig. 23.9A**) was treated appropriately with a single screw that did not cross the physis (**Fig. 23.9B**). Despite adequate surgery, partial growth arrest occurred at the medial aspect of the physis, while the lateral aspect continued to grow, with a resultant varus deformity (**Fig. 23.9C**). A corrective osteotomy to realign the ankle joint was required (**Fig. 23.9D**).

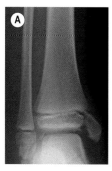
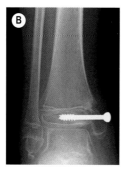
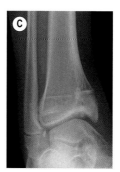
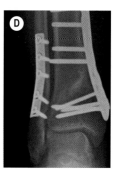

Fig. 23.9 Salter–Harris type III injury with partial growth arrest and subsequent osteotomy. See text for details.

## TYPES OF PAEDIATRIC FRACTURE

Children's bones are inherently more elastic (less brittle) than those of adults and can bend before fracturing completely. They have a thick periosteal sleeve that provides nutrition and mechanical support. Under a bending force, children's bones will progress through the following stages:

1. *Elastic deformation*: The bent bone returns to a normal shape when the deforming force is removed.

2. *Plastic deformation*: At higher load, the bones deform, although the cortices remain in continuity. The deformity remains after the force is removed.

3. *Torus (buckle) fracture*: With a greater load, failure occurs on the compression side of the bone, and the cortex buckles and fractures. The tension side of the bone remains in continuity, and the fracture remains stable (**Fig. 23.10**).

4. *Greenstick fracture*: Further loading causes failure of the tension side, as well as a buckle on the compression side (**Fig. 23.10**).

5. *Complete fracture*: This is loss of bone continuity on both the compression and tension sides. Note that even when the fracture progresses beyond greenstick to a complete fracture, the periosteum on the compression side usually remains intact, which may be invaluable when manipulating and immobilizing such fractures (**Fig. 23.10**).

## Fracture stability

An appreciation of fracture type and the implied state of the periosteum is crucial in understanding paediatric fracture management. Torus fractures are incomplete and are therefore intrinsically stable. Greenstick and complete fractures are unstable (**Fig. 23.11**), but the intact, loose, periosteum on the compression side of the fracture (A) is used to achieve fracture reduction (B), and to maintain this position using three-point cast moulding (C).

Simple transverse or short oblique fractures will not shorten under load and are termed length-stable (**Fig. 23.12A**). Comminuted and spiral fractures are length-unstable (**Fig. 23.12B**), and these cannot be held out to length with plaster or elastic intramedullary nails (see Fig. 23.8), and often require other forms of surgical stabilization.

## Avulsion (apophyseal) fractures

An apophysis is a secondary ossification centre that commonly has a ligament or muscle attachment. These are vulnerable to avulsion injury; the elbow, pelvis and proximal femur are common sites.

## Remodelling

An angulated paediatric fracture has a powerful potential for spontaneous correction by two mechanisms: realignment of the physis, and

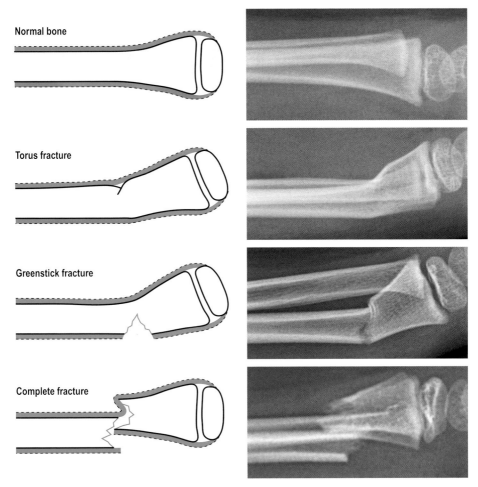

Normal bone

Torus fracture

Greenstick fracture

Complete fracture

Fig. 23.10 Bending fractures.

remodelling of metaphyseal or diaphyseal deformity (**Fig. 23.13**). The potential for children's bones to remodel gradually decreases as they approach skeletal maturity.

## Physeal realignment

The physis of a long bone is normally orientated orthogonally (at 90°) to the long axis of the bone. A malunited fracture, in which the physis is placed at an angle to the long axis, will cause a redistribution of load, with one side of the physis (the longer side) being placed under increased load, while the other (shorter) side comes under reduced load. The *Hueter–Volkmann Law* states that increased pressure on one part of the physis will retard its growth, while reduced pressure on another part will accelerate its growth. This leads to a gradual correction of the orientation of the physis (Fig. 23.13).

The physis will remodel best if the deformity is in the dominant plane of motion of the adjacent joint: for example, a sagittal (flexion/extension) deformity of the distal femur. There is very little ability to remodel a rotational deformity.

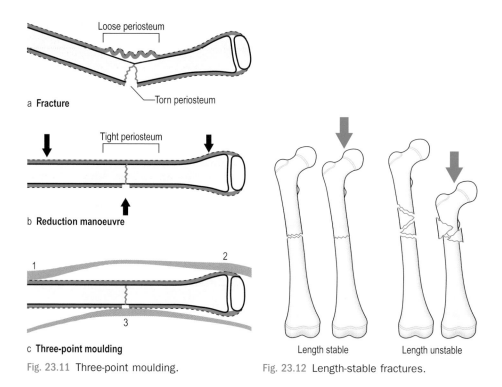

a **Fracture**

Loose periosteum

Torn periosteum

b **Reduction manoeuvre**

Tight periosteum

c **Three-point moulding**

Fig. 23.11 Three-point moulding.

Length stable        Length unstable

Fig. 23.12 Length-stable fractures.

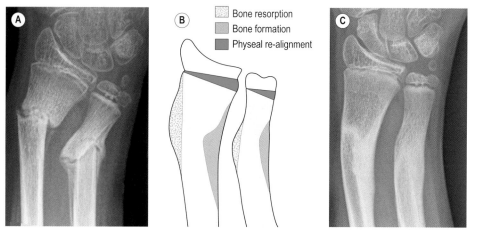

Bone resorption
Bone formation
Physeal re-alignment

Fig. 23.13 **A**, Malunion of a distal radius and ulnar fracture. **B**, Areas of bone under compression undergo bone formation whilst areas under tension undergo resorption (Wolff's Law). Differential growth in the physis results in realignment (Hueter Volkmann Law). **C**, the bones gradually remodel.

## Non-physeal remodelling

All bones undergo continuous remodelling in response to loading (Wolff's Law; p. 18), and this physiological process is helpful in remodelling a deformity after fracture. Angulation of a diaphyseal malunion results in increased mechanical loading and osteoblastic activity on the concave (compressed) side, resulting in bone formation, and increased osteoclastic activity on the convex (tension) side, resulting in bone resorption. The angulation thereby gradually appears to straighten (Fig. 23.13). This is a slower process than physeal realignment.

## Extent of remodelling

Remodelling is not entirely predictable but good potential occurs where there is:

- a younger age (at least 2 years before expected skeletal maturity)
- deformity in the plane of movement of the adjacent joint
- deformity close to a rapidly growing physis (e.g. proximal humerus, distal femur, distal radius; the physes at elbows and ankle are slower-growing and less able to remodel).

Angular deformity can correct at around 1° per month. The clinically apparent deformity will disappear before full radiological correction is seen.

## INTERPRETING PAEDIATRIC RADIOGRAPHS

Fracture identification can present a challenge to those unaccustomed to radiographs of the immature skeleton.

- *Clinical correlation*: It is crucial to correlate clinical findings with the images. A radiographic abnormality is unlikely to represent an acute fracture if the location in question is not tender.
- *Definition and contour*: The presence of the physis and various ossification centres can make it difficult to decide if a lucent line is pathological or physiological. Ossific nuclei will usually have a rounded, smooth appearance and physeal lines are usually broad and well defined. In contrast, fracture lines often show sharp or irregular angulation (**Fig. 23.14**)
- *Soft tissue signs*: Images may also show soft tissue swelling (**Fig. 23.15**) or abnormal fat–fluid levels, which can be more obvious than the bony injury (see Figs 10.7, 20.6). The presence of abnormal soft tissue signs should invite close scrutiny of the bony appearances or even further imaging.
- *Reference material*: Atlases of radiological variants should be readily available where children's radiographs are being viewed. This should avoid the need for requesting comparative radiographs of the unaffected limb.

## NEUROVASCULAR COMPLICATIONS

### Vascular injury

Peripheral pulses are often difficult to feel in small children, and vascular assessment relies more on the evaluation of colour, temperature and capillary refill. Acute ischaemia with a significant limb deformity requires urgent realignment of the limb, which must be carried out under procedural sedation without delay.

### Nerve injury

Young children often cannot comply with a full clinical assessment of motor and sensory function, in which case attention should be paid to objective features such as the absence of sweating or the passive position of the digits, which may betray neurological impairment. A relatively simple method of assessing the motor function of the three main nerves in the upper limb is shown in **Figure 23.16**. Motor testing in the lower limb, and sensory testing in both the upper and lower

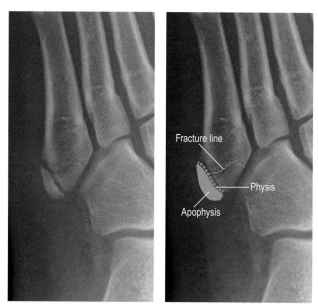

Fig. 23.14 Foot radiograph showing both physiological growth lines and a fracture line.

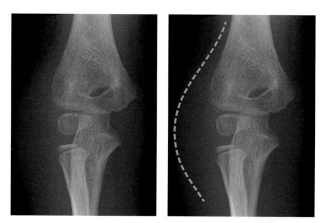

Fig. 23.15 Soft tissue swelling.

limbs, are the same as in adults (see Figures 3.17–3.22).

## NON-ACCIDENTAL INJURY

It is a sad fact that children can be the victims of physical and emotional abuse, often by those closest to them. Repeated abuse is not uncommon and 5% of affected children can die as a result. It is therefore of extreme importance that clinicians remain vigilant for the signs of non-accidental injury (NAI) and do not hesitate to escalate concerns through the appropriate pathways.

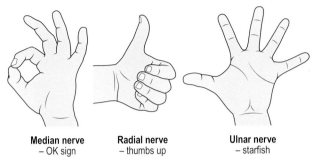

**Median nerve**
– OK sign

**Radial nerve**
– thumbs up

**Ulnar nerve**
– starfish

Fig. 23.16 Upper limb peripheral nerve: motor examination.

## History

NAI occurs across all demographic groups, with pre-school age children being most at risk. Features in the history that should raise suspicion include:

- delayed presentation
- inconsistent histories from carers, witnesses or the child
- multiple Emergency Department attendances
- history of child protection concerns – this is unlikely to be volunteered and should be checked in the child's records.

## Examination

Thorough physical examination is essential and the following findings raise concern:

- patterned or sharply defined bruising – e.g. fingertip- or implement-inflicted
- multiple bruising of different ages
- burns – especially multiple small burns suggestive of a cigarette tip
- subconjunctival haemorrhage – from shaking or choking
- intraoral or genitourinary injury
- bite marks.

## Radiological features

Specific skeletal injuries have an association with NAI and include:

- femoral fracture in pre-toddler-age children
- skull fracture
- rib fractures – especially when multiple
- metaphyseal corner or bucket-handle fractures
- coincidentally discovered, older, previously undiagnosed fractures.

Differential diagnoses for atypical fractures in children can include metabolic, genetic or congenital bone disease; however, these are complex to diagnose and should never be assumed to be the cause without proper investigation. Any suspicion of NAI mandates that the child be protected from further harm by being kept in hospital under supervision while senior and specialized help is sought.

## THE LIMPING CHILD

This is a common presentation to the Emergency Department and can be a diagnostic challenge. There is often no history of trauma but that does not exclude the possibility of injury, as children cannot be supervised at all times and may not admit to an accident. **Table 23.1** shows some of the possible diagnoses with associated features.

It is not uncommon to find no obvious cause for a limp and it may be appropriate to

**Table 23.1   Diagnosis of limp in a child**

| Cause | Typical features | For | Against |
|---|---|---|---|
| Toddler's fracture | Age 1–3 years<br>Should start to improve within 1 week of onset | Tibial tenderness<br>Radiograph may show fine spiral fracture line (**Fig. 23.17**) | Pyrexia<br>Abnormal bloods<br>No localizing signs at tibia |
| Irritable hip/transient synovitis | Age 3–10 yrs<br>History of preceding coryzal illness | Pyrexia <38°C<br>Child sore but well<br>Joint effusion on ultrasound | Pyrexia >38°C<br>C-reactive protein >20 mg/L<br>Abnormal full blood count<br>Limb pseudoparalysis |
| Septic arthritis | All ages<br>History 1–2 days<br>Ill child | C-reactive protein >20 mg/L<br>Abnormal FBC<br>Pyrexia >38°C<br>Limb pseudoparalysis<br>Joint effusion | Normal bloods >48 hrs after onset<br>No effusion on ultrasound >48 hrs after onset |
| Osteomyelitis/pyomyositis | All ages<br>History <1 week | As for septic arthritis | As for septic arthritis<br>Joint effusion possible but treat as septic arthritis if present |
| Perthes' disease | Age 3–10 yrs<br>History >2 weeks<br>Weight-bearing | Well child<br>Abnormal hip examination<br>Typical radiographic features | Abnormal bloods<br>Pyrexia |
| Slipped capital femoral epiphysis (SCFE) | Age typically 9–14 yrs<br>Thigh or knee pain (rather than hip pain)<br>Sudden or prolonged history | Abnormal hip examination with loss of internal rotation and abduction<br>Frog lateral hip radiograph abnormal (see Fig. 25.5) | Normal frog lateral hip radiograph<br>Abnormal bloods<br>Pyrexia |

*The ages given for the various causes of a limp represent typical ranges but it is possible for younger and older children to be affected by these pathologies.*

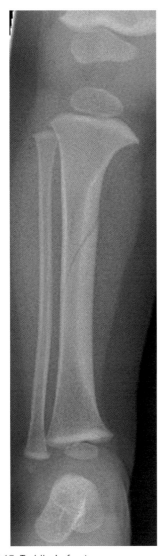

Fig. 23.17 Toddler's fracture.

discharge the child with simple analgesia and advice. It is suggested that the following criteria should be met before considering discharge:

- well child
- normal investigations (as above)
- no concern about abuse or neglect
- reliable carers who comprehend advice to return if the situation deteriorates.

## SHOULDER GIRDLE

### CLAVICLE

Clavicle injuries are common in childhood and may affect:

- *Medial clavicle*: Dislocation of the sternoclavicular joint is very rare but a disruption of the medial physis (a Salter–Harris I or II fracture) can occur. This physis does not close until the age of 25.
- *Mid-shaft*: Mid-shaft fractures are the most common.
- *Lateral clavicle*: Injuries of the lateral clavicle most commonly cause a physeal or metaphyseal fracture, leaving the acromioclavicular and coracoclavicular ligaments intact.

## Emergency Department management

### Clinical features

- In older children, the mechanism of injury is usually a sports-related fall.
- The full length of the clavicle should be palpated to localize tenderness and swelling (see Fig. 8.4).
- A sternoclavicular joint dislocation presents with medial swelling or loss of prominence.

### Radiological features

- *AP view of the clavicle*: This is usually adequate to confirm most clavicular fractures.
- *Ultrasound*: This can be used to look for physeal separation medially or laterally.
- *CT*: This may be required to demonstrate displacement of the medial end of the clavicle, which is poorly seen on plain radiographs

### Immobilization

A broad arm sling (see Fig. 4.1) provides definitive management of most clavicular shaft and physeal injuries.

## Orthopaedic management
### Non-operative

Children are allowed to move the affected limb as pain allows, and to wean themselves from the sling as soon as it is comfortable.

### Operative

Operative management is reserved for open fractures and might be considered in multiple trauma injuries in older children and adolescents. On occasion, a bony prominence causing skin problems may be excised later. Stabilization of lateral clavicular injuries is rare, as these are usually physeal or metaphyseal fractures that heal rapidly, leaving the ligaments intact.

A posteriorly displaced sternoclavicular dislocation will require reduction if there is dysphagia or dyspnoea (see Fig. 8.15).

### SCAPULA

Scapular fractures are very rare in children but can often be confused with the numerous secondary ossification centres seen in the immature scapula. As with adults, a true scapular fracture is indicative of significant trauma to the upper torso, head and neck.

### PROXIMAL HUMERAL FRACTURES

Greenstick fractures of the proximal humeral metaphysis and physeal injuries constitute the majority of injuries in this region. The remodelling potential of the proximal humerus is exceptional, allowing a high tolerance for displacement and angulation.

## Classification

The Salter–Harris classification (Fig. 23.3) is applied to injuries of the proximal humeral physis.

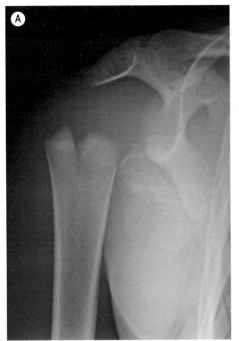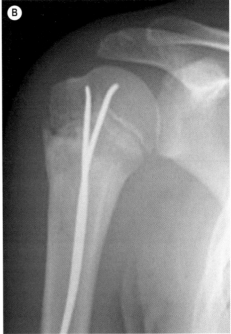

Fig. 24.1 **A**, Off-ended fracture dislocation of the proximal humerus. **B**, Treatment was with closed manipulation and intramedullary flexible nails introduced retrograde via an anterolateral approach.

## Emergency Department management

### Clinical features

- The patient often presents holding the arm, with localized pain and loss of function. Some swelling may be seen, with bruising developing later.

### Radiological features

- *Shoulder trauma series*: AP and axillary (or modified axial) radiographs are taken (see Fig. 8.7).
- *Ultrasound*: Under 2 years of age, an ultrasound is better at demonstrating the cartilaginous proximal humerus than plain radiography.

### Immobilization

Significant deformity, *including off-ended fractures*, can be accepted in most children (see below), and symptomatic treatment with a sling is usually all that is required (p. 76).

## Orthopaedic management

### Non-operative

Physeal and metaphyseal fractures can be expected to heal within 2–4 weeks, with full mobilization as soon as pain permits.

### Operative

Due to the remodelling potential in this area, surgery is rarely indicated. Off-ended proximal humeral fractures in children *over 10 years* are an exception and are treated with reduction and flexible intramedullary nailing (**Fig. 24.1**). Percutaneous k-wiring can be complicated by wire migration and is not recommended.

## GLENOHUMERAL DISLOCATION

Glenohumeral dislocation is very rare in children, occurring principally amongst adolescents. These injuries should be treated in the same way as adult ones (p. 146).

## HUMERAL CYSTS

The proximal humerus is the most common site for unicameral (Latin: *uni-*, 'one' and *camera*, 'chamber'), or simple, bone cysts. Unicameral bone cysts are predisposed to fracture and are often discovered after injury. Radiological features suggestive of bony cyst include (**Fig. 24.2**):

● lytic appearance
● well-defined margin
● cortical thinning.

Atypical features, such as poorly defined margins, soft tissue calcification or periosteal reaction, require further investigation with MRI to exclude more aggressive lesions or malignancy.

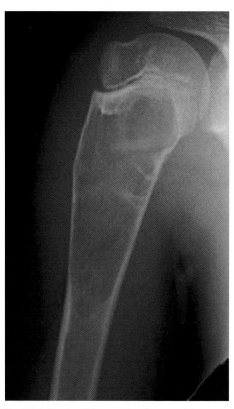

Fig. 24.2 Proximal humeral unicameral bone cyst.

## Management

Most fractures will heal with non-operative treatment, although some diaphyseal lesions may prove very unstable and merit intramedullary flexible nailing. It is a common misconception that fracture healing promotes resolution of the cyst when, in fact, 90% persist after fracture healing and remain vulnerable to further injury. Surgical ablation of the cyst by injection or curettage and grafting can be offered if the risk of further low-energy fracture is intolerable for the patient or incompatible with lifestyle choices such as contact sports.

## HUMERAL SHAFT FRACTURES

These are unusual in children and can almost always be managed with a u-slab or cast and sling (Fig. 4.8). Such fractures in infants have an association with *non-accidental injury* (p. 562).

## ELBOW

The elbow is a relatively common site of injury in childhood and can be complex to evaluate radiologically due to the various ossification centres. Careful clinical examination to locate precise areas of tenderness or swelling is helpful.

Anatomically, an important distinction lies in the structure of the condyles (Latin: 'knuckle') and epicondyles (Latin: *epi-*, 'upon'). In the adult, these are essentially one structure and form the medial and lateral prominences of the distal humerus. In the child, the condyles are in continuity with the humeral shaft while the epicondyles are separated from the shaft by a physis. Children can therefore suffer either condylar or epicondylar injuries.

The cardinal paediatric elbow injuries include:

● supracondylar fractures – the most common
● lateral condyle fractures
● medial condyle – rare
● medial epicondyle avulsion – often associated with elbow dislocation
● elbow dislocation
● radial head/neck fractures.

## Radiological assessment of the paediatric elbow

The normal radiological appearances of the elbow vary with age as ossification progresses. The acronym 'CRITOL' is useful (**Fig. 24.3**):

The *radiocapitellar line* (see Fig. 10.6) and *anterior humeral line* are important indicators of anatomical alignment. The *sail sign* (see Fig. 10.7) indicates the likelihood of a fracture being present, even if the fracture itself cannot be discerned on the radiograph.

- Skin puckering at the antecubital fossa suggests tethering of the skin by the proximal spike of the fracture (see Fig. 24.8).
- 5% will have an ipsilateral fracture, often of the distal radius.
- Neurovascular integrity of the limb should be verified. Up to 15% of type 3 supracondylar fractures present with neuropathy and 5% with significant vascular compromise.
- Compartment syndrome (p. 45) is a risk, although rare.

## SUPRACONDYLAR FRACTURES OF THE HUMERUS

This injury occurs from a fall on the outstretched arm. The fracture occurs in the thinnest portion of the bone between the coronoid and olecranon fossae.

## Classification

### Extension type

More than 90% of supracondylar fractures occur in extension. These are classified according to the modified *Gartland classification* (**Fig. 24.4**):

- *Type 1*: fracture of anterior cortex but no displacement.
- *Type 2*: fracture angulated but the posterior cortex of distal humerus remains intact.
- *Type 3*: fracture displaced (and often rotated) with no cortical contact.

### Flexion type

Less than 10% of supracondylar fractures are of the flexion type or are complex intracondylar fractures, and these are more challenging to treat (**Fig. 24.5**). There is no formal classification for these injuries.

## Emergency Department management

### Clinical features

- There is swelling and deformity of the elbow.
- Bruising is seen in the antecubital fossa.

### ✓ Key point

The radial pulse of a small child can be difficult to palpate and its *absence does not in itself indicate acute ischaemia*. It is more important to inspect the hand for signs of adequate perfusion:

- A *warm, pink hand* with capillary return of less than 3 seconds suggests good perfusion and there is therefore no acute threat to the limb. Timely, but not urgent, reduction is acceptable and the brachial artery does not need to be explored.
- A *cool, pale hand*, however, is an emergency and it is not helpful in this setting to spend time seeking the pulse with a Doppler probe when what is needed is urgent reduction of the fracture. If this cannot be carried out in theatre within an hour, it may be necessary to manipulate the arm under sedation in the Emergency Department to try to restore circulation. Return of good perfusion buys time, but the limb must be monitored vigilantly while definitive treatment is awaited. Failure to restore the circulation or subsequent deterioration after initial success is an indication to explore the brachial artery in combination with surgical reduction and stabilization of the fracture. Angiography is seldom used as the location of arterial injury is at the fracture site.

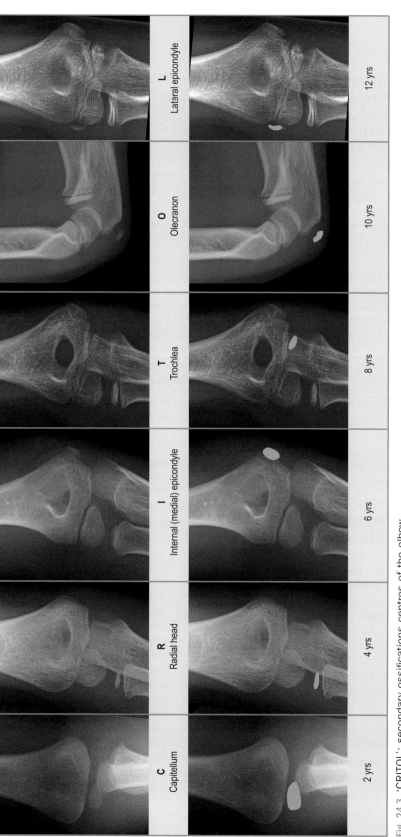

Fig. 24.3 'CRITOL': secondary ossifications centres of the elbow.

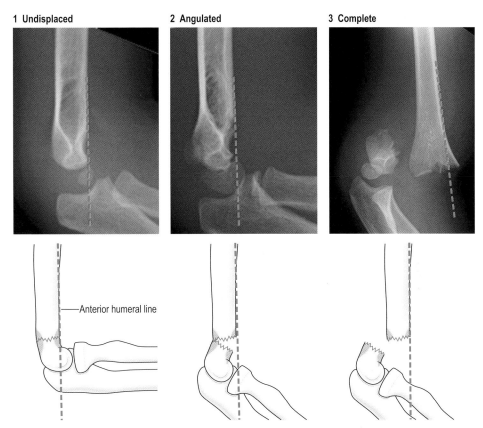

**1 Undisplaced**    **2 Angulated**    **3 Complete**

—Anterior humeral line

Fig. 24.4 The Gartland classification of supracondylar fractures.

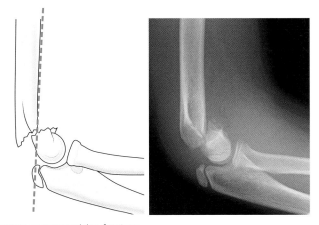

Fig. 24.5 Flexion-type supracondylar fracture.

### Initial reduction and immobilization

The priority for the obviously injured elbow is to provide analgesia and splintage. An above-elbow backslab can be applied (see Fig. 4.9) in the position in which the patient presents, which is often extension. Attempts to flex such a limb for the purposes of casting will be painful and can compromise neurovascular structures. Radiographs taken thereafter define management.

### Radiological features

● *AP and lateral views of the elbow.*

### Outpatient follow-up

● Type 1 extension fractures should be placed into a cast at 90–100° of elbow flexion.

### Inpatient referral

● Type 2 or 3 extension injuries and any flexion type injury should remain in the initial splint and be referred to the orthopaedic service.

## Orthopaedic management

### Non-operative

Type 1 extension fractures are removed from cast after 3 weeks and full mobilization is commenced.

### Operative

#### *Extension-type supracondylar fractures*

Type 2 fractures, where the distal humerus is extended behind the anterior humeral line, and all type 3 fractures, require manipulation under anaesthesia (MUA), pinning and casting for 3 weeks (see 'Surgical technique'). Some 90% should be amenable to closed reduction. Extensive swelling, bruising or puckering in the antecubital fossa or a long proximal, medial spike on radiograph (see Fig. 24.8) can be a warning of potential difficulties.

#### *Flexion-type supracondylar fractures*

Flexion-type fractures are reduced and pinned with the elbow in near-full extension. This is a more challenging procedure.

---

**SURGICAL TECHNIQUE: Reduction and fixation of a Gartland type 3 extension supracondylar humeral fracture**

#### Surgical set-up

The child is placed supine with an arm table. Ensure adequate AP and lateral images can be obtained without the arm being moved. This may require positioning younger children at 90° to the table with their legs on an extension attachment. This allows the affected limb to be positioned over the foot of the table, affording unimpeded access for the c-arm. An upper arm tourniquet is applied but not inflated unless converting to open reduction.

#### Closed reduction (Fig. 24.6)

1. *Traction*: With an assistant securing the proximal humerus, gentle but steady and continuous traction should be applied to the extended arm for 2 minutes. An AP view with the image intensifier at this point will show restoration of length and demonstrate any medial, lateral or rotational displacement of the distal fragment.
2. *Medial/lateral correction*: Medial or lateral translational displacement seen on the AP view should now be addressed with direct manipulation while maintaining longitudinal traction. Only proceed to step 3 when satisfactory alignment has been obtained on the AP view.
3. *Reduction of the extension*: The surgeon should keep hold of the wrist in one hand while placing his free hand around the patient's elbow with his thumb on the olecranon. The patient's elbow is then flexed gently while the surgeon's thumb

maintains pressure on the olecranon. The elbow should allow flexion beyond 100°. If it does not, this may indicate entrapment of tissues within the fracture. In this situation, the arm should be brought back out into extension and the antecubital fossa reinspected. If there is puckering, or a bone spike is palpable under the skin, an attempt should be made to 'milk' this gently to free up the soft tissues before repeating the reduction process from step 1. A lateral view is achieved by rotating the image intensifier (not the limb) through 90°. If this is unsatisfactory, then return to step 1.

If an adequate reduction is not achieved after two or three attempts, consider open reduction (see below).

### Pinning

Pinning following reduction is performed with the elbow supported in flexion (**Fig. 24.7A**). The fracture is held with two crossed medial and lateral k-wires, or with two or three laterally based wires (**Fig. 24.7B,C**).

- *Lateral wires* should be passed percutaneously through a stab incision to avoid dragging epithelial tissue into the wire tract.

- *Medial wires* must be placed via an open approach to avoid iatrogenic injury to the ulnar nerve. This is performed using an incision that is adequate for visualizing the medial epicondyle to ensure that the k-wire is placed directly on to bone. Soft tissue retraction must be used to prevent the rotating wire from wrapping adjacent structures around the wire and thus causing tension or entrapment of the ulnar nerve.

All wires should be passed at low revolutions to reduce the risk of thermal damage.

Once wires are seated, the fracture should be stressed gently in sagittal and coronal planes to check stability. If the fracture remains unstable, a third wire can be passed and/ or the other wires repositioned.

### Post procedure

An above-elbow backslab is applied with the arm in 80–90° of flexion (see Fig. 4.9), ensuring that good circulation in the fingers is maintained.

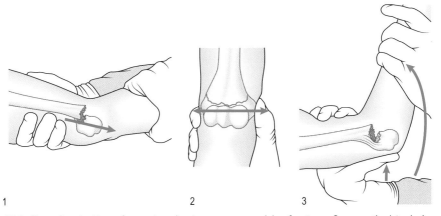

1                    2                    3

Fig. 24.6 Closed reduction of an extension-type supracondylar fracture. See surgical technique box for details.

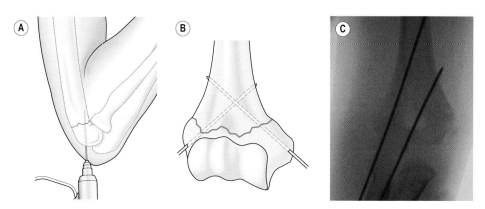

Fig. 24.7 K-wiring of a supracondylar fracture. See surgical technique box for details.

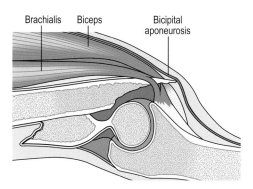

Fig. 24.8 Irreducible supracondylar fracture

### Open reduction of an extension supracondylar fracture

The options include a medial approach, lateral (Kocher) approach or anterior approach. Each has its own merits and selection will depend on fracture configuration, the presence or absence of neurovascular compromise, and the surgeon's familiarity with the approach.

### Anterior approach to the elbow

This approach allows good access to neurovascular structures and visualization of the proximal fracture fragment that has punctured through the brachialis and biceps, and lies beneath the bicipital aponeurosis (**Fig. 24.8**). It also leaves a scar that is relatively satisfactory cosmetically.

The incision is transverse at the flexor crease of the elbow and can be extended proximally along the medial border of biceps or distally along the medial border of brachioradialis

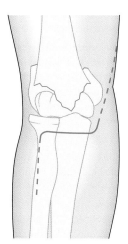

Fig. 24.9 Anterior approach to the elbow: incision.

(**Fig. 24.9**). Care must be taken with the incision, as neurovascular structures may be tented up over the fracture and be very near the skin. The lateral cutaneous nerve of the forearm is vulnerable at the lateral aspect of the incision. The proximal spike of the fracture is often identified easily, having punched through the brachialis and bicipital aponeurosis. Gentle dissection should expose the median nerve and brachial artery to ensure that they are not trapped by the fracture. After removal of interposed soft tissue, the fracture can be reduced with posteriorly directed pressure on the proximal fragment. This can be confirmed by palpation and radiographs, following which the fracture is stabilized as described above.

## COMPLICATIONS

### *Early*

Local    Infection: The exposed k-wire ends may become colonized or infected. This should be treated vigorously with antibiotics to prevent septic arthritis of the elbow

Neurapraxia: Injury to the median nerve should resolve within 10–12 weeks

Stiffness: Some early stiffness is normal but a functional range of motion should return within 6 weeks. Some minor loss of extension can persist

### *Late*

Local    Deformity: 5% of patients have some residual deformity. Very little remodelling is seen after the age of 5 years. Cubitus varus (gunstock) deformity is disfiguring, although not functionally problematic (**Fig. 24.10**). If the deformity is severe, then distal humeral osteotomy may be indicated for cosmetic reasons

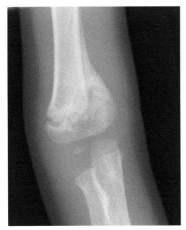 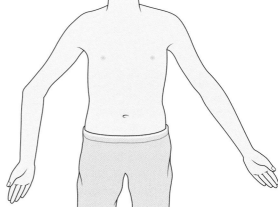

Fig. 24.10 Cubitus varus.

## LATERAL CONDYLAR FRACTURES

These represent 15% of paediatric elbow fractures and can be difficult to spot and easy to under-estimate. They are associated with significant deformity from malunion and the rare paediatric complication of non-union.

## Classification

The *Milch classification* describes the fracture in relation to the trochlear groove (**Fig. 24.11**):

● *Type 1*: The fracture line exits at or lateral to the capitotrochlear groove.

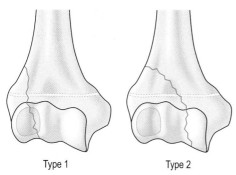

Type 1                Type 2

Fig. 24.11 Milch classification of lateral condylar fractures.

• *Type 2*: The fracture line exits though the trochlea, resulting in instability of the fracture, and often of the entire humero-ulnar joint.

## Emergency Department management

### Clinical features
• The patient presents with a painful elbow and is intolerant of movement.
• There is tenderness laterally.
• Lateral swelling may be seen, although this is often not obvious.
• A small lateral bruise can be present.

### Radiological features
• *AP and lateral views of the elbow*: These radiographs are usually sufficient but features can be subtle. Significant soft tissue swelling laterally is indicative of this injury, as is a posterior fat-pad sign (see Fig. 10.7).
• *Internal oblique view*: This is achieved by taking an AP view with the arm internally rotated by 30°. It is particularly useful in confirming the extent of displacement.
• *CT scan*: This is occasionally used where there is diagnostic uncertainty.

### Immobilization and outpatient follow-up
• Fractures with <2 mm of displacement on AP, lateral and oblique views are treated in an above-elbow cast and referred to fracture clinic. They must be seen within 5 days, as displacement identified after this time may be difficult to treat.

### Inpatient referral
• Fractures with >2 mm of displacement should be referred for surgical reduction and stabilization.

## Orthopaedic management
### Non-operative
Fractures with <2 mm of displacement are treated in an above-elbow cast for 3–4 weeks. They must be closely observed, with weekly radiographs out of cast until healed.

### Operative
Fractures with >2 mm of displacement should be reduced and stabilized. This can be done closed with percutaneous fixation in minimally displaced cases but open reduction is often needed to ensure restoration of the articular surface. A lateral or posterolateral approach can be used but stripping of the soft tissues from the back of the distal humerus must be avoided to prevent osteonecrosis of the capitellum. Stability can be conferred with diverging k-wires or a cannulated screw in the metaphyseal segment in older children. A cast is applied for 3 weeks before mobilization.

### COMPLICATIONS

*Later*

| | |
|---|---|
| Local | A lateral bump persists on the elbow in 50% but is of no functional significance. Osteonecrosis, malunion and non-union can occur but reasonable function can return in these situations without intervention. Late surgery is usually for cosmetic reasons |

## MEDIAL CONDYLAR FRACTURES

These are very unusual fractures but are intra-articular and must be differentiated from epicondylar injuries. They require reduction and stabilization if displaced.

## MEDIAL EPICONDYLAR FRACTURES

This is an apophyseal avulsion injury and is often associated with elbow dislocation (see **Fig. 24.12**). If the medial epicondyle cannot be seen on radiographs after elbow trauma in a child over 6 years old, then it may be incarcerated in the humero-ulnar joint (**Fig. 24.13**).

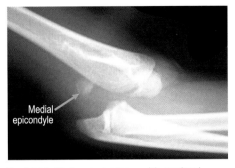

Fig. 24.12 Dislocated elbow with avulsed medial epicondyle.

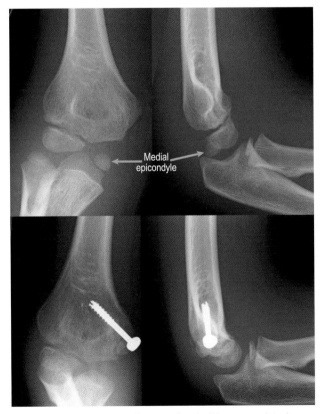

Fig. 24.13 Incarcerated medial epicondyle fracture fixed with a cannulated screw. (Compare with image of medial epicondyle, Fig. 24.3.)

### Non-operative

In the setting of a congruent elbow and a medial epicondylar fracture that is *not* incarcerated in the joint, conservative treatment in a cast or sling for 2 weeks is acceptable.

### Operative

If the fracture is incarcerated in the elbow joint, Roberts' manœuvre should be attempted. Under sedation or general anaesthetic, the elbow is extended, supinated and pulled into valgus. The wrist is then swiftly brought into extension, thus using the tension in the flexors to pull the medial epicondyle out of the joint. If this is unsuccessful, it will need to be retrieved via a medial surgical approach.

## ELBOW DISLOCATION

Closed reduction under general anaesthetic or sedation is usually successful (p. 209). Attention must be paid to the medial epicondyle to ensure it is not incarcerated in the joint (Fig. 24.13; see also above). A small proportion of elbow dislocations will require open reduction due to entrapment of capsular tissue or buttonholing of the distal humerus through anterior tissues. This can be carried out via a medial or anterior approach, as described on page 574 for open reduction of a supracondylar fracture. Following reduction, most children are more comfortable in a cast or backslab. Active mobilization is begun at 1–2 weeks.

## OLECRANON FRACTURES

The variable appearances of the olecranon apophysis can cause diagnostic uncertainty. Displaced fractures are operatively stabilized with tension band wiring (p. 203).

## RADIAL HEAD AND NECK FRACTURES

Fracture through the proximal radial epiphysis (head) is very unusual in children and most injuries in this region comprise fractures through the physis and/or metaphysis. The proximal radial epiphysis should be visible after the age of 4 or 5, and so its absence from the expected location on plain radiographs is abnormal.

## Emergency Department management

### Clinical features

- The patient will present with pain and stiffness in the elbow.
- There will be local tenderness but little swelling.

### Radiological features

- *AP and lateral views of the elbow*: These will show the fracture and an elevated fat pad. If there is insufficient elbow extension to obtain an AP view, then consider tilted views perpendicular to the proximal radius.
- *Ultrasound*: This can be useful to identify the radial head in the younger child.

### Immobilization and outpatient follow-up

- Radial neck fractures with an angulation of <45° can be treated with a cast for comfort and referred to fracture clinic.

### Inpatient referral

- Radial neck fractures with angulation >45° should be referred for reduction.

## Orthopaedic management

### Non-operative

Radial neck fractures with an angulation of <45° can be weaned from cast after 2 weeks and allowed progressive mobilization.

### Operative

Angulation >45° is an indication for intervention. Initially a closed reduction should be attempted, with recourse to percutaneous or open surgery if this is unsuccessful. Mobilization is instituted after 3 weeks in a cast.

1. *Closed reduction*: Apply direct pressure over the radial head while rotating the forearm in varying degrees of elbow flexion. This often achieves reduction to within acceptable parameters (i.e. <45° of angulation).
2. *K-wire insertion*: If closed reduction fails, a k-wire can be passed percutaneously to lever the radial head back into position.

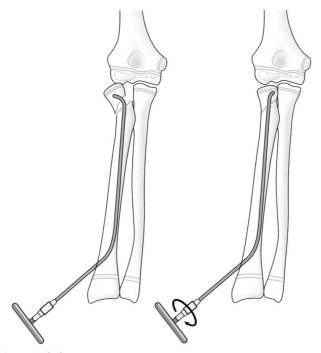

Fig. 24.14 Metaizeau technique.

3. *Metaizeau technique*: A 2-mm intramedullary flexible nail is passed retrograde from the distal radial styloid until the 'hockey stick' end engages the radial head and can reduce it with rotation of the nail (**Fig. 24.14**).

4. *Open reduction*: Open reduction via a Kocher's incision (see Fig. 10.18) carries a significant risk of osteonecrosis of the radial head and the risks and benefits should be considered carefully before proceeding. The radial head can be stabilized with antegrade k-wires.

## FOREARM

### MONTEGGIA FRACTURE DISLOCATION

Fracture patterns are similar to those in adults (see Figs 11.3 and 11.15) and are usually treated with surgical stabilization of the ulna with a plate or intramedullary device (**Fig. 24.15**). Children can also sustain a radial head

dislocation with plastic deformity of the ulna. The radiocapitellar line should be carefully scrutinized on AP and lateral radiographic views (see Fig. 10.6). A delay in the diagnosis of radiocapitellar dislocation is associated with poorer long-term results.

### ✓ Key point

Always examine the elbow and wrist in patients with forearm fractures, and obtain good-quality radiographs.

### GALEAZZI FRACTURE DISLOCATION

True Galeazzi injuries with disruption of the distal radioulnar joint (DRUJ) are most unusual in children, as the distal ulnar physis fails before the ligaments of the DRUJ. The combination of a distal radial fracture and ulnar physeal separation can be considered to be a

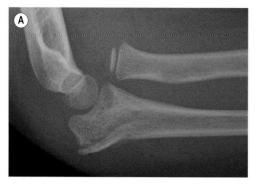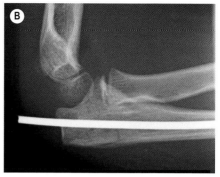

Fig. 24.15 Monteggia fracture treated with a TENS nail. **A**, Proximal ulnar fracture with dislocation of the radial head. **B**, Ulna and radial head both reduced.

paediatric Galeazzi variant. Reduction and k-wiring of the radial fracture usually constitute sufficient treatment.

## DIAPHYSEAL FRACTURES OF RADIUS AND ULNA

These are amongst the most common fractures encountered in children. The incidence peaks in the early teenage years. Most can be managed successfully with closed treatment and have good functional results.

## Classification

The AO system can be applied but simple descriptive terminology of location and fracture type is most commonly used. Incomplete, or greenstick, fractures should be recognized, as should plastic deformity (see Fig. 23.10).

## Emergency Department management

### Clinical features

- Diaphyseal forearm fractures are usually obvious clinically. The patient will present in distress with a clear deformity.

- Carefully inspect the forearm for any breaks in the skin. The forearm is the most common site for open fractures in children.

- A detailed assessment of the neurovascular status is mandatory.

- Compartment syndrome (p. 45) is rare but always a possibility, particularly with high-energy injuries.

### Radiological features

- *AP and lateral views of the forearm*: Both the elbow and wrist joints must be inspected carefully to ensure that the joints remain congruent.

### Immobilization and outpatient follow-up

- The limb should be splinted in an above-elbow backslab (see Fig. 4.9).

- Undisplaced fractures are referred to the fracture clinic.

### Inpatient referral

- Displaced fractures should be referred for potential manipulation or fixation.

- Emergency reduction of deformity should only be attempted if there are signs of acute neurovascular compromise. This is rare, even in the face of quite significant clinical deformity.

## Orthopaedic management

### Non-operative

Remodelling can resolve diaphyseal deformity if >2 years of growth remains, but the potential is less than it is for metaphyseal injuries (see Fig. 23.11). Indications for non-operative management include:

- <15° of angulation

- no malrotation or loss of the radial bow.

Residual angulation is less well tolerated in more proximal locations, and the threshold for

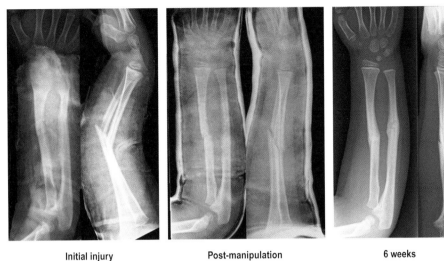

| Initial injury | Post-manipulation | 6 weeks |

Fig. 24.16 Conservative management of a both-bones forearm fracture.

## Table 24.1    Outpatient follow-up of diaphyseal radius and ulna fractures

| Age range | Follow-up |
| --- | --- |
| <5 years | Radiographs at 1 week for position check. Remove the cast after 3 weeks |
| 5–10 years | Radiographs at 1 week for position check. Remove the cast after 4 weeks |
| >10 years | Radiographs at 1 week then 2 weeks for position check. Remove the cast after 6 weeks |

All diaphyseal fractures should be radiographed to confirm healing at time of planned cast removal

manipulation should decrease accordingly. Angulation from malunion of the ulna is clinically very apparent but of less functional impact than malunion of the radius, which results in restriction of forearm rotation. If alignment and rotation are satisfactory, off-ended fractures can be accepted.

### Operative
*Closed reduction*
The great majority of displaced diaphyseal fractures can be successfully managed with closed reduction under general anaesthetic (**Fig. 24.16**). Greenstick fractures are usually

stable when treated in a cast using the principles of three-point moulding (see Fig. 23.11). Angulated, off-ended fractures will require an initial increase in the deformity to relax the intact periosteum, followed by longitudinal traction before reduction (see Fig. 4.4). The forearm should be cast in whatever position provides the best reduction.

**Table 24.1** summarizes follow-up required.

### Flexible intramedullary nailing
This technique is indicated in open fractures, Monteggia injuries, irreducible fractures and

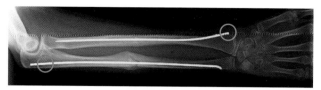

Fig. 24.17 TENS nailing of a both-bones forearm fracture. The orange circles demonstrate the nail entry points.

those with early loss of reduction (at the 1-week clinic review). It is usually carried out using flexible intramedullary nails in one or both bones (see 'Surgical technique' and **Fig. 24.17**). Postoperatively, a cast is often used for comfort for 3–4 weeks. The nails are usually removed after 3–6 months.

There are a number of important considerations in flexible intramedullary nailing of the forearm:

- Only one nail is required for each bone.
- It may be preferable to nail the most displaced/unstable bone first.
- It is acceptable to nail only one bone if the other is thought to be stable.

### Plate fixation

This is an alternative method but it is more invasive and carries a risk of later fracture at the ends of the plates in 5%.

### SURGICAL TECHNIQUE: Flexible intramedullary nailing of the radius and ulna

#### Surgical set-up

- The patient is placed supine with the arm extended on an arm table.
- An arm tourniquet is placed but only inflated if open reduction is required.
- Intravenous antibiotics are given at induction.

#### Nail selection

The diameter of the nail should not exceed 50% of the medullary diameter at the isthmus of the radius/ulna. The correct nail is usually between 1.5 and 2.5 mm in diameter.

#### Retrograde nailing of the radius

1. Incision: Make a 15-mm longitudinal incision in the mid-lateral line over the distal radius. The incision should start 1 cm proximal to the physis, as seen on fluoroscopy. Careful dissection down on to the underlying periosteum will avoid damage to the superficial radial nerve and tendons (**Fig. 24.18**).
2. Start point: Use a bone awl or 3.2-mm drill to create an entry point 1 cm proximal to the physis, on the radial aspect of the bone. Take care not to breach the opposite cortex.
3. Nail pre-bending: The nail must be bent to reproduce the radial bow. This can be guided by holding the nail over the forearm and taking an image with the nail superimposed over the radius.
4. Nail insertion: Using the nail holder/chuck, insert the nail through the entry point with the curved tip of the nail pointing into the bone. Once in, the nail should be rotated 180°. Using small, alternating rotations, advance the nail up to the fracture

site. Avoid hammering the nail, as it is likely to drive the nail out of the bone. Fracture apposition is achieved with closed manipulation and the nail is directed across the fracture site using the angle at the tip of the nail. The nail is progressed into the proximal segment, continuing up to the bicipital tuberosity.

5. Nail cutting: Withdraw the nail by 1 cm and then cut it, leaving approximately 15 mm of nail proud of the bone. Then tap in the nail using a punch and hammer, aiming to leave enough of it proud of the bone to allow removal but not so much as to cause skin irritation.

### Antegrade nailing of the ulna

1. Incision: Make a 15-mm incision over the proximal ulna on the radial side of the crest from the level of the coronoid back to the tip of the olecranon. Use blunt dissection to expose the periosteum.

2. Start point: The entry point for the ulnar nail is on the radial side of the proximal metaphysis at the level of the coronoid. Create an entry point, as described above using fluoroscopy, and feel to ensure the entry point is as close to the midline as possible.

3. Nail insertion: The nail is *not pre-bent*. Using the nail holder/chuck, insert the nail through the entry point, as described for insertion of the radial nail. Using small, alternating rotations, advance the nail up to the fracture site. Fracture reduction is achieved with closed manipulation and the nail is directed across the fracture site using the angle at the tip of the nail. The nail is progressed into the distal segment, continuing up to a point 1 cm proximal to the distal ulnar physis.

4. Cut the nail: Withdraw the nail by 1 cm and then cut it, leaving approximately 15 mm of nail proud of the bone. Then tap in the nail using a punch and hammer, aiming to leave enough of it proud of the nail to allow removal but not so much as to cause skin irritation.

### Postoperative management

After the wounds are sutured and dressed, an above-elbow backslab or cast can be applied to provide additional symptomatic relief for 2–3 weeks. Sports should be avoided until healing is confirmed radiographically. Note that healing of both bones is often asynchronous and it may take 2–3 months for full union to occur.

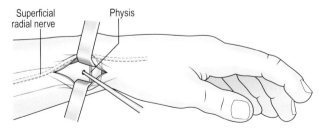

Fig. 24.18 Approach to the radial styloid.

## COMPLICATIONS

### Early

| | |
|---|---|
| Local | Re-fracture: This is the most common complication at around 5%, and resumption of sporting or other high-risk behaviours should be delayed for 2 months following cast removal |

### Late

| | |
|---|---|
| Local | Malunion should be observed in the short term, as remodelling often improves the appearance and function of the limb without the requirement for intervention. A plateau in recovery with residual unacceptable function or appearance is an indication for corrective osteotomy |

# WRIST

## FRACTURES OF THE DISTAL RADIUS AND ULNA

These fractures are amongst the most common ones of childhood. The majority are benign, as they benefit from close proximity to the swiftly growing physes of the distal radius and ulna with good remodelling potential (see Fig. 23.13). Most are pure metaphyseal fractures but physeal injuries are common and are usually Salter–Harris type II. Intra-articular fractures are rare.

## Classification

The Salter–Harris classification (see Fig. 23.3) is used for physeal injuries. A descriptive classification is adopted for non-physeal injuries.

## Emergency Department management

### Clinical features

- There is usually pain with associated swelling, tenderness and deformity of the wrist.
- A careful neurological assessment is important (see Fig. 23.16).

### Radiological features

- *AP and lateral views of the wrist*: Small cortical irregularities or bumps may be minor

buckle fractures (**Fig. 24.19**; see also Fig. 12.16).

### Immobilization and reassessment

A wrist backslab is applied (p. 68), followed by repeat radiographs and documentation of neurovascular examination.

### Outpatient referral

- Minor buckle fractures of the distal radius require only symptomatic treatment in a removable splint for 2–3 weeks. Formal follow-up is not necessary.

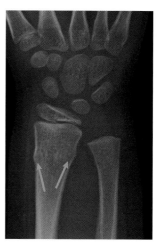

Fig. 24.19 Buckle fracture of the distal radius.

- Metaphyseal fractures with up to 30° of angulation should be referred to the fracture clinic.

## Orthopaedic management

### Non-operative

#### Minor buckle fractures of the distal radius

When only a cortical bump of the radial metaphysis is seen, with minimal or no angulation, then symptomatic treatment in a removable splint for 2–3 weeks is all that is required. Formal follow-up is not necessary.

#### Dorsally angulated fractures

Dorsal angulation or displacement is well tolerated cosmetically and functionally with up to 30° of dorsal tilt acceptable in younger children. Similarly, up to 50% of dorsal translation of a Salter–Harris II fracture will remodel fully in a year. A Colles-type cast (see p. 68) is acceptable for both metaphyseal and physeal fractures.

#### Volarly angulated fractures

Fractures with volar tilt are less acceptable cosmetically but still remodel well if 2 or more years of growth remain. An above-elbow cast is required for these angulated fractures and should be applied with the forearm in supination to overcome the deforming force of brachioradialis.

### Operative

#### Metaphyseal fractures

- Metaphyseal fractures with >30° of angulation.
- Off-ended metaphyseal fractures.

For displaced or angulated metaphyseal fractures, a closed manipulation and moulded cast are usually effective (p. 83), with radiographic review within 1 week to check for re-displacement. Off-ended metaphyseal fractures that have undergone closed reduction should be stabilized with a single k-wire passed in a retrograde manner through the radial styloid and across the fracture (**Fig. 24.20**).

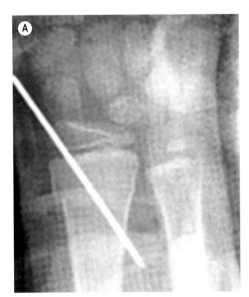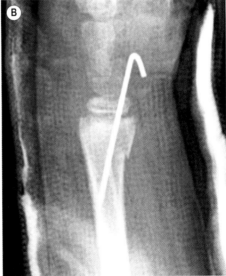

Fig. 24.20 Salter–Harris II fracture of the distal radius treated with a single k-wire. **A,** AP view. **B,** Lateral view.

**Table 24.2    Outpatient management of distal radius fractures**

| Age range | Follow-up |
|-----------|-----------|
| <5 years | Radiographs at 3–5 days. Cast for 3 weeks |
| 5–10 years | Radiographs at 3–5 days. Cast for 4 weeks |
| >10 years | Radiographs at 3–5 days. Cast for 5 weeks |

*Physeal fractures*
- Salter–Harris II fractures with >50% translation.

Physeal fractures should be manipulated and stabilized with one smooth k-wire passed through the radial styloid. These wires are usually removed at around 3 weeks without the need for anaesthetic. Physeal fractures should *not* be manipulated more than 5 days post injury, as this carries a high chance of growth plate injury.

Outpatient management is summarized in **Table 24.2**.

## HAND AND CARPUS

### CARPUS

Carpal fractures and dislocations similar to those seen in adults can be encountered but are rare in children.

### SCAPHOID

Scaphoid fractures are extremely rare under the age of 10 but often encountered by mid-adolescence. If the mechanism of injury and physical findings are suggestive of scaphoid injury, then the standard scaphoid series of radiographs should be obtained (see Fig. 12.10). In many children, the fracture is of the distal pole with a small, avulsed fragment. These injuries can be treated symptomatically with a wrist splint.

A more proximal fracture requires immobilization in a Colles-type cast or splint and review at 2 weeks. Most confirmed scaphoid fractures in children are minimally displaced and simple cast treatment for 4–8 weeks until healed is effective. In older children with higher-energy injuries, angulated or more displaced fractures may be seen and the principles of managing adult scaphoid fractures then apply.

## METACARPALS AND FINGERS
### General principles

Most children's hand fractures do not require anything more than supportive strapping or bracing for 1 or 2 weeks, and an early resumption of activity.

Most fractures can be adequately supported with buddy strapping, although a volar slab or malleable splint with the joints in the position of safety may be more comfortable, particularly for younger children (see Figs 13.10–13.13). A small number of children's hand and finger fractures do benefit from operative intervention: commonly, closed reduction and wiring. Hand fractures stabilize very quickly and reduction of finger fractures should be carried out within 3–5 days of injury.

### Specific fractures
#### Crush injuries
Crush injuries of the fingertips are very common and require good lavage. This can be done in the Emergency Department by bathing the finger in antiseptic solution. Antibiotics and tetanus cover are required. Minor angulations of the distal phalanx can be improved under inhaled nitrous oxide and oxygen, sedation or local block, followed by mallet splint support for 2 weeks (see Fig. 13.9).

#### Distal phalangeal fractures and nailbed injury
Simple fractures at the base of the distal phalanx can be reduced and splinted with a mallet splint under block. Significant nailbed damage requires treatment under general anaesthetic (see p. 285).

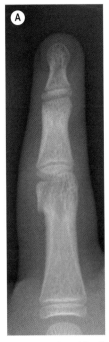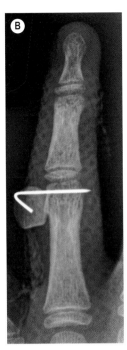

Fig. 24.21 Condylar fracture of the proximal phalanx treated with k-wire. **A**, The fracture is unstable and has displaced. **B**, The articular surface has been restored by closed fracture reduction and stabilization with transverse wire.

## Rotational injuries

Phalangeal and metacarpal fractures showing signs of malrotation (see Fig. 13.6) should be reduced. Most can be stabilized with buddy strapping augmented by a cast or splint. Only when reduction cannot be held in this way would a k-wire be placed across the fracture.

## Condylar fractures

Displaced or angulated condylar fractures will often result in significant deformity and are an indication for closed reduction and stabilization with a percutaneous k-wire (**Fig. 24.21**). Open reduction can cause physeal damage and stiffness, which are worse than a minor degree of residual deformity from an injury.

## Phalangeal neck fractures

Some angulation (<20°) of phalangeal neck fractures into flexion or extension can be accepted in children. Greater angulation can be reduced closed and splinted. Off-ended phalangeal neck fractures are more unstable and are likely to need k-wire fixation.

## Phalangeal base fractures

Phalangeal fractures angled in the coronal plane do not remodel, so very little angulation can be accepted. Reduction under local block is usually successful, using a pen in the web space as a fulcrum (see Fig. 13.26).

## PELVIS AND ACETABULUM

### PELVIC FRACTURES

Pelvic fractures are generally rare in the paediatric population, the most frequently encountered being the benign avulsion-type injuries seen in adolescents (see Fig. 15.14). These type A fractures usually require only symptomatic treatment with crutches, analgesia, and referral to fracture clinic. Very displaced, large avulsions (>2 cm) should be discussed with Orthopaedics, as fixation might be offered.

Fractures disrupting the pelvic ring are managed initially in the same way as adult injuries (p. 333). Remember that the child's pelvis is more elastic than the adult's, and it takes a proportionally higher transfer of energy to cause a fracture, with a greater risk of visceral injury. The vast majority of children's pelvic ring fractures are managed conservatively with a period of bed rest followed by assisted mobilization. Unstable fractures may be better treated with surgical stabilization in older children (>8 years) and is most appropriate in children who are approaching or have reached skeletal maturity.

### ACETABULAR FRACTURES

Acetabular fractures are an uncommon injury in childhood. The key difference between paediatric and adult acetabular fractures is that the triradiate cartilage of the immature pelvis is vulnerable, and injuries preferentially affect this susceptible physeal area. This can lead to premature physeal closure, leading to growth disturbance and progressive subluxation of the hip.

Fractures that are undisplaced or minimally (<2 mm) displaced can be treated conservatively, but require 4–8 weeks of non-weight-bearing, depending on age.

Displaced fractures may require treatment following the principles established for adult injuries (p. 344) aiming to restore joint congruity and hip stability. This includes the added challenge of restoring the alignment of the triradiate cartilage. If operative treatment is intended, it should be undertaken within a few days due to rapid healing of physeal injuries, which prevents reduction if there is a delay.

Consideration should be given to the later removal of metalwork that crosses the triradiate cartilage.

## HIP

### HIP FRACTURES

Hip fractures are not common in children and typically result from high-energy trauma, with a 30% associated risk of injury to the head, viscera or other extremity. Fractures from low-energy trauma suggest a pre-existing pathological process, such as a bone cyst, metabolic bone disease or neoplasia. Hip fractures are associated with a high rate of complications, including progressive deformity.

### Paediatric vascular anatomy of the hip

As in the adult hip, the vascular supply to the femoral head arises principally from the medial and (to a lesser extent) lateral circumflex femoral arteries, which feed the retinacular vessels to the epiphysis (see Fig. 17.04). These are of particular importance, as there is no intraosseous supply across the physis, and the ligamentum teres has a negligible contribution below the age of 8, and only 20% of the femoral head blood supply thereafter. Damage to the retinacular vessels therefore renders the epiphysis ischaemic.

## Classification

The Delbet classification has prognostic significance (**Fig. 25.1**):

- *Type I – Transphyseal fractures*: These may represent a severe slipped capital femoral epiphysis (see below) and consideration should be given to the risk factors for that condition (such as hypothyroidism, hypogonadism and renal disease). There is a very high rate of growth arrest and avascular necrosis (AVN).

- *Type II – Transcervical fractures*: These are the most common type of paediatric hip fracture. There is a high rate of AVN.

- *Type III – Basicervical fractures*: These have a lower rate of AVN.

- *Type IV – Intertrochanteric fractures*: These have the lowest rate of AVN, although type III and IV injuries are prone to varus malunion.

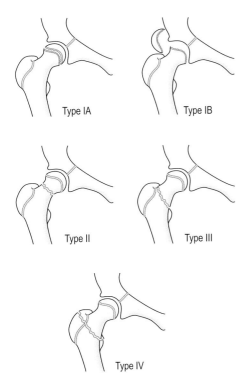

Fig. 25.1 Delbet classification of paediatric hip fractures.

## Emergency Department management

### Clinical features

- There is likely to have been a high-energy mechanism or a sporting injury.

- The patient will present in severe pain and resist any hip movement.

### Radiological features

- *AP and lateral radiographs of the hip* (not frog lateral).

- *MRI*: If the fracture appears pathological or a stress fracture is suspected, an MRI may be useful.

### Inpatient referral

- No form of cast or traction is required in the Emergency Department. The patient should be provided with analgesia and referred to Orthopaedics.

## Orthopaedic management

### Non-operative

Undisplaced or minimally displaced fractures in a toddler can be treated non-operatively in a spica cast for 3–4 weeks (**Fig. 25.2**).

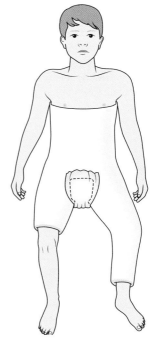

Fig. 25.2 Hip spica cast.

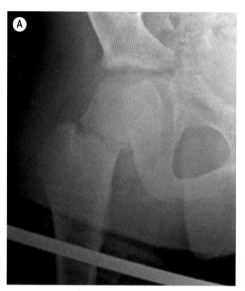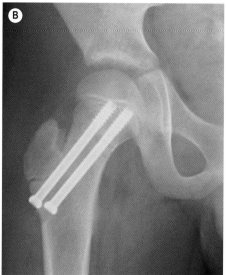

Fig. 25.3 **A**, Displaced Delbet type II femoral neck fracture. **B**, Treatment is with closed reduction and percutaneous cannulated screws that extend to, but do not cross, the physis.

## Operative

As for young adults, displaced hip fractures should be treated urgently (within 24 hours) in order to minimize the risk of AVN. The majority of childhood hip fractures are displaced and unstable, and require reduction and internal fixation. If closed reduction fails, then an open approach must be used to achieve satisfactory reduction. The anterior Smith-Peterson or anterolateral Watson Jones approaches are commonly used:

- *Type I fractures*: Fixation crosses the physis, but should be removed as soon as healing is satisfactory.
- *Type II and III fractures*: Fixation is best achieved with closed reduction and percutaneous fixation with cannulated screws that do not cross the physis (**Fig. 25.3**) (smooth pins in children <3 years).
- *Type IV* intertrochanteric fractures: These may be best fixed with specific paediatric hip plates.

## COMPLICATIONS

### *Later*

Local    Avascular necrosis: This is the most common and devastating complication of hip fracture

Premature physeal arrest: This may be complete or incomplete, leading to coxa breva, vara or valga

Non-union: This raises the possibility of underlying bone disease, or inadequate reduction or mechanical stability. Revision surgery may be advisable

## HIP DISLOCATION

Dislocation of the paediatric hip is not common but is associated with high-energy trauma in older children. In younger children, confusion can arise with developmental or neurological hip dislocation, but in these cases there will be radiological features of acetabular dysplasia and often a relevant medical history. Posterior dislocation is most common (>90%).

### Emergency Department management

#### Clinical features

- As there is generally a high-energy mechanism, other injuries must be excluded and formal primary and secondary surveys performed.
- The patient will present with the hip held in flexion, adduction and internal rotation (for a posterior dislocation).
- Assess the neurovascular state of the lower limb carefully, particularly the sciatic nerve, and exclude other associated injuries, especially femoral shaft fracture.

#### Radiological features

- AP view of the pelvis and lateral view of the hip.

#### Reduction

Closed reduction is performed without delay (see Fig. 17.37) but the vulnerability of the capital physis should be remembered. If closed reduction fails, an open reduction will be required. MRI or CT should be performed following reduction to exclude incarcerated intra-articular fragments. Surgical treatment is described on page 377.

## SLIPPED CAPITAL FEMORAL EPIPHYSIS

Slipped capital femoral epiphysis (SCFE) is the most common cause of hip morbidity in the adolescent. The incidence of SCFE is estimated at 1 per 10 000 but is more common in males and certain ethnic groups, such as those of African or Polynesian descent. SCFE typically occurs between the ages of 10 and 13 in girls and 11 and 14 in boys but is also seen in younger and older children. Although the cause of most SCFEs is never established, all patients, particularly those outside the typical demographic group, should be screened for hypothyroidism and renal failure.

### Classification

SCFE can be classified according to the timing of presentation – acute, chronic or acute on chronic – or the angle of the slip, as described by *Southwick* (**Fig. 25.4**). However, the most useful classification is that of *Loder*, which distinguishes stable from unstable slips:

- *Stable slips*: The child can weight-bear on presentation (with or without walking aids). The prognosis is generally good.
- *Unstable slips*: The child is unable to weight-bear (with or without walking aids). The prevalence of AVN is approximately 50%, leading to a poor outcome.

### Emergency Department management

#### Clinical features

- SCFE may present acutely, or with a history of days or even weeks of symptoms. Pain may be felt at the hip or groin but, not uncommonly, all the pain may be felt at the thigh or knee. The diagnosis can be delayed considerably (and potentially disastrously) if the assessment has been erroneously focused on the knee.
- The patient is likely to limp. Close observation of the patient lying supine may reveal increased external rotation of the affected leg at rest. An unstable SCFE will be painful on any movement of the hip. A stable SCFE will allow hip movement but there will be a subtle loss of internal rotation and abduction of the hip.
- Leg length difference can be very subtle in early SCFEs and is often missed.

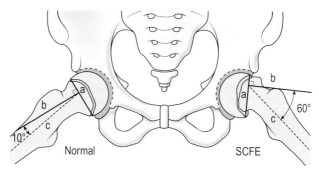

Fig. 25.4 Southwick slip angle. SCFE, Slipped capital femoral epiphysis. Construct three lines on the frog lateral: (a) between the anterior and posterior points of the physis, (b) a line drawn at 90° to (a), (c) the axis of the femur, and measure the angle between (b) and (c). The slip angle is the *difference* between the slipped and normal sides. (12° is taken as normal if both sides are involved.)

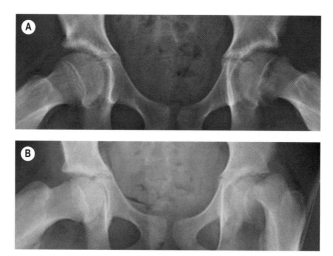

Fig. 25.5 Left-sided slipped capital femoral epiphysis. **A**, Mild. **B**, Severe.

## Radiological features

- *Frog lateral view of the pelvis* (**Fig. 25.5**): This is the crucial diagnostic view. A standard AP of the hips can fail to reveal subtle SCFEs and cannot exclude the diagnosis.

- *MRI*: More detailed imaging is not usually needed but axial MRI may assist in confirming the degree of slip.

### Inpatient referral

- A suspected case of SCFE must be referred as an inpatient to Orthopaedics.

## Orthopaedic management

### Non-operative

There is no role for non-operative management of SCFE, as further displacement is a significant risk.

### Operative

The primary aim of treatment is to prevent further displacement of the epiphysis. The majority of SCFEs with slip angles of up to 60° can be managed with in situ fixation with a single cannulated screw (**Fig. 25.6**).

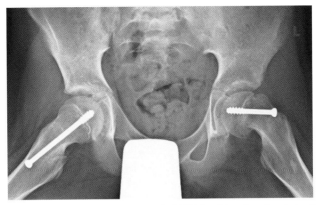

Fig. 25.6 Slipped capital femoral epiphysis. A left SCFE fixed in situ. Prophylactic fixation has been carried out on the right hip.

Controversy exists when managing the severely displaced, unstable SCFE. In the rare situation with a clear history of less then 24 hours since onset, then a closed reduction and fixation can be justified, although AVN is still a significant risk. More commonly, the history is longer and consideration should be given to referring these cases urgently to tertiary centres with a specialist interest in their management. The treatment options considered in these circumstances may include:

- attempted, partial closed reduction and screw fixation
- open procedures to achieve reduction, such as the modified Dunn or surgical dislocation technique

- later extracapsular osteotomies to try to reduce deformity; these have their own complications.

---

 **Key point**

---

Consideration should always be given to prophylactic fixation of the opposite hip due to the 30–60% risk of a contralateral SCFE in the future. SCFEs related to endocrinopathies or renal dysfunction should always include contralateral hip fixation as part of the treatment.

---

## COMPLICATIONS

### Later

Local        Avascular necrosis: This is encountered in 50% of unstable SCFEs

Chondrolysis: This stems from joint penetration following errors in screw placement

Subtrochanteric fracture: This may occur where the screw entry point has been placed below the level of the lesser trochanter

Loss of fixation or implant breakage

Degenerative arthritis: More severe slips have a greater risk; delay in diagnosis is related to increased slip severity

## FEMUR

### FEMORAL SHAFT FRACTURES

Femoral shaft fractures represent <2% of fractures in childhood but can be difficult to manage, clinically, socially and economically. They present in a bimodal distribution, with fractures occurring in early childhood, due to the relative weakness in cortical strength at that age, and then later in mid-adolescence, due largely to the high energy associated with road traffic accidents. At all ages, femoral shaft fractures are more common in boys, with an overall male to female ratio of $2.6:1$.

Other important causes of femoral shaft fractures include non-accidental injury (NAI) (p. 562) and pathological fracture. NAI has been shown to account for up to 50% of femoral fractures presenting below the age of 4, and should be actively ruled out if a child is below walking age. Pathological fractures can be due to generalized bone conditions such as osteogenesis imperfecta; osteopaenia related to chronic disease such as cerebral palsy; or a neoplastic lesion, either benign or malignant.

### Emergency Department management

#### Clinical features

- The history is commonly of a fall from a height, or a sporting or vehicle collision. Other injuries must be excluded by formal primary and secondary surveys, and appropriate fluid resuscitation should be started.
- The thigh will be deformed and swollen.
- A careful neurovascular assessment is required.

#### Immobilization

Reduce any gross deformity with splintage or traction (p. 389) under procedural sedation and analgesia prior to obtaining imaging.

#### Radiological features

- *AP and lateral views of the femur*: Plain radiographs should be taken, including the hip and the knee joint.

- *Hip or knee series*: If a proximal or distal extension is suspected, views centred over the affected joint will help to identify periphyseal or intra-articular involvement.
- *MRI*: If a pathological fracture is suspected, an MRI may be required.

## Orthopaedic management

The management strategy for a paediatric femoral shaft fracture is largely based on the child's age and weight. However, it will also take into consideration the wishes and social circumstances of the family, local expertise and equipment, and the potential drawbacks of prolonged hospitalization versus the complications associated with surgery. The options are summarized in **Table 25.1**.

### Non-operative

Children up to the age of 5 can usually be managed non-operatively. Considerable deformity is acceptable in anticipation of remodelling (**Table 25.2**).

- *Pavlik harness*: This is appropriate for children <6 months old. It is applied for 2–3 weeks. A spica cast is an alternative.
- *Gallows traction* (**Fig. 25.7**): This is used for children between the ages of 6 months and 18 months, and who weigh <12 kg. The traction is used for 2–3 weeks. Gallows traction should not be used in an older or heavier child, as perfusion to the foot may become compromised.
- *Balanced traction*: This is often used temporarily prior to the application of a spica cast (see Fig. 18.13 and p. 392).
- *Spica casts* (see Fig. 25.2): These are generally applied under a general anaesthetic with intraoperative imaging. A few days in traction prior to spica application can help reduce spasm, lower the risk of shortening in the spica, and allow time to evaluate the full circumstances of the injury. The results of spica treatment are generally good if attention is paid to cast application and the acceptable limits for reduction are known. Great care must be taken to avoid traction

**Table 25.1    Management options for paediatric femoral fractures**

| Age | Management options | Duration of treatment |
| --- | --- | --- |
| 0–6 months | Pavlik harness<br>Early spica cast | 2–3 weeks |
| 7 months to 5 years | Traction<br>Early spica cast<br>Delayed spica cast<br>External fixation (rare) | 1 week per year of age |
| 6–11 years | Flexible intramedullary nails<br>Plating<br>External fixation (rare) | Intramedullary devices can be removed after 9 months |
| >11 years | Flexible intramedullary nails<br>Plating<br>Lateral entry antegrade<br>  intramedullary nail<br>External fixation | Intramedullary devices can be removed after 9 months |

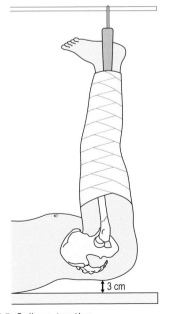

Fig. 25.7 Gallows traction.

on the proximal calf when attempting to restore length, as this can compromise calf circulation.

## Operative

For children over the age of 5 years, although traction and casting are effective, treatment times are often unacceptably long, and preference is usually towards operative fixation.

- *Flexible intramedullary nailing*: This is appropriate for a child weighing <45 kg (**Fig. 25.8**). Flexible nails are introduced into the medullary canal at the metaphysis to avoid iatrogenic injury to the physis. Two nails are used in combination so that there is symmetrical bracing, as each nail bears against the inner aspect of the cortex at three points.
- *Plating*: This is appropriate for a heavier child or for a fracture that is 'length-unstable' (comminuted or long spiral) (Fig. 23.12). Submuscular bridge plating has been shown to be an effective option (**Fig. 25.9**).

**Table 25.2    Acceptable limits of deformity when treating femoral fractures in children**

| Age | Coronal plane | Sagittal plane | Shortening |
| --- | --- | --- | --- |
| <2 years | 30° | 30° | 20 mm |
| 2–5 years | 15° | 30° | 20 mm |
| 5–10 years | 10° | 15° | 15 mm |
| >10 years | 5° | 10° | 10 mm |

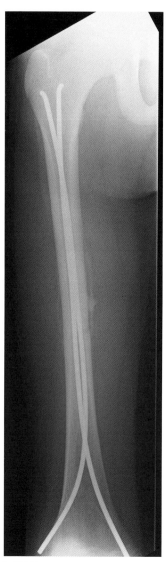

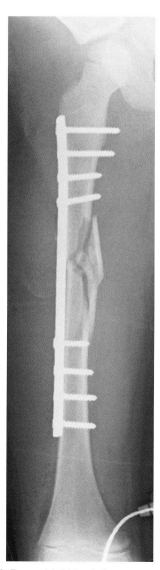

Fig. 25.8 TENS nailing of the femur.

Fig. 25.9 Femoral bridge plating.

- *Intramedullary nailing*: For a child approaching skeletal maturity, intramedullary nails have been developed with entry points placed lateral to the piriformis fossa to avoid iatrogenic damage to the retinacular vessels (see Fig. 17.4). The adult-style piriformis fossa entry nails must *not* be used due to the risk of femoral epiphyseal AVN. Only once a child has reached skeletal maturity can conventional adult intramedullary nails be used safely.

- *External fixation*: This may be preferred in the setting of severe soft tissue damage and when other strategies are not appropriate (see Fig. 18.27). This option is, however, associated with an increased risk of refracture.

## SURGICAL TECHNIQUE: Flexible nailing of femoral shaft fractures

### Note
This technique is not suitable for patients >45 kg.

### Set-up
- Use of a traction table is at the surgeon's discretion but can be helpful.

### Technique
- Select two identical flexible nails of 40% of the diameter of the femoral canal at its narrowest.
- Pre-bend the nails, planning for the apex of the curve to be at the level of the fracture. This can be achieved by taking images with the nails superimposed over the femur. Aim for an approximate 30° curve.

### Retrograde technique (Fig. 25.10)
This technique is suitable for diaphyseal fractures proximal to the distal metadiaphyseal junction. Fractures below this level should be addressed using an antegrade technique.

Identify the distal femoral physis on imaging. Mark the skin 3 cm proximal to the physis. Make a 2-cm incision starting at this mark and running distally on both the medial and lateral aspects of the distal thigh. Dissect down to bone and protect the soft tissues while creating an entry point in the bone 3 cm proximal to the physis on both the medial and lateral aspects of the distal femoral metaphysis. A bone awl or 4-mm drill can be used. Avoid diaphyseal entry points due to the risk of fracture.

Insert the nails and advance each with small, rotating movements up the medullary canal to the fracture. It can be difficult to advance the nails initially as they abut the opposite cortex. Avoid using a hammer at this point, as it may drive the nail through the cortex. Increasing the curve at the tip of the nail can help at this stage.

Once both nails are at, but not across, the fracture, the fracture should be reduced and each nail passed in small increments across into the proximal fragment. The nails should then be advanced so that the tips lie in the proximal metaphysis, ideally with some separation. The medial nail will attempt to advance up the femoral neck but be careful that it does not exit posteriorly as the femoral neck anteverts.

Withdraw the nails by 10 mm, cut them just below skin level, and then tap them back in by 10 mm or so until the distal ends of the nails are sufficiently buried to avoid skin irritation (check with knee flexed). Between 10 and 15 mm of nail should be left out of the bone to allow retrieval.

### Antegrade technique (Fig. 25.11)

This technique is for fractures at (or distal to) the distal metadiaphyseal junction.

The nails are inserted through two entry points 2-3 cm apart on the lateral femoral cortex just proximal to the level of the lesser trochanter. More distal entry points must be avoided due to the risk of subtrochanteric fracture. The same nail diameter is used as above but the method of pre-bending differs, as shown in **Figure 25.11**. The remainder of the technique is as described for retrograde insertion.

### Postoperative management

- Apply light dressings for 3–4 days.
- Encourage range of motion exercises for the hip and knee plus isometric muscle rehabilitation as soon as the patient is comfortable.
- Touch weight-bearing is allowed initially unless it is a length-unstable fracture.
- Progress to full weight-bearing when callus is seen.

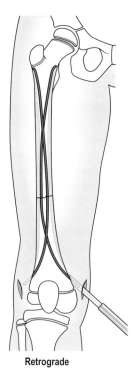

Retrograde

Fig. 25.10 Retrograde TENS femoral nail: correct positioning.

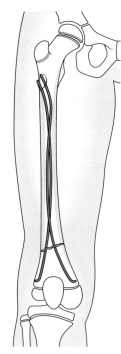

Fig. 25.11 Antegrade TENS femoral nail for a distal fracture.

# COMPLICATIONS

### Later

Local    Leg length discrepancy: This is common after femoral shaft fractures. Shortening will occur where there are off-ended fracture fragments but growth acceleration will occur in the first 18 months post injury. This can lead to length equalization or even overgrowth, and is allowed for with cast or traction as above

Malunion: This can occur but delayed or non-unions are very rare in most childhood femoral fractures (**Fig. 25.12**)

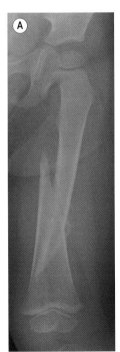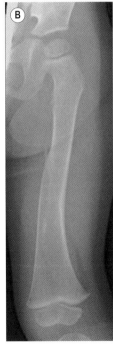

Fig. 25.12 Malunion. **A**, A valgus malunion of a mid-shaft femoral fracture in a 3-year-old treated on traction. **B**, One year later, significant remodelling has occurred.

# KNEE

## FRACTURES OF THE DISTAL FEMUR

Whilst representing <1% of childhood fractures, these injuries are important due to their association with growth disturbance, soft tissue and neurovascular injury.

## Classification

The Salter–Harris classification is readily applicable to and useful for these injuries.

## Emergency Department management

### Clinical features

- There is often a history of a sporting or high-energy injury.

- The knee will be swollen with a large haemarthrosis. Significant deformity may be seen if the fracture is displaced.

- The neurovascular anatomy is vulnerable as it crosses the knee (see Fig. 19.3); perform a careful assessment of the neurovascular state of the limb.

### Radiological features

- AP and lateral radiographs of the knee (**Fig. 25.13**).

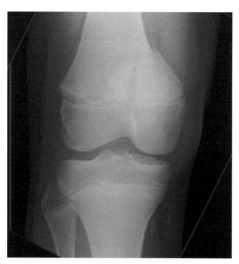

Fig. 25.13 Salter–Harris II fracture of the distal femur.

- *CT or MRI*: Axial imaging can be useful in evaluating intra-articular extension or concurrent soft tissue disruption in selected cases.

### Immobilization and referral

Reduce any gross deformity under procedural sedation and analgesia, particularly where there is neurovascular compromise. Traction is applied first to regain length. Gentle varus or valgus stress, and then flexion or extension, are then applied, depending on the direction of deformity. If reduction is difficult, do not force the fracture, as this may injure the physis. Perfecting the reduction may require a general anaesthetic or an open reduction. Apply a resting splint and provide analgesia before obtaining imaging.

## Orthopaedic management

### Non-operative

Undisplaced fractures can be managed in a cylinder cast but frequent radiographic review is needed to ensure there is no loss of position. In preschool-aged children, closed reduction and application of a cylinder cast, with some acceptance of residual angulation of up to 30° in the sagittal plane, is acceptable.

Angulation in the coronal plane, however, is not acceptable and requires operative reduction.

### Operative

In school-age children, the aim of treatment is an anatomical reduction of the articular surface (for Salter–Harris types III and IV), and reorientation of the physis, particularly aiming to avoid rotational or coronal plane deformity. Stabilization can be achieved with:

- *Screws*: These are effective for Salter–Harris types II, III and IV (**Fig. 25.14**). Transverse compression screws are used in the metaphysis and/or epiphysis. The screws must not cross the physis.

- *Crossed wires or Steinmann pins*: These are used for transverse fractures or if the fragments are too small to accommodate screws. The wires are passed retrograde through the condyles, traversing the physis, and aiming to cross above the fracture in the metaphysis (**Fig. 25.15**). This will require a low angle of entry with the pins to ensure good separation of the pins at the fracture site. Pins should be cut off to lie under the skin to reduce the risk of intra-articular sepsis.

A cylinder cast is then applied with the knee in slight flexion to decompress posterior structures. The cast is removed once callus is visible at 3–4 weeks.

## Complications

Good functional recovery is usually seen within 3 months. However, growth disturbance is encountered in up to 50% of these injuries and observation for 2 years is advisable.

## PATELLAR DISLOCATION

True patellar dislocation is relatively common in children and may result from a direct blow or, more commonly, a simple twisting movement. The diagnosis may be uncertain, as the patella has often reduced spontaneously by the time the child arrives in the Emergency Department. Minor forms of patellar instability, comprising abnormal patellar

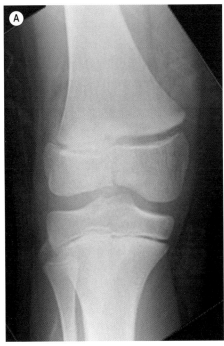
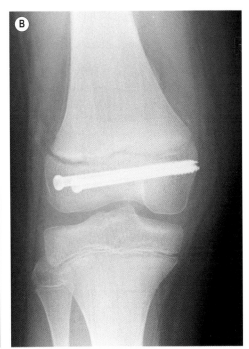

Fig. 25.14 Salter–Harris III fracture. **A**, Fracture of the distal femur. **B**, Fracture treated with partially threaded screws.

## ✓ Key point

The distal metaphysis is a common site for buckle fractures in children with neuromuscular disorders who are non-ambulatory. This area is vulnerable due to osteopaenia and the commonly associated fixed knee contractures. Patients may present with subtle signs, and a low threshold for imaging the distal femur is advisable in this setting. Confirmed fractures can be managed with a splint, slab or full cast, which should accommodate the knee flexion contracture. Deformity at the fracture can be accepted, as long as it will not interfere significantly with function later on. Care should be taken to protect pressure areas on the affected and contralateral limb, and splintage is removed as soon as early healing is detected.

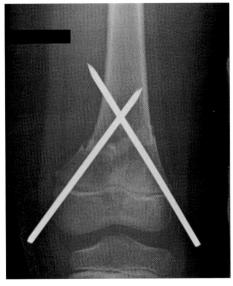

Fig. 25.15 Retrograde, crossed Steinmann pins for stabilization of a metaphyseal distal femoral fracture.

movement (patellofemoral maltracking) or partial dislocation (subluxation), are the most common cause of knee problems in children. There are usually complaints of 'locking', although on close questioning this is very rarely locking in the true orthopaedic sense of mechanical inability to straighten the knee. Similarly, there is usually a history of subjective instability, or the knee 'giving way', although again the knee is very rarely objectively unstable. The management is described on page 441.

## TIBIAL SPINE FRACTURE AND ANTERIOR CRUCIATE LIGAMENT DISRUPTION

See pages 430 and 432.

## PATELLAR FRACTURE

Patellar fractures in children display the same range of clinical and morphological features as adult fractures. An additional type, the *patellar sleeve fracture*, is unique to children. This is an avulsion fracture presenting with pain and swelling around the lower pole of the patella and inability to perform a straight leg raise. Sleeve fractures can be difficult to confirm on radiographs (**Fig. 25.16**) and ultrasound is helpful. A sleeve fracture fragment is usually too small to be fixed, and these injuries will usually require a suture technique to fix the patellar tendon back to the lower pole of the patella (p. 436). Knee movement should be restricted in a slightly flexed cast or hinged brace for 4 weeks postoperatively.

## PROXIMAL TIBIAL FRACTURES

Like distal femoral fractures, injuries of the proximal tibial physis are important because of the high rate of growth at this site (and hence likelihood of growth disorders), and the vulnerable neurovascular structures behind the knee.

Metaphyseal fractures of the proximal tibia can appear to be relatively benign in young children. Often, the fracture appears to be of greenstick type with an acceptable degree of angulation, meriting only a few weeks of cast immobilization. These fractures can, however, go on to develop progressive valgus over the ensuing 12–24 months. This is termed a *Cozen fracture* and is thought to be due to asymmetric overgrowth (**Fig. 25.17**). This rarely causes any functional issue and the majority remodel back to acceptable alignment over the next 2–3 years. Conservative management of the acquired deformity is therefore recommended. It is helpful to warn patients and carers that this might occur.

## Classification

Fractures involving the physis are described according to the Salter–Harris classification. Non-physeal injuries are described by fracture location, appearance, displacement and angulation.

## Emergency Department management

### Clinical features
- There may be a history of a high-energy motor vehicle collision or a fall from a height, but often the cause is a sporting injury.
- The patient will be unwilling to bear weight and may have a tense haemarthrosis.
- A careful neurovascular assessment should be undertaken.
- The limb should be splinted prior to obtaining radiographs.

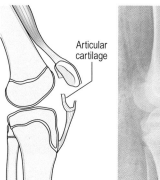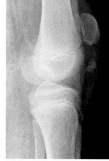

Articular cartilage

Fig. 25.16 Patellar sleeve fracture.

- Closed reduction in the Emergency Department is not warranted unless there is critical ischaemia.

### Radiographic features
- *AP and lateral knee radiographs.*
- *MRI*: This is occasionally useful in the assessment of associated soft tissue injuries.

## Orthopaedic management

### Non-operative
Non-operative management is appropriate for the majority of undisplaced injuries. Displaced fractures may be amenable to closed reduction

under anaesthesia. A full above-knee cast is maintained for 4–6 weeks, followed by active mobilization.

### Operative
Irreducible or persistently displaced fractures require open exploration. Often, the problem is found to be interposed periosteum. Fixation is with crossed wires or transverse compression screws.

## TIBIAL TUBEROSITY FRACTURES

Tibial tuberosity fractures are unusual and occur between the ages of 13 and 16, when the anterior tibial physis is closing and vulnerable. It is similar to, but should be distinguished from, Osgood–Schlatter disease – a chronic, painful but stable traction apophysitis.

## Classification (Fig. 25.18)

The *Watson Jones* classification is used:

- *Type I*: A fracture through the secondary ossification centre of the tibial tuberosity.
- *Type II*: A fracture through the physis of the tuberosity. The tuberosity epiphysis lifts anteriorly and proximally.
- *Type III*: A fracture that propagates from the tuberosity in a proximal and posterior direction so that it involves the articular portion of the proximal tibial epiphysis.

## Emergency Department management

### Clinical features
- The history is usually of an athletic boy, aged 14–16, who has had a sudden con-

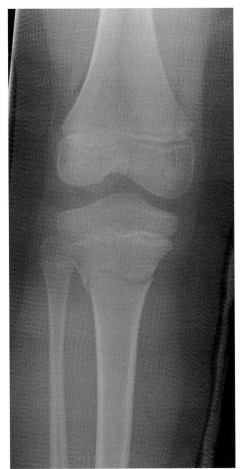

Fig. 25.17 Cozen fracture.

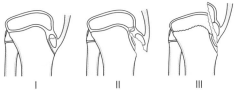

Fig. 25.18 Watson Jones classification of tibial tuberosity fractures.

traction of the quadriceps against resistance, such as when sprinting or kicking.

- There will be local pain and tenderness over the tuberosity, and often a palpable defect.
- There will be pain and weakness of knee extension, and an extensor lag.

### Radiological features

- *AP and lateral knee radiographs*: Ascertain the degree of involvement of the articular surface of the tibia.

### Immobilization

The knee should be placed in a backslab or knee extension splint for comfort, and the patient referred to Orthopaedics.

## Orthopaedic management

### Non-operative

Non-operative management is appropriate for minimally displaced injuries. An extension knee splint is worn for 4 weeks.

### Operative

Displaced tuberosity fractures are reduced and fixed surgically with compression screws across the physis in those approaching skeletal maturity. Knee movement is restricted in a brace for 4 weeks postoperatively.

### TIBIAL DIAPHYSEAL FRACTURES

The majority of these injuries in children occur in the distal third of the tibia from rotational force. This results in a spiral or oblique fracture. The fibula is intact in two-thirds of cases and this results in a risk of progressive displacement of the tibial fracture into varus in length-unstable patterns (oblique and spiral).

---

 **Key point**

Compartment syndrome is rare but can occur in children with tibial fractures. The risk factors and presenting features are the same as in adults. Compartment monitoring can be used in children at risk and prompt fasciotomy is required if the condition is diagnosed (p. 45).

## Emergency Department management

### Clinical features

- These fractures usually result from sports or motor vehicle collisions, and patients suffering high-energy mechanisms of injury should undergo full primary and secondary surveys.
- There is usually obvious deformity and swelling of the leg.
- The skin should be inspected for any breach or tension, and the distal neurovascular integrity should be assessed carefully.

### Radiological features

- *AP and lateral radiographs of the tibia*: These should include the knee and ankle.

### Reduction and immobilization

The tibia should be realigned under conscious sedation and analgesia to avoid vascular or skin compromise. An above-knee backslab should be applied (p. 562), and repeat radiographs obtained. The neurovascular status of the leg should be reviewed regularly. Refer to Orthopaedics.

## Orthopaedic management

### Non-operative

A certain degree of angulation and displacement can be accepted within the parameters shown in **Table 25.3**. Closed casting is sufficient to treat most tibial fractures in children. A long-leg cast with 15° of knee flexion is used for an initial period of 2–4 weeks, followed by conversion to a short-leg cast for a similar period. Radiographic surveillance is required for the first 3 weeks and cast wedging can be very effective between weeks 1 and 3 to correct minor losses of position (see Fig. 20.19 and p. 445). Care should be taken to evaluate rotation, as some fractures that initially appear to have displaced into varus may in fact have displaced into internal malrotation. Fractures in a poor position require manipulation under anaesthesia followed by casting.

## Table 25.3    Acceptable limits for tibial diaphyseal fracture deformity

|  | Age <8 years | Age ≥8 years |
|---|---|---|
| Shortening | 1 cm | 0.5 cm |
| Varus | 10° | 5° |
| Valgus | 10° | 5° |
| Anterior angulation | 10° | 5° |
| Posterior angulation | 10° | 5° |
| Rotation | 10° | 5° |

## Operative management

Surgical stabilization of tibial fractures is rarely required but is indicated following open fractures, failure of closed treatment, multiple injuries or situations where long-leg casting is impractical.

- *Flexible intramedullary nailing*: Two antegrade nails with a diameter of approximately 40% of the width of the medullary canal are used (**Fig. 25.19**). A short period of supplementary short-leg casting following nailing can provide additional symptomatic relief.

- *Plating*: This is rarely used for tibial diaphyseal fractures.

- *Intramedullary nailing*: Adult nailing systems that utilize a transphyseal proximal entry point should be avoided until a year before skeletal maturity due to the risk of growth arrest.

- *External fixation* (p. 467): This may be preferred in the setting of severe soft tissue damage and when the other strategies are not appropriate. This option is, however, associated with an increased risk of malunion and refracture.

### TODDLER'S FRACTURE

A twisting injury to the tibia in ambulant children under 3 years old can result in a minimally displaced spiral fracture (see Fig. 23.17). This

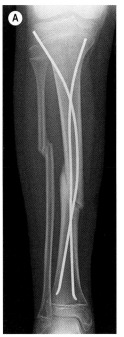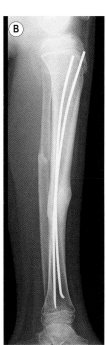

Fig. 25.19 TENS nailing of the tibia. This oblique fracture has united with acceptable minor valgus which will remodel. **A**, AP view, **B**, Lateral view.

may not be readily apparent on radiographs and is part of the differential diagnosis for the limping child. After exclusion of more serious possibilities, a suspected toddler's fracture can be treated with a long-leg cast for 2 weeks. A radiograph at the end of treatment will often show a healing fracture to confirm the diagnosis.

### DISTAL TIBIAL METAPHYSEAL FRACTURES

These fractures are prone to drift into recurvatum and can be difficult to control in a cast. Unlike with adults, it is permissible to place the child's foot in equinus for a few weeks if this is required to achieve or maintain neutral alignment of these distal fractures. More unstable fractures, often with medullary impaction, may need plating or percutaneous wire stabilization.

# ANKLE

## ANKLE FRACTURES

Ankle fractures are common injuries amongst children, and usually result from an indirect rotational force occurring during sport or a fall. The physes are weaker than the adjacent bones and ligaments, and paediatric ankle fractures tend to involve these. More complex transitional fractures occur in adolescents as a result of the gradual closure of the distal tibial physis from medially to laterally between the ages of 13 and 15.

## Classification

The *Dias and Tachdjian classification* (**Fig. 25.20**) is a modification of the Lauge Hansen classification, based on the position of the foot at the time of injury and the deforming force. The groups are:

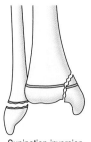

Supination-inversion

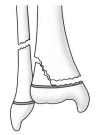

Pronation-eversion-external rotation

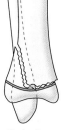

Supination-plantar flexion

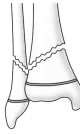

Supination-external rotation

Fig. 25.20 Dias–Tachdjian classification of ankle fractures.

1. *Supination–inversion* (SI) (**Fig. 25.21**):

   Stage 1: Avulsion injury to the fibula causing a Salter–Harris I fracture to the physis; this is the most common type of paediatric ankle fracture but may be difficult to diagnose, as the radiographs may look quite normal despite point tenderness at the fibular physis.

   Stage 2: Salter–Harris III or IV fracture at the medial malleolus; there is a high risk of growth disturbance.

2. *Pronation–eversion–external rotation* (PEER):

   Salter–Harris II fracture of the distal tibia with a lateral metaphyseal fragment.

   Greenstick metaphyseal–diaphyseal fibular fracture.

3. Supination–external rotation (SER):

   Stage 1: Salter–Harris II fracture of the distal tibia, with a posterolateral Thurston Holland fragment.

   Stage 2: Additional spiral fracture of the fibula.

4. *Supination–plantar flexion* (SPF):

   Salter-Harris II fracture of the distal tibial physis with a Thurston Holland fragment posteriorly, seen on the lateral radiograph.

5. *Axial compression*:

   Salter–Harris V injury to the distal tibia; these injuries are difficult to diagnose, and are suggested by gross swelling in the absence of other fracture patterns. Extended follow-up for 2 years is required to diagnose physeal arrest radiographically before a leg-length discrepancy or angular deformity arises.

6. *Adolescent variants*:

   Juvenile Tillaux – see below.

   Triplane fracture – see below.

## Emergency Department management

### Clinical features

● The patient will complain of pain and swelling around one or both malleoli and difficulty weight-bearing.

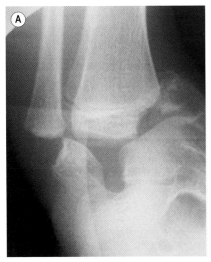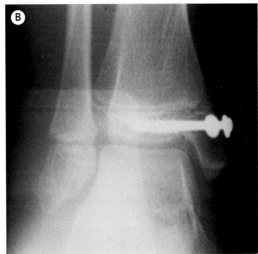

Fig. 25.21 Supination-inversion dislocation of the ankle. **A**, Salter–Harris type IV of the medial malleolus with Salter–Harris type I of the lateral malleolus. **B**, The fracture was reduced and fixed with cannulated screws.

- As for adult ankle injuries a full assessment must include palpation of the proximal fibula, base of fifth metatarsal and both malleoli to identify additional or alternative injuries (see Fig. 21.3), and a neurovascular assessment.

## Radiological features

- *Ankle series*: This includes AP, mortise and lateral radiographs.
- *CT*: This is highly useful in the evaluation of intra-articular fractures.

### Reduction and immobilization

Urgent reduction of gross deformity will be required if the skin or neurovascular supply is threatened. A below-knee backslab should then be applied.

### Outpatient follow-up

- Patients with undisplaced SH I–V fractures of the distal tibia and fibula can usually be discharged in a below-knee cast with advice to elevate the limb and avoid bearing weight until fracture clinic review in 1 week.

### Inpatient referral

- If there is displacement, extensive swelling or pain, then admission for bed rest and limb elevation in a well-padded backslab

may be more appropriate before applying the definitive cast.

## Orthopaedic management

### Non-operative management

- Patients with undisplaced SH I–V fractures of the distal tibia and fibula are treated in cast for 4–8 weeks, depending on age, with radiographic review at 1 week.
- More displaced SH I or II fractures (>10° valgus, >5° varus or >20° anterior or posterior tilt) of the distal tibia and/or fibula will require reduction, which can usually be achieved closed, followed by casting.

### Operative management

- Failure of closed reduction implies periosteal or muscle entrapment within the fracture. This can be removed surgically through a small open, direct approach.
- The transphyseal, intra-articular SH III and IV types must be anatomically reduced and stabilized with k-wires, cannulated screws or a combination of these, avoiding the fixation crossing the physis if possible (**Fig. 25.21**). Patients are managed in a cast or orthosis (moon boot), non-weight-bearing for 6 weeks postoperatively.

### Salter–Harris VI (lawnmower) injuries

Tissue loss over the medial malleolus from shearing on a road surface or rotary blade can result in loss of the medial portion of the distal tibia, the physis, and zone of Ranvier. These are severe injuries requiring meticulous debridement and often complex soft tissue procedures, and have a high risk of growth disturbance.

### Transitional fractures

These complex fractures occur in adolescents as a result of the gradual closure of the distal tibial physis from medially to laterally between the ages of 13 and 15. Only part of the physis remains structurally vulnerable, producing specific fracture patterns (**Fig. 25.22**).

### Tillaux fractures (see Fig. 21.17)

These are Salter–Harris type III fractures in children of 13–16 years, in whom the central and medial portions of the physis have already closed (see Fig. 25.22). The fracture is caused by the anterior inferior tibiofibular ligament (see Fig. 21.2) avulsing the remaining anterolateral corner of the distal tibial epiphysis (the tubercle of Chaput), which has not yet fused. These fractures are intra-articular; any displacement >2 mm requires reduction and wire or screw stabilization (see Fig. 21.17).

### Triplane fractures (Fig. 25.23)

This term encompasses a variety of multiplanar fractures involving the closing distal tibial physis (see Fig. 25.22). They therefore occur

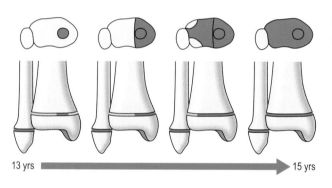

Fig. 25.22 Distal tibial physeal closure.

13 yrs ➡ 15 yrs

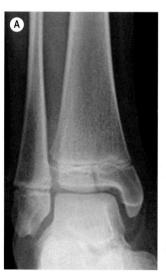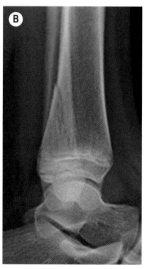

Fig. 25.23 Triplane fracture. **A**, AP view: note the appearance of a Salter–Harris type III injury. **B**, Lateral view: note the appearance of a Salter–Harris type II injury.

in adolescents, and radiographs of ankles in this age group must be scrutinized for these injuries. Be particularly suspicious of an apparent Salter–Harris II fracture of the tibia on the lateral radiograph. CT is almost invariably indicated if triplane fractures are suspected, in order to establish displacement and intra-articular involvement.

Fractures with <2 mm displacement can be treated in a long-leg cast, non-weight-bearing, for 3 weeks, then 3 weeks in a below-knee walking cast. A repeat CT is obtained at 1 week to ensure maintenance of position. Displacement of >2 mm merits reduction, which may be either closed, percutaneous or open with stabilization using combinations of wires and/or screws, depending on fracture pattern. If stabilization is good, then a short-leg cast can be used for 6 weeks until healing, with gradual reintroduction of weight-bearing.

## COMPLICATIONS

### Early

Local   Stiffness: This is less of a problem than in the adult but adolescents may require physiotherapy to assist recovery. Patients should be warned that some minor symptoms can persist for 12–18 months after ankle fracture

### Late

Local   Physeal arrest (p. 553): This may complicate all Salter–Harris types, III and IV being most at risk. Accurate reduction and anatomical healing may reduce but not abolish the risk of this complication. For this reason, all physeal ankle fractures should be followed up for 2 years (or until skeletal maturity if that is sooner) with 6-monthly radiographs. Signs of growth disturbance (p. 556) may prompt intervention before clinical deformity is apparent

## FOOT

The greatest challenge in treating the paediatric foot is the variation of radiological appearance with age. Multiple secondary ossification centres exist and a suitable reference atlas can be most helpful to differentiate between these and avulsion fractures (see Fig. 23.14).

## Classification

Classification is area-specific and uses adult classification systems with the addition of Salter–Harris for physeal injuries.

## Emergency Department management

### Clinical features

- The assessment of the foot is described on page 521.

- The foot in the younger child is very cartilaginous, and significant bone or joint disruption from trauma is rare. Soft tissue damage can be underestimated after crush or higher-energy injuries, and these may need admission for elevation and observation, even with apparently normal radiographs. Degloving of the skin is a possibility when the foot has been run over.

- In the older child and adolescent, more adult-type fractures are seen, although less frequently. Hindfoot and midfoot injuries, such as talar neck and calcaneal fractures, should be treated as in the adult. Midfoot disruptions, including Lisfranc fracture-dislocations, can be difficult to identify because the normal increased cartilage thickness gives the appearance of wider separation of the bones.

### Radiological features

- *Foot series* (AP, lateral and oblique plain radiographs): AP and lateral radiographs of the ankle are needed to evaluate the hindfoot.
- *CT*: This can be very helpful for diagnosing subtle fractures and evaluating displacement.

### Outpatient follow-up

- The vast majority of fractures are treated non-operatively in a cast for 2–6 weeks, depending on type and severity.

### Inpatient referral

- Crushing or high-energy involvement merits admission for elevation and observation, irrespective of bony injury.
- Open fractures require admission for formal lavage and debridement, although most open fractures of the lesser digits are usually amenable to lavage under local anaesthetic, antibiotic and tetanus cover, and outpatient management.

## Orthopaedic management

### Non-operative

The vast majority of paediatric foot fractures are managed non-operatively with strapping, bandaging and casting as required for comfort and mobility. Elevation during the first week is very important to aid reduction of the swelling, which is often significant. Cast change after a week may be needed once swelling has subsided. Mobilization is allowed as pain dissipates.

### Operative

Displaced fractures of the talus or calcaneus will require fixation in the same manner as for adults (p. 522). Lisfranc fracture-dislocations of the tarsometatarsal joint must be reduced and stabilized (p. 542). K-wires are often used in younger children but cannulated screws are more secure in the larger, more fully ossified foot. Operative management of fractures of the metatarsals and phalanges is indicated only for open injuries, or gross deformity that cannot be controlled with buddy strapping. Fixation is with retrograde k-wires, which are removed at 3 weeks.

## COMPLICATIONS

### *Early*

| Local | Infection: Infection of percutaneous k-wires occurs in around 5%. Removal of these wires at the earliest opportunity reduces the risk |

### *Late*

| Local | Avascular necrosis: AVN of the talus following talar neck fracture is rare in the paediatric population but has been reported |
| | Malunions: These may remodel to some extent but persistent deformity will be poorly tolerated in this high-demand age group |

# Index

Page numbers followed by 'f' indicate figures, 't' indicate tables, and 'b' indicate boxes.